A CONSUMER'S GUIDE TO PRESCRIPTION MEDICINES

Dr Barrington Cooper and Dr Laurence Gerlis
Consultant Pharmacist: Dawn Hurrell

With a Foreword by
TP Astill LLB, BPharmS, FRPharmS, FBIM
Director, National Pharmaceutical Association

- All commonly used medicines included
- All known side effects listed
- Key medical terms explained
- Easy-to-follow table of drug interactions
- Full listing of insulin products

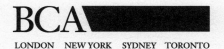

LONDON   NEW YORK   SYDNEY   TORONTO

Edited, designed, and produced by Curtis Garrett Limited
The Old Vicarage, Horton cum Studley, Oxford OX9 1BT

This edition published 1993 by BCA
By arrangement with Reed Consumer Books Limited
Michelin House, 81 Fulham Road, London SW3 6RB
and Auckland, Melbourne, Singapore and Toronto

A catalogue record for this book is available from the
British Library

CN 2820

Printed in Great Britain

Preface to the Second Edition

The acceptance this Guide has received since it was first published in 1990 has been gratifying. We offered information to patients that was previously not available to them and, as consumers, they have responded warmly to the book. Providing patients with information about their treatment has proved to be part of the new wave in medical care in which the person participates actively rather than passively accepting authority.

This fully revised second edition incorporates the hundreds of changes to prescription medicines which have occurred over the past three years. Many new products are included and many amendments have been made. The work of Dawn Hurrell has been invaluable in the preparation of this edition and, as a practising pharmacist, she underlines our belief in the team concept of medical treatment and in the importance of the pharmacist's role.

A Consumer's Guide to Prescription Medicines has been used by pharmacists to offer information to patients at the time the prescription is collected. In addition to the doctor/patient relationship, the pharmacist/patient interaction provides an opportunity to involve patients in the pharmaceutical aspects of their medical care.

It is our intention to continue to improve and update this book. Reader's enquiries have always been helpful, and they contribute to the interaction between patient and doctor. We see this book as an integral part of that relationship.

Dr Barrington Cooper and Dr Laurence Gerlis
21 Devonshire Place, London W1
1992

Preface to the First Edition

We have always felt that patient education is a vital part of the healing process in preventive and therapeutic medicine. Those patients who are best informed are also those for whom treatment is most likely to be successful.

The main purpose of this book is only to reinforce advice which a prescribing doctor has given already to a patient receiving that prescription. It confirms information about drug names and type, as well as the condition which is being treated.

As prescribing physicians, we have made a conscious effort to provide information without, in any way, undermining the vitally important doctor-patient relationship. Thus, we have excluded injectable preparations and a small number of other sensitive areas of information. Our decision to use brand and generic names is not a statement of medical politics, but it is designed to help people who may have medication prescribed in either way. New European laws on product liability require a physician to explain possible side effects to patients, and this book will, to some extent, fulfil this role. Thus, *A Consumer's Guide to Prescription Medicines* should also be a valuable aid to doctors who are prescribing the medications listed.

Dr Barrington Cooper and Dr Laurence Gerlis
21 Devonshire Place, London Wl
1989

Foreword

It is no exaggeration to say that the last fifty years have seen a revolution in pharmacy and medicine. In the 'good old days', the family doctor would write a prescription which was usually in the form of a recipe and, quite deliberately, in semi-legible handwriting so that the patient could not read it — just in case the patient was able to decipher the writing, the names of the ingredients were in abbreviated Latin! The pharmacist would look at the prescription, nod sagely, and disappear out of sight behind his dispensary screen to make the pills or to mix the ingredients of the ointment or medicine. The name of the product never appeared on the label because everyone, including most patients, felt that it was undesirable for ordinary people to know what had been prescribed. It can now be revealed that what was in the bottle was probably innocuous and pharmacologically ineffective. The curative power of medicine in those days derived in large measure from the mystery and mystique which surrounded its preparation, coupled always with the doctor's bedside manner and confident reassurance.

Since then, there has been an enormous increase in scientific knowledge, especially of the way in which chemical substances affect the organs of the human body and of the way in which the body itself works. Antibiotics and other anti-infective agents have also been discovered, with the result that many hitherto fatal diseases have either disappeared altogether or can now be cured easily. Those who criticize the pharmaceutical industry forget too readily the former ravages of tuberculosis, polio, meningitis, septicaemia, typhoid fever, endocarditis, and other killing and crippling diseases. Many people suffering from asthma, epilepsy, hormone deficiency, or allergy can now lead a normal life whereas they would previously have been severely handicapped, confined to a wheelchair, or dead at an early age. Modern advances in surgery, such as organ transplants, have also been made possible by the drugs which control the body's natural tendency to reject 'invaders'.

Alongside this pharmaceutical revolution, there has also been a consumer revolution. Nowadays, you want to **know** what kind of drugs you are taking, and rightly so. While some people may regret the passing of the age of medicinal mystique, most of us prefer to be told precisely what is wrong with us and what is being provided to put us right. We want to know what effect the medicine is likely to have, what side effects might occur, and what precautions we need to take to ensure that the medicine behaves as it should. The modern medicine is certainly a powerful weapon for good, but it is also often complex in its chemistry and formulation. It is important, therefore, that patients are properly informed about their medicines, not only for their own peace of mind, but also so that the product gives them the maximum possible benefit with the minimum risk of harm.

For these reasons, I welcome warmly this new book by Dr Cooper and Dr Gerlis. In simple language it tells us what we need to know about our prescribed medicines. It reinforces and supplements what we have been told by our doctor and pharmacist, it will help us to understand why a particular medicine has been selected; and it tells us how it should be used. As the authors emphasize in their introduction, the book is not intended to be a substitute for professional advice. You should not hesitate to talk to your doctor or pharmacist if you are in serious doubt about any aspect of your treatment. But this book is a very usable source of reference and will fill reassuringly many gaps in our knowledge. It will help to remove those little apprehensions which many of us feel when we leave the surgery with the prescription and the pharmacy with our medicine.

T P Astill LLB, BPharmS, FRPharmS, FBIM
Director, National Pharmaceutical Association

How the book works

Apart from injectables and a small number of other medicines and appliances, all medicines which may be commonly prescribed through the National Health Service or private practice in the United Kingdom should be found in this book. They are arranged in strict alphabetical order throughout with brand names, generic names, and any commonly used medical terms contained within the same sequence. There is also a chart to be found on page 709 which explains the way in which various drugs may interact with one another or with other substances such as alcohol. Some drugs are required to be prescribed by its generic, or scientific, name only and it is then up to the dispensing pharmacist to select a particular manufacturer's product. Other drugs are prescribed by a brand name. In this book, the main descriptions of any preparation are to be found under its commonly used brand name while the generic name will then cross refer to the main entry. In a small number of cases, where only a generic name exists, the main description will fall under that name.

Similarly, one particular medicine may be manufactured by more than one drug company under a variety of brand names. In such cases the authors have selected one preparation to be given the complete description, and then other preparations are, once again, cross-referred to the main entry. And, of course, the main entry also refers in its 'Other preparations' to any other manufacturer's version of the medicine. Thus, no matter what name has been used on the container of a medicine dispensed to a patient, it is a simple matter quickly to find a full description of the preparation. Note also that medicines included in the first edition of this book and which have subsequently been discontinued are still entered as headwords but with a note stating 'Product now discontinued'.

The name of the medicine is given in bold type at the beginning of each entry, with the name of the manufacturing company in brackets on the next line. A short paragraph then follows describing the medicine in terms of its appearance, strength where this is relevant, what kind of drug it is — eg antacid, and what it is used to treat — eg dyspepsia. The usual dose or dose range is given for the particular uses of the medicine, including any variations that may be required to treat children, the elderly, or in any other special circumstances. The next section indicates whether the drug is available through the NHS, by private prescription, or over the counter without any prescription being needed. Any possible side effects that the medicine might produce are explained as well as any cautionary advice in its use. It is clearly stated If a medicine is not to be used for particular groups of patients, such as pregnant women, or to treat certain conditions or states. And any known interactions with other medicines or substances such as alcohol are also indicated. The components of the preparation are given in terms of their scientific names, and any other preparations of these components are also included at the end of the entry.

How to use this book (including how *not* to use it)

When a doctor prescribes a medicine for a patient, then he or she will always explain carefully to the patient how it is to be used. Similarly, the pharmacist will always write instructions for the drug's dose on the container, and the name of the drug will also be clearly visible. If you look up the name in *A Consumer's Guide to Prescription Medicines*, you will be able to confirm that you have understood the doctor's instructions fully so that you can be confident you are making the best possible use of the medicine. It will also help you to anticipate and prepare for any possible side effects, and ensure that you are not taking anything else which perhaps the doctor was not made aware of and which might interact with the prescription. More importantly perhaps, the book will enable you to become better informed generally about the medicine(s) which has been prescribed to treat or prevent a particular condition.

A Consumer's Guide to Prescription Medicines is **not** a guide to self-prescription. Nor is it a 'home doctor'. The authors recognize clearly that it is the advice of the prescribing doctor, given after a careful investigation of the patient and his or her symptoms, that should always be followed by patients. If the information given in this book differs in any particular from the doctor's recommendations about a medicine, this must only be a basis for discussing such differences with the prescribing doctor or perhaps with the dispensing pharmacist.

The information contained in this book should not be followed in preference to the recommendations of the prescription even though it has been compiled by highly qualified physicians and a pharmacist using the most up-to-date sources. There are few doctors or pharmacists who do not welcome well-informed questioning by their patients, and it is the purpose of this book to add to the information already given by the prescribing physician in the surgery and on the product's labelling. On the other hand, the authors have chosen not to include the names and addresses of the manufacturers of the drugs described because it is the policy of most drug companies not to respond directly to enquiries concerning their medicines from individual patients; generally, they will refer such enquiries back to the general practitioner.

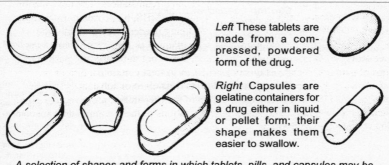

Left These tablets are made from a compressed, powdered form of the drug.

Right Capsules are gelatine containers for a drug either in liquid or pellet form; their shape makes them easier to swallow.

A selection of shapes and forms in which tablets, pills, and capsules may be supplied to help in their identification.

An annotated guide to understanding the entries

manufacturer's brand name or scientific name

manufacturer

general description including physical appearance, strength where appropriate, the type of drug, and the conditions it is used to treat

Depixol
(Lundbeck)

A yellow tablet supplied at a strength of 3 mg and used as a sedative to treat schizophrenia and other mental disorders, especially withdrawal or apathy.

dose range, including any variations for children or the elderly (note: this is for guidance only and you should always follow the physician's advice)

Dose: usually 1-3 tablets a day, up to a maximum of 6 tablets a day.
Availability: NHS and private prescription.

not all medicines are available through the National Health Service, while some are available over the counter without prescription

these are the most commonly noted side effects. In many cases, however, no side effects or only some will be experienced

Side effects: muscle spasms, restlessness, hands shaking, dry mouth, urine retention, palpitations, low blood pressure, weight gain, changes in libido, low body temperature, breast swelling, menstrual changes, jaundice, blood and skin changes, drowsiness, rarely fits.

circumstances where care should be exercised by certain groups of patients or those taking other medicines

Caution: in pregnant women, the elderly, and in patients suffering from kidney, liver, heart, or lung disease, Parkinson's disease, or anyone who is intolerant of those drugs taken by mouth.

Not to be used for: children, or for very excitable or overactive patients.

any groups of patients who should **not** take this medicine

these are substances, such as alcohol or foods, or other drugs with which this medicine should not usually be taken

Caution needed with: alcohol, tranquillizers, pain killers, ANTIHYPERTENSIVES, antidepressants, anticonvulsants, antidiabetic drugs, LEVODOPA.

the active ingredients of the medicine

Contains: FLUPENTHIXOL DIHYDROCHLORIDE.
Other preparations: Depixol Injection, Depixol-Conc, FLUANXOL (Lundbeck).

this lists other forms of the same medicine, or equivalent drugs from a different manufacturer (note: since the medicine may be of a different strength, the doses may be different)

(note: CAPITALS indicate a separate entry in the book)

AAA Spray
(Rhone-Poulenc Rorer)

An aerosol used as an antibacterial and local anaesthetic to treat sore throat, minor infections of the nose and throat.

Dose: 2 sprays every 2-3 hours up to a maximum of 16 sprays in 24 hours; children over 6 years half adult dose.
Availability: NHS, private prescription, over the counter.
Side effects:
Caution:
Not to be used for: children under 6 years.
Caution needed with:
Contains: BENZOCAINE, CETALKONIUM CHLORIDE.
Other preparations:

Abidec
(Warner-Lambert)

Drops used as a multivitamin preparation to treat vitamin deficiencies.

Dose: adults and children over 1 year 0.6 ml a day; infants under 1 year half adult dose.
Availability: NHS, private prescription, over the counter.
Side effects:
Caution:
Not to be used for:
Caution needed with: LEVODOPA.
Contains: CALCIFEROL, THIAMINE HYDROCHLORIDE, RIBOFLAVINE, PYRIDOXINE HYDROCHLORIDE, NICOTINAMIDE, ASCORBIC ACID.
Other preparations: Abidec Capsules (now discontinued).

Accupro
(Parke-Davis)

A brown, elliptical, triangular, or round tablet according to strengths 5 mg, 10 mg, and 20 mg, and used as an ACE INHIBITOR in addition to DIURETICS and DIGOXIN in the treatment of congestive heart failure and high blood pressure.

Dose: 2.5 mg a day at first, then usually 10-40 mg a day to a maximum 80 mg a day.
Availability: NHS and private prescription.
Side effects: headache, dizziness, inflammation of the nose, cough, upper respiratory tract infection, tiredness, nausea, stomach, abdominal,

chest, or muscle pain, low blood pressure, severe allergy.
Caution: in the elderly, and in patients suffering from kidney disease, some vascular diseases, and in those undergoing anaesthesia. The treatment should be started in hospital. Your doctor may advise blood and urine checks.
Not to be used for: children, pregnant women, nursing mothers, or for patients suffering from some heart valve diseases, some kidney disorders.
Caution needed with: some DIURETICS, some potassium supplements, NON-STEROIDAL ANTI-INFLAMMATORY DRUGS, TETRACYCLINES.
Contains: QUINAPRIL
Other preparations:

ACE inhibitor (angiotension converting enzyme inhibitor)
a drug which blocks the production of water-retaining hormones and thus functions as a DIURETIC. Example captopril *see* CAPOTEN.

---

acebutolol *see* **Secadrex, Sectral**

---

acematacin *see* **Emflex**

Acepril *see* **Capoten**
(Squibb)

---

acetazolamide *see* **Diamox, Diamox Sustets**

---

acetic acid *see* **Aci-Jel, Phytex**

---

acetohexamide *see* **Dimelor**

---

acetomenaphthone *see* **Ketovite**

Acetoxyl
(Stiefel)

A gel used as an antibacterial and skin softener to treat acne.

Dose: wash and dry the affected area and apply the gel once a day.
Availability: NHS, private prescription, over the counter.
Side effects: irritation, peeling.
Caution: keep out of the eyes, nose, and mouth; children should use the weaker gel; may bleach fabrics.
Not to be used for:
Caution needed with:
Contains: BENZOYL PEROXIDE.
Other preparations: ACNEGEL (Stiefel), BENOXYL (Stiefel), BENZAGEL (Bioglan), NERICUR (Schering), PANOXYL (Stiefel), QUINODERM (Quinoderm).

---

acetylcysteine *see* Fabrol, Ilube, Parvolex

Acezide *see* Capozide
(Squibb)

Achromycin capsules *see* Tetracycline
(Lederle)

Achromycin ointment
(Lederle)

An ointment used as an antibiotic to treat skin infections.

Dose: apply once a day or as needed.
Availability: NHS and private prescription.
Side effects: additional infection.
Caution: in patients suffering from liver or kidney failure, perforated ear drum.
Not to be used for: children or pregnant women.
Caution needed with: milk, minerals, contraceptive pill, ANTACIDS.
Contains: TETRACYCLINE hydrochloride.
Other preparations: Achromycin Ophthalmic Oil Suspension (for eye infections), Achromycin ear/eye ointment (for eye/outer ear infections).

Aci-Jel
(Cilag)

A jelly with applicator used as an antiseptic to treat non-specific vaginal infection.

Dose: 1 application into the vagina twice a day.
Availability: NHS, private prescription, over the counter.
Side effects: irritation and inflammation.
Caution: in pregnant women
Not to be used for: children.
Caution needed with:
Contains: ACETIC ACID.
Other preparations:

---

acipimox *see* Olbetam

---

acitretin *see* Neotigason

Acnecide *see* Acnegel
(Galderma)

Acnegel
(Stiefel)

A gel used as an antibacterial and skin softener to treat acne.

Dose: wash and dry the affected area and apply the gel once a day.
Availability: NHS, private prescription, over the counter.
Side effects: irritation, peeling.
Caution: keep out of the eyes, nose, mouth; may bleach fabrics.
Not to be used for:
Caution needed with:
Contains: BENZOYL PEROXIDE.
Other preparations: Acnegel Forte, ACETOXYL (Stiefel), ACNECIDE (Galderma), BENOXYL (Stiefel), BENZAGEL (Bioglan), NERICUR (Schering), PANOXYL (Stiefel), QUINODERM (Quinoderm).

Acnidazil
(Janssen)

A cream used as an antibacterial and skin softener to treat acne.

Dose: wash and dry the affected area, and apply the cream once a day for the first week, then twice a day for the next 4-8 weeks.
Availability: NHS, private prescription, over the counter.
Side effects: irritation, peeling.
Caution: keep out of the eyes, nose, mouth; may bleach fabrics.
Not to be used for:
Caution needed with:
Contains: MICONAZOLE NITRATE, BENZOYL PEROXIDE.
Other preparations:

---

acrivastine *see* **Semprex**

---

acrosoxacin *see* **Eradacin**

Actal
(Sterling Health)

A white tablet supplied at a strength of 360 mg and used as an ANTACID to treat indigestion, dyspepsia.

Dose: 1-2 tablets when needed.
Availability: private prescription and over the counter.
Side effects: sodium overload is possible.
Caution:
Not to be used for: children.
Caution needed with: TETRACYCLINE antibiotics, tablets which are coated to protect the stomach.
Contains: ALEXITOL SODIUM.
Other preparations: Actal Suspension (now discontinued).

Actidil — ANTIHISTAMINE tablet/elixir. Product now discontinued.

Actifed Compound
(Wellcome)

A linctus used as an ANTIHISTAMINE and SYMPATHOMIMETIC to treat cough, congestion.

Dose: adults 10 ml 3 times a day; children 2-5 years 2.5 ml 3 times a day, 6-12 years 5 ml 3 times a day.
Availability: private prescription and over the counter.
Side effects: drowsiness, reduced reactions, irregular or rapid heart rate, excitement.
Caution: in patients suffering from liver or kidney disease.
Not to be used for: children under 2 years, patients suffering from heart or thyroid disorders.
Caution needed with: alcohol, sedatives, some antidepressants (MAOIS and TRICYCLICS).
Contains: TRIPROLIDINE hydrochloride, PSEUDOEPHEDRINE hydrochloride, DEXTROMETHORPHAN hydrobromide.
Other preparations: Actifed Expectorant, Actifed Tablets, Actifed Syrup.

Actinac
(Roussel)

A lotion used as an antibacterial, STEROID, and skin softener to treat acne and associated disorders.

Dose: apply to the affected area night and morning for 4 days, then at night only for 3 weeks after the spots have gone.
Availability: NHS and private prescription.
Side effects: severe reddening of the skin.
Caution: in pregnant women. Remove jewellery before applying.
Not to be used for:
Caution needed with:
Contains: CHLORAMPHENICOL, HYDROCORTISONE acetate, BUTOXYETHYL NICOTINATE, ALLANTOIN, precipitated SULPHUR.
Other preparations:

Actonorm
(Wallace)

A white liquid supplied in 200 ml bottles and used as an ANTACID to treat indigestion, wind.

Dose: adults 5-20 ml after meals.
Availability: private prescription and over the counter.
Side effects: few; occasionally constipation or diarrhoea.
Caution:
Not to be used for: children.
Caution needed with: TETRACYCLINE antibiotics.
Contains: ALUMINIUM HYDROXIDE, MAGNESIUM HYDROXIDE, activated DIMETHICONE.
Other preparations: Actonorm powder.

Actraphane *see* **Insulin**
(Novo Nordisk)

Actrapid *see* **Insulin**
(Novo Nordisk)

Acupan
(3M Healthcare)

A white tablet supplied at a strength of 30 mg and used as an ANALGESIC to relieve pain.

Dose: 1-3 tablets 3 times a day.
Availability: NHS and private prescription.
Side effects: nausea, nervousness, dry mouth, dizziness.
Caution: in patients suffering from kidney or liver disease, pregnant women.
Not to be used for: patients with a history of convulsions or suffering from heart attack, children.
Caution needed with: MAOIS, ANTICHOLINERGICS, SYMPATHOMIMETICS, TRICYCLICS.
Contains: NEFOPAM hydrochloride.
Other preparations: Acupan Injection.

acyclovir *see* **Zovirax, Zovirax Ointment**

Adalat
(Bayer)

An orange, liquid-filled capsule supplied at strengths of 5 mg, 10 mg and used as an anti-anginal treatment for angina, Raynaud's phenomenon.

Dose: 10 mg 3 times a day at first, then according to response up to 60 mg a day with or after food. For Raynaud's phenomenon 10-20 mg mg 3 times a day with food or after meals.
Availability: NHS and private prescription.
Side effects: headache, flushes, fluid retention, dizziness, chest pain, rarely jaundice, gum swelling.
Caution: in patients with weak hearts, liver disease, or low blood pressure.
Not to be used for: children, pregnant women, nursing mothers, or patients suffering from severe low blood pressure.
Caution needed with: ANTIHYPERTENSIVES, CIMETIDINE, QUINIDINE.

Contains: NIFEDIPINE.
Other preparations: ADALAT RETARD (Bayer), BETA ADALAT (Bayer), CALCILAT (Eastern), CORACTEN (Evans Medical), NIFENSAR XL (Rhone-Poulenc Rorer).

Adalat Retard
(Bayer)

A pink/grey tablet supplied at strengths of 10 mg, 20 mg and used as an ANTIHYPERTENSIVE to treat high blood pressure.

Dose: 10-20 mg twice a day at first, adjust to 10-40 mg twice a day according to response.
Availability: NHS and private prescription.
Side effects: headache, flushes, fluid retention, dizziness,chest pain,gum swelling, rarely jaundice.
Caution: in patients with weak heart or liver disease.
Not to be used for: children, pregnant women, nursing mothers, or for patients suffering from severe low blood pressure.
Caution needed with: other ANTIHYPERTENSIVES, CIMETIDINE, QUINIDINE.
Contains: NIFEDIPINE.
Other preparations: Adalat LA (Bayer), BETA ADALAT (Bayer), CORACTEN (Evans Medical), NIFENSAR XL (Rhone-Poulenc Rorer).

Adcortyl
(Princeton)

A cream used as a STEROID treatment for dermatitis, psoriasis, external ear infections, sunburn, insect bites and stings.

Dose: apply to the affected area 2-4 times a day.
Availability: NHS and private prescription.
Side effects: fluid retention, suppression of adrenal glands, thinning of the skin may occur.
Caution: use for short periods of time only.
Not to be used for: patients suffering from acne or any other skin infections caused by tuberculosis, ringworm, viruses, or fungi, or continuously especially in pregnant women.
Caution needed with:
Contains: TRIAMCINOLONE ACETONIDE.
Other preparations: Adcortyl Ointment.

Adcortyl in Orabase
(Princeton)

A paste used as a STEROID treatment for mouth ulcers, mouth infections, gingivitis, lesions.

Dose: apply the paste to the affected area 2-4 times a day without rubbing in.
Availability: NHS and private prescription.
Side effects:
Caution: in pregnant women. Do not use for infants over extended periods.
Not to be used for: patients suffering from untreated mouth infections.
Caution needed with:
Contains: TRIAMCINOLONE ACETONIDE.
Other preparations:

Adifax
(Servier)

A white capsule supplied at a strength of 15 mg and used in addition to dietary measures in the treatment of severe obesity.

Dose: 1 capsule in the morning and 1 capsule in the evening at meal times.
Availability: NHS and private prescription.
Side effects: dry mouth, nausea, constipation, diarrhoea, drowsiness, dizziness, headache, frequency of urination.
Caution: treatment limited to 3 months, and withdrawn gradually.
Not to be used for: children, the elderly, pregnant women, nursing mothers, or for patients suffering from glaucoma, history of anorexia, mental illness, kidney or liver disease, drug or alcohol abuse.
Caution needed with: MAOIS, ANTIHYPERTENSIVES, antidiabetics, antidepressants, sedatives, other drugs used to reduce appetite.
Contains: DEXFENFLURAMINE
Other preparations:

Adizem *see* Tildiem
(Napp)

---

adrenal glands

the adrenal glands are organs situated above the kidneys which produce hormones, including STEROIDS.

---

adrenaline *see* **Brovon, Epifrin, Epinal, Eppy, Ganda, Medihaler-EPI, Min-i-jet Adrenaline, Rybarvin, Simplene**

Aerobec *see* **Becotide**
(3M Healthcare)

Aerolin Auto *see* **Ventolin**
(3M Healthcare)

Afrazine
(Schering-Plough)

A spray used as a SYMPATHOMIMETIC treatment for blocked nose.

Dose: adults and children over 5 years 2-3 sprays in each nostril twice a day.
Availability: private prescription and over the counter.
Side effects: itching nose, headache, sleeplessness, rapid heart rate.
Caution: in patients suffering from overactive thyroid gland, diabetes, coronary disease. Do not use for extended periods.
Not to be used for: children under 5 years.
Caution needed with: MAOIS.
Contains: OXYMETAZOLINE HYDROCHLORIDE.
Other preparations: Dristan (Whitehall), Vicks Sinex (Proctor and Gamble).

---

agar *see* **Agarol**

Agarol
(Warner-Lambert)

An emulsion used as a lubricant and stimulant to treat constipation.

Dose: children 5-12 years 5 ml at bedtime, adults 5-15 ml at bedtime.
Availability: private prescription and over the counter.
Side effects: allergies to phenolphthalein, blood or protein in the urine.
Caution: in patients with swallowing difficulties. Avoid prolonged use.
Not to be used for: children under 5 years.
Caution needed with:
Contains: LIQUID PARAFFIN, PHENOLPHTHALEIN, AGAR.

Other preparations:

Akineton
(Knoll)

A white, scored tablet supplied at a strength of 2 mg and used as an ANTICHOLINERGIC to treat Parkinson's disease.

Dose: ½ tablet twice a day at first, then increasing to a tablet 3 times a day, increasing again and then reducing.
Availability: NHS and private prescription.
Side effects: drowsiness, dry mouth, blurred vision.
Caution: in patients suffering from abnormal heart rhythm or heart attack, epilepsy, urinary obstruction.
Not to be used for: children or patients suffering from gastro-intestinal obstruction, glaucoma; pregnant women or nursing mothers.
Caution needed with: other anti-parkinson drugs, sedating drugs.
Contains: BIPERIDEN HYDROCHLORIDE.
Other preparations:

albendazole *see* Eskazole

Albucid
(Nicholas)

Drops used as a sulphonamide antibiotic to treat eye infections.

Dose: 2-4 drops into the eye every 2-6 hours.
Availability: NHS and private prescription.
Side effects: temporary irritation.
Caution:
Not to be used for:
Caution needed with:
Contains: SODIUM SULPHACETAMIDE.
Other preparations: Albucid Ointment (now discontinued).

alclometasone diproprionate *see* Modrasone

alcohol *see* Glykola, Labiton, Verdiviton

Alcopar
(Wellcome)

Dispersible granules in a sachet of 2.5 g and used as an anti-worm treatment for worms.

Dose: adults and children over 2 years 1 sachet dispersed in water; children under 2 years half adult dose.
Availability: NHS, private prescription, over the counter.
Side effects: stomach upset.
Caution:
Not to be used for: patients who are continuously vomiting.
Caution needed with:
Contains: BEPHENIUM HYDROXY-NAPHTHOATE.
Other preparations:

Alcos-Anal — ointment to treat haemorrhoids/anal itch. Product now discontinued.

Aldactide 50
(Gold Cross)

A buff tablet supplied at a strength of 50 mg and used as a diuretic to treat congestive heart failure.

Dose: adults 2-4 tablets a day; children 1.5-3 mg per kg bodyweight a day in divided doses.
Availability: NHS and private prescription.
Side effects: breast enlargement, stomach upset, drowsiness, rash, sensitivity to light, blood changes.
Caution: in pregnant women, young patients, and in patients suffering from liver or kidney disease, gout, or diabetes. Your doctor may advise regular blood tests.
Not to be used for: nursing mothers or for patients suffering from severe kidney failure, progressive kidney failure, raised potassium levels.
Caution needed with: potassium supplements, lithium, DIGOXIN, CARBENOXOLONE, ANTIHYPERTENSIVES, ACE INHIBITORS.
Contains: SPIRONOLACTONE, HYDROFLUMETHIAZIDE, (CO-FLUMACTANE).
Other preparations: Aldactide 25.

Aldactone
(Searle)

A buff tablet or a white tablet according to strengths of 25 mg, 50 mg, 100 mg and used as a diuretic to treat congestive heart failure, cirrhosis of the liver, fluid retention.

Dose: adults congestive heart failure 100 mg a day increasing to 400 mg a day, then 75-200 mg a day with food; children 3 mg per kg bodyweight a day in divided doses. For other conditions as advised by physician.
Availability: NHS and private prescription.
Side effects: breast enlargement, stomach upset, rash, drowsiness, headache, confusion.
Caution: in pregnant women or young patients, and in patients suffering from kidney or liver disease. Your doctor may advise regular blood tests.
Not to be used for: nursing mothers or for patients suffering from kidney failure or raised potassium levels.
Caution needed with: potassium supplements, CARBENOXOLONE, DIGITALIS, ACE INHIBITORS, ANTIHYPERTENSIVES.
Contains: SPIRONOLACTONE.
Other preparations: LARACTONE, SPIRETIC (DDSA), SPIROCTAN (MCP) SPIROLONE (Berk), SPIROSPARE (Ashbourne).

Aldomet
(MSD)

A yellow tablet supplied at strengths of 125 mg, 250 mg, 500 mg and used as an ANTIHYPERTENSIVE to treat high blood pressure.

Dose: adults 250 mg 2-3 times a day at first, adjust to a maximum of 3 g a day at 2-day intervals; children 10 mg per kg bodyweight a day at first in 2-4 divided doses.
Availability: NHS and private prescription.
Side effects: sleepiness, headache,weakness, depression, slow heart rate, congestion of the nose, dry mouth, stomach upset, jaundice, blood changes.
Caution: in patients suffering from certain types of anaemia, history of liver disease, kidney disease, or patients undergoing anaesthesia. Your doctor may advise regular blood tests.
Not to be used for: patients suffering from liver disease, depression, phaeochromocytoma (a disease of the adrenal glands).
Caution needed with: TRICYCLICS, MAOIS, other ANTIHYPERTENSIVES.
Contains: METHLYDOPA.
Other preparations: DOPAMET (Berk), MEDOMET (DDSA), METALPHA (Ashbourne).

---

alexitol sodium *see* **Actal, Droxalin**

alfacalcidol *see* **One-Alpha**

Algesal
(Duphar)

A cream used as an ANALGESIC rub to treat rheumatic conditions.

Dose: massage into the affected area 3 times a day.
Availability: NHS, private prescription, over the counter.
Side effects:
Caution: in pregnant women.
Not to be used for: children under 6 years.
Caution needed with:
Contains: DIETHYLAMINE SALICYLATE.
Other preparations: Lloyds cream (Seton).

Algicon
(Rhone-Poulenc Rorer)

A white tablet used as an ANTACID to treat heartburn, hiatus hernia, indigestion.

Dose: adults 1-2 tablets 4 times a day after meals and at night.
Availability: NHS, private prescription, over the counter.
Side effects: few; constipation or diarrhoea.
Caution: patients suffering from diabetes owing to sucrose content.
Not to be used for: children, or in kidney failure or severe debilitation.
Caution needed with: TETRACYCLINE antibiotics, tablets which are specially coated to protect the stomach.
Contains: MAGNESIUM ALGINATE, ALUMINIUM HYDROXIDE/MAGNESIUM CARBONATE, MAGNESIUM CARBONATE, POTASSIUM BICARBONATE.
Other preparations: Algicon Suspension.

alginic acid *see* **Gastrocote, Gastron, Gaviscon, Topal**

Algitec *see* Tagamet
(S K B)

Alimix *see* Prepulsid
(Janssen)

allantoin *see* **Actinac, Alphosyl, Alphosyl HC, Dermalex**

Allbee with C
(Whitehall)

A green/yellow capsule used as a multivitamin treatment for vitamin B and vitamin C deficiencies.

Dose: adults 1-3 capsules a day; children 1 capsule a day.
Availability: private prescription and over the counter.
Side effects:
Caution:
Not to be used for:
Caution needed with: LEVODOPA.
Contains: THIAMINE mononitrate, RIBOFLAVINE, PYRIDOXINE hydrochloride, NICOTINAMIDE, CALCIUM PANTOTHENATE, ASCORBIC ACID.
Other preparations: BC 500 (Whitehall).

Allegron
(Dista)

A white tablet or an orange, scored tablet according to strengths of 10 mg, 25 mg and used as a TRICYCLIC antidepressant to treat depression, bedwetting in children.

Dose: adults 20-40 mg a day at first in divided doses increasing to up to 100 mg a day as needed and then reducing to 30-75 mg a day; elderly 10 mg 3 times a day at first; children over 6 years 10-30 mg half an hour before bed time. Reduced doses in the elderly.
Availability: NHS and private prescription.
Side effects: dry mouth, constipation, urine retention, blurred vision, palpitations, drowsiness, sleeplessness, dizziness, hands shaking, low blood presure, weight change, skin reactions, jaundice or blood changes. Loss of sexual desire may occur.
Caution: in nursing mothers or in patients suffering from heart disease, thyroid disease, epilepsy, diabetes, glaucoma, urinary retention, adrenal tumour, some other psychiatric conditions. Your doctor may advise regular blood tests.
Not to be used for: children under 6 years, pregnant women, or for patients suffering from heart attacks, liver disease, heart block.
Caution needed with: alcohol, ANTICHOLINERGICS, ADRENALINE, MAOIS, BARBITU-RATES, other antidepressants, ANTIHYPERTENSIVES.
Contains: NORTRIPTYLINE HYDROCHLORIDE.
Other preparations: AVENTYL (Eli Lilly).

allopurinol *see* **Zyloric**

allyloestrenol *see* **Gestanin**

almasilate *see* **Malinal**

Almazine *see* **Ativan.** Product now discontinued.

Almodan *see* **Amoxil**
(Berk)

Alnide *see* **Mydrilate**
(Cusi)

aloin *see* **Alophen**

Alomide
(Galen)

Drops used to treat allergic conjunctivitis.

Dose: adults 1-2 drops in each eye 4 times a day; children over 4 years, as adult dose.
Availability: NHS and private prescription.
Side effects: irritation of the eye.
Caution: in pregnant women and nursing mothers.
Not to be used for: patients who wear soft contact lenses, or for children under 4 years.
Caution needed with:
Contains: LODOXAMIDE
Other preparations:

Alophen
(Warner-Lambert)

A brown pill used as a stimulant and ANTICHOLINERGIC to treat constipation.

Dose: adults 1-3 pills at bedtime.
Availability: private prescription and over the counter.
Side effects: allergy to PHENOLPHTHALEIN, skin rash, protein in the urine.
Caution:
Not to be used for: children or for patients suffering from glaucoma or inflammatory bowel disease.
Caution needed with:
Contains: ALOIN, PHENOLPHTHALEIN, IPECACUANHA, BELLADONNA EXTRACT.
Other preparations:

Aloral *see* **Zyloric.** Product now discontinued.

---

aloxiprin *see* **Palaprin Forte**

---

alpha-beta-pinenes *see* **Rowachol**

Alpha Keri
(Westwood)

A liquid used to treat dry, itchy skin conditions.

Dose: adults and children add 1-2 capsful to the bath, or rub a small amount on to wet skin; infants use half a capful per bath.
Availability: NHS, private prescription, over the counter.
Side effects:
Caution:
Not to be used for:
Caution needed with:
Contains: LIQUID PARAFFIN, LANOLIN OIL.
Other preparations:

Alphaderm
(Norwich Eaton)

A cream used as a STEROID and wetting agent to treat eczema, dermatitis.

Dose: wash and dry the affected area, and apply twice a day.
Availability: NHS and private prescription.

Side effects: fluid retention, suppression of adrenal glands. Thinning of the skin may occur.
Caution: use for short periods of time only.
Not to be used for: patients suffering from acne or any other skin infections caused by tuberculosis, ringworm, viruses, or fungi, or continuously especially in pregnant women.
Caution needed with:
Contains: HYDROCORTISONE, UREA.
Other preparations: CALMURID HC (Kabi Pharmacia), SENTIAL (Kabi Pharmacia).

Alphavase *see* Hypovase
(Ashbourne)

Alphodith *see* Anthranol
(Stafford-Miller)

Alphosyl
(Stafford-Miller)

A cream used as an anti-psoriatic to treat psoriasis.

Dose: massage thoroughly into the affected area 2-4 times a day.
Availability: NHS, private prescription, over the counter.
Side effects: irritation, sensitivity to light.
Caution:
Not to be used for: patients suffering from acute psoriasis.
Caution needed with:
Contains: COAL TAR EXTRACT, ALLANTOIN.
Other preparations: Alphosyl Lotion, Alphosyl 2-in-1 Shampoo. CLINITAR (Shire), GELCOTAR (Quinoderm), POLYTAR (Stiefel), PSORIDERM (Dermal), PSORIGEL (Galderma), T-GEL (Neutrogena).

Alphosyl HC
(Stafford-Miller)

A cream used as an anti-psoriatic and STEROID treatment for psoriasis.

Dose: apply to the affected area twice a day.
Availability: NHS and private prescription.
Side effects: thinning of the skin, fluid retention, suppression of adrenal

glands.

Caution: in pregnant women, and in patients on extended treatment —
withdraw gradually.

Not to be used for: children under 5 years, or for patients suffering from
acne or other skin infections unless otherwise directed, or continuously
especially in pregnancy.

Caution needed with:

Contains: COAL TAR EXTRACT, ALLANTOIN, HYDROCORTISONE.

Other preparations: TARCORTIN (Stafford-Miller).

---

alprazolam *see* Xanax

Alrheumat *see* Orudis
(Bayer)

Altacite Plus
(Roussel)

A white liquid used as an ANTACID and anti-wind preparation to treat wind,
indigestion, dyspepsia, and gastric ulcers.

Dose: adults 10 ml between meals and at bedtime; children 8-12 years
half adult dose.

Availability: NHS, private prescription, over the counter.

Side effects: few; occasional diarrhoea and constipation.

Caution:

Not to be used for: children under 8 years.

Caution needed with: TETRACYCLINE antibiotics, tablets which are coated to
protect the stomach.

Contains: HYDROTALCITE, activated DIMETHICONE (CO-SIMALCITE).

Other preparations: Altacite suspension and tablets (antacids only —
available on NHS prescription only if prescribed generically).

Alu-Cap
(3M Healthcare)

A green/red capsule supplied at a strength of 475 mg and used as an
ANTACID to treat hyperacidity, and to regulate blood phosphate levels in
patients with kidney failure.

Dose: adults 1 tablet 4 times a day and at bedtime (higher doses for

phosphate regulation).
Availability: NHS, private prescription, over the counter.
Side effects: few; occasional bowel disorders such as constipation.
Caution:
Not to be used for: children.
Caution needed with: TETRACYCLINE antibiotics, tablets which are coated to protect the stomach.
Contains: ALUMINIUM HYDROXIDE GEL.
Other preparations:

Aludrox
(Charwell)

A white gel used as an ANTACID to treat dyspepsia, hyperacidity.

Dose: 5-10 ml four times a day between meals and at bedtime (reduced doses for children).
Availability: NHS (when prescribed as a generic), private prescription, over the counter.
Side effects: occasionally constipation.
Caution:
Not to be used for: infants.
Caution needed with: TETRACYCLINE antibiotics, tablets which are coated to protect the stomach.
Contains: ALUMINIUM HYDROXIDE GEL.
Other preparations: tablets and other combination preparations including Aludrox SA (now discontinued).

Aluhyde
(Sinclair)

A white, scored tablet used as an antispasmodic and ANTACID to treat hyperacidity and intestinal spasm.

Dose: 2 tablets after meals.
Availability: private prescription and over the counter.
Side effects: occasionally constipation and blurred vision.
Caution: in patients suffering from prostate enlargement.
Not to be used for: children or for patients suffering from glaucoma.
Caution needed with: TETRACYCLINE antibiotics, tablets which are coated to protect the stomach.
Contains: ALUMINIUM HYDROXIDE GEL, MAGNESIUM TRISILICATE, BELLADONNA liquid extract.
Other preparations:

Aluline *see* **Zyloric.** Product now discontinued.

---

aluminium acetate *see* **aluminium acetate ear drops, aluminium acetate lotion, Xyloproct**

---

aluminium acetate ear drops

Drops supplied at strengths of 8% and 13%, and used as an astringent to treat inflammation of the outer ear.

Dose: insert directly into the ear or saturate a gauze wick and apply into the ear.
Availability: NHS, private prescription, over the counter.
Side effects:
Caution:
Not to be used for:
Caution needed with:
Contains: ALUMINIUM ACETATE.
Other preparations:

---

aluminium acetate lotion

A lotion used as an astringent to treat weeping eczema and wounds.

Dose: to be used undiluted as a wet dressing.
Availability: NHS, private prescription, over the counter.
Side effects:
Caution:
Not to be used for:
Caution needed with:
Contains: ALUMINIUM ACETATE.
Other preparations:

---

aluminium chlorhydroxide see **Medrone Lotion, Neo-Medrone Lotion**

---

aluminium chloride *see* **Anhydrol Forte**

---

aluminium hydroxide gel *see* **Alu-Cap, Aludrox, Aluhyde,**

29

Asilone, Diovol, Theodrox

aluminium hydroxide *see* **Actonorm, APP, Caved-S, Gastrocote, Gastron, Gelusil, Kolanticon, Loasid, Maalox, Mucaine, Polyalk, Topal,**

aluminium hydroxide/magnesium carbonate *see* **Algicon, Andursil**

aluminium oxide *see* **Andursil, Brasivol**

Alupent
(Boehringer Ingelheim)

An off-white, scored tablet supplied at a strength of 20 mg and used as an anti-asthma drug to treat bronchial spasm brought on by chronic bronchitis, asthma, emphysema.

Dose: adults 1 tablet 4 times a day; children use syrup.
Availability: NHS and private prescription.
Side effects: abnormal heart rhythm, tremor, nervous tension, headache, dilation of the veins, rapid heart rate.
Caution: in diabetics and patients suffering from high blood pressure.
Not to be used for: patients suffering from cardiac asthma, acute heart disease, overactive thyroid gland.
Caution needed with: MAOIS, TRICYCLICS, SYMPATHOMIMETICS.
Contains: ORCIPRENALINE SULPHATE.
Other preparations: Alupent Syrup, Alupent Aerosol.

Alupram *see* **Valium.** Product now discontinued.

Aluzine *see* **Lasix.** Product now discontinued.

Alvedon
(Novex)

A suppository used to treat pain and fever in children.

Dose: children aged 1-5 years, 1-2 suppositories up to 4 times a day.
Availability: NHS, private prescription, over the counter.
Side effects:
Caution: in patients suffering from kidney or liver damage.
Not to be used for: children under 1 year or over 5 years, adults.
Caution needed with: other preparations containing PARACETAMOL.
Contains: PARACETAMOL
Other preparations: CALPOL INFANT, DISPROL PAEDIATRIC, PALDESIC, PARACETA-
MOL PAEDIATRIC ELIXIR, SALZONE.

---

alverine citrate *see* **Spasmonal**

---

amantadine *see* **Symmetrel**

Ambaxin
(Upjohn)

An off-white, oblong, scored tablet supplied at a strength of 400 mg and
used as a broad-spectrum penicillin to treat respiratory, ear, nose, and
throat, skin, soft tissue, urinary tract, and venereal infections.

Dose: adults 1-2 tablets 2-3 times a day (higher doses in venereal infec-
tions); children over 5 years ½ tablet 3 times a day.
Availability: NHS and private prescription.
Side effects: allergy, stomach disturbances.
Caution: in patients suffering from kidney disease, severe liver disease,
glandular fever.
Not to be used for: children under 5 years.
Caution needed with:
Contains: BACAMPICILLIN hydrochloride.
Other preparations:

---

ambucetamide *see* **Femerital**

Amfipen *see* **ampicillin**
(Brocades)

Amilco *see* **Moduretic**
(Baker Norton)

Amilmaxco *see* **Moduretic**
(Ashbourne)

---

amiloride *see* **amiloride tablets, Burinex A, Frumil, Hypertane, Kalten, Lasoride, Moducren, Navispare, Normetic**

---

amiloride tablets

A yellow, diamond-shaped tablet supplied at a strength of 5 mg and used as a potassium-sparing DIURETIC to maintain potassium level when used with other DIURETICS.

Dose: 1-2 tablets a day at first, then up to 4 tablets a day if needed.
Availability: NHS and private prescription.
Side effects: stomach upset, rash.
Caution: in pregnant women or nursing mothers and in patients suffering from diabetes with a predisposition to high potassium levels, gout, liver or kidney disease. Your doctor may advise blood tests for potassium levels.
Not to be used for: children or for patients suffering from high potassium levels or progressive kidney failure.
Caution needed with: potassium supplements, potassium-sparing DIURETICS, ACE INHIBITORS.
Contains: AMILORIDE hydrochloride.
Other preparations: AMILOSPARE (Ashbourne), BERKAMIL (Berk), MIDAMOR (Morson).

Amilospare *see* **amiloride tablets**
(Ashbourne)

---

aminoglutethimide *see* **Orimeten**

---

aminophylline *see* **Pecram, Phyllocontin Continus, Theodrox**

---

amiodarone *see* **Cordarone X**

amitriptyline *see* **Domical, Elavil, Lentizol, Limbitrol 5, Triptafen, Tryptizol**

Amix *see* **Amoxil**
(Ashbourne)

amlodipine *see* **Istin**

ammonium chloride *see* **Benylin Expectorant, Guanor, Histalix**

Amnivent *see* **Phyllocontin Continus**
(Ashbourne)

amodiaquine *see* **Camoquin**

Amopen *see* **Amoxil**
(Yorkshire)

Amoram *see* **Amoxil**
(Eastern)

amorolfine *see* **Loceryl**

amoxapine *see* **Asendis**

Amoxidin *see* **Amoxil.** Product now discontinued.

Amoxil
(Bencard)

A maroon/gold capsule supplied at a strength of 250 mg, 500 mg and used as a broad-spectrum penicillin to treat respiratory, ear, nose, and throat, urinary, venereal, and soft tissue infections. Also for dental abscess, and to prevent infection of the heart during dental procedures

Dose: adults 250-500 mg 3 times a day; children half adult dose; infants under 6 months use Amoxil Paediatric Suspension.
Availability: NHS and private prescription.
Side effects: stomach upset, allergy.
Caution: in patients suffering from glandular fever.
Not to be used for: patients suffering from penicillin allergy.
Caution needed with:
Contains: AMOXYCILLIN trihydrate.
Other preparations: Amoxil Dispersible, Amoxil Syrup SF, Amoxil Paediatric Suspension, Amoxil 3g Sachet SF, Amoxil 750 mg Sachet SF, Amoxil Fiztab, AMOXIDIN, ALMODAN (Berk), AMIX (Ashbourne), AMOPEN (Yorkshire), AMORAM (Eastern), AMRIT (BHR), FLEMOXIN (Paines and Byrne).

---

amoxycillin *see* Amoxil, Augmentin

---

amphotericin *see* Fungilin, Fungilin Cream, Fungilin Lozenges

---

ampicillin capsules

A capsule supplied at strengths of 250 mg, 500 mg and used as a broad-spectrum penicillin to treat respiratory, ear, nose, and throat, and soft tissue infections. Also for urinary tract and venereal infections.

Dose: adults 250 mg-1 g 4 times a day; children half adult dose.
Availability: NHS and private prescription.
Side effects: stomach upset, allergy.
Caution: in patients suffering kidney disease, glandular fever.
Not to be used for: patients suffering from penicillin allergy.
Caution needed with:
Contains: AMPICILLIN.
Other preparations: Ampicillin Syrup, Ampicillin Injection, AMFIPEN (Brocades), AMPILAR, PENBRITIN (Beecham), RIMACILLIN (Rima), VIDOPEN (Berk).

---

ampicillin *see* ampicillin capsules, Ampiclox Neonatal Suspension, Magnapen, Neonatal, Penbritin, Vidopen

Ampiclox Neonatal
(Beecham)

A suspension used as a penicillin treatment for serious or mixed infections.

Dose: in young babies 0.6 ml every 4 hours; older children and adults treated by injection.
Availability: NHS and private prescription.
Side effects: allergy, stomach upset.
Caution: in patients suffering from glandular fever.
Not to be used for:
Caution needed with:
Contains: AMPICILLIN, CLOXACILLIN.
Other preparations: Ampiclox Injection.

Ampilar *see* **ampicillin. Product now discontinued.**

Amrit *see* Amoxil
(BHR)

---

amylobarbitone *see* Amytal, Sodium Amytal, Tuinal

Amytal
(Eli Lilly)

A white tablet supplied at a strength of 50 mg and used as a BARBITURATE to treat sleeplessness.

Dose: 100-200 mg before going to bed.
Availability: controlled drug; NHS and private prescription.
Side effects: drowsiness, hangover, dizziness, allergies, headache, confusion, excitement.
Caution: in patients suffering from liver, kidney, or lung disease. Dependence (addiction) may develop.
Not to be used for: children, young adults, pregnant women, nursing mothers, the elderly, patients with a history of drug or alcohol abuse, or

suffering from porphyria (a rare blood disorder), or in the management of pain.

Caution needed with: anticoagulants (blood-thinning drugs), alcohol, other tranquillizers, STEROIDS, the contraceptive pill, GRISEOFULVIN, RIFAMPICIN, PHENYTOIN, METRONIDAZOLE, CHLORAMPHENICOL.

Contains: AMYLOBARBITONE.

Other preparations: SODIUM AMYTAL (Eli Lilly).

Anacal
(Panpharma)

An ointment used as a soothing, anti-inflammatory treatment for haemorrhoids, anal fissure, anal itch.

Dose: adults and children over 5 years apply one or more times a day as required.
Availability: NHS, private prescription, over the counter.
Side effects:
Caution:
Not to be used for: children under 5 years.
Caution needed with:
Contains: HEPARINOID, LAUROMACROGOL.
Other preparations: Anacal Suppositories.

Anaflex Cream
(Geistlich)

A cream used as an antibacterial and antifungal treatment for skin infections.

Dose: apply the cream to the affected area 1-2 times a day.
Availability: NHS, private prescription, over the counter.
Side effects:
Caution:
Not to be used for:
Caution needed with:
Contains: POLYNOXYLIN.
Other preparations: Anaflex Lozenges, Anaflex Paste, Anaflex Powder, Anaflex Aerosol (all now discontinued).

Anaflex lozenges — treatment for mouth infections. Product now discontinued.

Anafranil
(Ciba-Geigy)

A yellow/caramel capsule, orange/caramel capsule, or blue/caramel capsule according to strengths of 10 mg, 25 mg, 50 mg and used as a TRICYCLIC antidepressant to treat depression, obsessions, phobias.

Dose: adults 10 mg at first increasing to 30-250 mg a day ; elderly 10 mg a day at first up to a maximum of 75 mg a day.
Availability: NHS and private prescription.
Side effects: dry mouth, constipation, urine retention, blurred vision, palpitations, drowsiness, sleeplessness, dizziness, low blood pressure, weight change, skin reactions, jaundice or blood changes, loss of libido may occur.
Caution: in nursing mothers or in patients suffering from heart disease, liver disease, thyroid disease, adrenal tumour, glaucoma, urine retention, epilepsy, diabetes, some other psychiatric conditions. Your doctor may advise regular blood tests.
Not to be used for: children, pregnant women, or for patients suffering from heart attacks, liver disease, heart block.
Caution needed with: alcohol, ANTICHOLINERGICS, ADRENALINE, BARBITURATES, MAOIS, other antidepressants, ANTIHYPERTENSIVES, CIMETIDINE, oestrogens, some local anaesthetics.
Contains: CLOMIPRAMINE hydrochloride.
Other preparations: Anafranil SR, Anafranil Injection, Anafranil Syrup.

---

analgesic

A preparation used to relieve pain. Example PARACETAMOL TABLETS.

Anapolon 50
(Syntex)

A white, scored tablet supplied at a strength of 50 mg and used as an anabolic STEROID treatment for certain types of anaemia.

Dose: adults 2-5 mg/kg body weight a day, reducing on improvement; children over 2 years 2-4 mg/kg body weight a day in divided doses.
Availability: NHS and private prescription.
Side effects: liver disease, jaundice, fluid retention, high calcium levels, masculinization and absence of menstruation in women.
Caution: in patients suffering from heart failure, enlarged prostate, diabetes. Your doctor may advise liver tests.
Not to be used for: children under 2 years, pregnant women, nursing mothers, or for patients with kidney or liver disease, breast cancer (in

men), or cancer of the prostate.
Caution needed with: other STEROIDS (corticosteroids), anticoagulants.
Contains: OXYMETHOLONE
Other preparations:

Androcur
(Schering)

A white, scored tablet supplied at a strength of 50 mg and used as an anti-androgen to treat severe hypersexuality and sexual deviation in men.

Dose: 1 tablet in the morning and 1 tablet in the evening.
Availability: NHS and private prescription.
Side effects: tiredness, depression, weight gain, breast enlargement, changes in hair pattern, osteoporosis.
Caution: in patients suffering from diabetes or liver disease. Patients must give consent to treatment. Your doctor may advise regular blood and sperm tests.
Not to be used for: men under 18 years or where bones and testes have not reached full development, or for patients suffering from acute liver disease, malignant or wasting disease, severe chronic depression, history of thrombosis or embolism.
Caution needed with: alcohol.
Contains: CYPROTERONE ACETATE.
Other preparations: CYPROSTAT (Schering).

Andursil — ANTACID and anti-wind preparation. Product now discontinued.
(Geigy)

---

anethol *see* **Rowatinex**

Angilol *see* **Inderal**
(DDSA)

Angiopine *see* **Adalat**
(Ashbourne)

Angiozem *see* Tildiem
(Ashbourne)

Anhydrol Forte
(Dermal)

A roll-on solution used to treat excessive sweating of the armpits, hands, or feet.

Dose: apply if necessary at night. Wash off in the morning. Children only to be treated on the feet.
Availability: NHS and private prescription.
Side effects:
Caution: in children. Avoid contact with clothes or jewellery. Ensure that area is dry and not shaved for 12 hours before or after use.
Not to be used for: inflamed and broken skin areas.
Caution needed with:
Contains: ALUMINIUM CHLORIDE.
Other preparations:

---

anise *see* simple linctus

Anquil
(Janssen)

A white tablet supplied at a strength of 0.25 mg and used as an antipsychotic drug for controlling unacceptable sexual behaviour.

Dose: 1-6 tablets a day in divided doses.
Availability: NHS and private prescription.
Side effects: muscle spasms, restlessness, hands shaking, dry mouth, urine retention, palpitations, low blood pressure, weight gain, changes in libido, low body temperature, breast swelling, menstrual changes, jaundice, blood and skin changes, stomach upset, drowsiness, rarely fits.
Caution: in nursing mothers, and in patients suffering from liver or kidney disease, epilepsy, or Parkinson's disease. Your doctor may advise regular blood and liver tests.
Not to be used for: children or for pregnant women.
Caution needed with: alcohol, tranquillizers, pain killers, ANTIHYPERTENSIVES, antidepressants, anticonvulsants, antidiabetic drugs, LEVODOPA.
Contains: BENPERIDOL.
Other preparations:

Antabuse
(CP Pharm)

A white, scored tablet supplied at a strength of 200 mg and used as an enzyme inhibitor, additional treatment for alcoholism.

Dose: initially as advised by doctor, reducing to ½ or 1 tablet a day for maintenance.
Availability: NHS and private prescription.
Side effects: drowsiness, tiredness, nausea, bad breath, reduced sex drive, rarely mental disturbances.
Caution: in patients suffering from liver, kidney, or breathing diseases, diabetes, epilepsy, drug addiction.
Not to be used for: children, pregnant women, or patients suffering from heart failure, coronary artery disease, mental disorders.
Caution needed with: alcohol, BARBITURATES, PARALDEHYDE, sedatives.
Contains: DISULFIRAM.
Other preparations:

---

antacid

A preparation which reduces the acid content of the stomach, used to relieve indigestion. Example MAGNESIUM TRISILICATE MIXTURE.

---

antazoline phosphate *see* Vasocon-A

---

antazoline sulphate *see* Otrivine-Antistin

Antepar — antiworm agent. Product now discontinued.

Antepsin
(Wyeth)

A white, oblong tablet supplied at a strength of 1 g and used as a cell-surface protector in the treatment of gastritis and ulcers.

Dose: adults 2 tablets twice a day in water.
Availability: NHS and private prescription.
Side effects: stomach upset, dry mouth, rash.
Caution: in kidney function impairment.

Not to be used for: children.
Caution needed with: TETRACYCLINE antibiotics, PHENYTOIN, DIGOXIN, CIMETIDINE.
Contains: SUCRALFATE.
Other preparations: Antepsin suspension.

Anthranol
(Stiefel)

An ointment used as an anti-psoriatic treatment for psoriasis.

Dose: apply in small amounts once a day at first, and then wash off after 10 minutes, then allowing 30 minutes before washing off.
Availability: NHS and private prescription.
Side effects: irritation and burning, allergy.
Caution: stains skin and clothing.
Not to be used for: patients suffering from acute or pustular psoriasis.
Caution needed with:
Contains: DITHRANOL.
Other preparations: ALPHODITH (Stafford-Miller), DITHROCREAM (Dermal), EXOLAN (Dermal), PSORADRATE (Norwich Eaton) — some available over the counter.

anthraquinone glycosides *see* Pyralvex

anticholinergic

a drug which blocks the action of acetyl choline, a nerve transmitter. Anticholinergics are used to reduce muscle spasm. The effects include dry mouth, difficulty passing urine, and possibly confusion. Example, HYOSCINE *see* Buscopan.

anticholinesterase

a drug which enhances the action of acetyl choline, a nerve transmitter. Example NEOSTIGMINE *see* Prostigmin.

antihistamine

A preparation which blocks the histamine response in the body which occurs during an allergic reaction. Antihistamines are used to treat all types of allergy (skin rashes, hay fever, etc). Example CHLORPHENIRAMINE *see* Piriton.

antihypertensive

A preparation used to lower blood pressure. Example ß-BLOCKERS *see* Inderal.

Antipressan *see* Tenormin
(Berk)

Antoin — ANALGESIC tablet. Product now discontinued.

Antraderm — treatment stick for psoriasis. Product now discontinued.

Anturan
(Ciba-Geigy)

A yellow tablet supplied at strengths of100 mg, 200 mg and used as a uric acid-lowering drug to treat gout, gouty arthritis, high uric acid levels.

Dose: 100-200 mg a day with food at first increasing to 600 mg a day over 2-3 weeks and then reduce to the minimum effective dose.
Availability: NHS and private prescription.
Side effects: acute gout, stones in the urinary tract, kidney colic, gastro-intestinal bleeding, kidney or liver disease, rash, blood changes.
Caution: in pregnant women, and in patients suffering from kidney disease, latent heart failure. Drink plenty of fluids. Your doctor may advise blood and kidney tests.
Not to be used for: children, patients with a history of peptic ulcer, severe liver or kidney disease, acute gout, blood disorders, allergies induced by anti-inflammatory drugs.
Caution needed with: salicylates, anticoagulants, HYPOGLYCAEMICS, SULPHONAMIDES, PENICILLINS, THEOPHYLLINE, PHENYTOIN.
Contains: SULPHINPYRAZONE.
Other preparations:

Anugesic-HC
(Warner)

A cream used as a soothing, antiseptic, STEROID treatment for haemorrhoids, anal itch, and other rectal disorders.

Dose: apply night and morning, and after passing motions.
Availability: NHS and private prescription.
Side effects: systemic corticosteroid effects (*see* Precortisyl).
Caution: do not use for prolonged periods; special care is required for
pregnant women.
Not to be used for: children or for patients suffering from tuberculous,
fungal, and viral infections.
Caution needed with:
Contains: PRAMOXINE hydrochloride, HYDROCORTISONE acetate, ZINC OXIDE,
PERU BALSAM, BENZYL BENZOATE, BISMUTH OXIDE.
Other preparations: Anugesic-HC suppositories.

Anusol
(Warner-Lambert)

A suppository used as a soothing, antiseptic, astringent treatment for
haemorrhoids, anal itch, and other rectal and anal disorders.

Dose: 1 suppository night and morning, and after passing motions.
Availability: NHS, private prescription, over the counter.
Side effects:
Caution:
Not to be used for: children.
Caution needed with:
Contains: BISMUTH SUBGALLATE, BISMUTH OXIDE, PERU BALSAM, ZINC OXIDE.
Other preparations: Anusol cream, Anusol ointment.

Anusol HC
(Warner)

A suppository used as a STEROID, antiseptic, astringent treatment for
haemorrhoids and inflammation of the anus and rectum.

Dose: 1 suppository night and morning after passing motions.
Availability: NHS and private prescription.
Side effects: systemic corticosteroid effects (*see* Precortisyl).
Caution: in pregnant women; do not use for prolonged periods.

Not to be used for: children or for patients suffering from tuberculous, fungal, and viral infections.
Caution needed with:
Contains: HYDROCORTISONE acetate, BENZYL BENZOATE, BISMUTH SUBGALLATE, BISMUTH OXIDE, RESORCINOL, PERU BALSAM, ZINC OXIDE.
Other preparations: Anusol HC ointment.

Anxon — tranquillizer. Product now discontinued.

Apisate
(Wyeth)

A yellow tablet used as an appetite suppressant to treat obesity.

Dose: 1 tablet a day early in the morning or mid-afternoon.
Availability: controlled drug. NHS and private prescription.
Side effects: tolerance, addiction, mental disturbances, sleeplessness, nervousness, agitation.
Caution: in women during the first three months of pregnancy, and in patients suffering from high blood pressure, angina, abnormal heart rhythm, peptic ulcer.
Not to be used for: children, the elderly, or patients suffering from arteriosclerosis, overactive thyroid, severe high blood pressure, glaucoma, or with a history of alcoholism, drug addiction, or mental illness.
Caution needed with: MAOIS, SYMPATHOMIMETICS, METHYLDOPA, GUANETHIDINE, psychotropics, or obesity drugs.
Contains: DIETHYLPROPION HYDROCHLORIDE, THIAMINE, RIBOFLAVINE, PYRIDOXINE, NICOTINAMIDE.
Other preparations: TENUATE DOSPAN (Merrell Dow)

APP
(Chancellor)

A powder used as an ANTACID to treat ulcers, indigestion, nausea, acidity.

Dose: adults 5 ml 3-4 times a day in liquid.
Availability: private prescription only.
Side effects: occasionally constipation.
Caution: in patients suffering from prostate enlargement.
Not to be used for: infants or for patients suffering from glaucoma, myaesthenia gravis.
Caution needed with:
Contains: PAPAVERINE, CALCIUM CARBONATE, ALUMINIUM HYDROXIDE, HOMATROPINE,

MAGNESIUM CARBONATE, BISMUTH CARBONATE.
Other preparations: APP tablets (also available over the counter).

Apresoline
(Ciba)

A yellow tablet or pink tablet according to strengths of 25 mg, 50 mg and used as a vasodilator in addition to DIURETICS and glycosides for the treatment of moderate to severe chronic heart failure, moderate to severe high blood pressure.

Dose: 25 mg 3 or 4 times a day at first increasing every second day to 50-75 mg 3 or 4 times a day if necessary; hypertension 25 mg twice times a day at first with a ß-BLOCKER and DIURETIC.
Availability: NHS and private prescription.
Side effects: rapid heart rate, headache, flushes, especially if more than 100 mg a day are taken; rarely liver damage, kidney disorders, changes in blood count, nerve disorders.
Caution: in nursing mothers and in patients suffering from coronary or cerebrovascular disease, kidney failure, liver disease.
Not to be used for: children, for patients suffering from certain heart diseases, or during the first half of pregnancy
Caution needed with: TRICYCLIC antidepressants, MAOIS, ANTIHYPERTENSIVES, tranquillizers.
Contains: HYDRALAZINE HYDROCHLORIDE.
Other preparations: Apresoline Injection.

Aprinox
(Boots)

A white tablet supplied at strengths of 2.5 mg, 5 mg and used as a DIURETIC to treat fluid retention, high blood pressure.

Dose: 5-10 mg each morning or each alternate day at first then 5-10 mg once or twice a week. High blood pressure 2.5-5 mg a day.
Availability: NHS and private prescription.
Side effects: low potassium levels, rash, sensitivity to light, blood changes, gout, tiredness.
Caution: in pregnant women, nursing mothers, the elderly and for patients suffering from diabetes, severe kidney or liver disease, or gout.
Not to be used for: children or for patients suffering from urine failure or severe or progressive kidney failure.
Caution needed with: LITHIUM, DIGOXIN, blood pressure-lowering drugs.
Contains: BENDROFLUAZIDE.
Other preparations: BERKOZIDE (Berk), CENTYL (Leo), NEO-NACLEX (Evans).

Apsifen *see* **Brufen**. Product now discontinued.

Apsin VK *see* **penicillin**. Product now discontinued.

Apsolol *see* **Inderal**
(APS)

Apsolox *see* **Trasicor**
(APS)

Aquasept
(Hough, Hoseason)

A solution used as a disinfectant for skin and body cleansing and disinfecting.

Dose: use as a soap.
Availability: NHS, private prescription, over the counter.
Side effects:
Caution: keep out of the eyes.
Not to be used for:
Caution needed with:
Contains: TRICLOSAN.
Other preparations: TRICLOSEPT.

---

aqueous cream BP

A cream used as an emollient to treat dry skin conditions.

Dose: apply as required.
Availability: NHS, private prescription, over the counter.
Side effects:
Caution:
Not to be used for:
Caution needed with:
Contains: aqueous cream BP.
Other preparations:

---

arachis oil *see* **Cerumol, Fletcher's Arachis Oil, Oilatum**

Aradolene — ANALGESIC rub to treat rheumatic conditions. Product now discontinued.

Arbralene *see* **Betaloc**
(Berk)

Arelix
(Hoechst)

A green/orange capsule supplied at a strength of 6 mg and used as a DIURETIC to treat high blood pressure.

Dose: 1-2 a day as a single morning dose.
Availability: NHS and private prescription.
Side effects: electrolyte imbalance.
Caution: in pregnant women, nursing mothers, or in patients suffering from liver or kidney disease, gout, diabetes, enlarged prostate, or impaired urination. Your doctor may advise regular bood tests.
Not to be used for: children or for patients suffering from cirrhosis of the liver.
Caution needed with: DIGOXIN, LITHIUM, aminoglycosides, cephalosporin antibiotics, blood pressure-lowering drugs, NON-STEROID ANTI-INFLAMMATORY DRUGS.
Contains: PIRETANIDE.
Other preparations:

Arobon — diarrhoea treatment. Product now discontinued.

aromatic oils *see* **Pavacol-D**

Arpicolin
(RP Drugs)

A syrup supplied at strengths of 2.5 mg/5 ml, 5 mg/5 ml and used as an ANTICHOLINERGIC treatment for Parkinson's disease.

Dose: 2.5-5 mg 3 times a day at first increasing every 2-3 days by 2.5-5 mg a day to a maximum of 30 mg a day.
Availability: NHS and private prescription.
Side effects: ANTICHOLINERGIC effects, confusion at high doses.
Caution: in patients suffering from heart problems, gastro-intestinal obstruction, glaucoma, enlarged prostate. The dosage should be reduced gradually.
Not to be used for: children or patients suffering from tardive dyskinesia (a movement disorder).
Caution needed with: PHENOTHIAZINES, ANTIHISTAMINES, antidepressants.
Contains: PROCYCLIDINE hydrochloride.
Other preparations: KEMADRIN (Wellcome).

Arpimycin *see* **Erythrocin**. Product now discontinued.

Artane
(Lederle)

A white, scored tablet supplied at strengths of 2 mg, 5 mg and used as an ANTICHOLINERGIC treatment for Parkinson's disease, drug-induced Parkinson's disease.

Dose: 1 mg on the first day, 2 mg second day, then increased by 2 mg a day every 3-5 days usually to 5-15 mg a day.
Availability: NHS and private prescription.
Side effects: ANTICHOLINERGIC effects, confusion and agitation at high doses.
Caution: in patients suffering from heart, kidney, or liver disease, enlarged prostate, glaucoma, or gastro-intestinal obstruction. Dose should be reduced gradually.
Not to be used for: children.
Caution needed with: PHENOTHIAZINES, ANTIHISTAMINES, antidepressants.
Contains: BENZHEXOL.
Other preparations: BENTEX, BROFLEX (Bio-Medical).

Arthrofen *see* **Brufen**
(Ashbourne)

Arthrosin *see* **Naprosyn**
(Ashbourne)

Arthroxen *see* **Naprosyn**
(Ashbourne)

Artracin *see* **Indocid**
(DDSA)

Arythmol
(Knoll)

A white tablet supplied in strengths of 150 mg, 300 mg and used as an anti-arrhythmic drug to treat heart rhythm disturbances

Dose: 150-300 mg 3 times a day.
Availability: NHS and private prescription.
Side effects: nausea, vomiting, dizziness, diarrhoea, constipation, headache, tiredness, skin rash, slow heart rate.
Caution: in the elderly, patients with pace makers, and in patients suffering from heart failure, liver and kidney disorders.
Not to be used for: children, pregnant women, or for patients suffering from uncontrolled heart failure, obstructive lung disease, electrolyte disturbances, some heart rhythm disturbances.
Caution needed with: other anti-arrhythmics, DIGOXIN, WARFARIN, CIMETIDINE, PROPANOLOL, METOPROLOL, RIFAMPICIN.
Contains: PROPAFENONE.
Other preparations:

Asacol
(S K B)

A red, coated, oblong tablet supplied at a strength of 400 mg and used as a salicylate to treat ulcerative colitis.

Dose: 3-6 tablets a day in divided doses.
Availability: NHS and private prescription.
Side effects: stomach disturbances, headache.
Caution: in patients suffering from kidney disease, raised blood urea, protein in the urine, and in pregnant women.
Not to be used for: children.
Caution needed with: LACTULOSE or any preparations that increase the acidity of the motions.
Contains: MESALAZINE.
Other preparations: Asacol suppositories, PENTASA (Brocades), SALOFALK (Thames).

Ascabiol
(Rhone-Poulenc Rorer)

An emulsion used as an insect-destroying drug to treat scabies, pediculosis.

Dose: as advised by doctor. (Infants and children use diluted preparation).
Availability: NHS, private prescription, over the counter.
Side effects: irritation.
Caution: keep out of the eyes.
Not to be used for:
Caution needed with:
Contains: BENZYL BENZOATE.
Other preparations:

---

ascorbic acid *see* **Abidec, Allbee with C, BC 500, BC 500 with Iron, Concavit, Fefol-Vit Spansule, Ferrograd C, Fesovit Spansule, Fesovit Z Spansule, Galfervit, Givitol, Irofol C, Ketovite, Lipoflavonoid, Multivite, Octovit, Oralcer, Orovite, Orovite 7, Polyvite, Pregnavite Forte F, Redoxon, Surbex T, Tonivitan, Uniflu and Gregovite C, Villescon, vitamins capsules.**

Asendis
(Novex)

A white, orange, blue, or white, hexagonal tablet according to strengths of 25 mg, 50 mg, 100 mg, 150 mg and used as a TRICYCLIC antidepressant to treat depression.

Dose: 100-150 mg a day increasing to 300 mg a day.
Availability: NHS and private prescription.
Side effects: ANTICHOLINERGIC effects, drowsiness, impotence, nausea, vomiting, breast enlargement, convulsions at high doses.
Caution: in the elderly, and in patients who are a suicide risk, or who are suffering from epilepsy, glaucoma, urine retention, confusion, agitation.
Not to be used for: pregnant women, nursing mothers, or for patients suffering from recent heart attack, heart block, heart rhythm disturbances, severe liver disease, mania.
Caution needed with: MAOIS, SYMPATHOMIMETICS, BARBITURATES, alcohol, ANTIHYPERTENSIVES, anaesthetics.
Contains: amoxapine.
Other preparations:

Aserbine
(Bencard)

A cream and solution used as a wound cleanser to treat varicose ulcers, burns, bed sores, and for cleansing of wounds.

Dose: wash the wound with the solution and apply cream twice a day.
Availability: NHS, private prescription, over the counter.
Side effects:
Caution: avoid the eyes.
Not to be used for:
Caution needed with:
Contains: MALIC ACID, BENZOIC ACID, SALICYLIC ACID, PROPYLENE GLYCOL.
Other preparations:

Asilone
(Crookes)

A white liquid used as an ANTACID, anti-wind preparation to treat gastritis, ulcers, dyspepsia, wind.

Dose: adults 5-10 ml before meals and at bedtime
Availability: NHS, private prescription, over the counter.
Side effects: occasionally constipation.
Caution:
Not to be used for: infants and children.
Caution needed with: tablets which are coated to protect the stomach.
Contains: activated DIMETHICONE, ALUMINIUM HYDROXIDE GEL, MAGNESIUM OXIDE.
Other preparations: Asilone suspension, Asilone tablets (not available on NHS), MAALOX PLUS (Rhone-Poulenc Rorer — tablets not available on NHS), INFACOL (Pharmax) — for infants. Also POLYCROL, SILOXYL, UNIGEST — all now discontinued..

Asmaven *see* Ventolin
(APS)

Aspav
(Roussel)

A white, dispersible tablet used as ANALGESIC to relieve pain after operations and pain associated with cancers for which surgery is inappropriate.

Dose: 1-2 tablets dispersed in water every 4-6 hours up to a maximum of 8 tablets in 24 hours.

Availability: NHS and private prescription.
Side effects: allergies, asthma, gastro-intestinal bleeding, constipation, nausea, confusion.
Caution: in pregnant women, women in labour, nursing mothers, the elderly, and in patients suffering from head injury, underactive thyroid gland, a history of bronchospasm or anti-inflammatory induced allergies, kidney or liver disease.
Not to be used for: children, women who may later become pregnant, unconscious patients, or patients suffering from respiratory depression, blocked airways, gastric ulcer, haemophilia.
Caution needed with: MAOIS, sedatives, anticoagulants, antidiabetic drugs, NON-STEROID ANTI-INFLAMMATORY DRUGS, uric acid-lowering drugs, METHOTREXATE, sulphonamide antibiotics.
Contains: ASPIRIN, PAPAVERETUM.
Other preparations:

Aspellin
(Fisons)

A liniment or a spray used as a topical ANALGESIC to treat muscular rheumatism, sciatica, lumbago, fibrositis.

Dose: massage gently into the affected area 3 times a day.
Availability: NHS, private prescription, over the counter.
Side effects: may be irritant.
Caution:
Not to be used for: areas near the eyes, or where the skin is broken or inflamed, or on membranes (such as the mouth).
Caution needed with:
Contains: ASPIRIN, MENTHOL, CAMPHOR, METHYL SALICYLATE.
Other preparations:

---

aspirin *see* **Antoin, Aspav, Aspellin, aspirin tablets, aspirin 75 mg tablets Claradin, Co-Codaprin Dispersible, Codis, Doloxene Co., Equagesic, Hypon, Migravess Forte, Nu-Seals Aspirin, Paynocil, Platet 300, Robaxisal Forte, Solprin, Trancoprin**

---

aspirin 75 mg tablets

A white tablet supplied at a strength of 75 mg and used to prevent heart attack or stroke, in patients known to be at risk.

Dose: 1-4 tablets a day (dissolved in water).
Availability: NHS, private prescription, over the counter.
Side effects: stomach upsets, allergy, asthma.
Caution: in pregnant women and in patients suffering from uncontrolled high blood pressure or asthma.
Not to be used for: children under 12 years, nursing mothers, or for patients suffering from haemophilia or stomach ulcer.
Caution needed with: anticoagulants, some antidiabetic drugs, anti-inflammatory agents, METHOTREXATE, SPIRONOLACTONE, STEROIDS, some uric-acid lowering drugs.
Contains: ASPIRIN
Other preparations:

---

aspirin tablets

A white tablet supplied at a strength of 300 mg and used as an ANALGESIC to relieve pain and reduce fever.

Dose: 1-3 tablets every 4-6 hours as needed to a maximum of 12 tablets a day.
Availability: NHS, private prescription, over the counter.
Side effects: stomach upsets, allergy, asthma.
Caution: in pregnant women, the elderly, or in patients with a history of allergy to aspirin, asthma, impaired kidney or liver function, indigestion.
Not to be used for: children, nursing mothers, or patients suffering from haemophilia, or ulcers.
Caution needed with: anticoagulants (blood-thinning drugs), some antidiabetic drugs, anti-inflammatory agents, METHOTREXATE, SPIRONOLACTONE, STEROIDS, some ANTACIDS, some uric acid-lowering drugs.
Contains: ASPIRIN.
Other preparations: Dispersible Aspirin, PLATET CLEARTAB (Nicholas), NU-SEALS ASPIRIN (Lilly).

---

astemizole *see* Hismanal

AT 10
(Sanofi Winthrop)

A solution used as a source of vitamin D to treat vitamin D deficiency.

Dose: 1-7 ml taken by mouth each week.
Availability: NHS, private prescription, over the counter.
Side effects: loss of appetite, listlessness, vertigo, stupor, nausea, urgent

need to urinate, thirst.

Caution: in pregnant women nursing mothers.Your doctor may advise that your calcium levels should be checked regularly.

Not to be used for: children.

Caution needed with: CHOLESTYRAMINE, some DIURETICS, DIGOXIN and similar drugs.

Contains: DIHYDROTACHYSTEROL.

Other preparations:

Atarax
(Pfizer)

An orange tablet or a green tablet according to strengths of 10 mg, 25 mg and used as an ANTIHISTAMINE to treat anxiety and itching.

Dose: anxiety 50-100 mg 4 times a day; itching 25 mg 1-4 times a day.

Availability: NHS and private prescription.

Side effects: drowsiness, ANTICHOLINERGIC effects, involuntary movements if a high dosage is taken.

Caution: in patients suffering from kidney disease. Patients should be warned of reduced judgement and abilities. Only to be used in children for itching (reduced doses).

Not to be used for: pregnant women.

Caution needed with: alcohol and sedatives.

Contains: HYDROXYZINE HYDROCHLORIDE.

Other preparations: Atarax Syrup, UCERAX (UCB).

Atenix *see* Tenormin
(Ashbourne)

Atenixco *see* Tenoretic, Tenoret-50
(Ashbourne)

---

atenolol *see* Antipressan, Atenix, Beta-Adalat, Kalten, Tenif, Tenoret 50, Tenoretic, Tenormin, Totamol, Vasaten

---

Atensine *see* Valium
(Berk)

Ativan
(Wyeth)

A blue, oblong, scored tablet or a yellow, oblong, scored tablet according to strengths of 1 mg, 2.5 mg and used as a tranquillizer to treat anxiety.

Dose: elderly 0.5-2 mg a day; adults 1-4 mg a day.
Availability: NHS (when prescribed as a generic) and private prescription.
Side effects: drowsiness, confusion, unsteadiness, stomach upset, low blood pressure, rash, changes in vision, changes in libido, retention of urine. Risk of addiction increases with dose and length of treatment. May impair judgement.
Caution: in the elderly, pregnant women, nursing mothers, in women during labour, and in patients suffering from lung disorders, kidney or liver disorders. Avoid long-term use and withdraw gradually.
Not to be used for: children, or for patients suffering from acute lung diseases, some chronic lung diseases, some obsessional and psychotic diseases.
Caution needed with: alcohol, other tranquillizers, anti-convulsants.
Contains: LORAZEPAM.
Other preparations: ALMAZINE.

Atromid-S
(ICI)

A red capsule supplied at a strength of 500 mg and used as a lipid-lowering agent to treat elevated cholesterol.

Dose: 20-30 mg per kg body weight a day in 2-3 divided doses after meals.
Availability: NHS and private prescription.
Side effects: stomach upset, gallstones, muscle aches.
Caution: in patients with low serum proteins. Your doctor may advise diet and other changes in lifestyle as well as regular blood tests.
Not to be used for: children, pregnant women, or for patients with a history of gall bladder problems or kidney or liver disease.
Caution needed with: anticoagulants, antidiabetic drugs, PHENYTOIN.
Contains: CLOFIBRATE.
Other preparations:

Atropine Minims
(SNP)

Drops used as an ANTICHOLINERGIC preparation for pupil dilation.

Dose: 1 drop into the eye as needed.
Availability: NHS and private prescription.
Side effects: stinging in the eye, dry mouth, blurred vision, intolerance of light, rapid heart rate, rarely psychological changes.
Caution:
Not to be used for: patients suffering from narrow angle glaucoma.
Caution needed with:
Contains: ATROPINE SULPHATE.
Other preparations: Atropine Eye Drops.

---

atropine methonitrate *see* **Brovon, Rybarvin**

---

atropine sulphate *see* **Atropine Minims, Diarphen, Isopto Atropine, Lomotil**

Atrovent
(Boehringer Ingelheim)

An inhaler used as an ANTICHOLINERGIC preparation to relieve blocked airways especially as a result of bronchitis.

Dose: adults 1-2 metered doses 3-4 times a day; children under 6 years 1 dose 3 times a day; 6-12 years 1-2 doses 3 times a day.
Availability: NHS and private prescription.
Side effects: dry mouth, constipation, retention of urine.
Caution: in patients suffering from enlarged prostate, glaucoma.
Not to be used for:
Caution needed with:
Contains: IPRATROPIUM BROMIDE.
Other preparations: Atrovent Forte Inhaler, Atrovent Solution.

Audax
(Napp Consumer)

Drops used as an ANALGESIC to relieve pain associated with acute inflammation of the outer or middle ear.

Dose: every four hours fill the ear with the liquid and plug it.
Availability: NHS, private prescription, over the counter.
Side effects:
Caution:

Not to be used for:
Caution needed with:
Contains: CHOLINE SALICYLATE.
Other preparations:

Audicort
(Lederle)

Drops used as an antibiotic and STEROID treatment for inflammation and infection of the outer ear.

Dose: 2-5 drops into the ear 3-4 times a day.
Availability: NHS and private prescription.
Side effects: additional infection, local irritation.
Caution: in pregnant women and nursing mothers.
Not to be used for: children or for patients suffering from viral lesions, tubercular skin diseases, or perforated ear drum.
Caution needed with:
Contains: TRIAMCINOLONE ACETONIDE, NEOMYCIN.
Other preparations:

Augmentin
(Beecham)

A white, oval tablet used as a broad-spectrum penicillin to treat respiratory, ear, nose, and throat, urinary tract, skin, and soft tissue infections.

Dose: 1-2 tablets 3 times a day for up to 14 days (children use suspension).
Availability: NHS and private prescription.
Side effects: penicillin allergy and stomach disturbances.
Caution: in pregnant women, nursing mothers, and in patients suffering from kidney or liver disease, glandular fever.
Not to be used for: patients suffering from penicillin allergy.
Caution needed with:
Contains: CLAVULANIC ACID, AMOXYCILLIN (CO-AMOXICLAV).
Other preparations: Augmentin Dispersible, Augmentin Intravenous, Augmentin Suspension.

Auralgicin — antibacterial ear drops. Product now discontinued.

Auraltone — ANALGESIC ear drops. Product now discontinued.

auranofin *see* **Ridaura**

A

Aureocort
(Lederle)

A cream used as a STEROID, antibacterial treatment for skin disorders where there is also inflammation and infection.

Dose: apply a small quantity of the cream to the affected area 2-3 times a day.
Availability: NHS and private prescription.
Side effects: fluid retention, suppression of adrenal glands. Thinning of the skin may occur.
Caution: use for short periods of time only.
Not to be used for: patients suffering from acne or any other skin infections caused by tuberculosis, ringworm, viruses, or fungi, or continuously especially in pregnant women.
Caution needed with:
Contains: TRIAMCINOLONE ACETONIDE, CHLORTETRACYCLINE HYDROCHLORIDE.
Other preparations: Aureocort Ointment.

Aureomycin Capsules
(Lederle)

A yellow capsule supplied at a strength of 250 mg and used as a tetracycline to treat infections.

Dose: 1-2 capsules 4 times a day.
Availability: NHS and private prescription.
Side effects: stomach disturbances, allergies, further infections.
Caution: in patients suffering from liver or kidney disease.
Not to be used for: children, nursing mothers, or for women in the latter half of pregnancy.
Caution needed with: milk, ANTACIDS, mineral supplements, contraceptive pill.
Contains: CHLORTETRACYCLINE.
Other preparations: AUREOMYCIN OINTMENT.

Aureomycin Ointment
(Lederle)

An ointment used as an antibiotic to treat eye and skin infections.

Dose: apply eye ointment into the eye every 2 hours, or skin ointment on gauze to the affected area once a day or as needed.
Availability: NHS and private prescription.
Side effects: additional infection.
Caution:
Not to be used for:
Caution needed with:
Contains: CHLORTETRACYCLINE HYDROCHLORIDE.
Other preparations: Aureomycin Cream, Aureomycin Eye Ointment.

Aventyl
(Eli Lilly)

A white/yellow capsule supplied at a strength of 10 mg, 25 mg and used as a TRICYCLIC antidepressant to treat depression, bed wetting in children.

Dose: adults 20-40 mg a day increasing to 100 mg a day if needed in divided doses, then usually 30-75 mg a day; elderly 10 mg 3 times a day at first; children over 6 years 10-35 mg ½ hour before bedtime.
Availability: NHS and private prescription.
Side effects: dry mouth, constipation, urine retention, blurred vision, palpitations, drowsiness, sleeplessness, dizziness, hands shaking, low blood presure, weight change, skin reactions, jaundice or blood changes, loss of libido may occur.
Caution: in nursing mothers or in patients suffering from heart disease, thyroid disease, epilepsy, diabetes, some other psychiatric conditions. Your doctor may advise regular blood tests.
Not to be used for: children under 6 years, pregnant women, or for patients suffering from heart attacks, liver disease, heart block.
Caution needed with: alcohol, ANTICHOLINERGICS, adrenaline, MAOIS, BARBITURATES, other antidepressants, ANTIHYPERTENSIVES, CIMETIDINE, oestrogens, some local anaestetics.
Contains: NORTRYPTILINE hydrochloride.
Other preparations: Aventyl Liquid (now discontinued).

Avloclor
(ICI)

A white, scored tablet supplied at a strength of 250 mg and used as an antimalarial, amoebicide preparation for the prevention of malaria, and the treatment of hepatitis, amoebiasis.

Dose: prevention of malaria adults 2 tablets on the same day once a week, children 5 mg per kg bodyweight once a week (start 2 weeks before entering endemic area, and continue for 4 weeks after leaving); treatment of hepatitis adults only 4 tablets a day for 2 days then 1 tablet twice a day for 2-3 weeks.

Availability: NHS, private prescription, over the counter (for prevention of malaria).

Side effects: headache, stomach upset, skin eruptions, hair loss, blurred vision, eye damage, blood disorders, loss of pigments.

Caution: in pregnant women, nursing mothers, and in patients suffering from porphyria (a rare blood disorder), kidney or liver disease, or psoriasis. Your doctor may advise regular eye tests before and during treatment.

Not to be used for:

Caution needed with:

Contains: CHLOROQUINE PHOSPHATE.

Other preparations: NIVAQUINE (Rhone-Poulenc Rorer)

Avomine
(Rhone-Poulenc Rorer)

A white, scored tablet supplied at a strength of 25 mg and used as an ANTIHISTAMINE treatment for travel sickness, nausea, vomiting, vertigo.

Dose: adults travel sickness 1 at bedtime before long journeys or 1-2 hours before short journeys, nausea 1 tablet 1-4 times a day; children 5-10 years half adults dose.

Availability: NHS, private prescription, over the counter.

Side effects: drowsiness, reduced reactions, rarely skin eruptions.

Caution: in pregnant women, and in patients suffering from liver or kidney disease.

Not to be used for: children under 5 years.

Caution needed with: alcohol, sedatives, and some antidepressants (MAOIS).

Contains: PROMETHAZINE THEOCLATE.

Other preparations:

Axid
(Eli Lilly)

A pale-yellow/ dark-yellow capsule supplied at a strength of 150 mg and 300 mg and used for treatment and prevention of ulcers and to treat gastro-oesophageal reflux.

Dose: ulcers: 300 mg in the evening or 150 mg twice a day; prevention: 150 mg in the evening for up to a year. Reflux: 150-300 mg twice a day for up to 12 weeks.

Availability: NHS and private prescription.

Side effects: headache, chest pain, muscle ache, fatigue, dreams, runny nose, sore throat, cough, itch, sweating, changes in liver enzymes.
Caution: in pregnant women and nursing mothers, and in patients suffering from impaired kidney and liver functions.
Not to be used for: children.
Caution needed with:
Contains: NIZATIDINE.
Other preparations:

---

azapropazone *see* **Rheumox**

---

azatadine *see* **Congesteze**

---

azatadine maleate *see* **Optimine**

---

azelaic acid *see* **Skinoren**

---

azelastine *see* **Rhinolast**

---

azithromycin *see* **Zithromax**

---

azlocillin *see* **Securopen**

---

bacampicillin hydrochloride *see* **Ambaxin**

---

bacitracin *see* **Cicatrin, Polybactrin, Polyfax, Tri-Cicatrin, Tribiotic**

---

baclofen *see* **Baclospas, Lioresal**

Baclospas *see* **Lioresal**
(Ashbourne)

Bacticlens — disinfectant solution. Product now discontinued.

Bactrim *see* **Septrin**

Bactroban Nasal
(Beecham)

An ointment used as an antibiotic to treat infections of the nose or skin.

Dose: apply 2-3 times a day for 5-7 days or up to 10 days for skin infections.
Availability: NHS and private prescription.
Side effects:
Caution: in patients suffering from kidney disease. Keep out of the eyes.
Not to be used for:
Caution needed with:
Contains: MUPIROCIN.
Other preparations: Bactroban Ointment.

Balmandol
(Smith and Nephew Pharm)

A liquid used to treat dry skin conditions, including eczema and dermatitis.

Dose: add 15-30 ml to the bath and soak for 10-15 minutes, or apply to wet skin after showering.
Availability: NHS, private prescription, over the counter.
Side effects:
Caution:
Not to be used for:
Caution needed with:
Contains: ALMOND OIL, LIQUID PARAFFIN.
Other preparations:

Balmosa
(Pharmax)

A cream used as an ANALGESIC rub to treat muscular rheumatism, fibrositis, lumbago, sciatica, unbroken chilblains.

Dose: massage into the affected area as needed.
Availability: NHS, private prescription , over the counter.
Side effects: may be irritant.
Caution:
Not to be used for: areas near the eyes, on broken or inflamed skin, or on membranes (such as the mouth).
Caution needed with:
Contains: MENTHOL, CAMPHOR, METHYL SALICYLATE, CAPSICUM OLEORESIN.
Other preparations:

Balneum Plus
(Merck)

A liquid used to treat itching and dry skin conditions.

Dose: 1-3 measures added to the bath; children use ¼-¾ measures.
Availability: NHS, private prescription, over the counter.
Side effects:
Caution:
Not to be used for:
Caution needed with:
Contains: SOYA OIL, LAUROMACROGOLS.
Other preparations: Balneum.

Balneum with Tar
(Merck)

A bath oil used as an emollient and anti-psoriatic to treat eczema, itchy or thickening skin disorders, psoriasis.

Dose: adults add 20 ml to the bath water; children over 2 years add 10 ml and use for a maximum of 6 weeks.
Availability: NHS, private prescription, over the counter.
Side effects:
Caution:
Not to be used for: for children under 2 years or for patients suffering from wet or weeping skin problems or where the skin is badly broken.
Caution needed with:
Contains: COAL TAR, SOYA OIL.
Other preparations: POLYTAR EMOLLIENT (Stiefel).

Baltar
(Merck)

A liquid used as an antipsoriatic treatment for psoriasis, dandruff, eczema, dermatoses of the scalp.

Dose: shampoo the hair with the liquid 1-3 times a week.
Availability: NHS, private prescription, over the counter.
Side effects:
Caution: keep out of the eyes.
Not to be used for: children under 2 years or for patients suffering from wet or weeping dermatoses, or where the skin is badly broken.
Caution needed with:
Contains: coal tar.
Other preparations: POLYTAR (Stiefel).

Banocide — anti-worm agent. Product now discontinued.

Baratol
(Monmouth)

A blue tablet or a green, scored tablet according to strengths of 25 mg, 50 mg and used as an ANTIHYPERTENSIVE to treat high blood pressure.

Dose: 25 mg twice a day at first increasing by 25-50 mg a day at two-weekly intervals to a maximum of 200 mg a day if needed in 2-3 divided doses.
Availability: NHS and private prescription.
Side effects: drowsiness, dry mouth, blocked nose, increase in bodyweight, inability to ejaculate.
Caution: in patients suffering from kidney or liver weakness, Parkinson's disease, epilepsy, depression; patients with weak hearts should be treated with DIGOXIN and DIURETICS.
Not to be used for: children or patients suffering from heart failure.
Caution needed with: MAOIS, ANTIHYPERTENSIVES.
Contains: INDORAMIN hydrochloride.
Other preparations: DORALESE (Bridge).

---

barbiturate

A sedative drug used to treat the most severe cases of sleeplessness and epilepsy. Examples AMYLOBARBITONE *see* Amytal, and PHENOBARBITONE.

Barquinol HC — STEROID, anti-infective skin cream. Product now discontinued.

Baxan
(Bristol-Myers Squibb)

A white capsule supplied at a strength of 500 mg and used as a cephalosporin antibiotic to treat respiratory, skin, and soft tissue infections, ear infections, urine infections.

Dose: adults 1-2 capsules twice a day; children under 1 year 25 mg per kg body weight a day in divided doses, 1-6 years 250 mg twice a day, over 6 years 500 mg twice a day.
Availability: NHS and private prescription.
Side effects: allergy, stomach disturbances.
Caution: in patients suffering from kidney disease or who are sensitive to penicillins.
Not to be used for:
Caution needed with: certain DIURETICS.
Contains: CEFADROXIL.
Other preparations: Baxan Suspension.

Baycaron
(Bayer)

A white, scored tablet supplied at a strength of 25 mg and used as a DIURETIC to treat high blood pressure, fluid retention.

Dose: 1-2 a day as a single dose in the morning for 10-14 days, then 1 a day or 1 every other day. (Up to 4 a day for fluid retention.)
Availability: NHS and private prescription.
Side effects: dyspepsia, nausea.
Caution: in pregnant women, nursing mothers, or in patients suffering from kidney or liver disease, diabetes, or gout.
Not to be used for: patients suffering from cirrhosis of the liver, severe kidney failure, Addison's disease, or severely raised calcium levels.
Caution needed with: DIGOXIN, LITHIUM, ANTIHYPERTENSIVES.
Contains: MEFRUSIDE.
Other preparations:

Bayolin
(Bayer)

A cream used as an ANALGESIC rub to treat rheumatism, fibrositis, lumbago, sciatica.

Dose: massage gently into the affected area 2-3 times a day.
Availability: NHS, private prescription , over the counter.
Side effects: may be irritant.
Caution:
Not to be used for: areas near the eyes, broken or inflamed skin, or on membranes (such as the mouth).
Caution needed with:
Contains: HEPARINOID, GLYCOL SALICYLATE, BENZYL NICOTINATE.
Other preparations:

BC 500
(Whitehall)

An orange, oblong tablet used as a multivitamin preparation to treat vitamin B and vitamin C deficiency, and to aid recovery from illness, long-term alcoholism, long-term antibiotic treatment.

Dose: 1 tablet a day.
Availability: private prescription and over the counter.
Side effects:
Caution:
Not to be used for: children.
Caution needed with: LEVODOPA.
Contains: THIAMINE mononitrate, RIBOFLAVINE, NICOTINAMIDE, PYRIDOXINE hydrochloride, CALCIUM PANTOTHENATE, ASCORBIC ACID, CYANOCOBALAMIN.
Other preparations:

BC 500 with Iron — vitamin and iron supplement. Product now discontinued.

Becloforte *see* **Becotide**
(A & H)

---

beclomethasone *see* **Aerobec, Beconase, Becotide, Propaderm, Ventide**

Becodisks *see* Becotide
(A & H)

Beconase
(A & H)

A powder in an aerosol or a suspension in an atomizer supplied at a strength of 50 micrograms and used as a STEROID to treat rhinitis, hay fever.

Dose: 2 sprays into each nostril twice a day.
Availability: NHS and private prescription.
Side effects: irritation of the nose, nose bleeds, disturbance of taste and smell.
Caution: in pregnant women, nursing mothers, in patients with nasal infections, and in patients transferring from STEROIDS taken by mouth.
Not to be used for: children under 6 years.
Caution needed with:
Contains: BECLOMETHASONE DIPROPRIONATE.
Other preparations: Beconase Aqueous.

Becosym
(Roche Nicholas)

A brown tablet used as a source of B vitamins to treat B vitamin deficiencies.

Dose: adults 1-3 tablets a day; children use syrup.
Availability: NHS (when prescribed as a generic), private prescription, over the counter.
Side effects:
Caution:
Not to be used for:
Caution needed with: LEVODOPA.
Contains: THIAMINE, RIBOFLAVINE, NICOTINAMIDE, PYRIDOXINE.
Other preparations: Becosym Syrup (not available on NHS), Becosym Forte Tablets (not available on NHS).

Becotide
(A & H)

An aerosol supplied at a strength of 50 micrograms, 100 micrograms, 200 micrograms and used as a STEROID to treat bronchial asthma.

Dose: adults 400 micrograms a day in 2-4 doses, up to 800 micrograms a day in severe cases; children up to 400 micrograms a day.
Availability: NHS and private prescription.
Side effects: hoarseness, thrush.
Caution: in pregnant women, in patients transferring from STEROIDS taken by mouth, or in patients suffering from tubercular lungs.
Not to be used for:
Caution needed with:
Contains: BECLOMETHASONE.
Other preparations: AEROBEC AUTOHALER (3M Healthcare), BECLOFORTE (A & H), BECODISKS (A & H).

Bedranol SR *see* Inderal LA
(Lagap)

---

belladonna *see* Alophen, Aluhyde, Bellocarb, Carbellon

Bellocarb
(Sinclair)

A beige tablet used as an ANTACID and anti-spasm treatment for bowel spasm, ulcers, dyspepsia.

Dose: 1-2 tablets, crushed and chewed, 4 times a day.
Availability: over the counter and private presecription.
Side effects: occasionally constipation.
Caution: in patients with enlarged prostate, heart, kidney, or liver problems.
Not to be used for: patients suffering from glaucoma.
Caution needed with:
Contains: BELLADONNA, MAGNESIUM TRISILICATE, MAGNESIUM CARBONATE.
Other preparations:

Bendogen *see* Esbatal
(Lagap)

---

bendrofluazide *see* Aprinox, bendrofluazide tablets, Berkozide, Centyl, Centyl-K, Corgaretic 40, Inderetic, Neo-Naclex, Neo-Naclex-K, Prestim, Tenavoid

bendrofluazide tablets

A white tablet or a white, scored tablet according to strengths of 2.5 mg, 5 mg used to treat fluid retention and high blood pressure.

Dose: fluid retention 5-10 mg a day or every other day; high blood pressure 2.5-5 mg a day.
Availability: NHS and private prescription.
Side effects: low potassium levels, rash, sensitivity to light, blood changes, gout, tiredness
Caution: in pregnant women, nursing mothers, or in patients suffering from liver or kidney disease, diabetes, gout.
Not to be used for: children or for patients suffering from kidney failure or severe kidney failure, Addison's disease, or porphyria (abnormal red blood cells).
Caution needed with: DIGOXIN, LITHIUM, ANTIHYPERTENSIVES.
Contains: BENDROFLUAZIDE.
Other preparations: APRINOX (Boots), BERKOZIDE (Berk), CENTYL (Leo), NEO-NACLEX (Evans).

Benemid
(MSD)

A white, scored tablet supplied at a strength of 500 mg and used as a uric acid-lowering agent to to treat gout, hyperuricaemia, and to prolong the activity of some antibiotics..

Dose: ½ tablet twice a day for the first 7 days then 1 tablet twice a day. (4 a day if used with antibiotics, and reduced doses for children.)
Availability: NHS and private prescription.
Side effects: headache, stomach upset, frequent urination, hypersensitivity, sore gums, flushes, acute gout, kidney stones, kidney colic.
Caution: in pregnant women and in patients with kidney disease or a history of peptic ulcer. Drink plenty of fluids.
Not to be used for: children (except with antibiotics), patients suffering from blood changes, kidney uric acid stones, or to start treatment during an acute attack.
Caution needed with: salicylates, PYRAZINAMIDE, sulphonamides, ß-lactam antibiotics, INDOMETHACIN, METHOTREXATE, some antidiabetic drugs.
Contains: PROBENECID.
Other preparations:

Benerva
(Roche)

A white tablet supplied in strengths of 25 mg, 50 mg, 100 mg, 300 mg and used as a source of vitamin B1 to treat beri-beri, neuritis.

Dose: 25-50 mg a day.
Availability: NHS (when prescribed as a generic), private prescription, over the counter.
Side effects:
Caution:
Not to be used for: children.
Caution needed with:
Contains: THIAMINE hydrochloride.
Other preparations: Benerva Compound.

Benoral
(Sanofi Winthrop)

A white, oblong tablet supplied at a strength of 750 mg and used as an ANALGESIC for the relief of pain, fever, rheumatoid arthritis, osteoarthritis, pain in bones or muscles.

Dose: 2 tablets 3 times a day.
Availability: NHS, private prescription, over the counter.
Side effects: stomach upsets, allergy, asthma.
Caution: in the elderly, in pregnant women, and in patients with a history of allergy to aspirin or asthma, or who are suffering from impaired kidney or liver function, indigestion.
Not to be used for: children, nursing mothers, haemophiliacs, or patients suffering from ulcers.
Caution needed with: anticoagulants (blood-thinning drugs), some antidiabetic drugs, anti-inflammatory agents, METHOTREXATE, SPIRONOLACTONE, STEROIDS, some ANTACIDS, some uric acid-lowering drugs.
Contains: BENORYLATE.
Other preparations: Benoral Suspension, Benoral Sachets.

benorylate *see* **Benoral**

Benoxyl 20 — antibacterial treatment for skin ulcers. Product now discontinued.

Benoxyl 5
(Stiefel)

A cream used as an antibacterial and skin softener to treat acne.

Dose: wash and dry the affected area, then apply once a day.
Availability: NHS, private prescription, over the counter.
Side effects: irritation, peeling.
Caution: keep out of the eyes, nose, and mouth. May bleach fabrics.
Not to be used for:
Caution needed with:
Contains: BENZOYL PEROXIDE.
Other preparations: Benoxyl 10 Lotion, (Benoxyl with Sulphur — now discontinued), ACETOXYL (Stiefel), ACNEGEL (Stiefel), ACNECIDE (Galderma), BENZAGEL (Bioglan), NERICUR (Schering), PANOXYL (Stiefel), QUINODERM (Quinoderm).

---

benperidol *see* **Anquil**

---

benserazide hydrochloride *see* **Madopar**

Bentex *see* **Artane.** Product now discontinued.

Benylin Expectorant
(Warner-Lambert)

A syrup used as an ANTIHISTAMINE, expectorant, and sputum softener to treat cough, bronchial congestion.

Dose: adults 5-10 ml every 2-3 hours; children 1-5 years 2.5 ml every 3-4 hours, 6-12 years 5 ml every 3-4 hours.
Availability: private prescription and over the counter.
Side effects:
Caution:
Not to be used for: children under 1 year.
Caution needed with:
Contains: DIPHENHYDRAMINE HYDROCHLORIDE, AMMONIUM CHLORIDE, SODIUM CITRATE, MENTHOL.
Other preparations: Benylin Paediatric, Benylin with Codeine (Benylin Decongestant — now discontinued).

Benzagel
(Bioglan)

A white gel supplied at a strength of 5% or 10 % and used as an antibacterial and skin softener to treat acne.

Dose: (start with the 5% strength gel) wash and dry the affected area, then apply 1-2 times a day.
Availability: NHS, private prescription, over the counter.
Side effects: irritation, peeling.
Caution: keep out of the eyes, nose, and mouth. May bleach fabrics.
Not to be used for:
Caution needed with:
Contains: BENZOYL PEROXIDE.
Other preparations: ACETOXYL (Stiefel), ACNEGEL (Stiefel), ACNECIDE (Galderma), BENOXYL (Stiefel), BENZAGEL (Bioglan), NERICUR (Schering), PANOXYL (Stiefel), QUINODERM (Quinoderm).

---

benzalkonium chloride *see* **Callusolve, Capitol, Conotrane, Drapolene, Ionax, Ionil T, Roccal, Timodine, Torbetol**

---

benzathine penicillin *see* **Penidural**

---

benzhexol *see* **Artane**

---

benzocaine *see* **AAA Spray, Auralgicin, Auraltone, Intralgin, Medilave, Merocaine, Rybarvin, Transvasin, Tyrozets**

---

benzoic acid *see* **Aserbine, Malatex**

---

benzoic acid compound ointment BP

An ointment used as an antifungal preparation to treat infections such as ringworm.

Dose: apply twice a day.
Availability: NHS, private prescription, over the counter.
Side effects:

Caution:
Not to be used for:
Caution needed with:
Contains: BENZOIC ACID, SALICYLIC ACID, EMULSIFYING OINTMENT.
Other preparations:

benzoyl peroxide *see* **Acetoxyl, Acnegel, Acnidazil, Benoxyl 5, Benzagel, Nericur, Panoxyl, Quinoderm Cream, Quinoped, Theraderm**

benzthiazide *see* **Dytide, Decaserpyl Plus**

benztropine *see* **Cogentin**

benzydamine *see* **Difflam, Difflam Oral Rinse**

benzyl benzoate *see* **Anugesic-HC, Anusol HC, Ascabiol**

benzyl nicotinate *see* **Bayolin, Salonair**

bephenium hydroxy-naphthoate *see* **Alcopar.**

Berkamil *see* **Amiloride**
(Berk)

Berkatens *see* **Cordilox**
(Berk)

Berkmycen *see* **Tetracycline**
(Berk)

Berkolol see Inderal
(Berk)

Berkozide see bendrofluazide
(Berk)

Berotec
(Boehringer Ingelheim)

An aerosol supplied at a strength of 0.1 mg and 0.2 mg and used as a broncho-dilator to treat bronchial asthma, emphysema, bronchitis.

Dose: adults 1-2 sprays 3 times a day up to a maximum of 2 sprays every 6 hours; children 1 spray 3 times a day up to a maximum of 2 spray every 6 hours (using lower strength only).
Availability: NHS and private prescription.
Side effects: headache, dilation of the blood vessels, nervous tension.
Caution: in pregnant women and in patients suffering from heart disease, angina, abnormal heart rhythms, high blood pressure, overactive thyroid gland.
Not to be used for:
Caution needed with: SYMPATHOMIMETICS.
Contains: FENOTEROL hydrobromide.
Other preparations: Berotec Nebuliser Solution.

Beta-Adalat
(Bayer)

A reddish-brown capsule used to treat high blood pressure, angina.

Dose: adults 1 capsule a day increasing to 2 capsules a day if necessary; elderly no more than 1 capsule a day.
Availability: NHS and private prescription.
Side effects: flushing, headache, dizziness, dry eyes, skin rash, fluid retention, jaundice, gum swelling.
Caution: in patients under anaesthesia or those with weak heart, lung, kidney or liver disease, diabetes.
Not to be used for: children, pregnant women, nursing mothers, or for patients suffering from heart block, failure, or shock.
Caution needed with: CIMETIDINE, QUINIDINE, other heart drugs.
Contains: ATENOLOL, NIFEDIPINE.
Other preparations: TENIF (Stuart).

beta-blocker (ß-blocker)

a drug which blocks some of the effects of adrenaline in the body. Beta-blockers are used to treat angina, high blood pressure, and other conditions. Example PROPANOLOL *see* Inderal.

Beta-Cardone
(Evans)

A green tablet, pink tablet, or white tablet according to strengths of 40 mg, 80 mg, 200 mg and used as a ß-BLOCKER to treat angina, high blood pressure, heart rhythm disturbance, and as an additional treatment for overactive thyroid.

Dose: heart rhythm disturbance40 mg 3 times a day for 7 days, then 120-240 mg a day in single or divided doses. For angina 80 mg twice a day for 7-10 days, then 200-600 mg a day in single or divided doses. High blood pressure 80 mg twice a day for 7-10 days, then 200-600 mg a day. Overactive thyroid 120-240 mg a day.
Availability: NHS and private prescription.
Side effects: cold hands and feet, sleep disturbances, slow heart rate, tiredness, wheezing, heart failure, stomach upset, dry eyes, rash.
Caution: in pregnant women, nursing mothers, and in patients suffering from diabetes, kidney or liver disorders, asthma. May need to be withdrawn before surgery. Withdraw gradually. Your doctor may advise additional treatment with DIURETICS or DIGOXIN.
Not to be used for: children or for patients suffering from heart block or failure, asthma.
Caution needed with: VERAPAMIL, CLONIDINE withdrawal, some anti-arrhythmic drugs and anaesthetics, some ANTIHYPERTENSIVES, CIMETIDINE, sedatives, SYMPATHOMIMETICS, INDOMETHACIN, antidiabetics, ERGOTAMINE.
Contains: SOTALOL HYDROCHLORIDE.
Other preparations: SOTACOR (Bristol-Myers Squibb).

Beta-Prograne *see* Inderal LA
(Tillomed)

Betadine Gargle and Mouthwash
(Napp)

A solution used as an antiseptic to treat inflammation of the mouth and pharynx brought on by thrush and other bacterial infections.

Dose: Wash out the mouth or gargle with the diluted or undiluted solution up to 4 times a day.
Availability: NHS, private prescription, over the counter.
Side effects: rarely local irritation and sensitivity.
Caution:
Not to be used for: children under 6 years.
Caution needed with:
Contains: POVIDONE-IODINE.
Other preparations: BETASEPT GARGLE AND MOUTHWASH (Napp).

Betadine Ointment
(Napp)

An ointment used as an antiseptic to treat ulcers.

Dose: apply to the affected area and cover once a day.
Availability: NHS, private prescription, over the counter.
Side effects: rarely irritation.
Caution: in patients sensitive to iodine.
Not to be used for:
Caution needed with:
Contains: POVIDONE-IODINE.
Other preparations:

Betadine Pessaries
(Napp)

A pessary and applicator supplied at a strength of 200 mg and used as an antiseptic to treat inflammation of the vagina.

Dose: 1 pessary to be inserted into the vagina night and morning for at least 14 days.
Availability: NHS, private prescription, over the counter.
Side effects: irritation and sensitivity.
Caution:
Not to be used for: children.
Caution needed with:
Contains: POVIDONE-IODINE.
Other preparations: Betadine Vaginal Gel, Betadine VC Kit.

Betadine Scalp and Skin Cleanser
(Napp)

A solution used as an antiseptic and detergent to treat acne, seborrhoeic scalp and skin disorders.

Dose: use as a shampoo or apply directly to the skin and then cleanse properly.
Availability: NHS, private prescription, over the counter.
Side effects: rarely irritation or sensitivity.
Caution:
Not to be used for: children under 2 years.
Caution needed with:
Contains: POVIDONE-IODINE.
Other preparations: Betadine Skin Cleanser, Betadine Shampoo, BETASEPT ACNE WASH (Napp), BETASEPT SHAMPOO (Napp).

Betadine Dry Powder Spray
(Napp)

A spray used as an antiseptic to treat infected cuts, wounds, and burns.

Dose: spray on to the affected area once a day or as needed until the area is covered with powder.
Availability: NHS, private prescription, over the counter.
Side effects:
Caution: keep out of the eyes.
Not to be used for: patients suffering from non-toxic colloid goitre.
Caution needed with:
Contains: POVIDONE-IODINE.
Other preparations: Betadine Antiseptic Paint, Betadine Antiseptic Solution, Betadine Alcoholic Solution, Betadine Surgical Scrub.

Betadur CR *see* Inderal LA
(Monmouth)

Betagan
(Allergan)

Drops used as a ß-BLOCKER to treat glaucoma and high blood pressure in the eye.

Dose: 1 drop once or twice a day.
Availability: NHS and private prescription.
Side effects: eye irritation, headache, dizziness, systemic ß-BLOCKER effects (*see* Blocadren).

Caution: in nursing mothers, and in patients suffering from diabetes or breathing problems.
Not to be used for: children, pregnant women, and in patients suffering from asthma or some heart disorders, heart failure.
Caution needed with: RESERPINE, ß-BLOCKERS taken by mouth.
Contains: LEVOBUNOLOL
Other preparations:

---

betahistine dihydrochloride *see* Serc

---

betaine hydrochloride *see* Kloref

Betaloc
(Astra)

A white, scored tablet supplied at strengths of 50 mg, 100 mg and used as a ß-BLOCKER to treat angina, high blood pressure, and as additional treatment for overactive thyroid, migraine, and heart rhythm defects.

Dose: for angina and heart rhythm defects 50-100 mg 2-3 times a day. High blood pressure 50 mg twice a day at first increasing to 400 mg a day if needed in 1 or 2 doses. Overactive thyroid 50 mg 4 times a day. Migraine 100-200 mg a day.
Availability: NHS and private prescription.
Side effects: cold hands and feet, sleep disturbances, slow heart rate, tiredness, wheezing, heart failure, stomach upset, dry eyes, rash.
Caution: in pregnant women, nursing mothers, and in patients suffering from diabetes, kidney or liver disorders. May need to be withdrawn before surgery. Withdraw gradually. Your doctor may advise additional treatment with DIGOXIN and DIURETICS.
Not to be used for: children or for patients suffering from heart block or failure, asthma.
Caution needed with: VERAPAMIL, antidiabetics, CLONIDINE withdrawal, some anti-arrhythmic drugs and anaesthetics, some ANTIHYPERTENSIVES, ERGOTAMINE, CIMETIDINE, sedatives, SYMPATHOMIMETICS, INDOMETHACIN.
Contains: METOPROLOL TARTRATE.
Other preparations: Betaloc injection, Betaloc-SA, ARBRALENE (Berk), LOPRESSOR (Ciba-Geigy), MEPRANIX (Ashbourne).

---

betamethasone *see* Betnelan, Betnesol, Betnesol Drops,

Betnovate, Betnovate Rectal, Bextasol, Diprosalic, Fucibet, Vista-Methasone

Betasept *see* Betadine
(Napp)

betaxolol *see* Betoptic, Kerlone

bethanechol *see* Myotonine

bethanidine *see* Esbatal

Betim *see* Blocadren
(Leo)

Betnelan
(Evans)

A white, scored tablet supplied at a strength of 0.5 mg and used as a STEROID to treat severe asthma, allergies, rheumatoid arthritis, collagen diseases.

Dose: adults 1-10 tablets a day, then reduce as needed; children 1-7 years quarter to half adult dose, 7-12 years half to three-quarters adult dose.
Availability: NHS and private prescription.
Side effects: high blood sugar, thin bones, mood changes, ulcers.
Caution: in pregnant women, in patients who have had recent bowel surgery, or who are suffering from inflamed veins, psychiatric disorders, virus infections, some cancers, some kidney diseases, thinning of the bones, ulcers, tuberculosis, other infections, high blood pressure, glaucoma, epilepsy, diabetes, underactive thyroid, liver disease, stress. Withdraw gradually.
Not to be used for:
Caution needed with: PHENYTOIN, PHENOBARBITONE, EPHEDRINE, RIFAMPICIN, DIURETICS, ANTICHOLINESTERASES, DIGOXIN, antidiabetic agents, anticoagulants, NON-STEROID ANTI-INFLAMMATORY DRUGS.

Contains: BETAMETHASONE.
Other preparations: BETNESOL (Evans).

B

Betnesol Tablets
(Evans)

A pink, scored tablet supplied at a strength of 0.5 mg and used as a STEROID to treat severe asthma, allergies, rheumatoid arthritis, collagen diseases.

Dose: adults 1-10 tablets a day, then reduce as needed; children 1-7 years quarter to half adult dose, 7-12 years half to three-quarters adult dose.
Availability: NHS and private prescription.
Side effects: high blood sugar, thin bones, mood changes, ulcers.
Caution: in pregnant women, in patients who have had recent bowel surgery, or who are suffering from inflamed veins, psychiatric disorders, virus infections, some cancers, some kidney diseases, thinning of the bones, ulcers, tuberculosis, other infections, high blood pressure, glaucoma, epilepsy, diabetes, underactive thyroid, liver disease, stress. Withdraw gradually.
Not to be used for:
Caution needed with: PHENYTOIN, PHENOBARBITONE, EPHEDRINE, RIFAMPICIN, DIURETICS, ANTICHOLINESTERASES, DIGOXIN, antidiabetic agents, anticoagulants, NON-STEROID ANTI-INFLAMMATORY DRUGS.
Contains: BETAMETHASONE SODIUM PHOSPHATE.
Other preparations: Betnesol Injection, Betnesol-N, betnesol drops.

Betnesol Drops
(Evans)

Drops used as a STEROID to treat inflammation of the ear, nasal passages, or eyes where infection is not present. (Use Betnesol-N for infected conditions.)

Dose: 2-3 drops into each nostril or ear every 2-3 hours, or 1-2 drops into the eye every 1-2 hours.
Availability: NHS and private prescription.
Side effects: sensitivity, resistance to neomycin (with Betnesol-N), thining of the cornea, cataract, rise in the eye pressure.
Caution: do not use for longer than is necessary especially in pregnancy.
Not to be used for: patients suffering from viral, tubercular, or fungal conditions of the nose, ear, or eye, dendritic ulcer, glaucoma, or where soft contact lenses are worn. Betnesol-N not to be used on perforated ear

drum.
Caution needed with:
Contains: BETAMETHASONE SODIUM PHOSPHATE.
Other preparations: Betnesol-N, Betnesol Ointment, Betnesol-N Ointment, BETNESOL TABLETS.

Betnovate
(Glaxo)

A cream or ointment used as a STEROID to treat psoriasis, eczema, external ear and other skin disorders, dermatitis. (Use Betnovate-N and Betnovate-C for infected conditions.)

Dose: apply a small quantity of the cream to the affected area 2-3 times a day.
Availability: NHS and private prescription.
Side effects: fluid retention, suppression of adrenal glands, thinning of the skin may occur.
Caution: use for short periods of time only.
Not to be used for: patients suffering from acne or any other skin infections caused by tuberculosis, ringworm, viruses, or fungi, or continuously especially in pregnant women.
Caution needed with:
Contains: BETAMETHASONE valerate.
Other preparations: Betnovate RD, Betnovate Scalp Application, Betnovate-N, Betnovate-C, DIPROSONE (Schering-Plough). Also LOTRIDERM (Schering-Plough) — with CLOTRIMAZOLE for infected conditions.

Betnovate Rectal
(Glaxo)

An ointment with applicator used as a STEROID, local anaesthetic treatment for haemorrhoids and mild proctitis.

Dose: apply 2 or 3 times a day at first and then reduce.
Availability: NHS and private prescription.
Side effects: systemic corticosteroid effects (*see* Precortisyl).
Caution: do not use for prolonged periods; care for pregnant women.
Not to be used for: children or for patients suffering from tuberculous, bacterial, fungal, or viral infections.
Caution needed with:
Contains: BETAMETHASONE valerate, PHENYLEPHRINE hydrochloride, LIGNOCAINE hydrochloride.
Other preparations:

Betoptic
(Alcon)

Drops used as a ß-BLOCKER to treat hypertension of the eyes, glaucoma.

Dose: 1 drop into the eye twice a day.
Availability: NHS and private prescription.
Side effects: temporary discomfort, rarely reduction in the sensitivity of the cornea, reddening, staining, or inflammation of the cornea.
Caution: in patients with a history of blocked airways disease, diabetes, overactive thyroid, or who are under general anaesthetic.
Not to be used for: children, or for patients using soft contact lenses or suffering from some heart diseases.
Caution needed with:
Contains: BETAXOLOL hydrochloride.
Other preparations:

Bextasol — STEROID inhaler to treat asthma. Product now discontinued.

---

bezafibrate *see* Bezalip-Mono

Bezalip-Mono
(Boehringer-Mannheim)

A white tablet supplied at a strength of 400 mg and used as a lipid-lowering drug to treat high blood lipids.

Dose: 1 tablet a day after food at night or in the morning.
Availability: NHS and private prescription.
Side effects: stomach upset, muscle aches, rash.
Caution: in patients with kidney disease. Your doctor may advise change in diet or lifestyle.
Not to be used for: children, pregnant women, nursing mothers, or for patients suffering from severe kidney or liver disease.
Caution needed with: anticoagulants, antidiabetics, MAOIS.
Contains: BEZAFIBRATE.
Other preparations: Bezalip.

BiNovum
(Cilag)

A white tablet and a peach tablet used as an oestrogen, progestogen contraceptive.

Dose: 1 tablet a day for 21 days starting on day 1 of the period.
Availability: NHS and private prescription.
Side effects: enlarged breasts, bloating and fluid retention, cramps, leg pains, mood change, reduction in sexual desire, headaches, nausea, vaginal erosion, discharge, and bleeding, weight gain, skin changes.
Caution: in patients suffering from high blood pressure, diabetes, vascular disorders, asthma, depression, kidney disease, multiple sclerosis, womb diseases. Your doctor may advise you not to smoke, to have regular examinations. You should stop treatment at the first sign of serious symptoms such as severe headache or jaundice. Treatment should be stopped before surgery.
Not to be used for: pregnant women, or for patients suffering from sickle-cell anaemia, history of heart disease or thrombosis, liver disorders, some cancers, undiagnosed vaginal bleeding, some ear, skin, and kidney disorders.
Caution needed with: RIFAMPICIN, TETRACYCLINES, GRISEOFULVIN, BARBITURATES, PHENYTOIN, PRIMIDONE, CARBAMAZEPINE, ETHOSUXIMIDE, CHLORAL HYDRATE, DICHLORALPHENAZONE.
Contains: ETHINYLOESTRADIOL, NORETHISTERONE.
Other preparations:

Biogastrone
(Sanofi Winthrop)

A white, scored tablet supplied at a strength of 50 mg and used as an anti-ulcer treatment for stomach ulcers.

Dose: 2 tablets 3 times a day after food for 7 days followed by reduced-dose maintenance therapy.
Availability: NHS and private prescription.
Side effects: fluid retention, low potassium levels, high blood pressure.
Caution: in patients suffering from sodium or water retention.
Not to be used for: children, the elderly, pregnant women, or for patients with heart, kidney, or liver problems or low potassium levels.
Caution needed with: DIGOXIN, DIURETICS.
Contains: CARBENOXOLONE.
Other preparations: Duogastrone for duodenal ulcers (now discontinued). PYROGASTRONE (Sanofi) containing ALUMINIUM HYDROXIDE, SODIUM ALGINATE, and POTASSIUM BICARBONATE for reflux and oesophagitis. BIOPLEX (Thames) for mouth ulcers.

Biophylline
(Delandale)

A syrup used as a broncho-dilator to treat bronchial spasm.

Dose: adults 5-10 ml every 6-8 hours; children 2-6 years 2.5 ml every 6-8 hours, 6-12 years 2.5-5 ml every 6-8 hours.
Availability: NHS, private prescription, over the counter.
Side effects: rapid heart rate, stomach upset, headache, sleeplessness, nausea, abnormal rhythms.
Caution: in the elderly, pregnant women, nursing mothers, and in patients suffering from heart or liver disease, or peptic ulcer.
Not to be used for:
Caution needed with: CIMETIDINE, ERYTHROMYCIN, CIPROFLOXACIN, INTERFERON, DIURETICS, STEROIDS, some other broncho-dilators.
Contains: THEOPHYLLINE hydrate.
Other preparations: LASMA (Pharmax), NUELIN (3M Healthcare), PRO-VENT (Wellcome), SLO-PHYLLIN (Lipha), THEODUR (Astra), UNIPHYLLIN (Napp).

Bioplex *see* Biogastrone
(Thames)

Bioral
(Sterling Health)

A gel used as a cell-surface protector to treat mouth ulcers.

Dose: apply after meals and at bed time.
Availability: NHS, private prescription, over the counter.
Side effects:
Caution:
Not to be used for:
Caution needed with:
Contains: CARBENOXOLONE sodium.
Other preparations: BIOPLEX (Thames).

Biorphen
(Bioglan)

A solution to be taken by mouth, supplied at a concentration of 25 mg/5 ml and used as an ANTICHOLINERGIC preparation to treat Parkinson's disease.

Dose: 30 ml a day at first in divided doses increasing every 2-3 days by 5-10 ml to up to 60 ml a day.

Availability: NHS and private prescription.
Side effects: euphoria, ANTICHOLINERGIC effects, confusion, agitation, rash.
Caution: in patients with heart disorders or gastro-intestinal blockage.
Dose should be reduced slowly.
Not to be used for: patients suffering from glaucoma, enlarged prostate,
some movement disorders.
Caution needed with: PHENOTHIAZINES, ANTIHISTAMINES, antidepressants.
Contains: ORPHENADRINE.
Other preparations: DISIPAL (Brocades).

---

biotin *see* Ketovite

---

biperiden hydrochloride *see* Akineton

---

bisacodyl

A tablet supplied at a strength of 5 mg and used as a stimulant to treat
constipation.

Dose: children under 10 years 1 tablet at night, adults and children over
10 years 2 tablets at night (increased to 4 tablets if necessary).
Availability: NHS, private prescription, over the counter.
Side effects: abdominal cramp.
Caution: avoid prolonged use.
Not to be used for: patients suffering from intestinal blockage.
Caution needed with: no ANTACIDS should be taken within 1 hour.
Contains: bisacodyl.
Other preparations: Bisacodyl Suppositories, DULCOLAX (Windsor).

---

bismuth carbonate *see* APP

---

bismuth oxide *see* Anugesic-HC, Anusol, Anusol HC

---

bismuth subgallate *see* Anusol, Anusol HC

---

bismuth subnitrate *see* Roter, Caved S

bisoprolol fumarate *see* **Emcor, Monocor**

BJ6 *see* hypromellose eye drops
(Martindale, Thornton & Ross)

B

Blocadren
(MSD)

A blue, scored tablet supplied at a strength of 10 mg and used as a ß-
BLOCKER to treat angina, high blood pressure, migraine, and as a treatment
following heart attack.

Dose: following heart attack ½ tablet twice a day for 2 days, then 1 tablet
twice a day. For angina ½ tablet 2-3 times a day at first increasing if
required by 1-1½ tablets a day every 3 days. For high blood pressure 1
tablet a day at first increasing to a maximum of 6 tablets a day if needed.
For migraine 1-2 tablets once a day.
Availability: NHS and private prescription.
Side effects: cold hands and feet, sleep disturbances, slow heart rate,
tiredness, wheezing, heart failure, stomach upset, dry eyes, rash.
Caution: in pregnant women, nursing mothers, and in patients suffering
from diabetes, kidney or liver disorders. May need to be withdrawn before
surgery. Withdraw gradually. Your doctor may advise additional treatment
with DIGOXIN and DIURETICS.
Not to be used for: children, or for patients suffering from heart block or
failure, asthma.
Caution needed with: VERAPAMIL, CLONIDINE withdrawal, some anti-
arrhythmic drugs and anaesthetics, some ANTIHYPERTENSIVES, ERGOTAMINE,
antidiabetics, CIMETIDINE, sedatives, SYMPATHOMIMETICS, INDOMETHACIN.
Contains: TIMOLOL MALEATE.
Other preparations: BETIM (Leo).

Bocasan
(Oral-B)

A sachet of white granules used as a disinfectant to treat gingivitis, mouth
infections.

Dose: dissolve a sachet of granules in warm water and rinse out the
mouth 3 times a day after meals.
Availability: NHS, private prescription, over the counter.
Side effects:
Caution:

86

Not to be used for: patients suffering from kidney disease.
Caution needed with:
Contains: SODIUM PERBORATE MONOHYDRATE, SODIUM HYDROGEN TARTRATE.
Other preparations:

Bolvidon
(Organon)

A white tablet supplied at a strength of 10 mg, 20 mg, and 30 mg and used as tetracyclic antidepressant to treat depression.

Dose: adults 30-40 mg a day at first, increasing gradually if needed to 90 mg a day; elderly up to 30 mg a day at first.
Availability: NHS and private prescription.
Side effects: drowsiness, bone marrow depression, possibility of jaudice, hypomania or convulsions when the drug should be withdrawn.
Caution: in pregnant women, the elderly, and in patients suffering from epilepsy, enlarged prostate, or heart attacks. Your doctor may advise regular blood tests.
Not to be used for: children, nursing mothers, or for patients suffering from mania or severe liver disease.
Caution needed with: MAOIS, alcohol, anticoagulants.
Contains: MIANSERIN HYDROCHLORIDE.
Other preparations: NORVAL (Bencard).

---

boric acid *see* **Phytex**

---

borneol *see* **Rowachol, Rowatinex**

Bradilan
(Napp)

A white tablet supplied at a strength of 250 mg and used as a vasodilator to treat peripheral vascular problems including intermittent difficulty walking, night cramps, chilblains, Raynaud's phenomenon (spasm of the arteries), some brain disorders. Also used to control high blood lipids.

Dose: 2-4 tablets 3 times a day.
Availability: NHS, private prescription, over the counter.
Side effects: flushes.
Caution:

Not to be used for: children.
Caution needed with:
Contains: NICOFURANOSE.
Other preparations:

Bradosol
(Zyma)

A white lozenge supplied at a strength of 0.5 mg and used as a disinfectant to treat infections of the mouth and throat.

Dose: 1 lozenge to be sucked every 2-3 hours.
Availability: NHS, private prescription, over the counter.
Side effects:
Caution:
Not to be used for:
Caution needed with:
Contains: DOMIPHEN BROMIDE.
Other preparations: Bradosol Plus.

---

bran see Fybranta

Brasivol
(Stiefel)

A paste used as an abrasive to treat acne (Available in two grades.).

Dose: wet the area then rub in vigorously for 15-20 seconds, rinse and
repeat 1-3 times a day. (Start with Grade 1 and progress if necessary to
Grade 2.)
Availability: NHS, private prescription, over the counter.
Side effects:
Caution:
Not to be used for: patients suffering from visible superficial arteries or
veins on the skin.
Caution needed with:
Contains: aluminium oxide.
Other preparations:

Brelomax
(Abbott)

A white, scored tablet supplied at a strength of 2 mg, and used as a broncho-dilator to prevent and control bronchial spasm in conditions where airways are obstructed (such as asthma).

Dose: adults,1 tablet 2-3 times a day; children 10-12 years, ½-1 tablet twice a day.)
Availability: NHS and private prescription.
Side effects: low potassium levels, shaking, rapid or forceful heartbeat, mild headache, or nervous tension.
Caution: in patients suffering from diabetes, overactive thyroid, high blood pressure, epilepsy or heart/circulation disorder.
Not to be used for: children under 10 years, or for patients suffering from kidney or liver failure, other liver disorders.
Caution needed with: STEROIDS, THEOPHYLLINE.
Contains: TULOBUTEROL.
Other preparations:

Brevinor
(Syntex)

A white tablet used as an oestrogen, progestogen contraceptive.

Dose: 1 tablet a day for 21 days starting on day 5 of the period.
Availability: NHS and private prescription.
Side effects: enlarged breasts, bloating and fluid retention, cramps, leg pains, mood change, reduction in sexual desire, headaches, nausea, vaginal erosion, discharge, and bleeding, weight gain, skin changes.
Caution: in patients suffering from high blood pressure, diabetes, vascular disorders, asthma, depression, kidney disease, multiple sclerosis, womb diseases. Your doctor may advise you not to smoke, to have regular examinations. You should stop treatment at the first sign of serious symptoms such as severe headache or jaundice. Treatment should be stopped before surgery.
Not to be used for: pregnant women, or for patients suffering from sickle-cell anaemia, history of heart disease or thrombosis, liver disorders, some cancers, undiagnosed vaginal bleeding, some ear, skin, and kidney disorders.
Caution needed with: RIFAMPICIN, TETRACYCLINES, GRISEOFULVIN, BARBITURATES, PHENYTOIN, PRIMIDONE, CARBAMAZEPINE, ETHOSUXIMIDE, CHLORAL HYDRATE, DICHLORALPHENAZONE.
Contains: ETHINYLOESTRADIOL, NORETHISTERONE.
Other preparations: OVYSMEN (Cilag).

Bricanyl
(Astra)

A white, scored tablet supplied at a strength of 5 mg and used as a broncho-dilator to treat bronchial spasm brought on by asthma, bronchitis, or emphysema.

Dose: adults 1 tablet twice a day or every 8 hours; children under 7 years use syrup, 7-15 years half adult dose.
Availability: NHS and private prescription.
Side effects: shaking of the hands, dilation of the blood vessels, tension, headache.
Caution: in pregnant women and in diabetics, or in patients suffering from high blood pressure, abnormal heart rhythms, heart muscle disorders, overactive thyroid gland, angina.
Not to be used for:
Caution needed with: SYMPATHOMIMETICS.
Contains: TERBUTALINE SULPHATE.
Other preparations: Bricanyl SA, Bricanyl Syrup, Bricanyl Inhaler, Bricanyl Spacer Inhaler, Bricanyl Refill Canister, Bricanyl Turbohaler, Bricanyl Respirator Solution, Bricanyl Respules, Bricanyl Injection, MONOVENT (Lagap).

Bricanyl Expectorant — broncho-dilator and expectorant. Product now discontinued.

---

brilliant green *see* Variclene

Britiazim
(Thames)

A white tablet supplied at a strength of 60 mg and used as a calcium antagonist to treat angina.

Dose: 1 tablet 3 times a day increasing if required to up to 6 a day in divided doses; elderly 1 twice a day at first.
Availability: NHS and private prescription.
Side effects: slow heart rate, fluid retention, nausea, rash, headache.
Caution: your doctor may advise regular monitoring of heart rate, especially in elderly patients or in patients suffering from kidney or liver problems.
Not to be used for: children or for pregnant women, or in patients suffering from severe heart conduction defects.

Caution needed with: ß-BLOCKERS, DIGOXIN.
Contains: DILTIAZEM HYDROCHLORIDE.
Other preparations: ADIZEM (Napp), ANGIOZEM (Ashbourne), TILDIEM (Lorex).

Brocadopa *see* **Larodopa**
(Brocades)

Broflex *see* **Artane**
(Bioglan)

bromazepam *see* **Lexotan**

bromocriptine mesylate *see* **Parlodel**

brompheniramine *see* **Dimotane Expectorant, Dimotane Plus, Dimotapp LA**

Bronchilator — broncho-dilator aerosol. Product now discontinued.

Bronchodil
(ASTA Medica)

An aerosol supplied at a strength of 0.5 mg and used as a broncho-dilator to treat bronchial asthma, bronchitis, emphysema.

Dose: adults 1-2 sprays every 3-6 hours; children over 6 years 1 spray every 3-6 hours.
Availability: NHS and private prescription.
Side effects: shaking of hands, nervous tension, headache, dilation of the blood vessels.
Caution: in pregnant women and in patients suffering from heart muscle disorders, angina, high blood pressure, abnormal heart rhythms, overactive thyroid gland.
Not to be used for: children under 6 years.
Caution needed with: SYMPATHOMIMETICS.
Contains: REPROTEROL HYDROCHLORIDE.

Other preparations: (Bronchodil Tablets, Bronchodil Respirator Solution — all now discontinued.)

Brovon
(Torbet)

A solution used as a broncho-dilator to treat bronchial spasm brought on by chronic bronchitis, bronchial asthma, emphysema.

Dose: inhale 1-2 times a day and once at night.
Availability: NHS and private prescription (availability limited to certain named patients).
Side effects: nervousness, tremor, dry mouth, abnormal heart rhythms.
Caution: in patients suffering from diabetes.
Not to be used for: children or for patients suffering from heart disease, high blood pressure, overactive thyroid gland.
Caution needed with: sympathomimetics.
Contains: ADRENALINE, ATROPINE METHONITRATE, PAPAVERINE HYDROCHLORIDE.
Other preparations:

Broxil — penicillin treatment for infections. Product now discontinued.

Brufen
(Boots)

A magenta-coloured, oval tablet supplied at strengths of 200 mg, 400 mg, 600 mg and used as a NON-STEROID ANTI-INFLAMMATORY DRUG to treat pain, rheumatoid arthritis, ankylosing spondylitis, osteoarthritis, sero-negative arthritis, peri-articular disorders, soft tissue injuries.

Dose: adults 1200-1800 mg a day in divided doses, to a maximum of 2400 mg a day; children use syrup.
Availability: NHS and private prescription.
Side effects: dyspepsia, stomach bleeding, rash, rarely low blood platelet levels.
Caution: in pregnant women, the elderly, and in patients suffering from asthma or allergy to aspirin or anti-inflammatory drugs, or liver, kidney, or heart disease.
Not to be used for: patients suffering from peptic ulcer.
Caution needed with:
Contains: IBUPROFEN.
Other preparations: Brufen Granules, Brufen Syrup, Brufen Retard, APSIFEN (APS), ARTHROFEN (Ashbourne), EBUFAC (DDSA), FENBID (S K B),

IBRUFHALAL (Halal), IBUMED (Medipharma Labs), ISISFEN (Isis), JUNIFEN (Boots), LIDIFEN (Berk), MOTRIN (Upjohn), PAXOFEN, RIMAFEN (Rima). Other brands are available over the counter (200 mg strength only)

Buccastem
(Reckitt & Colman)

A pale-yellow tablet supplied at a strength of 3 mg and used as an ANTIHISTAMINE treatment for vertigo as a result of Ménière's disease or labyrinthitis, nausea, vomiting, migraine.

Dose: 1-2 tablets twice a day allowed to dissolve between the upper lip and gum.
Availability: NHS and private prescription.
Side effects: low blood pressure especially in elderly or dehydrated patients, drowsiness, ANTICHOLINERGIC effects, sleeplessness, skin reactions.
Caution: in pregnant women or nursing mothers.
Not to be used for: children or for patients suffering from kidney or liver disease, blood changes, epilepsy, Parkinson's disease, prostate enlargement, glaucoma.
Caution needed with: alcohol, sedatives, alpha-blockers.
Contains: PROCHLORPERAZINE MALEATE.
Other preparations: STEMETIL (Rhone-Poulenc Rorer), VERTIGON (S K B).

buclizine hydrochloride *see* **Migraleve**

budesonide *see* **Preferid, Pulmicort, Rhinocort**

bufexamac *see* **Parfenac**

bumetanide *see* **Burinex, Burinex A, Burinex K**

buprenorphine *see* **Temgesic**

Burinex
(Leo)

A white, scored tablet supplied at strengths of 1 mg, 5 mg and used as a DIURETIC to treat fluid retention associated with congestive heart failure, liver and kidney disease, including the nephrotic syndrome.

Dose: 1 mg a day according to patient's response.
Availability: NHS and private prescription.
Side effects: low blood potassium, stomach discomfort, rash, cramps, blood changes, breast enlargement.
Caution: in pregnant women, nursing mothers, and in patients suffering from kidney or liver damage, diabetes, gout, enlarged prostate, or impaired urination. Your doctor may advise that potassium supplements may be needed.
Not to be used for: children or patients suffering from cirrhosis of the liver.
Caution needed with: LITHIUM, DIGOXIN, ANTIHYPERTENSIVES, some antibiotics.
Contains: BUMETANIDE.
Other preparations: Burinex Liquid, Burinex Injection, Burinex A, BURINEX K.

Burinex A
(Leo)

A cream, oval, scored tablet used as a DIURETIC.

Dose: 1-2 tablets a day.
Availability: NHS and private prescription.
Side effects: stomach upset, cramp, rash, blood changes.
Caution: in pregnant women, nursing mothers, and in patients suffering from diabetes, gout, enlarged prostate, problems in passing urine. Your doctor may advise regular blood tests.
Not to be used for: children, or for patients suffering from liver or kidney disease, adrenal gland disorder, high potassium levels or other body fluid imbalance.
Caution needed with: some DIURETICS, potassium supplements, ACE INHIBITORS, LITHIUM, some antibiotics, DIGOXIN, ANTIHYPERTENSIVES.
Contains: BUMETANIDE, AMILORIDE.
Other preparations:

Burinex K
(Leo)

A white, egg-shaped tablet used as a DIURETIC/potassium supplement to treat fluid retention associated with congestive heart failure, liver disease, and kidney disease where potassium supplement is required.

Dose: 1-4 tablets a day.
Availability: NHS and private prescription.
Side effects: rash, cramps, stomach discomfort, blood changes, breast enlargement.
Caution: in pregnant women, nursing mothers, and in patients suffering from enlarged prostate, or impaired urination, kidney or liver disease, gout, diabetes.
Not to be used for: children, or for patients suffering from raised potassium levels, Addison's disease, liver cirrhosis.
Caution needed with: LITHIUM, DIGOXIN, ANTIHYPERTENSIVES, some DIURETICS, some antibiotics.
Contains: BUMETANIDE, POTASSIUM CHLORIDE.
Other preparations:

Buscopan
(Boehringer Ingelheim)

A white tablet supplied at a strength of 10 mg and used as an anti-spasm treatment for bowel spasm, painful periods.

Dose: adults painful periods 2 tablets 4 times a day for 5 days starting 2 days before the period begins; bowel spasm children 6-12 years 1 tablet 3 times a day, adults 2 tablets 4 times a day.
Availability: NHS, private prescription, over the counter.
Side effects: blurred vision, confusion, dry mouth.
Caution:
Not to be used for: patients with glaucoma, inflammatory bowel disease, intestinal obstruction, or enlarged prostate.
Caution needed with:
Contains: HYOSCINE BUTYLBROMIDE.
Other preparations:

---

buserelin *see* Suprecur, Suprefact

Buspar
(Bristol-Myers Squibb)

A white, oval tablet supplied at a strength of 5 mg and used as a tranquillizer for the short-term treatment of anxiety.

Dose: 1 tablet 2-3 times a day increasing every 2-3 days to a maximum of

9 tablets a day.
Availability: NHS and private prescription.
Side effects: dizziness, headache, nervousness, rarely rapid heart rate, chest pain, confusion, dry mouth, tiredness.
Caution: in patients with a history of kidney or liver disease.
Not to be used for: children, pregnant women, nursing mothers, or for patients suffering from severe kidney or liver disease, epilepsy.
Caution needed with:
Contains: BUSPIRONE HYDROCHLORIDE.
Other preparations:

---

buspirone *see* **Buspar**

---

butobarbitone *see* **Soneryl**

---

butoxethyl nicotinate *see* **Actinac**

---

butoxyethyl nicotinate *see* **Finalgon**

---

butriptyline *see* **Evadyne**

Cacit
(Norwich Eaton)

A pink effervescent tablet used as a calcium supplement to treat calcium deficiency and thinning of the bones.

Dose: 1-6 tablets a day, dissolved in water.
Availability: NHS, private prescription, over the counter.
Side effects: nausea, vomiting, constipation, loss of appetite, abdominal and bone pain, thirst, increased urine output, weak muscles.
Caution: in patients suffering from kidney disorder or with a history of kidney stones.
Not to be used for: patients suffering from high calcium levels in the blood or urine.
Caution needed with: TETRACYCLINES, VITAMIN D.
Contains: CALCIUM CARBONATE.

Other preparations: CALCICHEW (Shire), CITRICAL (Shire).

---

cade oil *see* Polytar Liquid

---

cadexomer iodine *see* Iodosorb

Cafadol
(Typharm)

A yellow, scored tablet used as an ANALGESIC to relieve pain including period pain.

Dose: adults 2 tablets every 3-4 hours; children 5-12 years half adult dose.
Availability: private prescription and over the counter.
Side effects:
Caution: in patients with liver or kidney disease.
Not to be used for: children under 5 years.
Caution needed with: other medicines containing paracetamol.
Contains: PARACETAMOL, CAFFEINE.
Other preparations:

Cafergot
(Sandoz)

A white tablet used as an ergot preparation to treat migraine.

Dose: 1-2 tablets at the beginning of a migraine attack to a maximum of 4 tablets a day. Do not repeat within 4 days.
Availability: NHS and private prescription.
Side effects: nausea, muscular pain, abdominal pain, reduced circulation, weak legs.
Caution:
Not to be used for: children, pregnant women, nursing mothers, or in patients suffering from coronary, peripheral, or occlusive vascular disease, severe high blood pressure, kidney or liver disease, sepsis.
Caution needed with: ERYTHROMYCIN, ß-BLOCKERS.
Contains: ERGOTAMINE tartrate, CAFFEINE.
Other preparations: Cafergot Suppositories, LINGRAINE (Sanofi Winthrop), MEDIHALER-ERGOTAMINE (3M Healthcare), MIGRIL (Wellcome).

---

caffeine *see* **Antoin, Cafadol, Cafergot, Doloxene Co., Glykola, Hypon, Labiton, Migril, Parahypon, Pardale, Propain, Solpadeine, Syndol, Uniflu and Gregovite C**

Calabren *see* **Daonil**
(Berk)

---

calamine *see* **calamine and coal tar ointment, calamine lotion**

---

calamine and coal tar ointment BP

An ointment used to treat chronic eczema and psoriasis.

Dose: apply 1-3 times a day.
Availability: NHS, private prescription, over the counter.
Side effects: irritation, acne-like skin eruptions, sensitivity to light.
Caution: avoid broken or inflamed skin. Stains hair, skin, and fabrics.
Not to be used for:
Caution needed with:
Contains: CALAMINE, strong COAL TAR solution, ZINC OXIDE, WHITE SOFT PARAFFIN, hydrous WOOL FAT.
Other preparations:

---

calamine lotion BP

A lotion used to treat itchy skin conditions.

Dose: apply when required.
Availability: NHS, private prescription, over the counter.
Side effects:
Caution:
Not to be used for:
Caution needed with:
Contains: CALAMINE.
Other preparations: aqueous calamine cream BP, oily calamine lotion BP 1980, calamine ointment BP.

Calcichew
(Shire)

A white, chewable tablet supplied at a strength of 500 mg and used as a calcium supplement to treat calcium deficiency, and regulate blood phosphate levels in patients with kidney failure.

Dose: 1 tablet chewed 2-3 times a day.
Availability: NHS, private prescription, over the counter.
Side effects: constipation, wind.
Caution:
Not to be used for: patients suffering from overactive parathyroid glands, severe kidney disease, decalcifying tumours.
Caution needed with: TETRACYCLINES.
Contains: CALCIUM CARBONATE.
Other preparations: Calcichew D3, CACIT (Norwich Eaton), CITRICAL (Shire).

---

calciferol *see* **Abidec, Calciferol tablets, Calcimax, Chocovite, Concavit, Multivite, Orovite 7, Polyvite, Pregnavite Forte F, Tonivitan**

---

calciferol tablets

Tablets used as a vitamin D$_2$ supplement to prevent vitamin D deficiency.

Dose: 0.01-2.5 mg (400-100 000 units) a day, depending on condition.
Availability: NHS, private prescription, over the counter.
Side effects: loss of appetite, nausea, vomiting, diarrhoea, weight loss, excessive urine output, sweating, headache, thirst, vertigo, raised calcium and phosphate levels, lack of energy.
Caution: in infants. Patients receiving high doses may need regular blood tests.
Not to be used for: patients suffering from high calcium levels in the blood.
Caution needed with:
Contains: CALCIFEROL.
Other preparations: calciferol injection. (Many compound vitamin preparations available over the counter contain small quantities of CALCIFEROL.)

Calcilat *see* **Adalat**
(Eastern)

Calcimax
(Wallace)

A brown syrup used as a calcium and vitamin supplement to treat calcium deficiency where vitamins are also needed.

Dose: adults 20 ml 2-3 times a day; children 5-10 ml 3 times a day.
Availability: private prescription and over the counter.
Side effects:
Caution:
Not to be used for: patients suffering from overactive parathyroid glands, severe kidney disease, decalcifying tumours.
Caution needed with:
Contains: CALCIUM GLYCINE HYDROCHLORIDE, CALCIFEROL, THIAMINE, RIBOFLAVINE, PYRIDOXINE, CYANOCOBALAMIN, NICOTINAMIDE, CALCIUM PANTOTHENATE.
Other preparations:

---

calcipotriol *see* Dovonex

Calcisorb
(3M Healthcare)

A powder in a sachet of 4.7 g and used as an ion-exchange compound to treat raised calcium levels in the urine, recurring kidney stones, osteopetrosis.

Dose: adults 1 sachet dispersed in water with meals or sprinkled on to food 3 times a day; children 2 sachets a day in 3 divided doses with food.
Availability: NHS, private prescription, over the counter.
Side effects: diarrhoea.
Caution: treatment of children should be monitored, and the treatment should be accompanied by a low-calcium diet with foods rich in oxalates.
Not to be used for: pregnant women, nursing mothers, or for patients suffering from kidney disease, congestive heart disease, or any other conditions in which a low-sodium diet is needed.
Caution needed with:
Contains: SODIUM CELLULOSE PHOSPHATE.
Other preparations:

---

calcitriol *see* Rocaltrol

---

calcium carbonate *see* APP, Cacit, Citrical, Calcichew,

Gaviscon, Titralac

---

calcium chloride *see* Glandosane

---

calcium folinate *see* Refolinon, Rescufolin

---

calcium gluconate *see* Chocovite

---

calcium glycerophosphate *see* Glykola, Metatone, Tonivitan A & D, Tonivitan B, Verdiviton

---

calcium glycine hydrochloride *see* Calcimax

---

calcium hydrogen phosphate *see* Octovit

---

calcium lactate gluconate *see* Sandocal

---

calcium oxytetracycline *see* Trimovate

---

calcium pantothenate *see* Allbee with C, BC 500, BC 500 with Iron, Calcimax, Concavit, Ketovite, Polyvite

---

calcium phosphate *see* Pregnavite Forte F

---

calcium polystyrene *see* Calcium Resonium

Calcium Resonium
(Sanofi Winthrop)

A powder used as an ion-exchange resin to treat raised potassium levels.

Dose: adults 15 g 3-4 times a day; children 1 g per kg body weight a day in divided doses.
Availability: NHS, private prescription, over the counter.
Side effects: hypercalcaemia (raised calcium levels).
Caution: potassium and calcium levels should be checked.
Not to be used for: for patients suffering from overactive parathyroid glands, multiple myeloma (a bone marrow tumour), sarcoidosis (a disease causing raised calcium levels), certain forms of cancer with kidney failure and hypercalcaemia (raised calcium levels).
Caution needed with:
Contains: CALCIUM POLYSTYRENE SULPHONATE.
Other preparations:

Calcium Sandoz *see* Sandocal
(Sandoz)

---

calcium sulphaloxate *see* Enteromide

Callusolve
(Dermal)

A paint used as a skin softener to treat warts.

Dose: apply 4-5 drops of the paint to the wart, cover for 24 hours, rub away the treated part, and repeat the process.
Availability: NHS, private prescription, over the counter.
Side effects:
Caution: apply only to warts and avoid healthy skin.
Not to be used for: for treating warts on the face or anal and genital areas.
Caution needed with:
Contains: BENZALKONIUM CHLORIDE-BROMINE.
Other preparations:

Calmurid HC
(Kabi Pharmacia)

A cream used as a STEROID, wetting agent and skin softener to treat dry hyperkeratotic eczema and other skin disorders.

Dose: wash and dry the affected area, and apply twice a day.
Availability: NHS and private prescription.
Side effects: fluid retention, suppression of adrenal glands, thinning of the skin may occur.
Caution: use for short periods of time only.
Not to be used for: patients suffering from acne or any other skin infections caused by tuberculosis, ringworm, viruses, or fungi, or continuously especially in pregnant women.
Caution needed with:
Contains: HYDROCORTISONE, UREA, LACTIC ACID.
Other preparations: ALPHADERM (Norwich Eaton), SENTIAL HC (Kabi Pharmacia).

Calpol Infant
(Wellcome)
A suspension supplied at a strength of 120 mg/5 ml and used as an ANALGESIC to relieve pain.
Dose: under 3 months 2.5 ml 4 times a day; 3 months-1 year 2.5-5 ml 4 times a day; 1-6 years 5-10 ml 4 times a day.
Availability: NHS, private prescription, over the counter.
Side effects:
Caution: in patients suffering from kidney or liver disease.
Not to be used for: infants under 2 months.
Caution needed with: other medicines containg paracetamol.
Contains: PARACETAMOL.
Other preparations: Calpol Six Plus (prescribed as a generic), DISPROL PAEDIATRIC (Reckitt & Coleman), PALDESIC (RP Drugs), PANALEVE (Pinewood, prescribed as a generic), PARACETAMOL PAEDIATRIC ELIXIR, SALZONE (Wallace).

Calthor — penicillin treatment for infections. Product now discontinued.

CAM
(Rybar)
A syrup used as a broncho-dilator to treat bronchial spasm.

Dose: adults 20 ml 3-4 times a day; children under 2 years 2.5 ml 3-4 times a day, 2-4 years 5 ml 3-4 times a day, over 4 years 10 ml 3-4 times a day.
Availability: NHS, private prescription, over the counter.
Side effects: nervousness, sleeplessness, restlessness, dry mouth, cold hands and feet, abnormal heart rhythms.

Caution: in patients suffering from diabetes.
Not to be used for: infants under 3 months or for patients suffering from heart disease,high blood pressure, overactive thyroid gland.
Caution needed with: MAOIS
Contains: EPHEDRINE HYDROCHLORIDE.
Other preparations:

C Camcolit
(Norgine)

A white, scored tablet supplied at strengths of 250 mg, 400 mg and used as a LITHIUM salt to treat mania, manic depression, aggressive and self-injuring behaviour.

Dose: your doctor may advise a blood test to check correct dose.
Availability: NHS and private prescription.
Side effects: nausea, diarrhoea, shaking hands, muscular weakness, brain and heart disturbances, weight gain, fluid retention, overactive or underactive thyroid gland, thirst, frequent urination, skin reactions.
Caution: patients should be treated in hospital at first.
Not to be used for: children, pregnant women, nursing mothers, or for patients suffering from kidney or heart disease, Addison's disease, underactive thyroid gland, disturbed sodium balance.
Caution needed with: DIURETICS, NON-STEROID ANTI-INFLAMMATORY DRUGS, CARBAMAZEPINE, FLUPENTHIXOL, METHYLDOPA, PHENYTOIN, HALOPERIDOL.
Contains: LITHIUM carbonate.
Other preparations:

Camoquin — antimalarial treatment. Product now discontinued.

---

camphene *see* **Rowachol, Rowatinex**

---

camphor *see* **Aradolene, Aspellin, Balmosa, Salonair**

Canesten
(Bayer)

A solution used as an antifungal treatment for fungal inflammation and infection of the outer ear, skin, and nails.

Dose: 2-3 applications a day until 14 days after the symptoms have gone.
Availability: NHS, private prescription, over the counter.
Side effects: local irritation, allergy.
Caution:
Not to be used for:
Caution needed with:
Contains: CLOTRIMAZOLE, POLYETHYLENE GLYCOL solution.
Other preparations: Canesten Spray, Canesten Powder, MASNODERM
(Cusi).

Canesten 1
(Bayer)

A white, vaginal tablet plus applicator supplied at a strength of 500 mg and
used as an antifungal, antibacterial treatment for vaginal infections.

Dose: 1 tablet inserted into the vagina at night.
Availability: NHS, private prescription, over the counter.
Side effects: mild burning or irritation, allergy.
Caution:
Not to be used for: children.
Caution needed with:
Contains: CLOTRIMAZOLE.
Other preparations: Canesten 10% VC, Canesten Vaginal Tablets,
Canesten Cream, Canesten Duopak, Canesten Vaginal Cream.

Canesten-HC
(Bayer)

A cream used as a STEROID, antifungal, antibacterial treatment for fungal
skin infections where there is also inflammation.

Dose: apply to the affected area twice a day.
Availability: NHS and private prescription.
Side effects: fluid retention, suppression of adrenal glands, thinning of the
skin may occur.
Caution: use for short periods of time only.
Not to be used for: patients suffering from acne or any other skin infec-
tions caused by tuberculosis, ringworm, viruses, or fungi, or continuously
especially in pregnant women.
Caution needed with:
Contains: CLOTRIMAZOLE, HYDROCORTISONE.
Other preparations:

Cantil
(Boehringer Mannheim)

A yellow tablet supplied at a strength of 25 mg and used as an anti-spasm treatment for bowel spasm.

Dose: adults 1-2 tablets 3 or 4 times a day.
Availability: NHS and private prescription.
Side effects: blurred vision, stomach upset, dry mouth, retention of urine, rapid heart rate, flushing, dizziness, weakness, insomnia.
Caution: enlarged prostate gland.
Not to be used for: patients suffering from glaucoma.
Caution needed with: TRICYCLIC antidepressants, some tranquillizers, ANTIHISTAMINES.
Contains: MEPENZOLATE BROMIDE.
Other preparations: (Cantil Elixir — now discontinued.)

Capasal
(Dermal)

A shampoo used as an emollient and skin softener to treat psoriasis or seborrhoeic dermatitis of the scalp, cradle cap.

Dose: use as a shampoo, daily if necessary.
Availability: NHS, private prescription, over the counter.
Side effects:
Caution:
Not to be used for:
Caution needed with:
Contains: SALICYCLIC ACID, COCONUT OIL, distilled COAL TAR.
Other preparations:

Capitol
(Dermal)

A gel used as an antibacterial treatment for dandruff and other similar scalp disorders.

Dose: use as a shampoo.
Availability: NHS, private prescription, over the counter.
Side effects:
Caution:
Not to be used for:
Caution needed with:
Contains: BENZALKONIUM CHLORIDE.
Other preparations:

Caplenal *see* Zyloric
(Berk)

Capoten
(Squibb)

A mottled white, scored tablet, a mottled white, square tablet, or a mottled white, oval tablet according to strengths of 12.5 mg, 25 mg, 50 mg and used as an ACE INHIBITOR in addition to DIURETICS and DIGOXIN in the treatment of severe congestive heart failure, high blood pressure.

Dose: adults 6.25 mg or 12.5 mg at first then 25 mg 2-3 times a day up to a maximum of 150 mg a day; children as advised by physician. For moderate to mild high blood pressure 12.5 mg twice a day then 25 mg twice a day increasing to 50 mg twice a day at 2-4 week intervals if needed. Severe high blood pressure 12.5 mg twice a day at first, then 50 mg 3 times a day if needed.
Availability: NHS and private prescription.
Side effects: rash, loss of taste, rarely a cough, blood changes, protein in the urine.
Caution: in patients suffering from kidney disease, auto-immune diseases, or patients undergoing anaesthesia, immune suppressant treatment, or who are taking leucopenic drugs. Your doctor may advise regular blood tests.
Not to be used for: pregnant women, nursing mothers, or for patients suffering from some heart valve diseases , kidney disease.
Caution needed with: potassium-sparing DIURETICS, potassium supplements, NON-STEROID ANTI-INFLAMMATORY DRUGS, vasodilators, CLONIDINE, ALLOPURINOL, PROCAINAMIDE, PROBENECID, immunosuppressants.
Contains: CAPTOPRIL.
Other preparations: ACEPRIL (Squibb).

Capozide
(Squibb)

A white, scored tablet used as a DIURETIC/ACE INHIBITOR combination to treat high blood pressure.

Dose: 1-2 tablets a day.
Availability: NHS and private prescription.
Side effects: protein in the urine, low blood pressure, rash, loss of taste, blood changes, sensitivity to light, tiredness, rarely a cough.
Caution: in patients undergoing anaesthesia, immune suppressant treatment, or leucopenic drugs and those suffering from kidney disease,

auto-immune diseases, diabetes, gout, liver disease.
Not to be used for: children, pregnant women, nursing mothers or for patients suffering from some heart valve diseases, kidney disease.
Caution needed with: LITHIUM, NON-STEROID ANTI-INFLAMMATORY DRUGS, ALLOPURINOL, PROCAINAMIDE, PROBENECID, immunosuppressants, vasodilators, CLONIDINE, potassium-sparing DIURETICS, potassium supplements, ANTIHYPERTENSIVES.
Contains: CAPTOPRIL, HYDROCHLOROTHIAZIDE.
Other preparations: Capozide LS, ACEZIDE (Squibb).

Caprin
(Monmouth)

A pink tablet supplied at a strength of 324 mg and used as an ANALGESIC to treat rheumatic and associated conditions, and to reduce risk of heart attack.

Dose: for pain 3 tablets 3-4 times a day; to reduce risk of heart attack 1 tablet a day.
Availability: NHS, private prescription, over the counter.
Side effects: stomach upsets, allergy, asthma.
Caution: in the elderly, pregnant women, patients with a history of allergy to aspirin or asthma, or who are suffering from impaired liver or kidney function.
Not to be used for: children, nursing mothers, or patients suffering from haemophilia or ulcers.
Caution needed with: anticoagulants, some antidiabetic drugs, anti-inflammatory drugs, METHOTREXATE, SPIRONOLACTONE, STEROIDS, some ANTAC-IDS, some uric acid-lowering drugs.
Contains: ASPIRIN.
Other preparations: ASPIRIN TABLETS, NU-SEALS ASPIRIN (Lilly).

capsicum oleoresin *see* Aradolene, Balmosa, Cremalgin

captopril *see* Capoten, Capozide

Carace
(Morson)

A blue, oval tablet, a white, oval, scored tablet, a yellow, oval, scored tablet, or an orange, oval, scored tablet according to strengths of 2.5 mg, 5 mg, 10 mg, 20 mg and used as an ACE INHIBITOR to treat congestive heart failure in addition to DIURETICS and/or DIGOXIN; high blood pressure.

Dose: 2.5 mg once a day at first, increasing to 5-20 mg a day over 2-4 weeks. For high blood pressure 2.5 mg once a day at first, increasing to 10-20 mg once a day and a maximum of 40 mg a day.
Availability: NHS and private prescirption.
Side effects: low blood pressure, kidney failure, swelling, rash, dizziness, headache, diarrhoea, cough, tiredness, palpitations, chest pains, weakness.
Caution: in nursing mothers and in patients suffering from kidney disease, severe congestive heart failure, or undergoing anaesthesia.
Not to be used for: children, pregnant women, or for patients suffering from some heart valve or lung diseases, or some types of fluid retention.
Caution needed with: potassium-sparing DIURETICS, potassium supplements, INDOMETHACIN, LITHIUM, ANTIHYPERTENSIVES.
Contains: LISINOPRIL.
Other preparations: ZESTRIL (ICI).

Carace Plus
(Thomas Morson)

A yellow, hexagonal, scored tablet used as an ACE INHIBITOR and DIURETIC to treat high blood pressure.

Dose: 1-2 tablets a day.
Availability: NHS and private prescription.
Side effects: dizziness, headache, cough, tiredness, low blood pressure, severe allergy, nausea, diarrhoea, impotence.
Caution: in patients undergoing surgery or anaesthesia, or suffering from body fluid imbalance, heart or circulatory disorder, liver or kidney disease, gout, high uric acid levels, diabetes.
Not to be used for: pregnant women, nursing mothers, children, or for patients suffering from reduced urine output or who have previously suffered severe allergic reaction to ACE INHIBITORS
Caution needed with: potassium supplements, LITHIUM, NON-STEROID ANTI-INFLAMMATORY DRUGS, antidiabetics.
Contains: LISINOPRIL, HYDROCHLOROTHIAZIDE.
Other preparations: ZESTORETIC (ICI).

---

carbachol *see* carbachol tablets, Isopto Carbachol

---

carbachol tablets

Tablets supplied at a strength of 2 mg and used to treat urine retention after surgical procedures.

Dose: 1 tablet 3 times a day, half an hour before food.
Availability: NHS and private prescription.
Side effects: nausea, vomiting, sweating, blurred vision, heartbeat irregularities, colic.
Caution:
Not to be used for: pregnant women, or patients suffering from blockage in the intestine or urinary tract, asthma, irregular heartbeat, overactive thyroid, recent heart attack, epilepsy, low blood pressure, Parkinson's diseas, stomach ulcer, or where increased muscle activity in the urinary tracts could be harmful.
Caution needed with:
Contains: CARBACHOL.
Other preparations: carbachol injection,

Carbalax
(Pharmax)

A suppository used to treat constipation, local anal conditions.

Dose: 1 suppository 30 minutes before evacuation required.
Availability: NHS, private prescription, over the counter.
Side effects:
Caution:
Not to be used for: children.
Caution needed with:
Contains: SODIUM BICARBONATE, ANYHDROUS SODIUM ACID PHOSPHATE.
Other preparations:

carbamazepine *see* Tegretol

carbaryl *see* Carylderm, Clinicide, Derbac-C, Suleo-C

Carbellon
(Torbet)

A black tablet used as an anti-spasm, anti-wind, ANTACID preparation to treat acidity, ulcers, food poisoning.

Dose: children over 6 years 2 tablets 3 times a day; adults 2-4 tablets 3 times a day.
Availability: over the counter and private prescription.
Side effects: occasionally constipation.
Caution:
Not to be used for: patients suffering from glaucoma, pyloric stenosis, enlarged prostate.
Caution needed with:
Contains: MAGNESIUM HYDROXIDE, CHARCOAL, PEPPERMINT OIL.
Other preparations:

C

---

carbenoxolone *see* **Biogastrone, Bioplex, Bioral**

---

carbidopa monohydrate *see* **Sinemet**

---

carbimazole *see* **Neo-Mercazole**

---

carbinoxamine *see* **Davenol**

Carbo-Cort
(Lagap)

A cream used as a STEROID, anti-psoriatic treatment for eczema, lichen planus (a rare skin disorder).

Dose: apply to the affected area 2-3 times a day.
Availability: NHS and private prescription.
Side effects: fluid retention, suppression of adrenal glands, thinning of the skin may occur.
Caution: use for short periods of time only
Not to be used for: patients suffering from acne or any other skin infections caused by tuberculosis, ringworm, viruses, or fungi, or continuously especially in pregnant women.
Caution needed with:
Contains: HYDROCORTISONE, COAL TAR SOLUTION.
Other preparations: ALPHOSYL HC (Stafford Miller), TARCORTIN (Stafford Miller).

Carbo-Dome
(Lagap)

A cream used as an anti-psoriatic treatment for psoriasis.

Dose: apply to the affected area 2-3 times a day.
Availability: NHS, private prescription, over the counter.
Side effects: irritation, sensitivity to light.
Caution:
Not to be used for: patients suffering from acute psoriasis.
Caution needed with:
Contains: coal tar.
Other preparations: CLINITAR (Shire), GELCOTAR (Quinoderm), PSORIDERM (Dermal), PSORIGEL (Galderma).

---

carbocisteine *see* Mucodyne

Carbomix
(Penn)

Granules used as an adsorbent to treat acute poisoning, overdose of drugs.

Dose: adults dissolve the contents of the bottle in water and take by mouth as soon as possible after poisoning; children usually half adult dose.
Availability: NHS, private prescription, over the counter.
Side effects:
Caution: your doctor may advise additional treatment for certain overdoses.
Not to be used for:
Caution needed with: antidotes or emetics taken by mouth.
Contains: activated CHARCOAL.
Other preparations:

---

carboxymethylcellulose *see* Glandosane

Cardene
(Syntex)

A blue/white or blue/pale-blue capsule according to strengths of 20 mg, 30 mg and used as an anti-anginal, ANTIHYPERTENSIVE drug to treat chronic stable angina, high blood pressure.

Dose: 20 mg 3 times a day increasing after not less than 3 day intervals to 30 mg 3 times a day or as required. Not more than 120 mg a day.
Availability: NHS and private prescription.
Side effects: chest pain, dizziness, headache, swelling of lower limbs, flushing, feeling warm, palpitations and nausea.
Caution: in patients suffering from weak heart, congestive heart failure, or liver or kidney disease.
Not to be used for: children, pregnant women, nursing mothers, or for patients suffering from some heart valve diseases.
Caution needed with: DIGOXIN, CIMETIDINE.
Contains: NICARDIPINE hydrochloride.
Other preparations: Cardene SR.

Cardiacap *see* **Mycardol.** Product now discontinued.

Cardinol *see* **Inderal**
(CP Pharmaceuticals)

Cardura
(Pfizer)

A white five-sided tablet, a white egg-shaped tablet, or a white square tablet according to strengths of 1 mg, 2 mg, 4 mg and used as a selective alpha-blocker to treat high blood pressure.

Dose: 1 mg once a day at first increasing after 1-2 weeks if needed to 2 mg once a day and then 4 mg once a day, up to a maximum of of 16 mg a day.
Availability: NHS, private prescription.
Side effects: low blood pressure on standing, vertigo, dizziness, headache, tiredness, weakness, fluid retention.
Caution: in pregnant women.
Not to be used for: children or nursing mothers.
Caution needed with:
Contains: DOXAZOSIN.
Other preparations:

---

carfecillin *see* **Uticillin**

Carisoma
(Pharmax)

A white tablet supplied at strengths of 125 mg, 350 mg and used as a sedative to treat muscle and bone problems associated with muscle spasm.

Dose: elderly 125 mg 3 times a day; adults 350 mg 3 times a day.
Availability: NHS and private prescription.
Side effects: drowsiness, dizziness, nausea, lassitude, flushes, headache, constipation, rash.
Caution: in patients suffering from kidney or liver disease, or a history of alcoholism or drug addiction. Avoid long-term treatment and withdraw gradually.
Not to be used for: children, pregnant women, nursing mothers, or for patients suffering from acute intermittent porphyria (a rare blood disorder).
Caution needed with: sedatives, anticoagulants, STEROIDS, the contraceptive pill, PHENYTOIN, GRISEOFULVIN, RIFAMPICIN, PHENOTHIAZINES, TRICYCLICS.
Contains: CARISOPRODOL.
Other preparations:

---

carisoprodol *see* **Carisoma**

---

carmellose sodium *see* **Orabase**

---

carteolol hydrochloride *see* **Cartrol, Teoptic**

Cartrol
(Sanofi Winthrop)

A white tablet supplied at a strength of 10 mg and used as a ß-BLOCKER to treat angina.

Dose: 1-3 tablets a day.
Availability: NHS and private prescription.
Side effects: cold hands and feet, sleep disturbance, slow heart rate, tiredness, wheezing, heart failure, stomach upset, dry eyes, skin rash.
Caution: in pregnant women, nursing mothers, and in patients suffering from diabetes, kidney or liver disorders, asthma. May need to be withdrawn before surgery. Withdraw gradually. Your doctor may advise additional treatment with DIURETICS or DIGOXIN.

Not to be used for: children or for patients suffering from heart block or failure.

Caution needed with: VERAPAMIL, CLONIDINE withdrawal, some anti-arrhythmic drugs, some anaesthetics, RESERPINE, some ANTIHYPERTENSIVES, ERGOTAMINE, CIMETIDINE, sedatives, SYMPATHOMIMETICS, INDOMETHACIN, antidiabetics.

Contains: CARTEOLOL HYDROCHLORIDE.

Other preparations:

Carylderm
(Napp Consumer)

A lotion used as a pediculicide to treat lice in the head and pubic areas.

Dose: rub into the hair and allow to dry, then shampoo.
Availability: NHS, private prescription, over the counter.
Side effects:
Caution: keep out of the eyes. Flammable liquid — do not dry hair with hair dryer.
Not to be used for:
Caution needed with:
Contains: CARBARYL.
Other preparations: Carylderm Liquid Shampoo, clinicide (DeWitt), DERBAC-C (Napp), SULEO-C (Napp).

Catapres
(Boehringer Ingelheim)

A white tablet scored on one side supplied at strengths of 0.1 mg, 0.3 mg and used to treat high blood pressure.

Dose: 0.05-0.1 mg 3 times a day increasing every second or third day.
Availability: NHS and private prescription.
Side effects: drowsiness, dry mouth, dizziness, fluid retention.
Caution: in nursing mothers, in patients suffering from depression or peripheral vascular disease, and where ß-BLOCKERS are being withdrawn.
Not to be used for: children.
Caution needed with: TRICYCLICS, some alpha-blockers, other ANTIHYPERTENSIVES, sedatives.
Contains: CLONIDINE hydrochloride.
Other preparations: Catapres Perlongets, Catapres Injection.

Caved-S
(Farmitalia)

A brown tablet used as a cell-surface protector and ANTACID to treat peptic ulcer.

Dose: adults 2 tablets chewed between meals.
Availability: NHS, private prescription, over the counter.
Side effects: few; occasionally constipation.
Caution:
Not to be used for: children.
Caution needed with: TETRACYCLINE antibiotics.
Contains: LIQUORICE EXTRACT, ALUMINIUM HYDROXIDE, MAGNESIUM CARBONATE, SODIUM BICARBONATE, BISMUTH SUBNITRATE.
Other preparations: RABRO.

Ce-Cobalin *see* **Cytacon.** Product now discontinued.

Ceanel Concentrate
(Quinoderm)

A liquid used as an antibacterial, antifungal treatment for psoriasis, seborrhoeic inflammation of the scalp.

Dose: use as a shampoo 3 times a week at first and then twice a week or apply directly to other areas of skin as needed.
Availability: NHS, private prescription, over the counter.
Side effects:
Caution: keep out of the eyes.
Not to be used for:
Caution needed with:
Contains: PHENYLETHYL ALCOHOL, CETRIMIDE, UNDECANOIC ACID.
Other preparations:

Cedilanid — heart muscle stimulator. Product now discontinued.

Cedocard
(Farmitalia)

A white, pink, blue, or green scored tablet according to strengths of 5 mg, 10 mg, 20 mg, and 40 mg and used as a NITRATE treatment for severe congestive heart failure and angina.

Dose: heart failure 10-40 mg 3-4 times a day; angina 5-40 mg 3-4 times a day.
Availability: NHS, private prescription, over the counter.
Side effects: headache, flushes, dizziness.
Caution:
Not to be used for: children or for patients suffering from severe low blood pressure, heart shock, severe anaemia, brain haemorrhage.
Caution needed with:
Contains: ISOSORBIDE DINITRITE.
Other preparations: Cedocard I.V., IMTACK (Astra), ISORDIL (Monmouth), VASCARDIN (Nicholas).

C

Cedocard Retard
(Farmitalia)

A yellow scored tablet or an orange scored tablet according to strengths of 20 mg, 40 mg and used as a NITRATE treatment for angina.

Dose: 20-80 mg morning and evening.
Availability: NHS, private prescription, over the counter.
Side effects: headache, flushes, dizziness.
Caution:
Not to be used for: children, or for patients suffering from severe low blood pressure, heart shock, severe anaemia, brain haemorrhage..
Caution needed with:
Contains: ISOSORBIDE DINITRATE.
Other preparations: ISOKET RETARD (Schwarz), ISORDIL (Monmouth), SONI-SLO (Lipha), SORBICHEW (Stuart), IMTACK (Astra), SORBID-SA (Stuart), SORBITRATE (Stuart), VASCARDIN (Nicholas).

cefaclor *see* **Distaclor**

cefadroxil *see* **Baxan**

cefixime *see* **Suprax**

cefuroxime axetil *see* **Zinnat**

Celance
(Lilly)

An ivory, green, or pink, rectangular, scored tablet according to strengths of 0.05 mg, 0.25 mg, 1 mg, and used as an antiparkinsonian drug as an additional treatment for Parkinson's disease.

Dose: Initially 0.05 mg a day for 2 days, then gradually increasing to a maximum of 5 mg a day.
Availability: NHS and private prescription.
Side effects: hallucinations, confusion, movement disorder, drowsiness, low blood pressure, heartbeat abnormalities, nausea, dyspepsia, inflammation of the nose, breathing difficulty, double vision.
Caution: in pregnant women, nursing mothers, and in patients suffering from heart disease, abnormal heart rhythm, or with a history of hallucinations. Treatment should be withdrawn gradually.
Not to be used for: children.
Caution needed with: other similar antiparkinsonian drugs, ANTIHYPERTENSIVES, anticoagulants.
Contains: PERGOLIDE MESYLATE.
Other preparations:

Celectol
(Rhone-Poulenc Rorer)

A yellow, heart-shaped, scored tablet supplied at a strength of 200 mg and used as a ß-BLOCKER to treat high blood pressure.

Dose: 1-2 tablets a day in the morning 30 minutes before food.
Availability: NHS and private prescription.
Side effects: cold hands and feet, sleep disturbance, slow heart rate, tiredness, wheezing, heart failure, stomach upset, dry eyes, skin rash.
Caution: in pregnant women, nursing mothers, and in patients suffering from diabetes, kidney or liver disorders, asthma. May need to be withdrawn before surgery. Withdraw gradually. Your doctor may advise additional treatment with DIURETICS or DIGOXIN.
Not to be used for: children or for patients suffering from heart block or failure.
Caution needed with: VERAPAMIL, CLONIDINE withdrawal, some anti-arrhythmic drugs, some anaesthetics, RESERPINE, some ANTIHYPERTENSIVES, ERGOTAMINE, CIMETIDINE, sedatives, SYMPATHOMIMETICS, INDOMETHACIN, antidiabetics.
Contains: CELIPROLOL.
Other preparations:

Celevac
(Monmouth)

A pink tablet supplied at a strength of 500 mg and used as an adsorbent and bulking agent to treat constipation, colostomy control, diarrhoea, ulcerative colitis, diverticular disease, obesity.

Dose: to treat constipation adults 3-6 tablets night and morning with at least 300 ml liquid; to treat diarrhoea adults 3-6 tablets night and morning with little liquid; to treat obesity 3 tablets with liquid 30 minutes before a meal or when hungry; children in proportion to the dosage for a 70 kg adult.
Availability: NHS, private prescription, over the counter.
Side effects:
Caution: if treating diarrhoea, do not drink for 30 minutes before and after each dose.
Not to be used for: treating obesity in children or for patients suffering from blocked intestine.
Caution needed with:
Contains: METHYLCELLULOSE.
Other preparations: (Celevac granules — now discontinued), NILSTIM.

---

celiprolol *see* **Celectol**

---

cellulose *see* **Nilstim**

Centyl
(Leo)

A white tablet or a white, scored tablet according to strengths of 2.5 mg, 5 mg and used as a DIURETIC to treat fluid retention, high blood pressure, toxaemia of pregnancy.

Dose: adults 5-10 mg every morning at first, then 2.5-10 mg a day; children in proportion to dose for 70 kg adult.
Availability: NHS and private prescription.
Side effects: low blood potassium, rash, sensitivity to light, blood changes, gout, tiredness.
Caution: in pregnant women, nursing mothers, and in patients suffering from liver or kidney disease, gout, diabetes. Potassium supplements may be necessary. Your doctor may advise blood tests.
Not to be used for: patients suffering from severe kidney failure.
Caution needed with: LITHIUM, DIGOXIN, ANTIHYPERTENSIVES.

Contains: BENDROFLUAZIDE.
Other preparations: APRINOX (Boots), BENDROFLUAZIDE TABLETS, BERKOZIDE (Berk), NEO-NACLEX (Evans).

Centyl-K
(Leo)

A green, egg-shaped tablet used as a DIURETIC to treat fluid retention, high blood pressure, toxaemia of pregnancy, where a potassium supplement is needed; also prevention of recurring calcium kidney stones.

Dose: 2-4 tablets a day in the morning at first, then 1-4 a day or every other day; for kidney stones 2-3 tablets a day.
Availability: NHS and private prescription.
Side effects: rash, sensitivity to light, blood changes, gout, tiredness.
Caution: in pregnant women, nursing mothers, and in patients suffering from diabetes, kidney or liver disease, and gout.
Not to be used for: children or for patients suffering from severe kidney failure, Addison's disease, or raised potassium levels.
Caution needed with: LITHIUM, DIGOXIN, ANTIHYPERTENSIVES, some other DIURETICS.
Contains: BENDROFLUAZIDE, POTASSIUM CHLORIDE.
Other preparations: NEO-NACLEX K (Goldcrest).

---

cephalexin *see* Ceporex, Keflex

---

cephradine *see* Velosef

Ceporex
(Glaxo)

A pink tablet supplied at strengths of 250 mg, 500 mg, 1 g and used as a cephalosporin antibiotic to treat respiratory, skin, and soft tissue infections, ear infections, urinary infections, gonorrhoea.

Dose: adults and children over 7 years 1-2 g a day in 2-4 divided doses; children under 3 months 62.5-125 mg twice a day, 4 months- 2 years 250-500 mg a day, 3-6 years 500 mg-1 g a day, in 2-4 divided doses.
Availability: NHS and private prescription.
Side effects: allergy,stomach disturbances.
Caution: in patients suffering from kidney disease or who are very

sensitive to penicillins.
Not to be used for:
Caution needed with: loop DIURETICS (such as FRUSEMIDE).
Contains: CEPHALEXIN.
Other preparations: Ceporex Capsules, Ceporex Syrup, Ceporex Suspension, Ceporex Paediatric Drops, KEFLEX (Lilly).

---

ceratonia *see* **Arobon**

Cerebrovase *see* **Persantin**

Cerumol
(LAB)

Drops used as a wax softener to remove wax from the ears.

Dose: 5 drops into the ear twice a day for 3 days may enable syringing to be avoided.
Availability: NHS, private prescription, over the counter.
Side effects:
Caution:
Not to be used for: inflammation of the outer ear, dermatitis, eczema, perforated ear drum.
Caution needed with:
Contains: PARADICHLOROBENZENE, CHLORBUTOL, ARACHIS OIL.
Other preparations:

Cesamet
(Eli Lilly)

A blue/white capsule supplied at a strength of 1 mg and used as an anti-emetic drug to treat nausea and vomiting brought on by cytotoxic drugs.

Dose: 1-2 capsules the night before and again 1-3 hours before taking the first dose of the cytotoxic drug, up to a maximum of 6 capsules a day.
Availability: NHS and private prescription.
Side effects: drowsiness, reduced reactions, confusion, blurred vision, brain disturbances, low blood pressure, rapid heart rate, dry mouth, loss of appetite, stomach cramps.
Caution: in pregnant women, patients with a history of mental disorders, or patients suffering from severe liver disease.

Not to be used for:
Caution needed with: sedatives, alcohol, narcotic ANALGESICS.
Contains: NABILONE.
Other preparations:

---

cetalkonium chloride *see* **AAA Spray, Teejel**

Cetavlex
(ICI)

A cream used as an antiseptic to treat minor cuts and wounds, nappy rash.

Dose: apply as needed.
Availability: NHS, private prescription, over the counter.
Side effects:
Caution:
Not to be used for:
Caution needed with:
Contains: CETRIMIDE.
Other preparations:

Cetavlon PC — disinfectant shampoo used to treat dandruff. Product now discontinued.

---

cetirizine dihydrochloride *see* **Zirtek**

---

cetomacrogol *see* **Diprobase, Lipobase**

---

cetostearyl alcohol *see* **Diprobase, Lipobase, Unguentum Merck**

Cetriclens *see* **Savlodil.** Product now discontinued.

---

cetrimide *see* **Ceanel, Cetavlex, Cetavlon PC, Cetriclens,**
122

Cradocap, Drapolene,Savloclens, Savlodil, Savlon Hospital Concentrate, Tisept, Torbetol, Travasept 100

---

cetyl alcohol/coal tar distillate *see* **Pragmatar**

---

cetylpyridinium *see* **Medilave, Merocaine, Merocet**

---

chamomile *see* **Kamillosan**

---

charcoal *see* **Carbellon, Carbomix, Medicoal**

Chemotrim Paediatric *see* **Septrin**
(RP Drugs)

Chendol Tablets
(CP Pharmaceuticals)

An orange, scored tablet supplied at a strength of 250 mg and used as a bile acid to dissolve non-calcified gallstones.

Dose: 3-4 tablets a day.
Availability: NHS and private prescription.
Side effects: diarrhoea, itch.
Caution: monitor effects on liver function.
Not to be used for: children, women who are not taking contraceptive precautions, or for patients suffering from chronic liver disease or inflammatory intestinal disease.
Caution needed with: the contraceptive pill.
Contains: CHENODEOXYCHOLIC ACID.
Other preparations: Chendol Capsules. CHENOFALK (Thames).

---

chenodeoxycholic acid *see* **Chendol Tablets, Lithofalk**

Chenofalk *see* **Chendol Tablets**
(Thames)

Chloractil *see* **Largactil**
(DDSA)

---

choral hydrate *see* **Noctec, Welldorm**

---

chloramphenicol *see* **Actinac, chloramphenicol ear drops, chloramphenicol eye drops, Chloramphenicol Minims, Chloromycetin, Chloromycetin Hydrocortisone, Chloromycetin Ointment**

---

chloramphenicol ear drops

Drops used as an antibiotic to treat bacterial infection of the outer ear.

Dose: apply 2-3 times a day.
Availability: NHS and private prescription.
Side effects: allergy.
Caution: avoid prolonged use.
Not to be used for:
Caution needed with:
Contains: CHLORAMPHENICOL.
Other preparations:

---

chloramphenicol eye drops *see* Chloramphenicol Minims

Chloramphenicol Minims
(SNP)

Drops used as an antibiotic to treat bacterial infections of the eye.

Dose: adults 1 or more drops into the eye as needed; children 1 drop into the eye as needed.
Availability: NHS and private prescription.
Side effects: local allergy, bone marrow suppression.
Caution: remove contact lenses before using.
Not to be used for:
Caution needed with:
Contains: CHLORAMPHENICOL.
Other preparations: Chloramphenicol Eye Drops, CHLOROMYCETIN (Parke-Davis).

Chlorasept 2000
(Baxter)

A solution used as a disinfectant for cleansing wounds.

Dose: use as needed.
Availability: NHS and private prescription.
Side effects:
Caution:
Not to be used for:
Caution needed with:
Contains: chlorhexidine acetate.
Other preparations:

Chloraseptic
(Procter and Gamble)

A solution supplied with a spray and used as a disinfectant to treat sore throat, mouth ulcers, minor mouth and gum infections.

Dose: adults 5 sprays every 2 hours as needed or gargle or rinse mouth with solution diluted with equal amount of water; children 6-12 years 3 sprays every 2 hours as needed or rinse out mouth.
Availability: NHS, private prescription, over the counter.
Side effects:
Caution:
Not to be used for: children under 6 years, or for patients suffering from epiglottitis.
Caution needed with:
Contains: PHENOL, SODIUM PHENOLATE.
Other preparations: Chloraseptic Lozenges, Chloraseptic Mouthwash and Gargle.

Chlorasol
(Seton)

A solution in a sachet used as a disinfectant for cleaning and removing dead skin from ulcers.

Dose: apply to the affected areas as needed.
Availability: NHS, private prescription, over the counter.
Side effects: irritation.
Caution: keep away from the eyes and the clothes; throw away any remaining solution immediately.
Not to be used for: internal use.

Caution needed with:
Contains: SODIUM HYPOCHLORITE.
Other preparations:

---

chlorbutol *see* **Auralgicin, Cerumol, Eludril, Monphytol**

---

chlordiazepoxide *see* **Librium, Limbitrol 5, Tropium**

---

chlorhexidine *see* **Bacticlens, Cetriclens, Chlorasept 2000, Corsodyl, CX Powder, Eludril, Hibiscrub, Hibisol, Hibitane, Naseptin, Nystaform, Nystaform-HC, pHiso-Med, Rotersept, Savloclens, Savlodil, Savlon Hospital Concentrate, Tisept, Travasept 100, Unisept**

---

chlormethiazole edisylate *see* **Heminevrin.**

---

chlormezanone *see* **Lobak, Trancopal,Trancoprin**

---

chloroform suspension *see* **Glykola**

Chloromycetin
(Parke-Davis)

A white/grey capsule supplied at a strength of 250 mg and used as an antibiotic to treat typhoid, influenzae meningitis, severe infections.

Dose: adults and children over 2 weeks 50 mg per kg body weight a day in divided doses every 6 hours; children under 2 weeks half adult dose.
Availability: NHS and private prescription.
Side effects: blood changes, stomach disturbances, allergies, nerve inflammation.
Caution: your doctor may advise regular blood tests.
Not to be used for: minor infections or for prevention.
Caution needed with: anticoagulants, anticonvulsants, PARACETAMOL.
Contains: CHLORAMPHENICOL.
Other preparations: Chloromycetin Palmitate Suspension, CHLOROMYCETIN

Chloromycetin Eye Ointment
(Parke-Davis)

An ointment used as an antibiotic to treat bacterial conjunctivitis.

Dose: apply the ointment into the eye every 3 hours or more often if needed and continue until 2 days after the symptoms have gone.
Availability: NHS and private prescription.
Side effects: rarely bone marrow suppression.
Caution:
Not to be used for:
Caution needed with:
Contains: CHLORAMPHENICOL.
Other preparations: Chloromycetin Redidrops, chloramphenicol eye ointment, CHLORAMPHENICOL MINIMS (SNP).

Chloromycetin Hydrocortisone
(Parke-Davis)

An ointment used as an antibiotic, STEROID to treat eye infections.

Dose: apply into the eye up to once an hour depending on the severity of the infection.
Availability: NHS and private prescription.
Side effects: rise in eye pressure, thinning cornea, cataract, rarely bone marrow suppression.
Caution: in infants and pregnant women; do not use for extended periods.
Not to be used for: patients suffering from glaucoma, viral, fungal, or weeping infections.
Caution needed with:
Contains: CHLORAMPHENICOL, HYDROCORTISONE.
Other preparations:

chlorophenoxyethanol *see* **Phytocil**

chloroquine *see* **Avloclor, Nivaquine**

chlorothiazide *see* **Saluric**

chlorpheniramine maleate *see* **Expulin, Expurhin, Galpseud Plus, Haymine, Piriton, Rimarin**

chlorpromazine *see* **Largactil**

chlorpropamide *see* **Diabinese**

chlorquinaldol *see* **Locoid C**

chlortetracycline *see* **Aureocort, Aureomycin, Aureomycin Ointment**

chlorthalidone *see* **Hygroton, Hygroton K, Kalspare, Lopresoretic, Tenoret 50, Tenoretic**

Chlorthymol *see* **Alcos-Anal**

Chocovite
(Torbet)

A buff-coloured tablet used as a calcium and vitamin D_2 supplement to treat calcium deficiency.

Dose: 1-3 tablets sucked 3 times a day.
Availability: private prescription and over the counter.
Side effects:
Caution:
Not to be used for:
Caution needed with:
Contains: CALCIUM GLUCONATE, CALCIFEROL.
Other preparations:

cholecalciferol *see* **Octovit**

Choledyl
(Warner)

A pink tablet or a yellow tablet according to strengths 100 mg, 200 mg and used as a broncho-dilator to treat bronchial spasm brought on by chronic bronchitis or asthma.

Dose: adults 100-400 mg 4 times a day; children 3-6 years use syrup, 6-12 years 100 mg 3-4 times a day.
Availability: NHS, private prescription , over the counter.
Side effects: rapid heart rate, sleeplessness, nausea, change in heart rhythms, stomach upset.
Caution: in pregnant women, nursing mothers, and in patients suffering from heart or liver disease or peptic ulcer. Diabetics should avoid syrup.
Not to be used for: children under 3 years.
Caution needed with: CIMETIDINE, ERYTHROMYCIN, CIPROFLOXACIN, INTERFERON, STEROIDS, DIURETICS, some other broncho-dilators.
Contains: CHOLINE THEOPHYLLINATE.
Other preparations: Choledyl Syrup.

---

cholestyramine *see* **Questran**

---

choline bitartrate *see* **Lipoflavonoid, Lipotriad**

---

choline chloride *see* **Ketovite**

---

choline magnesium trisalicylate *see* **Trilisate**

---

choline salicylate *see* **Audax, Teejel**

---

choline theophyllinate *see* **Choledyl**

Chymocyclar *see* **Tetracycline.** Product now discontinued.

Chymoral Forte — enzyme to treat inflammatory swelling. Product now discontinued

---

chymotrypsin *see* **Chymoral Forte**

Cicatrin
(Wellcome)

A cream used as an aminoglycoside antibiotic to treat skin infections.

Dose: apply to the affected area up to 3 times a day.
Availability: NHS and private prescription.
Side effects: hearing damage, sensitization.
Caution: where there are large areas of damaged skin.
Not to be used for:
Caution needed with:
Contains: NEOMYCIN SULPHATE, BACITRACIN ZINC, L-CYSTEINE, GLYCINE, DL-THREONINE.
Other preparations: Cicatrin Aerosol, Cicatrin Powder.

---

ciclacillin *see* **Calthor**

Cidomycin Cream
(Roussel)

A cream used as an aminoglycoside antibiotic to treat burns, wounds, and skin infections including impetigo.

Dose: apply to the affected area 3-4 times a day.
Availability: NHS and private prescription.
Side effects: hearing damage, sensitization.
Caution: where there are large areas of damaged skin.
Not to be used for:
Caution needed with:
Contains: GENTAMICIN sulphate.
Other preparations: GENTICIN CREAM (Nicholas), Cidomycin Ointment.

Cidomycin Drops
(Roussel)

Drops used as an antibiotic to treat infections of the outer ear or eye.

Dose: 2-4 drops into the ear 3-4 times a day and at night, or 1-3 drops into the eye 3-4 times a day.
Availability: NHS and private prescription.
Side effects: additional infection.
Caution:
Not to be used for: patients suffering from perforated ear drum.
Caution needed with:
Contains: GENTAMICIN sulphate.
Other preparations: Cidomycin Eye Ointment, GARAMYCIN (Schering-Plough), GENTICIN (Nicholas).

---

cilazapril *see* **Vascace**

Cilest
(Ortho)

A blue tablet used as an oestrogen, progestogen contraceptive.

Dose: 1 tablet a day for 21 days, starting on day 1 of period.
Availability: NHS and private prescription.
Side effects: enlarged breasts, bloating and fluid retention, cramps, leg pains, mood change, reduction in sexual desire, headaches, nausea, vaginal erosion, discharge and bleeding, weight gain, skin changes.
Caution: in patients suffering from high blood pressure, diabetes, vascular disorders, asthma, depression, kidney disease, multiple sclerosis, womb diseases. Your doctor may advise you not to smoke, and to have regular examinations. You should stop treatment at the first sign of serious symptoms such as severe headache or jaundice. Treatment should be stopped before surgery.
Not to be used for: pregnant women, or for patients suffering from sickle-cell anaemia, history of heart disease or thrombosis, liver disorders, some cancers, undiagnosed vaginal bleeding, some ear, skin and kidney disorders.
Caution needed with: RIFAMPICIN, TETRACYCLINES, GRISEOFULVIN, BARBITURATES, PHENYTOIN, PRIMIDONE, CARBAMAZEPINE, ETHOSUXIMIDE, CHLORAL HYDRATE, DICHLORALPHENAZONE.
Contains: ETHINYLOESTRADIOL, NORGESTIMATE.
Other preparations:

---

cimetidine *see* **Tagamet**

cinchocaine *see* **Nupercainal, Proctosedyl, Scheriproct, Ultraproct, Uniroid**

---

cineole *see* **Copholco, Copholcoids, Rowachol, Rowatinex, Tercoda, Terpoin**

---

cinnarizine *see* **Stugeron, Stugeron Forte**

Cinobac
(Eli Lilly)

A green/orange capsule supplied at a strength of 500 mg and used as a quinolone antibiotic to treat infections of the urinary tract.

Dose: 1 capsule twice a day for 7-14 days; for prevention 1 at night.
Availability: NHS and private prescription.
Side effects: allergy, brain and stomach disturbances.
Caution: in patients suffering from kidney disease, or with a history of liver disease.
Not to be used for: children, pregnant women, nursing mothers or for patients suffering from severe kidney disease.
Caution needed with: anticoagulants, THEOPHYLLINE.
Contains: CINOXACIN.
Other preparations:

---

cinoxacin *see* **Cinobac**

---

ciprofibrate *see* **Modalim**

---

ciprofloxacin *see* **Ciproxin**

Ciproxin
(Bayer)

Tablets supplied at strengths of 250 mg, 500 mg, and used as an antibiotic to treat infections of the ear, nose, throat, urinary system, respiratory system, skin, soft tissues, bone, joints, stomach, and gonorrhoea (a venereal disease), and major infections.

Dose: 250-750 mg twice a day.
Availability: NHS and private prescription.
Side effects: stomach and intestinal disturbances, dizziness, headache, tiredness, confusion, convulsions, rash, pain in the joints, changes in blood, liver, or kidneys, blurred vision, rapid heart rate.
Caution: in patients suffering from severe kidney disease or with a history of convulsions. Plenty of liquid should be drunk.
Not to be used for: children, growing youngsters unless absolutely necessary, and pregnant women or nursing mothers.
Caution needed with: THEOPHYLLINE, ANTACIDS, alcohol, anticoagulants, NON-STEROID ANTI-INFLAMMATORY DRUGS, CYCLOSPORIN.
Contains: CIPROFLOXACIN.
Other preparations: Ciproxin Infusion.

---

cisapride *see* Prepulsid

---

citric acid *see* Effercitrate, Mictral, Rehidrat, simple linctus

---

Citrical
(Shire)

Orange-flavoured granules supplied in sachets of 500 mg and used as a calcium supplement to treat calcium deficiency.

Dose: 1 sachet dissolved in water up to 3 times a day.
Availability: NHS, private prescription, over the counter.
Side effects: constipation, wind.
Caution:
Not to be used for: children or for patients suffering from overactive parathyroid gland, decalcifying tumours, severe kidney failure.
Caution needed with: TETRACYCLINES.
Contains: CALCIUM CARBONATE.
Other preparations: CACIT (Norwich Eaton), CALCICHEW (Shire).

---

citrus fibre *see* Proctofibe

Claradin *see* **aspirin tablets.** Product now discontinued.

clarithromycin *see* **Klaricid**

Clarityn
(Schering-Plough)

A white, oval, scored tablet supplied at a strength of 10 mg and used as an ANTIHISTAMINE treatment for allergic rhinitis and other allergies.

Dose: 1 tablet a day (children use syrup).
Availability: NHS and private prescription.
Side effects: tiredness, headache, nausea.
Caution:
Not to be used for: children under 2 years, pregnant women, or nursing mothers.
Caution needed with:
Contains: LORATADINE.
Other preparations: Clarityn Syrup.

clavulanic acid *see* **Augmentin**

clemastine *see* **Tavegil**

Climagest
(Sandoz)

16 grey/blue tablets and 12 white tablets used as an oestrogen and progestogen treatment for menopausal symptoms.

Dose: 1 grey/blue tablet for 16 days followed by 1 white tablet for the next 12 days. Begin on day 1 of period if present.
Availability: NHS and private prescription.
Side effects: enlarged breasts, bloating and fluid retention, cramps, leg pains, mood change, reduction in sexual desire, headaches, nausea, vaginal erosion, discharge and bleeding, weight gain, skin charges.
Caution: in patients suffering from high blood pressure, diabetes, vascular disorders, asthma, depression, kidney disease, multiple sclerosis, womb diseases. Your doctor may advise you not to smoke, and to have regular examinations. You should stop treatment at the first sign of serious symptoms such as severe headache or jaundice. Treatment should be stopped before surgery.
Not to be used for: pregnant women, or for patients suffering from sickle-

cell anaemia, history of heart disease or thombosis, liver disorders, some cancers, undiagnosed vaginal bleeding, some ear, skin, and kidney disorders.

Caution needed with: RIFAMPICIN, TETRACYCLINES, GRISEOFULVIN, BARBITURATES, PHENYTOIN, PRIMIDONE, CARBAMAZEPINE. ETHOSUXIMIDE, CHLORAL HYDRATE, DICHLORALPHENAZONE.

Contains: OESTRADIOL VALERATE, NORETHISTERONE.

Other preparations:

C

Climaval
(Sandoz)

A grey-blue or blue tablet supplied at a strength of 1 mg, 2 mg and used as an oestrogen to treat menopausal symptoms in women who have had a hysterectomy.

Dose: 1-2 mg a day. May be taken continuously for up to 24 months.

Availability: NHS and private prescription.

Side effects: enlarged breasts, fluid retention, headache, nausea, vaginal bleeding, weight gain, skin changes, liver disorders, jaundice, rashes, vomiting.

Caution: in patients suffering from high blood pressure, diabetes, heart disease, vascular disorders, asthma, kidney disease, epilepsy, migraine, womb diseases, thyroid disorder. Your doctor may advise you to have regular examinations.

Not to be used for: the elderly (except for control of post-menopausal symptoms), pregnant women, nursing mothers, or for patients suffering from sickle-cell anaemia, history of heart disease or thombosis, liver disorders, some cancers, undiagnosed vaginal bleeding, some ear, skin and kidney disorders, jaundice, porphyria (a rare blood disorder), brain blood-vessel disease.

Caution needed with: DIURETICS, ANTIHYPERTENSIVES, drugs which induce liver enzymes (e.g. BARBITURATES, CARBAMAZEPINE, PHENYTOIN, RIFAMPICIN).

Contains: OESTRADIOL VALERATE.

Other preparations: PROGYNOVA (Schering), ZUMENON (Duphar).

clindamycin *see* Dalacin C, Dalacin T

Clinicide
(De Witt)

A liquid used as a pediculicide to treat lice of the head and pubic areas.

Dose: apply to the hair and allow to dry, then shampoo the following day.
Availability: NHS, private prescription, over the counter.
Side effects:
Caution: *keep out of the eyes.*
Not to be used for:
Caution needed with:
Contains: CARBARYL.
Other preparations: CARYLDERM (Napp), DERBAC-C (Napp), SULEO-C (Napp).

Clinitar Cream
(Shire)

A cream used as an antipsoriatic treatment for psoriasis, eczema.

Dose: apply to the affected area 1-2 times a day.
Availability: NHS, private prescription, over the counter.
Side effects: sensitivity to light.
Caution:
Not to be used for: patients suffering from pustular psoriasis.
Caution needed with:
Contains: COAL TAR EXTRACT.
Other preparations: Clinitar Shampoo, ALPHOSYL (Stafford-Miller), GELCOTAR (Quinoderm), PSORIDERM (Dermal), PSORIGEL (Galderma), T-GEL (Neutrogena), (Clinitar Gel — now discontinued).

Clinium — calcium antagonist to treat angina. Product now discontinued.

Clinoril
(MSD)

A hexagonal, yellow, scored tablet supplied at strengths of 100 mg, 200 mg and used as a NON-STEROID ANTI-INFLAMMATORY DRUG to treat rheumatoid arthritis, osteoarthritis, ankylosing spondylitis, acute gouty arthritis, other joint disorders.

Dose: 200 mg twice a day with drink or food.
Availability: NHS and private prescription.
Side effects: stomach pain, dyspepsia, rash, dizziness, buzzing in the ears, breathing difficulties, changes in the blood, urine, eyesight, heart rhythm disturbance, high blood sugar, kidney stones. Withdraw if fever or liver disorders occur.
Caution: in the elderly, and in patients with a history of stomach haemorrhage or ulcer, kidney or liver disease, or heart failure.

Not to be used for: children, pregnant women, nursing mothers, or for patients suffering from anti-inflammatory or aspirin induced allergy, peptic ulcer, or stomach bleeding.
Caution needed with: DIMETHYL SULPHOXIDE, ASPIRIN, anticoagulants, DIFLUSINAL, antidiabetics.
Contains: SULINDAC.
Other preparations:

---

clioquinol *see* **Barquinol HC, Haelan-C, Locorten-Vioform, Oralcer, Vioform-Hydrocortisone**

---

clobazam *see* **Frisium**

---

clobetasol propionate *see* **Dermovate**

---

clobetasone butyrate *see* **Eumovate Cream, Eumovate Drops, Trimovate**

---

clofazimine *see* **Lamprene**

---

clofibrate *see* **Atromid-S, Modalim**

Clomid
(Marion Merrell Dow)

A pale-yellow, scored tablet supplied at a strength of 50 mg and used as an anti-oestrogen treatment for sterility caused by failure of ovulation.

Dose: 1 tablet a day for five days starting on the fifth day of the period.
Availability: NHS and private prescription.
Side effects: enlargement of the ovaries, hot flushes, uncomfortable abdomen, blurred vision.
Caution:
Not to be used for: children, pregnant women, or for patients suffering from liver disease, large ovarian cyst, womb cancer.
Caution needed with:

Contains: CLOMIPHENE CITRATE.
Other preparations: SEROPHENE (Serono).

---

clomiphene citrate *see* **Clomid, Serophene**

---

clomipramine hydrochloride *see* **Anafranil**

---

clomocycline *see* **Megaclor**

---

clonazepam *see* **Rivotril**

---

clonidine *see* **Catapres, Dixarit**

---

clopamide *see* **Viskaldix**

Clopixol
(Lundbeck)

A pink tablet, light-brown tablet, or brown tablet according to strengths of 2 mg, 10 mg, 25 mg and used as a tranquillizer to treat mental disorders especially schizophrenia.

Dose: 20-30 mg a day at first, then usually 20-50 mg a day up to a maximum of 150 mg a day.
Availability: NHS and private prescription.
Side effects: muscle spasms, restlessness, hands shaking, dry mouth, urine retention, palpitations, low blood pressure, weight gain, changes in libido, low body temperature, breast swelling, menstrual changes, jaundice, blood and skin changes, drowsiness, rarely fits.
Caution: in pregnant women, nursing mothers, in the elderly who should take smaller dosage, and in patients suffering from Parkinson's disease, kidney, liver, or heart disease, or breathing disorders.
Not to be used for: children or for patients suffering from acute opiate, alcohol, or BARBITURATE poisoning, advanced kidney, liver, or heart disease, senility, apathy, or withdrawal, Parkinson's disease, severe arteriosclerosis, or for anyone who is intolerant of these drugs taken by mouth.

Caution needed with:
Contains: ZUCLOPENTHIXOL hydrochloride.
Other preparations: Clopixol Injection, Clopixol-Conc.

---

clorazepate potassium *see* Tranxene

---

clotrimazole *see* Canesten, Canesten 1, Canesten-HC, Lotriderm

---

cloxacillin *see* Orbenin, Ampiclox Neonatal Suspension

Clozaril
(Sandoz)

A yellow, scored tablet supplied at strengths of 25 mg, 100 mg, and used as a sedative to treat schizophrenia.

Dose: 25-50 mg on first day, increasing to a maximum of 900 mg a day. Usual maintenance dose 150-300 mg a day.
Availability: NHS and private prescription.
Side effects: blood changes, drowsiness, watering of the mouth, rapid heart beat, tiredness, dizziness, headache, difficulty in passing urine, stomach upset, change in electrical activity of the brain and heart, temporary upset of automatic body functions.
Caution: in the elderly, and in patients with a history of epilepsy or suffering from enlarged prostate, glaucoma, liver disease,.or intestinal abnormality. Patients should report any symptoms of infection. Your doctor may advise regular blood tests.
Not to be used for: children, pregnant women, nursing mothers, or for patients suffering from severe kidney or liver disease, alcoholism, drug intoxication, drowsiness or reduced reactions, or for those in a coma or having a history of drug-induced blood disorder.
Caution needed with: other drugs which cause blood disorder, some sedatives, alcohol, MAOIS, ANTICHOLINERGICS, drugs which lower blood pressure.
Contains: CLOZAPINE.
Other preparations:

---

co-amilofruse *see* Frumil, Lasoride

co-amilozide *see* **Moduretic, Hypertane**

---

co-amoxiclav *see* **Augmentin**

---

co-beneldopa *see* **Madopar**

Co-Betaloc
(Astra)

A white, scored tablet used as a ß-BLOCKER and DIURETIC combination to treat high blood pressure.

Dose: 1-3 tablets a day in single or divided doses.
Availability: NHS and private prescription.
Side effects: cold hands and feet, sleep disturbances, slow heart rate, tiredness, wheezing, heart failure, stomach upset, dry eyes, rash.
Caution: in pregnant women, nursing mothers, or patients suffering from asthma, diabetes, kidney or liver disorders. May need to be withdrawn before surgery. Withdraw gradually. Your doctor may advise addititional treatment with DIURETICS and DIGOXIN.
Not to be used for: children or patients suffering from heart block or failure.
Caution needed with: VERAPAMIL, CLONIDINE withdrawal, some anti-arrhythmic drugs and anaesthetics, RESERPINE, some ANTIHYPERTENSIVES, ERGOTAMINE, CIMETIDINE, antidiabetics, sedatives, SYMPATHOMIMETICS, INDOMETHACIN.
Contains: METOPROLOL tartrate, HYDROCHLOROTHIAZIDE.
Other preparations: Co-Betaloc SA.

Co-careldopa *see* Sinemet

Co-Codamol

A tablet used as an ANALGESIC to relieve pain.

Dose: adults 1-2 tablets every 4-6 hours to a maximum of 8 tablets a day; children 7-12 years ½-1 tablet every 4-6 hours to a maximum of 4 tablets a day.
Availability: NHS, private prescription, over the counter
Side effects:

Caution: in patients suffering from kidney or liver disease.
Not to be used for: children under 7 years.
Caution needed with: other medicines containing PARACETAMOL.
Contains: CODEINE PHOSPHATE, PARACETAMOL.
Other preparations: Co-Codamol Dispersible, PANADEINE (Sterling Health), PARACODOL (Fisons) — all available on NHS only when prescribed as generics.

Co-Codaprin Dispersible

A dispersible tablet used as an ANALGESIC to relieve pain.

Dose: 1-2 tablets in water every 4-6 hours as needed.
Availability: NHS, private prescription, over the counter.
Side effects: stomach upsets, allergy, asthma.
Caution: in the elderly, pregnant women, in patients with a history of allergy to ASPIRIN or asthma, or who are suffering from impaired kidney or liver function.
Not to be used for: children, nursing mothers, or for patients suffering from haemophilia, ulcers.
Caution needed with: anticoagulants, some antidiabetic drugs, anti-inflammatory agents, METHOTREXATE, SPIRONOLACTONE, STEROIDS, some uric acid-lowering drugs.
Contains: ASPIRIN, CODEINE PHOSPHATE.
Other preparations: Co-Codaprin, CODIS (Reckitt and Coleman) — all available on NHS only when prescribed as generics.

Co-Danthramer *see* Codalax

Co-Danthrusate

Capsules used as a stimulant and faecal softener to treat constipation.

Dose: adults 1-3 capsules at night; children over 6 years 1 capsule at night.
Availability: NHS and private prescription.
Side effects: red colour in urine.
Caution: in pregnant women and nursing mothers.
Not to be used for: children under 6 years, or for patients with blocked intestine.
Caution needed with:
Contains: DANTHRON, DOCUSATE sodium.
Other preparations: NORMAX (Evans) — available on NHS only when

prescribed as a generic.

co-dydramol

A tablet used as an opiate ANALGESIC to control pain.

Dose: 1-2 tablets every 4-6 hours up to a maximum of 8 tablets a day.
Availability: NHS, private prescription, over the counter.
Side effects: constipation, nausea, headache.
Caution: in pregnant women, the elderly, and in patients suffering from allergies, kidney or liver disease, or underactive thyroid.
Not to be used for: children or patients suffering from respiratory depression or blocked airways.
Caution needed with: alcohol, sedatives, other medicines containing PARACETAMOL.
Contains: DIHYDROCODEINE tartrate, PARACETAMOL.
Other preparations: PARAMOL (Napp) — only available on NHS if prescribed as a generic.

co-fluampicil *see* Magnapen

co-flumactane *see* Aldactide

co-phenotrope *see* Lomotil

co-prenozide *see* Trasidrex

co-proxamol

A tablet used as an opiate ANALGESIC to control pain.

Dose: 2 tablets 3-4 times a day.
Availability: NHS and private prescription.
Side effects: tolerance, dependence, drowsiness, constipation, dizziness, nausea, rash.
Caution: in pregnant women, the elderly, and in patients suffering from liver or kidney disease.
Not to be used for: children.

Caution needed with: alcohol, sedatives, anti-convulsant drugs, anticoagulants, other medicines containing PARACETAMOL.
Contains: DEXTROPROPOXYPHENE hydrochloride, PARACETAMOL.
Other preparations: COSALGESIC (Cox), DISTALGESIC (Dista) — all available on NHS only when prescribed as generics.

---

co-simalcite *see* Altacite Plus

---

co-tenidone *see* Tenoret-50, Tenoretic

---

co-trimoxazole *see* Septrin

---

coal tar extract *see* Alphosyl, Alphosyl HC, Clinitar Cream, Polytar, T Gel, Tarcortin

---

coal tar *see* Balneum with Tar, Baltar, calamine and coal tar ointment, Capasal, Carbo-Cort, Carbo-Dome, coal tar paste, coal tar and salicylic acid ointment, Cocois, Gelcosal, Gelcotar, Genisol, Ionil T, Meditar, Polytar, Polytar Emollient, Psoriderm, Psorigel, Psorin

---

coal tar paste BP

A paste used to treat chronic eczema and psoriasis.

Dose: apply 1-3 times a day.
Availability: NHS, private prescription, over the counter.
Side effects: irritation, acne-like skin eruptions, sensitivity to light.
Caution: avoid broken or inflamed skin.
Not to be used for:
Caution needed with:
Contains: strong COAL TAR solution, compound ZINC paste,
Other preparations: ZINC AND COAL TAR PASTE BP.

---

coal tar and salicylic acid ointment BP

An ointment used to treat chronic eczema and psoriasis.

Dose: apply 1-3 times a day.
Availability: NHS, private prescription, over the counter.
Side effects: irritation, acne-like skin eruptions, sensitivity to light.
Caution: avoid broken or inflamed skin. Stains skin, hair, and fabrics.
Not to be used for:
Caution needed with:
Contains: COAL TAR, SALICYLIC ACID, emulsifying wax, WHITE SOFT PARAFFIN, COCONUT OIL, POLYSORBATE 80, LIQUID PARAFFIN.
Other preparations:

Cobadex
(Cox)

A cream used as a STEROID treatment for skin disorders, itch of the anus and vulva.

Dose: apply a small quantity to the affected area 2-3 times a day.
Availability: NHS and private prescription.
Side effects: fluid retention, suppression of adrenal glands, thinning of the skin may occur.
Caution: use for short periods of time only.
Not to be used for: patients suffering from acne or any other skin infections caused by tuberculosis, ringworm, viruses, or fungi, or continuously especially in pregnant women.
Caution needed with:
Contains: HYDROCORTISONE, DIMETHICONE.
Other preparations:

Cobutolin — broncho-dilator to treat bronchial spasm. Product now discontinued.

Cocois
(Bioglan)

An ointment used for dry and scaly scalp conditions.

Dose: apply at night. Remove by washing in the morning.
Availability: NHS, private prescription, over the counter.
Side effects:
Caution:
Not to be used for:

Caution needed with:
Contains: COAL TAR SOLUTION, SALICYLIC ACID, SULPHUR, COCONUT OIL.
Other preparations: compound coconut oil ointment (Ung Cocois Co.)

---

coconut oil *see* **Capasal, coal tar and salicylic acid ointment, Cocois.**

Codafen Continus
(Napp)

A pink/white, capsule-shaped tablet used as an ANALGESIC and NON-STEROID ANTI-INFLAMMATORY DRUG to treat pain associated with arthritis, rheumatism, and other conditions, and to treat soft tissue injuries and musculo-skeletal disorders.

Dose: 1-3 tablets every 12 hours.
Availability: NHS and private prescription.
Side effects: stomach upset and bleeding, stomach ulcer, headache, dizziness, drowsiness, blurred vision, liver or kidney disorder, blood changes.
Caution: in pregnant women and in patients suffering from kidney, liver, or heart disorder, underactive thyroid gland, low blood pressure, head injury, raised pressure in the brain, or with a history of asthma or allergy to ASPIRIN or anti-inflammatory drugs.
Not to be used for: children, or patients suffering from breathing difficulty, chronic constipation, or stomach ulcer (including those with a history of stomach ulcer).
Caution needed with: MAOIS, sedatives, some DIURETICS, anticoagulants.
Contains: CODEINE PHOSPHATE, IBUPROFEN.
Other preparations:

Codalex
(Napp)

A liquid used as a laxative to treat constipation in the elderly, and in patients with heart failure or coronary thrombosis, or caused by ANALGESICS.

Dose: adults 5-10 ml at night; children 2.5-5 ml at night.
Availability: NHS and private prescription.
Side effects: colouring of urine and skin around the anus.
Caution: in pregnant women and incontinent patients.
Not to be used for: infants in nappies or patients suffering from intestinal blockage or pain in the abdomen.

Caution needed with:
Contains: POLOXAMER 188, DANTHRON (CO-DANTHRAMER).
Other preparations: Codalax Forte.

---

codeine linctus *see* Galcodine

---

codeine phosphate *see* Antoin, Co-Codamol, Co-Codaprin Dispersible, codeine tablets, Codafen, Codis, Diarrest, Galcodine, Medocodene, Migraleve, Panadeine, Paracodol, Parahypon, Parake, Pardale, Phensedyl, Propain, Solpadeine, Solpadol, Syndol, Tercoda, Terpoin, Tylex, Uniflu and Gregovite C.

---

codeine tablets

A tablet supplied at strengths of 15 mg, 30 mg, 60 mg and used as an opiate ANALGESIC to treat pain.

Dose: adults 10-60 mg every 4 hours as needed to a maximum of 200 mg a day; children 1-12 years 3 mg per kg body weight a day in divided doses.
Availability: NHS and private prescription.
Side effects: tolerance, dependence, drowsiness, dry mouth, blurred vision, constipation.
Caution: in women in labour, the elderly, or in patients suffering from overactive thyroid gland or liver disease.
Not to be used for: infants under 1 year or for patients suffering from respiratory depression or blocked airways.
Caution needed with: MAOIS, sedatives.
Contains:
Other preparations: codeine phosphate syrup.

---

codergocrine mesylate *see* Hydergine

Codis
(Reckitt & Colman)

A white, dispersible tablet used as an opiate ANALGESIC to control pain and reduce fever.

Dose: 1-2 tablets dispersed in water every 4 hours to a maximum of 8 tablets in 24 hours.
Availability: NHS (when prescribed as a generic), private prescription, over the counter.
Side effects: stomach upsets, allergy, asthma.
Caution: in the elderly, pregnant women, and in patients with a history of allergy to ASPIRIN or asthma, or who are suffering from impaired liver or kidney function, indigestion.
Not to be used for: children, nursing mothers, or patients suffering from haemophilia, ulcers.
Caution needed with: anticoagulants, some antidiabetic drugs, anti-inflammatory agents, METHOTREXATE, SPIRONOLACTONE, STEROIDS, some uric acid-lowering drugs.
Contains: ASPIRIN, CODEINE PHOSPHATE.
Other preparations: CO-CODAPRIN DISPERSIBLE.

Cogentin
(MSD)

A white, quarter-scored tablet supplied at a strength of 2 mg and used as an ANTICHOLINERGIC treatment for Parkinson's disease.

Dose: adults ¼ tablet a day at first increasing by ¼ tablet a day every 5-6 days to a maximum of 3 tablets a day; children 3-12 years as advised by physician.
Availability: NHS and private prescription.
Side effects: ANTICHOLINERGIC effects, confusion, agitation, and rash at high doses.
Caution: in patients suffering from rapid heart rate, enlarged prostate, glaucoma, stomach blockage. Dose should be reduced gradually.
Not to be used for: infants under 3 years or for patients suffering from certain movement disorders.
Caution needed with: ANTIHISTAMINES, antidepressants, some tranquillizers.
Contains: BENZTROPINE MESYLATE.
Other preparations: Cogentin Injection.

---

colchicine tablets

Tablets supplied at a strength of 500 micrograms and used to treat gout, or to prevent attacks while other therapy is initiated.

Dose: treatment, 2 tablets initially, then 1 every 2-3 hours until relief is obtained or until vomiting/diarrhoea occurs, or until a total of 20 tablets has been taken. The course should not be repeated within 3 days. Preventive

dose, 1 tablet 2-3 times a day.
Availability: NHS and private prescription.
Side effects: nausea, vomiting, abdominal pain, diarrhoea, bleeding in the stomach or intestine, rash, kidney damage, hair loss, blood disorders, nerve inflammation.
Caution: in pregnant women, nursing mothers, and in patients suffering from stomach, intestinal, or kidney disorder.
Not to be used for: children.
Caution needed with:
Contains: colchicine.
Other preparations:

Colestid
(Upjohn)

Granules in sachets containing 5 g used as a lipid-lowering agent to reduce lipids.

Dose: 5-30 g a day in 1-2 divided doses in fluid.
Availability: NHS and private prescription.
Side effects: constipation.
Caution: in pregnant women, nursing mothers. Vitamin A, D, and K supplements should be taken.
Not to be used for: patients suffering from complete biliary blockage.
Caution needed with: DIGOXIN, antibiotics, DIURETICS. Take any other drugs 1 hour before or 4 hours after Colestid.
Contains: COLESTIPOL.
Other preparations:

---

colestipol *see* **Colestid**

Colifoam
(Stafford-Miller)

Foam supplied in an aerosol and used as a STEROID treatment for ulcerative colitis and other bowel inflammations.

Dose: 1 application once or twice a day for 2 or 3 weeks followed by reduced applications.
Availability: NHS and private prescription.
Side effects: high blood sugar, thin bones, mood changes, ulcers.
Caution: in pregnant women and in patients suffering from severe ulcerative disease. Do not use for prolonged periods.

Not to be used for: children or for patients suffering from obstruction, abscess, fresh intestinal surgery, tuberculous, fungal or viral infections.
Caution needed with:
Contains: HYDROCORTISONE acetate.
Other preparations: HYDROCORTISONE SUPPOSITORIES.

Colofac
(Duphar)

A white tablet supplied at a strength of 135 mg and used as an anti-spasm treatment for bowel spasm.

Dose: adults 1 tablet 3 times a day, children over 10 years only adult dose. Take the dose 20 minutes before a meal.
Availability: NHS and private prescription.
Side effects:
Caution:
Not to be used for:
Caution needed with:
Contains: MEBEVERINE hydrochloride.
Other preparations: Colofac liquid.

Cologel — bulking agent to treat constipation. Product now discontinued.

Colpermin
(Farmitalia)

A blue capsule used as an antispasm treatment for irritable bowel syndrome.

Dose: adults 1-2 capsules 3 times a day, 30 minutes before meals.
Availability: NHS, private prescription, over the counter.
Side effects: heartburn, allergy, rash, headache, irregular heartbeat, tremor, loss of co-ordination.
Caution: must not be broken or chewed.
Not to be used for: children.
Caution needed with:
Contains: PEPPERMINT OIL.
Other preparations: MINTEC (Bridge).

Colven
(Rekitt & Colman)

Sachets used as an antispasmodic and bulking agent to treat irritable bowel syndrome.

Dose: 1 sachet twice a day in water before meals.
Availability: NHS and private prescription.
Side effects:
Caution:
Not to be used for: children, or for patients suffering from bowel obstruction, or kidney or heart disorders.
Caution needed with:
Contains: MEBEVERINE hydrochloride, ISPAGHULA husk.
Other preparations:

Combantrin
(Pfizer)

An orange tablet supplied at a strength of 125 mg and used as an anti-worm agent to treat worms.

Dose: adults and children over 6 months 10 mg per kg body weight in one dose.
Availability: NHS and private prescription.
Side effects: rash, stomach and brain disturbances.
Caution: in patients suffering from liver disease.
Not to be used for:
Caution needed with:
Contains: PYRANTEL EMBONATE.
Other preparations:

Comixco *see* Septrin
(Ashbourne)

Comox *see* **Septrin.** Product now discontinued.

Complement Continus
(Napp)

A yellow tablet supplied at a strength of 100 mg and used as a source of vitamin B_6 to treat vitamin B_6 deficiency including that developed by the contraceptive pill.

Dose: 1 tablet a day.

Availability: private prescription and over the counter.
Side effects:
Caution:
Not to be used for: children.
Caution needed with: LEVODOPA.
Contains: PYRIDOXINE hydrochloride.
Other preparations:

Comprecin
(Parke-Davis)

A blue, oval tablet supplied at a strength of 200 mg and used as an antibiotic to treat general and urinary infections.

Dose: 1-2 tablets twice a day for up to 14 days.
Availability: NHS and private prescription.
Side effects: nausea, vomiting, dizziness, altered taste, headache, indigestion, rash, stomach pain, tiredness, rapid heart rate, sleeplessness, seizures, shaking of the hands.
Caution: the elderly, and in patients with a history of epilepsy or impaired circulation to the brain, or suffering from kidney disease.
Not to be used for: children, pregnant women, or nursing mothers.
Caution needed with: THEOPHYLLINE, WARFARIN, FENBUFEN.
Contains: ENOXACIN.
Other preparations:

Concavit
(Wallace)

A capsule used as a multivitamin treatment for vitamin deficiencies.

Dose: 1 capsule a day.
Availability: private prescription, over the counter.
Side effects:
Caution: in pregnant women.
Not to be used for:
Caution needed with: LEVODOPA.
Contains: VITAMIN A, THIAMINE, RIBOFLAVINE, PYRIDOXINE, CYANOCOBALAMIN, ASCORBIC ACID, CALCIFEROL, VITAMIN E, NICOTINAMIDE, CALCIUM PANTOTHENATE.
Other preparations: Concavit Drops, Concavit Syrup.

Concordin
(MSD)

A pink tablet or a white tablet according to strengths of 5 mg, 10 mg and used as a TRICYCLIC antidepressant to treat depression.

Dose: adults 15-60 mg a day in divided doses at first; elderly 5 mg 3 times a day at first.
Availability: NHS and private prescription.
Side effects: dry mouth, constipation, urine retention, blurred vision, palpitations, drowsiness, sleeplessness, dizziness, hands shaking, low blood presure, weight change, skin reactions, jaundice or blood changes, loss of libido may occur.
Caution: in nursing mothers or in patients suffering from heart disease, thyroid disease, epilepsy, diabetes, adrenal tumour, urinary retention, glaucoma, some other psychiatric conditions. Your doctor may advise regular blood tests.
Not to be used for: children, pregnant women, or for patients suffering from heart attacks, liver disease, heart block.
Caution needed with: alcohol, ANTICHOLINERGICS, ADRENALINE, MAOIS, BARBITU-RATES, other antidepressants, ANTIHYPERTENSIVES, CIMETIDINE, oestrogens, some local anaesthetics.
Contains: PROTRYPTILINE hydrochloride.
Other preparations:

Condyline
(Brocades)

A solution with applicators used to treat warts on the penis and the external female genitalia.

Dose: apply twice a day for 3 days and repeat after 7 days if needed. Maximum treatment period 5 weeks.
Availability: NHS and private prescription.
Side effects: irritation.
Caution:
Not to be used for: children or on open wounds.
Caution needed with:
Contains: PODOPHYLLOTOXIN.
Other preparations: WARTICON (Janssen).

Congesteze — ANTIHISTAMINE/SYMPATHOMIMETIC treatment for allergic rhinitis. Product now discontinued.

---

conjugated oestrogens *see* **Premarin, Prempak-C**

Conotrane
(Boehringer Ingelheim)

A cream used as an antiseptic for protecting the skin from water, nappy rash, bed sores.

Dose: apply to the affected area several times a day.
Availability: NHS, private prescription, over the counter.
Side effects:
Caution:
Not to be used for:
Caution needed with:
Contains: BENZALKONIUM CHLORIDE, DIMETHICONE.
Other preparations:

Conova 30
(Gold Cross)

A white tablet used as an oestrogen, progestogen contraceptive.

Dose: 1 tablet a day for 21 days starting on day 5 of the period.
Availability: NHS and private prescription.
Side effects: enlarged breasts, bloating and fluid retention, cramps, leg pains, mood change, reduction in sexual desire, headaches, nausea, vaginal erosion, discharge, and bleeding, weight gain, skin changes.
Caution: in patients suffering from high blood pressure, diabetes, vascular disorders, asthma, depression, kidney disease, multiple sclerosis, womb diseases. Your doctor may advise you not to smoke, to have regular examinations. You should stop treatment at the first sign of serious symptoms such as severe headache or jaundice. Treatment should be stopped before surgery.
Not to be used for: pregnant women, or for patients suffering from sickle-cell anaemia, history of heart disease or thrombosis, liver disorders, some cancers, undiagnosed vaginal bleeding, some ear, skin, and kidney disorders.
Caution needed with: RIFAMPICIN, TETRACYCLINES, GRISEOFULVIN, BARBITURATES, PHENYTOIN, PRIMIDONE, CARBAMAZEPINE, ETHOSUXIMIDE, CHLORAL HYDRATE, DICHLORALPHENAZONE.
Contains: ETHINYLOESTRADIOL, ETHYNODIOL diacetate.
Other preparations:

Controvlar — oestrogen/progesterone treatment for menstrual problems. Product now discontinued.

Copholco
(Fisons)

A linctus used as an opiate, expectorant to treat laryngitis, inflammation of the windpipe.

Dose: adults 10 ml 4-5 times a day; children over 5 years 2.5-5 ml 3 times a day.
Availability: private prescription and over the counter.
Side effects: constipation.
Caution: in patients suffering from asthma.
Not to be used for: children under 5 years, or for patients suffering from liver disease.
Caution needed with: MAOIS.
Contains: PHOLCODINE, MENTHOL, CINEOLE, TERPIN HYDRATE.
Other preparations:

Copholcoids
(Fisons)

A black pastille used as an opiate, expectorant to treat dry cough.

Dose: adults 1-2 pastilles sucked 3-4 times a day; children over 5 years 1 pastille sucked 3 times a day.
Availability: private prescription and over the counter.
Side effects: constipation.
Caution: in patients suffering from asthma.
Not to be used for: children under 5 years or for patients suffering from liver disease.
Caution needed with: MAOIS.
Contains: PHOLCODINE, MENTHOL, CINEOLE, TERPIN HYDRATE.
Other preparations:

copper acetate *see* Cuplex

copper sulphate *see* Folicin, Tonivitan A & D

Coracten *see* Adalat
(Evans)

Cordarone X
(Sanofi Winthrop)

A white, scored tablet supplied at strengths of 100 mg, 200 mg and used as an anti-arrhythmic drug to treat heart rhythm disturbances.

Dose: adults 200 mg 3 times a day for 7 days, then 200 mg twice a day for 7 days, and 200 mg a day thereafter; children as advised by the physician.
Availability: NHS and private prescription.
Side effects: corneal deposits, sensitivity to light, pulmonary alveolitis, nervous system, liver, heart, eye, and thyroid effects.
Caution: in pregnant women and in patients suffering from heart failure or allergy to iodine. Your doctor may advise thyroid, eyes, heart, and liver tests.
Not to be used for: nursing mothers or for patients suffering from cardiac shock, some types of heart block, thyroid disease.
Caution needed with: calcium antagonists, anticoagulants taken by mouth, SS-BLOCKERS, DIGOXIN, anaesthetics, drugs to treat abnormal heart rhythm.
Contains: AMIODARONE hydrochloride.
Other preparations: Cordarone X Intravenous.

Cordilox
(Baker Norton)

A yellow tablet supplied at strengths of 40 mg, 80 mg, 120 mg and used as a calcium antagonist to treat angina, high blood pressure, heart rhythm disturbances.

Dose: heart rhythm distrubance: adults 40-120 mg 3 times a day; children under 2 years 20 mg 2-3 times a day; children over 2 years 40-120 mg 2-3 times a day. For angina 120 mg 3 times a day. For high blood pressure 160 mg twice a day; reduced doses for children.
Availability: NHS and private prescription.
Side effects: constipation, flushes.
Caution: in patients suffering from some types of heart conduction block or failure, liver or kidney disease, slow heart rate, or low blood pressure.
Not to be used for: patients suffering from severe heart conduction block, very slow heart rates.
Caution needed with: SS-BLOCKERS, QUINIDINE, DIGOXIN.
Contains: VERAPAMIL hydrochloride.
Other preparations: Cordilox I.V., GEANGIN (Cusi), SECURON (Knoll), UNIVER (Rhone-Poulenc Rorer), BERKATENS (Berk).

Cordilox 160
(Baker-Norton)

A yellow tablet supplied at a strength of 160 mg and used as a calcium antagonist to treat high blood pressure.

Dose: adults 1 tablet twice a day; children up to 10 mg per kg body weight a day in divided doses.
Availability: NHS and private prescription.
Side effects: constipation, flushes.
Caution: in patients suffering from some types of heart conduction block or failure, liver or kidney disease, slow heart rate, low blood pressure.
Not to be used for: patients suffering from severe heart conduction block, very slow heart rates.
Caution needed with: SS-BLOCKERS, QUINIDINE, DIGOXIN.
Contains: VERAPAMIL hydrochloride.
Other preparations: BERKATENS (Berk), GEANGIN (Cusi), SECURON (Knoll), UNIVER (Rhone-Poulenc Rorer).

Corgard
(Squibb)

A pale-blue tablet supplied at strengths of 40 mg, 80 mg and used as a ß-BLOCKER to treat heart rhythm disturbances, angina, high blood pressure, additional treatment in thyroid disease, migraine.

Dose: 40 mg a day at first increasing to 160 mg a day as required. A maximum of 240 mg a day is used in the treatment of angina. High blood pressure 80 mg a day at first, then 80-240 mg a day. Thyroid disease 80-160 mg once a day. Migraine 40 mg once a day at first, increasing to 80-160 mg a day as needed.
Availability: NHS and private prescription.
Side effects: cold hands and feet, sleep disturbances, slow heart rate, tiredness, wheezing, heart failure, stomach upset, dry eyes, rash.
Caution: in pregnant women, nursing mothers, and in patients suffering from diabetes, kidney or liver disorders, asthma. May need to be withdrawn before surgery. Withdraw gradually. Your doctor may advise additional treatment with DIURETICS or DIGOXIN.
Not to be used for: children or for patients suffering from heart block or failure.
Caution needed with: VERAPAMIL, CLONIDINE withdrawal, some anti-arrhythmic drugs and anaesthetics, RESERPINE, some ANTIHYPERTENSIVES, ERGOTAMINE, antidiabetics, CIMETIDINE, sedatives, SYMPATHOMIMETICS, INDOMETHACIN.
Contains: NADOLOL.
Other preparations:

Corgaretic 40
(Squibb)

A white, mottled, scored tablet used as a ß-BLOCKER/thiazide DIURETIC combination drug to treat high blood pressure.

Dose: 1-2 tablets a day.
Availability: NHS and private prescription.
Side effects: cold hands and feet, sleep disturbances, slow heart rate, tiredness, wheezing, heart failure, stomach upset, low blood potassium, rash, sensitivity to light, blood changes, gout, dry eyes.
Caution: in pregnant women or nursing mothers, or patients suffering from asthma, gout, diabetes, kidney or liver disorders. May need to be withdrawn before surgery. Withdraw gradually. Your doctor may advise additional treatment with DIGOXIN or DIURETICS.
Not to be used for: children or for patients suffering from heart block or failure, severe kidney failure, or liver disease.
Caution needed with: VERAPAMIL, CLONIDINE withdrawal, some anti-arrhythmic drugs and anaesthetics, RESERPINE, antidiabetics, CIMETIDINE, sedatives, SYMPATHOMIMETICS, INDOMETHACIN, LITHIUM, DIGOXIN, some ANTIHYPERTENSIVES, ERGOTAMINE, other DIURETICS.
Contains: NADOLOL, BENDROFLUAZIDE.
Other preparations: Corgaretic 80.

C

Corlan
(Evans)

A pellet supplied at a strength of 2.5 mg and used as a STEROID to treat mouth ulcers.

Dose: 1 pellet allowed to dissolve in the mouth touching the ulcer.
Availability: NHS and private prescription.
Side effects:
Caution: in pregnant women.
Not to be used for: patients suffering from untreated mouth infections.
Caution needed with:
Contains: HYDROCORTISONE.
Other preparations:

Coro-Nitro
(Boehringer Mannheim)

An aerosol used as a NITRATE for the treatment and prevention of angina.

Dose: 1-2 sprays under the tongue before exertion or when an attack begins to a maximum of 3 doses per attack.
Availability: NHS, private prescription, over the counter.
Side effects: headache, flushes, dizziness.
Caution: do not inhale spray.
Not to be used for: children.
Caution needed with:
Contains: GLYCERYL TRINITRATE.
Other preparations: DEPONIT (Schwarz), GLYTRIN (Sanofi-Winthrop), NITROCONTIN (Asta), NITRO-DUR (Schering-Plough), NITROLINGUAL (Lipha), PERCUTOL (Cusi), SUSCARD BUCCAL (Pharmax), SUSTAC (Pharmax), TRANSIDERM-NITRO (CIBA).

Corsodyl
(ICI)

A solution used as an antibacterial treatment for gingivitis, mouth ulcers, thrush, and for mouth hygiene.

Dose: rinse with 10 ml for 1 minute twice a day.
Availability: NHS, private prescription, over the counter.
Side effects: local irritation, stained tongue or teeth, may affect taste.
Caution:
Not to be used for:
Caution needed with:
Contains: CHLORHEXIDINE GLUCONATE.
Other preparations: Corsodyl Gel, Corsodyl Spray.

Cortelan *see* **Cortisyl.** Product now discontinued.

Cortenema *see* **Colifoam.** Product now discontinued.

cortisone *see* **Cortisyl**

Cortistab *see* **Cortisyl**
(Boots)

Cortisyl
(Roussel)

A white tablet supplied at strength of 25 mg and used as a STEROID to treat Addison's disease, and as replacement therapy after removal of the adrenal glands.

Dose: usually 12.5-37.5 mg a day, up to a maximum of 300 mg a day.
Availability: NHS and private prescription.
Side effects: high blood pressure, fluid retention, potassium loss, muscle weakness, weight gain, high blood sugar levels, thinning of bones, mood changes, stomach ulcer.
Caution: in pregnant women, in patients who have had recent bowel surgery, or who are suffering from inflamed veins, psychiatric disorders, virus infections, some cancers, some kidney diseases, thinning of the bones, ulcers, tuberculosis, other infections, high blood pressure, glaucoma, epilepsy, diabetes, underactive thyroid, liver disease, stress. Withdraw gradually.
Not to be used for: children.
Caution needed with: PHENYTOIN, PHENOBARBITONE, EPHEDRINE, RIFAMPICIN, DIURETICS, ANTICHOLINESTERASES, DIGOXIN, antidiabetic drugs, anticoagulants, NON-STEROID ANTI-INFLAMMATORY DRUGS.
Contains: CORTISONE ACETATE.
Other preparations: CORTISTAB (Boots) - additionally recommended to treat inflammation in allergic, rheumatic, and collagen diseases.

Cortucid — antibiotic/STEROID treatment for eye inflammation. Product now discontinued.

Corwin
(Stuart)

A yellow tablet supplied at a strength of 200 mg and used as a heart muscle stimulant to treat heart failure.

Dose: 1 tablet twice a day.
Availability: NHS and private prescription.
Side effects: stomach upset, headache, dizziness, muscle cramp, palpitations, rash.
Caution: in patients suffering from some lung and kidney disease, heart muscle and valve disease.
Not to be used for: children, pregnant women, nursing mothers, or patients suffering from sudden heart failure, rapid heart rate, low blood pressure, fluid retention.

Caution needed with:
Contains: XAMOTEROL fumarate.
Other preparations:

Cosuric *see* **Zyloric**
(DDSA)

Cosylan — cough suppressant. Product now discontinued.

Cotazym — pancreatic enzyme. Product now discontinued.

Coversyl
(Servier)

A white tablet supplied at strengths of 2 mg, 4 mg and used as an ACE INHIBITOR to treat high blood pressure, or as an additional treatment for congestive heart failure.

Dose: initially 2 mg a day, increasing to 4-8 mg a day; elderly 2 mg a day.
Availability: NHS and private prescription.
Side effects: rash, itching, flushing, severe allergy, low blood pressure, alteration of taste, nausea, stomach pain, tiredness, feeling of being unwell, headache, mild cough, blood changes, protein in the urine.
Caution: in patients suffering from kidney disease, or undergoing surgery or anaesthesia.
Not to be used for: children, pregnant women, or nursing mothers.
Caution needed with: other ANTIHYPERTENSIVES, potassium supplements, some DIURETICS, LITHIUM, antidepressants.
Contains: PERINDOPRIL TERTBUTYLAMINE.
Other preparations:

Cradocap — antiseptic shampoo to treat cradle cap/scurf. Product now discontinued.

Cremalgin
(Rhone-Poulenc Rorer)

A balm used as an ANALGESIC rub to treat rheumatism, fibrositis, lumbago,

160

sciatica.

Dose: massage into the affected area 2-3 times a day.
Availability: NHS, private prescription, over the counter.
Side effects: may be irritant.
Caution:
Not to be used for: areas near the eyes, or on broken or inflamed skin, or on membranes (such as the mouth).
Caution needed with:
Contains: METHYL NICOTINATE, GLYCOL SALICYLATE, CAPSICUM OLEORESIN.
Other preparations:

Creon
(Duphar)

A brown/yellow capsule used to supply pancreatic enzymes in the treatment of pancreatic exocrine insufficiency.

Dose: 1-2 capsules with meals.
Availability: NHS, private prescription, over the counter.
Side effects: perianal irritation.
Caution:
Not to be used for:
Caution needed with:
Contains: PANCREATIN.
Other preparations: COTAZYM, NUTRIZYM GR (Merck), PANCREASE (Cilag), PANCREX V (Paines and Byrne).

Cromogen *see* Intal
(Baker-Norton)

---

crotamiton *see* Eurax, Eurax-Hydrocortisone

---

crystal violet paint BP 1980

A purple solution used as a disinfectant to treat burns, boils, ulcers, and some skin infections, where the skin is not broken.

Dose: use undiluted as directed.
Availability: NHS, private prescription, over the counter.
Side effects:
Caution: stains skin and clothing.

Not to be used for: application to mucous membranes.
Caution needed with:
Contains: crystal violet (GENTIAN VIOLET).
Other preparations:

Cuplex
(SNP)

A gel used as a skin softener to treat warts, corns, and callouses.

Dose: at night apply 1-2 drops of gel to the wart after soaking in water and drying, remove the film in the morning and repeat the process, rubbing the area with a pumice stone between treatments.
Availability: NHS, private prescription, over the counter.
Side effects:
Caution: do not apply to healthy skin.
Not to be used for: warts on the anal or genital areas.
Caution needed with:
Contains: SALICYLIC ACID, LACTIC ACID, COPPER ACETATE.
Other preparations: DUOFILM (Stiefel), SALACTOL (Dermal), SALATAC (Dermal).

CX Powder
(Bio-Medical)

A powder used as a disinfectant to clean and disinfect the skin and prevent infection.

Dose: apply to the affected area 3 times a day.
Availability: NHS, private prescription, over the counter.
Side effects:
Caution:
Not to be used for:
Caution needed with:
Contains: CHLORHEXIDINE acetate.
Other preparations:

cyanocobalamin *see* BC 500, Calcimax, Cobalin, Concavit, Cytacon, Ketovite, Octovit, Verdiviton

cyclandelate *see* Cyclobral, Cyclospasmol

cyclizine *see* **Diconal, Migril, Valoid**

Cyclo-Progynova 1 mg
(Schering)

A beige tablet and a brown tablet used as an oestrogen and progestogen treatment for senile vaginitis, post-menopausal osteoporosis, menopausal symptoms.

Dose: 1 beige tablet a day for 11 days then 1 brown tablet a day for 10 days followed by 7 days without tablets. Begin on the fifth day of the period if present.
Availability: NHS and private prescription.
Side effects: enlarged breasts, bloating and fluid retention, cramps, leg pains, mood change, reduction in sexual desire, headaches, nausea, vaginal erosion, discharge, and bleeding, weight gain, skin changes.
Caution: in patients suffering from high blood pressure, diabetes, vascular disorders, asthma, depression, kidney disease, multiple sclerosis, womb diseases. Your doctor may advise you not to smoke, to have regular examinations. You should stop treatment at the first sign of serious symptoms such as severe headache or jaundice. Treatment should be stopped before surgery.
Not to be used for: pregnant women, or for patients suffering from sickle-cell anaemia, history of heart disease or thrombosis, liver disorders, some cancers, undiagnosed vaginal bleeding, some ear, skin, and kidney disorders.
Caution needed with: DIURETICS, ANTIHYPERTENSIVES, and drugs that change liver enzymes.
Contains: OESTRADIOL valerate; OESTRADIOL valerate and LEVONORGESTREL.
Other preparations: Cyclo-Progynova 2 mg.

---

cyclobarbitone *see* **Phanodorm**

Cyclocaps *see* Ventolin Rotocaps
(Pharbita)

Cyclobral — vasodilator to treat vascular disorders. Product now discontinued.

---

cyclofenil *see* **Rehibin**

Cyclogest
(Hoechst)

A suppository supplied at strengths of 200 mg, 400 mg and used as a progesterone treatment for premenstrual syndrome, puerperal depression.

Dose: 200-400 mg 1-2 times a day in the rectum or the vagina from the twelfth or fourteenth day of the cycle until the period begins.
Availability: NHS and private prescription.
Side effects: altered menstrual pattern, soreness, diarrhoea, wind.
Caution: in patients suffering from liver disease. Avoid contact with barrier contraceptives.
Not to be used for: children or for patients suffering from abnormal vaginal bleeding or a history of thromboembolic conditions.
Caution needed with:
Contains: PROGESTERONE.
Other preparations:

Cyclohaler *see* Ventolin
(Pharbita)

cyclopenthiazide *see* **Navidrex, Navidrex-K, Navispare**

Cyclopentolate Minims
(SNP)

Drops used as an ANTICHOLINERGIC agent in ophthalmic procedures.

Dose: 1 or more drops into the eye as needed.
Availability: NHS and private prescription.
Side effects:
Caution:
Not to be used for: patients suffering from narrow angle glaucoma.
Caution needed with:
Contains: CYCLOPENTOLATE HYDROCHLORIDE.
Other preparations: ALNIDE (Cusi), MYDRILATE (Boehringer Ingelheim).

cyclopentolate hydrochloride *see* **Cyclopentolate, Mydrilate**

Cyclospasmol — vasodilator to treat vascular disorders. Product now discontinued.

---

cyclosporin *see* **Sandimmun**

Cyklokapron
(Kabi)

A white, oblong, scored tablet supplied at a strength of 500 mg and used as a blood-clotting agent to treat menorrhagia and other heavy bleeding states.

Dose: 2-3 tablets 3-4 times a day for 3-4 days for a maximum of 3 cycles, or as advised by doctor.
Availability: NHS and private prescription.
Side effects: stomach upset.
Caution: in patients with kidney disease, haematuria in haemophilia. Your doctor may advise some patients to have regular eye tests.
Not to be used for: patients with a history of thrombosis.
Caution needed with:
Contains: TRANEXAMIC ACID.
Other preparations: Cyklokapron Injection, Cyklokapron Syrup.

---

cyproheptadine hydrochloride *see* **Periactin**

---

cyproterone acetate *see* **Androcur, Dianette**

Cystrin
(Farmitalia)

A white tablet supplied at strengths of 3 mg, 5 mg and used as an anti-spasmodic and ANTICHOLINERGIC treatment for incontinence, urgency or frequency of urination, or night-time incontinence in children.

Dose: adults, 5 mg 2-3 times a day, to a maximum of 20 mg a day; children over 5 years, 3 mg a day, increasing to 5 mg 2-3 times a day if needed.
Availability: NHS and private prescription.
Side effects: ANTICHOLINERGIC effects, flushing of the face.
Caution: in pregnant women, and in patients suffering from liver or kidney

disease, heart disorders, overactive thyroid, enlarged prostate, hiatus hernia or existing disturbance of normal bodily functions.

Not to be used for: children under 5 years, nursing mothers, or for patients suffering from blockage in the bowel or bladder, severe ulcerative colitis, other intestinal disorders, myaesthenia gravis, or glaucoma.

Caution needed with: sedatives, AMANTADINE, LEVODOPA, DIGOXIN, TRICYCLIC antidepressants, other ANTICHOLINERGICS.

Contains: OXYBUTYNIN HYDROCHLORIDE.

Other preparations: DITROPAN (Smith and Nephew).

Cytacon
(Evans)

A white tablet supplied at a strength of 50 micrograms as a source of vitamin B$_{12}$ to treat undernourishment, vitamin deficiencies, some types of anaemia, vitamin B$_{12}$ deficiency after stomach surgery.

Dose: adults 1-3 tablets a day up to a maximum of six tablets a day for pernicious anaemia; children use liquid.

Availability: private prescription and over the counter.

Side effects: rarely allergy.

Caution:

Not to be used for:

Caution needed with: PARA-AMINOSALICYLIC ACID, METHYLDOPA, COLCHICINE, CHOLESTYRAMINE, NEOMYCIN, BIGUANIDES, POTASSIUM CHLORIDE, CIMETIDINE.

Contains: CYANOCOBALAMIN.

Other preparations: Cytacon Liquid.

Cytotec
(Searle)

A white, hexagonal tablet supplied at a strength of 200 micrograms and used as a prostaglandin for the prevention and treatment of ulcers caused by anti-inflammatory drugs.

Dose: 4 tablets a day with meals and at bedtime for 4-8 weeks; prevention 1 tablet 2-4 times a day.

Availability: NHS and private prescription.

Side effects: diarrhoea, abdominal pain, stomach upset, menstrual disturbance, vaginal bleeding, rash, dizziness.

Caution: in patients suffering from circulatory disorders of the brain, heart, or peripheral vessels. Women of child-bearing age must use contraception.

Not to be used for: nursing mothers, pregnant women, or those planning a pregnancy.

Caution needed with:
Contains: MISOPROSTOL.
Other preparations:

---

d-alpha-tocopheryl acetate *see* Vita-E

---

d-panthenol *see* Verdiviton

Daktacort
(Janssen)

A cream used as a STEROID, antifungal, and antibacterial treatment for skin infections where there is also inflammation.

Dose: apply to the affected area 2-3 times a day.
Availability: NHS and private prescription.
Side effects: fluid retention, suppression of adrenal glands, thinning of the skin may occur.
Caution: use for short periods of time only.
Not to be used for: patients suffering from acne or any other skin infections caused by tuberculosis, ringworm, viruses, or fungi, or continuously especially in pregnant women.
Caution needed with:
Contains: MICONAZOLE nitrate, HYDROCORTISONE.
Other preparations: Daktacort Ointment.

Daktarin Tablets
(Janssen)

A white, quarter-scored tablet supplied at a strength of 250 mg and used as an antifungal treatment for stomach and mouth and throat infections, and as an additional treatment in the prevention of re-infection of the vagina and vulva.

Dose: adults 1 tablet 4 times a day; children use Oral Gel.
Availability: NHS and private prescription.
Side effects: stomach discomfort, phlebitis, itch, fever, diarrhoea, rash, vomiting, flushes.
Caution: in pregnant women.
Not to be used for:
Caution needed with: anticoagulants, anticonvulsants, antidiabetic drugs,

AMPHOTERICIN B.
Contains: MICONAZOLE.
Other preparations: DAKTARIN ORAL GEL (also available over the counter),
Daktarin Injection.

Daktarin Cream
(Janssen)

A cream used as an antifungal treatment for infections of the skin and
nails.

Dose: apply 1-2 times a day until 10 days after the wounds have healed.
Availability: NHS, private prescription, over the counter.
Side effects:
Caution:
Not to be used for:
Caution needed with:
Contains: MICONAZOLE nitrate.
Other preparations: Daktarin Twin Pack, Daktarin Spray Powder,
Daktarin Powder.

Daktarin Oral Gel
(Janssen)

A gel supplied at a strength of 25 mg and used as an antifungal treatment
for fungal infections of the mouth and pharynx.

Dose: adults hold 5-10 ml of gel in the mouth 4 times a day; children
under 2 years use 2.5 ml gel twice a day, 2-6 years 5 ml gel twice a day,
over 6 years 5 ml gel 4 times a day.
Availability: NHS, private prescription, over the counter.
Side effects: mild stomach upset.
Caution:
Not to be used for:
Caution needed with: WARFARIN.
Contains: MICONAZOLE.
Other preparations:

Dalacin C
(Upjohn)

A lavender capsule or a maroon/lavender capsule according to strengths
of 75 mg, 150 mg and used as an antibiotic treatment for serious infections.

Dose: adults150-450 mg every 6 hours; children under 12 years use Dalacin C Paediatric.
Availability: NHS and private prescription.
Side effects: stomach disturbances including colitis, jaundice, blood disorders.
Caution: in patients suffering from kidney or liver disease. The treatment should be stopped if diarrhoea and colitis develop.
Not to be used for: patients suffering from sensitivity to LINCOMYCIN.
Caution needed with: some drugs used during anaesthesia.
Contains: CLINDAMYCIN hydrochloride.
Other preparations: Dalacin C Paediatric, Dalacin C Phosphate.

Dalacin T
(Upjohn)

A solution used as an antibiotic treatment for acne.

Dose: apply to the affected area twice a day for up to 12 weeks.
Availability: NHS and private prescription.
Side effects: dry skin, inflammation, inflammation of the follicles, possible diarrhoea or colitis.
Caution: keep out of the eyes, mouth, and nose.
Not to be used for: patients sensitive to LINCOMYCIN.
Caution needed with: skin-softening agents.
Contains: CLINDAMYCIN phosphate.
Other preparations: Dalacin T Lotion.

Dalivit Drops
(Paines & Byrne)

Drops used as a multivitamin preparation in the prevention and treatment of vitamin deficiency.

Dose: 0-1 year 7 drops a day, over 1 year 14 drops a day.
Availability: NHS, private prescription, over the counter.
Side effects:
Caution:
Not to be used for: pregnant women.
Caution needed with: LEVODOPA.
Contains: VITAMIN A, ERGOCALCIFEROL, THIAMINE, RIBOFLAVINE, PYRIDOXINE, ASCORBIC ACID, NICOTINAMIDE.
Other preparations:

Dalmane
(Roche)

A grey/yellow capsule or a black/grey capsule according to strengths of 15 mg, 30 mg and used as a sleeping capsule for the short-term treatment of sleeplessness where sedation during the day does not cause difficulty.

Dose: elderly 15 mg before going to bed; adults 15-30 mg before going to bed.
Availability: private prescription only.
Side effects: light headedness, lack of co-ordination, confusion, vertigo, stomach upset, low blood pressure, rash, changes in vision and libido, retention of urine. Risk of addiction.
Caution: in the elderly, nursing mothers, pregnant women, and in patients suffering from lung, kidney, or liver disorders. Avoid long-term use.
Not to be used for: children or for patients suffering from lung disease or some obsessional and psychotic disorders.
Caution needed with: alcohol, other tranquillizers, anticonvulsants.
Contains: FLURAZEPAM.
Other preparations:

---

danazol *see* Danol

Daneral SA
(Hoechst)

An orange tablet supplied at a strength of 75 mg and used as an ANTIHISTAMINE treatment for allergies.

Dose: 1-2 tablets at night.
Availability: NHS, private prescription, over the counter.
Side effects: drowsiness, reduced reactions.
Caution: in nursing mothers.
Not to be used for: children.
Caution needed with: sedatives, MAOIS, alcohol.
Contains: PHENIRAMINE MALEATE.
Other preparations:

Danol
(Sanofi Winthrop)

A white/ grey or white/pink capsule according to strengths of 100 mg, 200 mg and used as a gonadotrophin release inhibitor to treat endometriosis (a womb and menstrual disorder), heavy periods, non-malignant breast disorders, premenstrual syndrome.

Dose: 200-800 mg a day in divided doses.
Availability: NHS and private prescription.
Side effects: nausea, dizziness, rash, backache, flushing, muscle spasm, male hormone effects, fluid retention, headache, emotional disturbance.
Caution: in patients suffering from epilepsy, migraine, diabetes, a tendency to gain weight, high blood pressure or other circulatory disorders.
Not to be used for: children, pregnant women, nursing mothers, or for patients suffering from porphyria (a rare blood disorder), kidney, liver, or heart disease, blocked blood vessels, some tumours, undiagnosed vaginal bleeding.
Caution needed with: contraceptive pill, anticoagulants, anticonvulsants, antidiabetics, ANTIHYPERTENSIVES, CYCLOSPORIN, STEROIDS.
Contains: DANAZOL.
Other preparations:

D

---

danthron *see* **Codalax, Co-Danthrusate, Normax**

Dantrium
(Norwich Eaton)

An orange/light brown capsule supplied at strengths of 25 mg, 100 mg and used as a muscle relaxant to treat chronic or severe spasticity associated with a stroke, multiple sclerosis, injury to the spinal cord, cerebral palsy.

Dose: 25 mg a day at first increasing as needed to a maximum of 100 mg 4 times a day.
Availability: NHS and private prescription.
Side effects: weakness, tiredness, drowsiness, diarrhoea.
Caution: in pregnant women and in patients suffering from lung or heart disease. Your doctor may advise that your liver should be checked before and 6 weeks after treatment.
Not to be used for: children or for patients suffering from liver disease or where spasticity is useful for movement.
Caution needed with: alcohol, sedatives.
Contains: DANTROLENE SODIUM.
Other preparations:

---

dantrolene sodium *see* **Dantrium**

Daonil

(Hoechst)

A white, oblong, scored tablet supplied at a strength of 5 mg and used as an antidiabetic drug to treat diabetes.

Dose: 1 tablet a day at breakfast at first increasing if needed by ½-1 tablet a day every 7 days to a maximum of 3 tablets a day.
Availability: NHS and private prescription.
Side effects: allergy including skin rash.
Caution: in the elderly and in patients suffering from kidney failure.
Not to be used for: children, pregnant women, nursing mothers, during surgery, or for patients suffering from juvenile diabetes, liver or kidney impairment, hormone disorders, stress, infections.
Caution needed with: ß-BLOCKERS, MAOIS, STEROIDS, DIURETICS, alcohol, the contraceptive pill, anticoagulants, lipid-lowering agents, ASPIRIN, antibiotics (RIFAMPICIN, sulphonamides antibiotics, CHLORAMPHENICOL), GLUCAGON, cyclophosphamide.
Contains: GLIBENCLAMIDE.
Other preparations: Semi-Daonil, CALABREN (Berk), DIABETAMIDE (Ashbourne), EUGLUCON (Roussel), LIBANIL (APS), MALIX.

---

dapsone tablets

A tablet supplied at strengths of 50 mg, 100 mg and used as an anti-leprotic treatment for leprosy.

Dose: 1-2 mg per kg body weight a day.
Availability: NHS and private prescription.
Side effects: liver disease, nausea, headache, dizziness, rapid heart rate, sleeplessness, rash, blood changes.
Caution: in pregnant women and in patients suffering from heart or lung disease, anaemia, glucose 6PD deficiency (an inherited disorder). This treatment should only be given under specialist advice.
Not to be used for: patients suffering from porphyria (a rare blood disorder).
Caution needed with: RIFAMPICIN, PROBENECID.
Contains: DAPSONE.
Other preparations:

---

dapsone *see* dapsone tablets, Maloprim

Daranide
(MSD)

A yellow, scored tablet supplied at a strength of 50 mg used as a fluid balance medication in additonal treatment for glaucoma.

Dose: 2-4 tablets at first then 2 tablets every 12 hours, reducing to ½-1 tablet 1-3 times a day.
Availability: NHS and private prescription.
Side effects: stomach upset, loss of weight, constipation, frequent need to urinate, headache, itch, lassitude, prickly sensation, blood changes.
Caution: in pregnant women. Potassium supplements may be needed.
Not to be used for: children or for patients suffering from liver or kidney disease, adrenocortical weakness, low sodium or potassium levels, severe blockage of the lungs.
Caution needed with: STEROIDS, ACTH, DIGOXIN, antidiabetic drugs, anticoagulants, local anaesthetics, SALICYLATES, anticonvulsants, TRIMETHOPRIM.
Contains: DICHLORPHENAMIDE.
Other preparations:

Daraprim
(Wellcome)

A white, scored tablet supplied at a strength of 25 mg and used as an antimalarial drug for the prevention of malaria.

Dose: adults and children over 10 years 1 tablet a week; children 5-10 years half adult dose. Continue for 4 weeks after leaving area.
Availability: NHS, private prescription, over the counter.
Side effects: rash, anaemia.
Caution: in pregnant women, nursing mothers, and in patients suffering from liver or kidney disease.
Not to be used for: children under 5 years.
Caution needed with: CO-TRIMOXAZOLE, LORAZEPAM.
Contains: PYRIMETHAMINE.
Other preparations: FANSIDAR (Roche), MALOPRIM (Wellcome).

Davenol
(Whitehall)

A linctus used as an ANTIHISTAMINE, SYMPATHOMIMETIC, and opiate preparation to treat cough.

Dose: adults 5-10 ml 3-4 times a day; children no more than 5 ml 3-4 times a day.

Availability: private prescription and over the counter.
Side effects: constipation, drowsiness, reduced reactions, anxiety, hands shaking, irregular or rapid heart rate, dry mouth, excitement, rarely skin eruptions.
Caution: in patients suffering from asthma, kidney disease, diabetes.
Not to be used for: children under 5 years or for patients suffering from liver disease, heart or thyroid disorders.
Caution needed with: MAOIS, alcohol, sedatives, TRICYCLICS.
Contains: CARBINOXAMINE MALEATE, EPHEDRINE HYDROCHLORIDE, PHOLCODINE.
Other preparations:

D DDAVP
(Ferring)

Nasal drops supplied in a dropper bottle and used as a hormone to treat diabetes insipidus (a fluid balance disorder).

Dose: adults 0.1-0.2 ml once or twice a day into the nose; children 0.05-0.1 ml once or twice a day.
Availability: NHS and private prescription.
Side effects:
Caution: pregnant women and in patients suffering from high blood pressure.
Not to be used for:
Caution needed with:
Contains: DESMOPRESSIN.
Other preparations:

De-Nol
(Brocades)

A white liquid used as a cell-surface protector to treat gastric and duodenal ulcer.

Dose: adults 10 ml diluted with 15 ml water twice a day 30 minutes before meals.
Availability: NHS, private prescription, over the counter.
Side effects: black colour to tongue and stools.
Caution:
Not to be used for: children or for patients suffering from kidney failure.
Caution needed with:
Contains: TRI-POTASSIUM DICITRATO BISMUTHATE.
Other preparations: De-Noltab.

De-Noltab *see* De-Nol

Debrisan
(Kabi Pharmacia)

A powder used as an absorbant to treat weeping wounds including ulcers.

Dose: wash the wound with a saline solution and, without drying first, coat with 3 mm of powder, and cover with a perforated plastic sheet; repeat before the sheet is saturated.
Availability: NHS, private prescription, over the counter.
Side effects:
Caution:
Not to be used for:
Caution needed with:
Contains: DEXTRANOMER.
Other preparations: Debrisan Paste, Debrisan Pads.

---

debrisoquine sulphate *see* Declinax

Decadron
(MSD)

A white, scored tablet supplied at a strength of 0.5 mg and used as a STEROID treatment for rheumatic or inflammatory conditions, allergy.

Dose: as prescribed by your doctor.
Availability: NHS and private prescription.
Side effects: high blood sugar, thin bones, mood changes, ulcers.
Caution: in pregnant women, in patients who have had recent bowel surgery, or who are suffering from inflamed veins, psychiatric disorders, virus infections, some cancers, some kidney diseases, thinning of the bones, ulcers, tuberculosis, other infections, high blood pressure, glaucoma, epilepsy, diabetes, underactive thyroid, liver disease, stress. Withdraw gradually.
Not to be used for:
Caution needed with: PHENYTOIN, PHENOBARBITONE, EPHEDRINE, RIFAMPICIN, DIURETICS, ANTICHOLINESTERASES, DIGOXIN, antidiabetic agents, anticoagulants, NON-STEROID ANTI-INFLAMMATORY DRUGS.
Contains: DEXAMETHASONE.
Other preparations:

Decaserpyl
(Roussel)

A white, scored tablet or a pink, scored tablet according to strengths of 5 mg, 10 mg and used as an ANTIHYPERTENSIVE drug to treat high blood pressure.

Dose: 10 mg 3 times a day at first, increasing by 5-10 mg a day at 7-day intervals if needed, up to 50 mg a day maximum.
Availability: NHS and private prescription.
Side effects: lethargy, vertigo, tremor, stomach upset, blocked nose.
Caution: in pregnant women, nursing mothers.
Not to be used for: children or for patients with a history of depression, active peptic ulcer, ulcerative colitis, severe kidney disease, Parkinson's disease.
Caution needed with: anticonvulsants.
Contains: METHOSERPIDINE.
Other preparations:

Decaserpyl Plus — ANTIHYPERTENSIVE to treat high blood pressure. Product now discontinued.

Declinax
(Roche)

A white, scored tablet supplied at a strength of 10 mg, and used as an ANTIHYPERTENSIVE drug to treat high blood pressure.

Dose: 10-20 mg once or twice a day at first, increasing to 120 mg a day if needed.
Availability: NHS and private prescription.
Side effects: low blood pressure when standing up, general feeling of being unwell, headache, failure of ejaculation.
Caution: in patients suffering from kidney disease.
Not to be used for: for children or for patients suffering from phaeochromocytoma (a disease of the adrenal glands) or recent heart attack.
Caution needed with: TRICYCLIC antidepressants, SYMPATHOMIMETICS.
Contains: DEBRISOQUINE SULPHATE.
Other preparations:

Decortisyl
(Roussel)

A white, scored tablet supplied at a strength of 5 mg and used as a STEROID treatment for rheumatic conditions, allergies.

Dose: adults 4-8 tablets a day in divided doses reducing by ½-1 tablet every 3-4 days to 1-4 tablets a day; children 1-7 years quarter to half adult dose, 7-12 years half to three-quarters adult dose.
Availability: NHS and private prescription.
Side effects: high blood sugar, thin bones, mood change, ulcers.
Caution: in pregnant women, in patients who have had recent bowel surgery, or who are suffering from inflamed veins, psychiatric disorders, virus infections, some cancers, some kidney diseases, thinning of the bones, ulcers, tuberculosis, other infections, high blood pressure, glaucoma, epilepsy, diabetes, underactive thyroid, liver disease, stress. Withdraw gradually.
Not to be used for:
Caution needed with: PHENYTOIN, PHENOBARBITONE, EPHEDRINE, RIFAMPICIN, DIURETICS, ANTICHOLINESTERASES, DIGOXIN, antidiabetic agents, anticoagulants, NON-STEROID ANTI-INFLAMMATORY DRUGS.
Contains: PREDNISONE.
Other preparations:

---

dehydrocholic acid tablets

Tablets supplied at a strength of 250 mg, and used as a treatment after surgery on the bile duct, to wash away gall stones.

Dose: 1-3 tablets 3 times a day
Availability: NHS and private prescription.
Side effects:
Caution:
Not to be used for: children, or for patients suffering from blocked bile duct or chronic liver disease.
Caution needed with:
Contains: dehydrocholic acid.
Other preparations:

Deltacortril
(Pfizer)

A brown tablet or a red tablet according to strengths of 2.5 mg, 5 mg and used as a STEROID treatment for collagen and allergic conditions.

Dose: 5-60 mg a day and then reduce to minimum effective dose.
Availability: NHS and private prescription.
Side effects: high blood sugar, thin bones, mood changes, ulcers.

Caution: in pregnant women, in patients who have had recent bowel surgery, or who are suffering from inflamed veins, psychiatric disorders, virus infections, some cancers, some kidney diseases, thinning of the bones, ulcers, tuberculosis, other infections, high blood pressure, glaucoma, epilepsy, diabetes, underactive thyroid, liver disease, stress. Withdraw gradually.
Not to be used for: infants under 1 year.
Caution needed with: PHENYTOIN, PHENOBARBITONE, EPHEDRINE, RIFAMPICIN, DIURETICS, ANTICHOLINESTERASES, DIGOXIN, antidiabetic agents, anticoagulants, NON-STEROID ANTI-INFLAMMATORY DRUGS.
Contains: PREDNISOLONE.
Other preparations: DELTASTAB (Boots), PRECORTISYL (Roussel), PREDNESOL (Glaxo), SINTISONE.

Deltastab *see* Precortisyl
(Boots)

---

demeclocycline *see* Ledermycin

Demix-100 *see* Vibramycin
(Ashbourne)

Depixol
(Lundbeck)

A yellow tablet supplied at a strength of 3 mg and used as a sedative to treat schizophrenia and other mental disorders, especially withdrawal or apathy.

Dose: usually 1-3 tablets a day, up to a maximum of 6 tablets a day.
Availability: NHS and private prescription.
Side effects: muscle spasms, restlessness, hands shaking, dry mouth, urine retention, palpitations, low blood pressure, weight gain, changes in libido, low body temperature, breast swelling, menstrual changes, jaundice, blood and skin changes, drowsiness, rarely fits.
Caution: in pregnant women, the elderly, and in patients suffering from kidney, liver, heart, or lung disease, Parkinson's disease, or anyone who is intolerant of those drugs taken by mouth.
Not to be used for: children, or for very excitable or overactive patients.
Caution needed with: alcohol, tranquillizers, pain killers,

ANTIHYPERTENSIVES, antidepressants, anticonvulsants, antidiabetic drugs, LEVODOPA.
Contains: FLUPENTHIXOL DIHYDROCHLORIDE.
Other preparations: Depixol Injection, Depixol-Conc, FLUANXOL (Lundbeck).

Deponit
(Schwarz)

Self-adhesive patches supplied in strengths of 5 mg, 10 mg and used as a NITRATE preparation for the prevention of angina.

Dose: apply a 5 mg patch at first increasing to 10 mg if required with each subsequent patch applied to a different part of the skin.
Availability: NHS, private prescription, over the counter.
Side effects: headache, rash, dizziness.
Caution: reduce use of this treatment by replacing with oral nitrates.
Not to be used for: children.
Caution needed with:
Contains: GLYCERYL TRINITRATE.
Other preparations: CORO-NITRATE (Boehringer Mannheim), GLYTRIN (Sanofi-Winthrop), NITROCONTIN (ASTA), NITRO-DUR (Schering-Plough), NITROLINGUAL (Lipha), PERCUTOL (Cusi), SUSCARD BUCCAL (Pharmax), SUSTAC (Pharmax), TRANSIDERM NITRO (CIBA).

---

dequalinium chloride *see* Labosept

Derbac-C Shampoo
(Napp)

A shampoo used as a pediculicide to treat head lice.

Dose: use as a shampoo, applying twice and then leaving the second treatment for 5 minutes before rinsing and drying. Repeat twice at 3-day intervals.
Availability: NHS, private prescription, over the counter.
Side effects:
Caution: keep out of the eyes.
Not to be used for: infants under 6 months.
Caution needed with:
Contains: CARBARYL.
Other preparations: Derbac-C Liquid, CARYLDERM (Napp), CLINICIDE (De Witt), SULEO-C (Napp).

Derbac-M
(Napp)

A liquid used as a pediculicide and scabicide to treat scabies, lice of the head and pubic areas.

Dose: apply liberally and then shampoo after 24 hours.
Availability: NHS, private prescription, over the counter.
Side effects:
Caution: keep out of the eyes.
Not to be used for: infants under 6 months.
Caution needed with:
Contains: MALATHION.
Other preparations: PRIODERM (Napp), SULEO-M (Napp).

Dermacort *see* hydrocortisone
(Panpharma)

Dermalex
(Sanofi Winthrop)

A lotion used as an antiseptic emollient to prevent and treat rashes (including incontinence rash) and to prevent bedsores.

Dose: apply sparingly every 4-6 hours.
Availability: NHS, private prescription, over the counter.
Side effects:
Caution:
Not to be used for:
Caution needed with:
Contains: SQUALENE, HEXACHLORAPHANE, ALLANTOIN.
Other preparations:

Dermonistat *see* **Daktarin.** Product now discontinued.

Dermovate
(Glaxo)

A cream used as a STEROID treatment for psoriasis, eczema, other skin disorders where there is inflammation

Dose: apply a small quantity to the affected area once or twice a day for

up to 4 weeks.
Availability: NHS and private prescription.
Side effects: fluid retention, suppression of adrenal glands, thinning of the skin may occur.
Caution: adults check after 4 weeks; children check after 1 week; use for short periods of time only.
Not to be used for: patients suffering from acne or any other skin infections caused by tuberculosis, ringworm, viruses, or fungi, or continuously especially in pregnant women.
Caution needed with:
Contains: CLOBETASOL PROPIONATE.
Other preparations: Dermovate Ointment, Dermovate Scalp Application, Dermovate-NN (for infected conditions).

D

Deseril
(Sandoz)

A white tablet supplied at a strength of 1 mg and used as an anti-spasmodic treatment for diarrhoea associated with carcinoid disease, migraine, severe headache.

Dose: for diarrhoea 12-20 tablets a day in divided doses. For migraine 1-2 tablets 3 times a day with food.
Availability: NHS and private prescription.
Side effects: nausea and other stomach disturbances, drowsiness, dizziness, fluid retention, arterial spasm, retroperitonital, pleural, and heart valve fibrosis (membrane thickening), leg cramps, weight gain, rash, hair loss, disturbance of nervous system.
Caution: in patients suffering from or with a history of stomach ulcer.
Not to be used for: children, pregnant women, nursing mothers, or patients suffering from severe high blood pressure, collagen disorders, coronary, peripheral, or occlusive vascular disease, liver or kidney disease, weight loss, sepsis, lung disease.
Caution needed with: medicines affecting blood vessels, ERGOTAMINE.
Contains: METHYSERGIDE.
Other preparations:

desipramine *see* **Pertofran**

desmopressin *see* **DDAVP, Desmospray**

Desmospray
(Ferring)

A nasal spray used as a hormone treatment for cranial diabetes insipidus, primary bedwetting, testing kidney function.

Dose: adults diabetes insipidus 1-2 sprays into the nose once or twice a day, kidney testing 2 sprays into each nostril; children diabetes insipidus as adult, kidney testing 1-15 years 1 spray into each nostril. Adults and children over 5 years primary bed wetting 1-2 sprays into each nostril before going to bed, for up to 3 months.
Availability: NHS and private prescription.
Side effects:
Caution: in pregnant women and in patients suffering from kidney disease, cardiovascular disease. Patients should not drink excessively after testing.
Not to be used for: children under 5 years (bedwetting).
Caution needed with:
Contains: DESMOPRESSIN.
Other preparations:

---

desogestrel *see* **Marvelon, Mercilon**

---

desonide *see* **Tridesilon**

---

desoxymethasone *see* **Stiedex**

Destolit
(Marion Merrell Dow)

A white, scored tablet supplied at a strength of 150 mg and used as a bile acid to dissolve gallstones.

Dose: 3-4 tablets a day in divided doses after meals with 1 dose always after the evening meal. Continue for 3-4 months after stones dissolve.
Availability: NHS and private prescription.
Side effects:
Caution:
Not to be used for: children, for women who are not taking contraceptive precautions, or for patients with a non-functioning gall bladder, active stomach ulcers, liver or certain diseases of the intestine.

Caution needed with: the contraceptive pill, oestrogens, treatments to reduce cholesterol levels.
Contains: URSODEOXYCHOLIC ACID.
Other preparations: URSOFALK (Thames).

Deteclo *see* Tetracycline
(Lederle)

Dexa-Rhinaspray
(Boehringer Ingelheim)

An aerosol used as a STEROID, antibiotic, and SYMPATHOMIMETIC treatment for allergic rhinitis.

Dose: adults 1 spray into each nostril no more than 6 times a day; children over 5 years 1 spray into each nostril no more than twice a day.
Availability: NHS and private prescription.
Side effects: itching nose.
Caution: do not use for extended periods.
Not to be used for: children under 5 years.
Caution needed with:
Contains: TRAMAZOLINE HYDROCHLORIDE, DEXAMETHASONE-21 ISONICOTINATE, NEOMYCIN sulphate.
Other preparations:

---

dexamethasone *see* Decadron, Maxidex, Maxitrol, Oradexon, Otomize, Sofradex, Sofradex Ointment

---

dexamethasone-21 isonicotinate *see* Dexa-Rhinaspray

---

dexamphetamine *see* Dexedrine

Dexedrine
(Evans)

A white, scored tablet supplied at a strength of 5 mg and used as a SYMPATHOMIMETIC to stimulate the central nervous system.

Dose: adults 1 tablet twice a day at first increasing every 7 days by 2 tablets a day to a maximum of 12 tablets a day; children 3-5 years ½ tablet a day at first increasing every 7 days by ½ tablet a day, 6-12 years 1-2 tablets a day at first increasing every 7 days by 1 tablet a day to a maximum of 4 tablets a day.

Availability: controlled drug, NHS and private prescription.

Side effects: sleeplessness, restlessness, slowing of growth, euphoria, mood change, dry mouth, loss of appetite, stomach upset, sweating, rapid heart rate, raised blood pressure, addiction.

Caution: in pregnant women.

Not to be used for: infants under 3 years, for patients with a history of drug abuse, or for patients suffering from cardiovascular disease, overactive thyroid gland, hyperexcitability, glaucoma.

Caution needed with: MAOIS, GUANETHIDINE.

Contains: DEXAMPHETAMINE sulphate.

Other preparations:

---

dexfenfluramine *see* **Adifax**

---

dextran *see* **Tears Naturale**

---

dextranomer *see* **Debrisan**

---

dextrin *see* **Nulacin**

---

dextromethorphan *see* **Actifed Compound, Cosylan, Lotussin**

---

dextromoramide tartrate *see* **Palfium**

---

dextropropoxyphene *see* **Co-proxamol, Doloxene, Doloxene Co.**

DF 118 *see* **dihydrocodeine tablets.** Product now discontinued

---

DHC Continus
(Napp)

A white capsule supplied at a strength of 60 mg, 90 mg, and 120 mg and used as an opiate to control pain associated with cancer.

Dose: 60-120 mg every 12 hours.
Availability: NHS and private prescription.
Side effects: constipation, nausea, headache, vertigo.
Caution: in the elderly, pregnant women, and in patients suffering from kidney or liver disease, allergy, underactive thyroid.
Not to be used for: children or for patients suffering from respiratory depression or blocked airways.
Caution needed with: alcohol, MAOIS, sedatives.
Contains: DIHYDROCODEINE tartrate.
Other preparations: DIHYDROCODEINE TABLETS.

Diabetamide *see* Daonil
(Ashbourne)

Diabinese
(Pfizer)

A white, scored tablet supplied at strengths of 100 mg, 250 mg and used as an antidiabetic treatment for diabetes.

Dose: 100-250 mg a day with breakfast, to a maximum of 500 mg a day.
Availability: NHS and private prescription.
Side effects: allergy, including skin rash.
Caution: in the elderly and in patients suffering from kidney failure.
Not to be used for: children, pregnant women, nursing mothers, during surgery, or for patients suffering from juvenile diabetes, liver or kidney disorders, stress, infections.
Caution needed with: ß-BLOCKERS, MAOIS, STEROIDS, DIURETICS, alcohol, anticoagulants, lipid-lowering agents, ASPIRIN, some antibiotics (RIFAMPICIN, sulphonamides, CHLORAMPHENICOL), GLUCAGON, cyclophosphamide, the contraceptive pill.
Contains: CHLORPROPAMIDE.
Other preparations: GLYMESE (DDSA).

Dialar *see* diazepam
(Lagap)

185

Diamicron
(Servier)

A white, scored tablet supplied at a strength of 80 mg and used as an anti-diabetic treatment for diabetes.

Dose: ½-1 tablet a day increasing if needed to a maximum of 4 a day in 2 divided doses.
Availability: NHS and private prescription.
Side effects: allergy, including skin rash.
Caution: in the elderly and in patients suffering from kidney failure.
Not to be used for: children, pregnant women, nursing mothers, during surgery, or for patients suffering from juvenile diabetes, liver or kidney disorders, stress, infections.
Caution needed with: ß-BLOCKERS, MAOIS, STEROIDS, DIURETICS, alcohol, anticoagulants, lipid-lowering agents, ASPIRIN, some antibiotics (RIFAMPICIN, sulphonamides, CHLORAMPHENICOL), GLUCAGON, cyclophosphamide, the contraceptive pill.
Contains: GLICLAZIDE.
Other preparations:

Diamox
(Storz)

A white, scored tablet supplied at a strength of 250 mg and used as a fluid balance drug to treat congestive heart failure, fluid retention, toxaemia of pregnancy, premenstrual tension, epilepsy, glaucoma.

Dose: 250-375 mg a day or every other day in the morning at first; for PMT 125-375 mg a day beginning 5-10 days before menstruation. For epilepsy adults 1-4 tablets a day in divided doses; children under 2 years 125 mg a day, 2-12 years 125-750 mg a day in divided doses. For glaucoma 1-4 tablets a day.
Availability: NHS and private prescription.
Side effects: flushing, thirst, headache, drowsiness, increased urination, pins and needles, blood changes, excitement, rash.
Caution: care in pregnant women and for patients suffering from gout or diabetes. Your doctor may advise that potassium supplements may be needed, and that blood, fluids, and electrolytes should be checked regularly.
Not to be used for: patients suffering from one form of glaucoma, some kidney conditions, adrenal insufficiency, low sodium or potassium levels.
Caution needed with: TRIMETHOPRIM, antidiabetics, anticoagulants taken by mouth.
Contains: ACETAZOLAMIDE.
Other preparations: Diamox Parenteral, Diamox SR.

Diamox Sustets *see* Diamox
(Storz)

Dianette
(Schering)

A beige tablet used as an anti-androgen and oestrogen to treat severe acne in women, hairiness.

Dose: 1 tablet a day for 21 days beginning on day 5 of the cycle, then 7 days without tablets.
Availability: NHS and private prescription.
Side effects: enlarged breasts, bloating and fluid retention, cramps, leg pains, mood change, reduction in sexual desire, headaches, nausea, vaginal erosion, discharge, and bleeding, weight gain, skin changes. The tablet also functions as an oral contraceptive.
Caution: in patients suffering from high blood pressure, diabetes, vascular disorders, asthma, depression, kidney disease, multiple sclerosis, womb diseases. Your doctor may advise you not to smoke, to have regular examinations. You should stop treatment at the first sign of serious symptoms such as severe headache or jaundice. Treatment should be stopped before surgery.
Not to be used for: children, males, pregnant women, or for patients suffering from sickle-cell anaemia, history of heart disease or thrombosis, liver disorders, some cancers, undiagnosed vaginal bleeding, some ear, skin, and kidney disorders.
Caution needed with: RIFAMPICIN, TETRACYCLINES, GRISEOFULVIN, BARBITURATES, PHENYTOIN, PRIMIDONE, CARBAMAZEPINE, ETHOSUXIMIDE, CHLORAL HYDRATE, DICHLORALPHENAZONE.
Contains: CYPROTERONE ACETATE, ETHINYLOESTRODIOL.
Other preparations:

Diarphen *see* Lomotil
(Mepra-Pharm)

Diarrest
(Galen)

A liquid supplied in 200 ml bottles and used as an opiate, anti-spasmodic, and electrolyte to treat diarrhoea.

Dose: adults 20 ml 4 times a day with water; children under 4 years as advised by manufacturer; children 4-5 years 5 ml 4 times a day; children 6-

9 years 10 ml 4 times a day; children 10-13 years 15 ml 4 times a day.
Availability: NHS and private prescription.
Side effects: sedation.
Caution: in patients suffering from thyroid disease, heart failure, kidney or liver disease, glaucoma, ulcerative colitis.
Not to be used for: patients suffering from pseudomembranous colitis (a bowel disorder), diverticular disease.
Caution needed with: MAOIS.
Contains: CODEINE PHOSPHATE, DICYCLOMINE HYDROCHLORIDE, POTASSIUM CHLORIDE, SODIUM CHLORIDE, SODIUM CITRATE.
Other preparations:

D

Diatensic *see* **Aldactane.** Product now discontinued.

---

diazepam tablets

A tablet supplied at strengths of 2 mg, 5 mg, 10 mg and used as a tranquillizer to treat anxiety.

Dose: elderly 3-15 mg a day; adults 6-30 mg a day; children 1-5 mg a day.
Availability: NHS and private prescription.
Side effects: drowsiness, confusion, unsteadiness, low blood pressure, rash, changes in vision, changes in libido, retention of urine. Risk of addiction increases with dose and length of treatment. May impair judgement.
Caution: in the elderly, pregnant women, nursing mothers, in women during labour, and in patients suffering from lung disorders, kidney or liver disorders. Avoid long-term use and withdraw gradually.
Not to be used for: children, or for patients suffering from acute lung diseases, some chronic lung diseases, some obsessional and psychotic diseases.
Caution needed with: alcohol, other tranquillizers, anticonvulsants.
Contains: diazepam.
Other preparations: diazepam suppositories, ATENSINE (Berk), DIALAR (Lagap), RIMAPAM (Rima), STESOLID (CP Pharmaceuticals), TENSIUM (DDSA), VALIUM (Roche) — all available on NHS only if prescribed as generics. Diazemuls (Dumex).

---

diazoxide *see* **Eudemine**

Dibenyline
(S K B)

A red/white capsule supplied at a strength of 10 mg and used as an anti-adrenaline drug to treat high blood pressure associated with phaeochromocytoma (a disease of the adrenal glands).

Dose: adults 1 capsule a day at first increasing by 1 capsule a day as necessary; children 1-2 mg per kg bodyweight per day in divided doses.
Availability: NHS and private prescription.
Side effects: low blood pressure when standing, dizziness, rapid heart rate, failure of ejaculation.
Caution: in patients suffering from congestive heart failure, cardiovascular or kidney disease. The drug has been shown to cause cancer in rodents.
Not to be used for: patients suffering strokes or heart attacks.
Caution needed with:
Contains: PHENOXYBENZAMINE.
Other preparations:

---

dichlorphenamide *see* Daranide

---

diclofenac sodium *see* Voltarol

Diclozip *see* Voltarol
(Ashbourne)

Diconal
(Wellcome)

A pink, scored tablet used as an opiate and anti-emetic to control pain.

Dose: 1 tablet at first and then as advised by physician.
Availability: controlled drug, NHS and private prscription.
Side effects: tolerance, dependence, drowsiness, dry mouth, blurred vision.
Caution: in pregnant women and in patients suffering from liver or kidney disease.
Not to be used for: children or for patients suffering from respiratory depression or blocked airways.
Caution needed with: MAOIS, alcohol, sedatives.
Contains: DIPIPANONE HYDROCHLORIDE, CYCLIZINE HYDROCHLORIDE.
Other preparations:

dicyclomine *see* **Diarrest, Kolanticon, Merbentyl**

Dicynene
(Delandale)

An oval, white tablet supplied at a strength of 500 mg and used as a blood-clotting agent to treat heavy periods and other bleeding disorders.

Dose: 500 mg every 4-6 hours.
Availability: NHS and private prescription.
Side effects: headache, rash, nausea.
Caution:
Not to be used for: children.
Caution needed with:
Contains: ETHAMSYLATE.
Other preparations: Dicynene Injection.

Didronel
(Norwich Eaton)

A white, rectangular tablet supplied at a strength of 200 mg and used as a calcium-lowering agent to treat Paget's disease, high calcium levels in cancer.

Dose: Paget's disease 5 mg per kg body weight a day as 1 dose 2 hours before food; high calcium levels 20 mg per kg body weight a day for 30-90 days.
Availability: NHS and private prescription.
Side effects: nausea, diarrhoea, metallic or altered taste.
Caution: in pregnant women, nursing mothers, and in patients suffering from enterocolitis. Kidney function should be checked regularly, and calcium and vitamin D levels should be maintained.
Not to be used for: children or for patients suffering from severe kidney disease.
Caution needed with:
Contains: ETIDRONATE DISODIUM.
Other preparations: DIDRONEL PMO (Norwich Eaton) — contains calcium supplement and used to treat osteoporosis.

Didronel PMO *see* Didronel
(Norwich Eaton)

dienoestrol *see* **Hormofemin, Ortho Dienoestrol**

---

diethylamine salicylate *see* **Algesal, Aradolene**

---

diethylcarbamazine *see* **Banocide**

---

diethylpropion hydrochloride *see* **Apisate, Tenuate Dospan**

Difflam
(3M Healthcare)

A cream used as an anti-inflammatory and ANALGESIC rub to relieve muscular and skeletal pain.

Dose: massage gently into the affected area 3-6 times a day.
Availability: NHS, private prescription , over the counter.
Side effects: may be irritant.
Caution:
Not to be used for: areas near the eyes or on broken or inflamed skin, or on membranes (such as the mouth).
Caution needed with:
Contains: BENZYDAMINE HYDROCHLORIDE.
Other preparations:

Difflam Oral Rinse
(3M Healthcare)

A solution used as an ANALGESIC and anti-inflammatory treatment for painful inflammations of the throat and mouth.

Dose: rinse or gargle with 15 ml every 90 minutes-3 hours.
Availability: NHS, private prescription, over the counter.
Side effects: numb mouth.
Caution:
Not to be used for: children.
Caution needed with:
Contains: BENZYDAMINE HYDROCHLORIDE.
Other preparations: Difflam Spray.

Diflucan
(Pfizer)

A blue/white, blue, or purple-white capsule according to strengths of 50 mg,150 mg, 200 mg and used as an antifungal treatment for vaginal or oral thrush, and general fungal infections.

Dose: 50 mg a day or 150 mg as a single dose for vaginal thrush; 50-100 mg a day for oral thrush; up to 400 mg a day for general infections
Availability: NHS and private prescription.
Side effects: stomach upset.
Caution: in patients suffering from kidney disease where more than a single dose is prescribed.
Not to be used for: children, pregnant women, or nursing mothers.
Caution needed with: anticoagulants, antidiabetics taken by mouth, THEOPHYLLINE, CYCLOSPORIN, PHENYTOIN, RIFAMPICIN.
Contains: fluconazole.
Other preparations: Diflucan Oral Suspension.

---

diflucortolone valerate *see* Nerisone

---

diflunisal *see* Dolobid

---

digitoxin tablets

Tablets supplied at a strength of 100 micrograms and used as a heart muscle stimulant similar to DIGOXIN treatment, especially for heart failure, abnormal rhythms.

Dose: adults ½-2 tablets a day.
Availability: NHS and private prescription.
Side effects: loss of appetite, nausea, vomiting, diarrhoea, stomach pain, disturbance of vision, headache, tiredness, confusion, deliirium, hallucinations, heart disturbances.
Caution: in the elderly, and in patients suffering from underactive thyroid, kidney damage, or recent heart attack.
Not to be used for: patients suffering from some types of heart disorder.
Caution needed with: NON-STEROID ANTI-INFLAMMATORY DRUGS, CHOLESTYRAMINE, COLESTIPOL, RIFAMPICIN, anti-epileptics, BARBITURATES, SS-BLOCKERS, calcium supplements, DIURETICS, AMINOGLUTETHIMIDE, CARBENOXOLONE, SUCRALFATE.
Contains: DIGITOXIN.
Other preparations:

digoxin *see* **Lanoxin**

---

dihydrocodeine *see* **co-dydramol, DF 118, DHC Continus, dihydrocodeine tablets, Paramol, Remedeine**

---

dihydrocodeine tablets

A white tablet supplied at a strength of 30 mg and used as an opiate to control pain; for cough use elixir.

Dose: adults1 tablet every 4-6 hours after meals; children 4-12 years 0.5-1 mg per kg body weight every 4-6 hours.
Availability: NHS and private prescription.
Side effects: constipation, nausea, headache, vertigo, vomiting, dizziness.
Caution: in pregnant women, the elderly, and in patients suffering from liver or kidney disease, allergy, underactive thyroid gland.
Not to be used for: children under 4 years, or for patients suffering from respiratory depression or blocked airways.
Caution needed with: alcohol, sedatives, maois.
Contains: DIHYDROCODEINE tartrate.
Other preparations: DHC CONTINUS (Napp).

---

dihydrotachysterol *see* **AT 10, Tachyrol**

---

diltiazem *see* **Britiazim, Tildiem**

Dimelor — antidiabetic treatment. Product now discontinued.

---

dimenhydrenate *see* **Dramamine**

---

dimethicone *see* **Actonorm, Altacite Plus, Andursil, Asilone, Cobadex, Conotrane, Diovol, Kolanticon, Loasid, Timodine**

---

dimethindene *see* **Fenostil Retard, Vibrocil**

dimethyl sulphoxide *see* **Herpid, Virudox**

Dimetriose
(Roussel)

A white capsule used to treat endometriosis (a womb and menstrual disorder).

Dose: 1 capsule twice a week, on days 1 and 4 of cycle, then on the same 2 days each week for the rest of the treatment.
Availability: NHS and private prescription.
Side effects: vaginal bleeding (spotting), acne, weight gain, stomach upset, cramp, depression, voice changes, hair growth.
Caution: in patients suffering from diabetes or high blood lipids. Ensure effective contraception (barrier methods must be used).
Not to be used for: children, pregnant women, nursing mothers, or for patients with heart, kidney, or liver disorder, blood vessel disease, or disturbance of metabolism.
Caution needed with: anticonvulsants, the contraceptive pill,. RIFAMPICIN.
Contains: GESTRINONE.
Other preparations:

Dimotane Expectorant
(Whitehall)

A liquid used as an ANTIHISTAMINE, expectorant, and SYMPATHOMIMETIC treatment for cough.

Dose: adults 5-10 ml 3 times a day; children 2-6 years 2.5 ml 3 times a day, 7-12 years 5 ml 3 times a day.
Availability: private prescription and over the counter.
Side effects: anxiety, hands shaking, rapid or abnormal heart rate, dry mouth, brain stimulation, drowsiness.
Caution: in patients suffering from diabetes.
Not to be used for: children under 2 years, or for patients suffering from cardiovascular problems, overactive thyroid gland.
Caution needed with: MAOIS, TRICYCLICS, sedatives, alcohol, ANTICHOLINERGICS.
Contains: BROMPHENIRAMINE maleate, GUAIPHENESIN, PSEUDOEPHEDRINE hydrochloride.
Other preparations: Dimotane Co, Dimotane Co Paediatric.

Dimotane Plus
(Wyeth)

A liquid used as an ANTIHISTAMINE and SYMPATHOMIMETIC treatment for allergic rhinitis.

Dose: adults 10 ml 3 times a day; children 6-12 years 5 ml 3 times a day.
Availability: NHS, private prescription, over the counter.
Side effects: drowsiness, reduced reactions, rarely stimulant effects.
Caution: in nursing mothers and in patients suffering from bronchial asthma, diabetes.
Not to be used for: patients suffering from glaucoma, comatose states, brain damage, epilepsy, retention of urine, cardiovascular problems, overactive thyroid.
Caution needed with: sedatives, MAOIS, TRICYCLICS, ANTICHOLINERGICS, alcohol.
Contains: BROMPHENIRAMINE maleate, PSEUDOEPHEDRINE hydrochloride.
Other preparations: Dimotane Plus Paediatric, Dimotane Plus LA, Dimotane LA, Dimotane Tablets, Dimotane Elixir.

D

Dimotapp LA
(Whitehall)

A brown tablet used as an ANTIHISTAMINE and SYMPATHOMIMETIC treatment for catarrh, allergic rhinitis, sinusitis.

Dose: adults 1 tablets night and morning; children use elixir.
Availability: private prescription and over the counter.
Side effects: drowsiness, reduced reactions, rarely stimulant effects.
Caution: in nursing mothers and in patients suffering from bronchial asthma, diabetes.
Not to be used for: patients suffering from glaucoma, comatose states, brain damage, epilepsy, retention of urine, cardiovascular problems, overactive thyroid.
Caution needed with: sedatives, MAOIS, TRICYCLICS, ANTICHOLINERGICS, alcohol.
Contains: BROMPHENIRAMINE maleate, PHENYLEPHRINE hydrochloride, PHENYLPROPANOLAMINE hydrochloride.
Other preparations: Dimotapp Elixir, Dimotapp Elixir Paediatric.

Dindevan
(Evans)

A white or a green, scored tablet according to strengths of 10 mg, 25 mg, 50 mg and used as an anticoagulant to prevent blood from clotting.

Dose: 200 mg a day at first, 100 mg the following day, then 50-150 mg a day.
Availability: NHS and private prescription.
Side effects: rash, fever, white cell count changes, diarrhoea, hepatitis, kidney damage, discoloration of urine.
Caution: in elderly and very ill patients, and for patients suffering from high blood pressure, weight changes, kidney disease, vitamin K deficiency.
Not to be used for: children, within 24 hours of surgery or labour, for pregnant women, nursing mothers, and for patients suffering from severe liver or kidney disease or haemorrhagic conditions.
Caution needed with: NON-STEROID ANTI-INFLAMMATORY DRUGS, antidiabetics, sulphonamides, QUINIDINE, antibiotics, PHENFORMIN, CIMETIDINE, drugs affecting the liver chemistry, STEROIDS.
Contains: PHENINDIONE.
Other preparations:

Dioctyl
(Medo)

A yellow tablet supplied at a strength of 100 mg and used as a faecal softener to treat constipation.

Dose: adults up to 500 mg a day in divided doses; children over 2 years 12.5-25 mg 3 times a day; 6 months-2 years 12.5 mg 3 times a day using syrup.
Availability: NHS, private prescription, over the counter.
Side effects:
Caution:
Not to be used for:
Caution needed with:
Contains: DOCUSATE SODIUM.
Other preparations: Dioctyl paediatric syrup, Dioctyl syrup.

Dioctyl Ear Drops
(Medo)

Drops used as a wax softener to remove ear wax.

Dose: 4 drops into the ear twice a day and plug with cotton wool.
Availability: NHS, private prescription, over the counter.
Side effects:
Caution:
Not to be used for: patients suffering from perforated ear drum.

Caution needed with:
Contains: SODIUM DOCUSATE, POLYETHYLENE GLYCOL.
Other preparations: WAXSOL (Norgine).

Dioderm *see* hydrocortisone cream
(Dermal)

Dioralyte
(Rhone-Poulenc Rorer)

Plain, citrus-, or blackcurrant-flavoured powder supplied as sachets and used as a fluid and electrolyte replacement to treat acute watery diarrhoea including gastroenteritis.

Dose: 1-2 sachets in 200-400 ml water after each occasion of diarrhoea; infants substitute equivalent volume of reconstituted powder to feeds; children 1 sachet after each occasion of diarrhoea.
Availability: NHS, private prescription, and over the counter.
Side effects:
Caution:
Not to be used for:
Caution needed with:
Contains: SODIUM CHLORIDE, POTASSIUM CHLORIDE, SODIUM BICARBONATE, GLUCOSE.
Other preparations: Dioralyte Effervescent, ELECTROLADE (Nicholas); GLUCO-LYTE (Cupal); REHIDRAT (Searle).

Diovol
(Pharmax)

A white suspension used as an ANTACID and anti-wind preparation to treat ulcers, hiatus hernias, wind, and acidity.

Dose: adults 5-10 ml 3 times a day.
Availability: NHS, private prescription, over the counter.
Side effects: occasionally constipation.
Caution:
Not to be used for: children.
Caution needed with: TETRACYCLINE antibiotics, tablets which are coated to protect the stomach.
Contains: ALUMINIUM HYDROXIDE, MAGNESIUM HYDROXIDE, DIMETHICONE.
Other preparations:

Dipentum
(Kabi Pharmacia)

A caramel-coloured capsule supplied at a strength of 250 mg used as a salicylate to treat ulcerative colitis.

Dose: 4-12 capsules a day with food.
Availability: NHS and private prescription.
Side effects: stomach upset, rash, headache, joint pains.
Caution:
Not to be used for: children, pregnant women, or for patients suffering from ASPIRIN allergy or kidney disease.
Caution needed with:
Contains: OLSALAZINE SODIUM.
Other preparations:

---

diphenhydramine *see* **Benylin Expectorant, Guanor, Histalix, Lotussin, Propain, Uniflu and Gregovite C**

---

diphenoxylate *see* **Lomotil**

---

diphenylpyraline *see* **Eskornade Spansule, Histryl Spansule, Lergoban**

---

dipipanone *see* **Diconal**

---

dipivefrin *see* **Propine**

---

dipotassium hydrogen phosphate *see* **Glandosane**

Diprobase
(Schering-Plough)

A cream used as an emollient to soften skin along with, or as an alternative to, STEROID preparations.

Dose: apply sparingly when required.

Availability: NHS, private prescription, over the counter.
Side effects:
Caution:
Not to be used for:
Caution needed with:
Contains: LIQUID PARAFFIN, WHITE SOFT PARAFFIN, CETOMACROGOL, CETOSTEARYL ALCOHOL.
Other preparations: Diprobase Ointment, LIPOBASE (Brocades), ULTRABASE (Schering).

Diprobath
(Schering-Plough)

A bath emulsion used to treat dry skin conditions.

Dose: adults, 2½ capfuls added to the bath, and soak for 20 minutes; children, 1 capful per bath.
Availability: NHS, private prescription, over the counter.
Side effects:
Caution:
Not to be used for:
Caution needed with:
Contains: light LIQUID PARAFFIN, ISOPROPYL MYRISTATE.
Other preparations: HYDROMOL (Quinoderm).

Diprosalic
(Schering-Plough)

An ointment used as a STEROID and skin softener to treat hard skin and dry skin disorders.

Dose: apply lightly to the affected area 1-2 times a day.
Availability: NHS and private prescription.
Side effects: fluid retention, suppression of adrenal glands, thinning of the skin may occur.
Caution: use for short periods of time only.
Not to be used for: patients suffering from acne or any other skin infections caused by tuberculosis, ringworm, viruses, or fungi, or continuously especially in pregnant women.
Caution needed with:
Contains: BETAMETHASONE DIPROPIONATE, SALICYLIC ACID.
Other preparations: Diprosalic Scalp Application.

D

Diprosone *see* **Betnovate**
(Schering-Plough)

---

dipyridamole *see* **Persantin**

Dirythmin SA
(Astra)

A white tablet supplied at a strength of 150 mg and used as an anti-arrhythmic drug to treat abnormal heart rhythm.

Dose: 2 tablets every twelve hours but no more than 6 tablets a day.
Availability: NHS and private prescription.
Side effects: ANTICHOLINERGIC effects.
Caution: in pregnant women, and in patients suffering from mild heart block, enlarged prostate, glaucoma, retention of urine, low potassium levels, heart failure, kidney or liver failure.
Not to be used for: children or for patients suffering from some types of heart block, heart muscle disease or shock.
Caution needed with: other similar drugs, ß-BLOCKERS, potassium-lowering drugs, ANTICHOLINERGICS.
Contains: DISOPYRAMIDE PHOSPHATE.
Other preparations: ISOMIDE (Monmouth), RYTHMODAN (Roussel).

Disadine DP *see* **Betadine Spray**. Product now discontinued.

Disalcid
(3M Healthcare)

An orange/grey capsule supplied at a strength of 500 mg and used as an ANALGESIC to treat osteoarthritis, rheumatoid arthritis, other joint disorders.

Dose: 4 capsules a day at first in divided doses before or with food, then 2 capsules 3-4 times a day with last dose at bed time if needed.
Availability: NHS and private prescription.
Side effects: stomach upsets, allergy, asthma.
Caution: in the elderly, pregnant women, in patients with a history of allergy to aspirin, asthma, or who are suffering from impaired liver or kidney function, indigestion.
Not to be used for: children, nursing mothers, or for patients suffering from haemophilia, ulcers.

Caution needed with: anticoagulants, some antidiabetic drugs, anti-inflammatory agents, METHOTREXATE, SPIRONOLACTONE, STEROIDS, some uric acid-lowering drugs.
Contains: SALSALATE.
Other preparations:

Disipal
(Brocades)

A yellow tablet supplied at a strength of 50 mg and used as an ANTICHOLINERGIC drug to treat Parkinson's disease.

Dose: 1 tablet 3 times a day at first increasing by 1 tablet a day every 2-3 days usually to 2-6 tablets a day and a maximum of 8 tablets a day.
Availability: NHS and private prescription.
Side effects: euphoria, ANTICHOLINERGIC effects, and confusion, agitation, and rash at high dose.
Caution: in patients suffering from heart problems or stomach obstruction. Reduce dose slowly.
Not to be used for: patients suffering from glaucoma, enlarged prostate, some movement disorders.
Caution needed with: PHENOTHIAZINES, ANTIHISTAMINES, antidepressants.
Contains: ORPHENDRINE hydrochloride.
Other preparations: Disipal Injection, BIORPHEN (Bioglan).

---

disopyramide *see* Dirythmin, Rythmodan

Disprol Paed
(Reckitt & Colman)

A suspension supplied at a strength of 120 mg/ 5 ml and used as an ANALGESIC to relieve pain and fever in children.

Dose: under 3 months 2.5 ml 4 times a day if needed, 3 months-1 year 2.5-5 ml 4 times a day if needed, 1-6 years 5-10 ml 4 times a day if needed, 6-12 years 10-20 ml 4 times a day if needed.
Availability: NHS, private prescription, over the counter.
Side effects:
Caution: in children suffering from liver or kidney disease.
Not to be used for: infants under 2 months.
Caution needed with: other medicines containing PARACETAMOL.
Contains: PARACETAMOL.
Other preparations: CALPOL (Wellcome), PALDESIC (RP Drugs), PANALEVE

(Pinewood — available on NHS if prescribed as a generic), PARACETAMOL
PAEDIATRIC ELIXIR.

Distaclor
(Dista)

A violet/white or violet/grey capsule supplied at strengths of 250 mg and 500 mg, and used as an antibiotic to treat ear, urinary, respiratory, soft tissue, and skin infections.

Dose: adults and children over 5 years 250 mg every 8 hours to a maximum of 4 g a day; children under 5 years reduced doses.
Availability: NHS and private prescription.
Side effects: allergy, stomach disturbances.
Caution: in patients suffering from kidney disease or who are very sensitive to penicillin.
Not to be used for:
Caution needed with: anticoagulants.
Contains: CEFACLOR.
Other preparations: Distaclor Suspension.

Distalgesic *see* Co-Proxamol
(Dista)

Distamine
(Dista)

A white tablet or a white, scored tablet according to strengths of 50 mg, 125 mg, 250 mg and used as an anti-arthritic drug and binding agent to treat severe active rheumatoid arthritis, cystinuria, Wilson's disease (inherited disorders), heavy metal poisoning, liver disease.

Dose: adults 125-250 mg a day for 4 weeks increasing by same amount at 4-12 week intervals, usually to 500-750 mg a day or a maximum of 1.5 g a day; elderly 50-125 mg a day at first increasing to a maximum of 1 g a day; children 50 mg a day for 4 weeks, increasing every 4 weeks to a usual dose of 15-20 mg per kg body weight a day. Or as advised.
Availability: NHS and private prescription.
Side effects: nausea, anorexia, fever, rash, loss of taste, blood changes, blood or protein in the urine, kidney changes, muscle disease.
Caution: in nursing mothers and in patients suffering from kidney disease, sensitivity to penicillin. Your doctor may advise that your blood and urine should be checked regularly.

Not to be used for: pregnant women or for patients suffering from lupus erythematosus, agranulocytosis, thrombocytopenia (rare blood and multi-system disorders).
Caution needed with: gold salts, anti-malaria or cytotoxic drugs, PHENYLBUTAZONE.
Contains: PENICILLAMINE.
Other preparations: PENDRAMINE (Asta).

Distaquaine V-K
(Dista)

A white, scored tablet supplied at a strength of 250 mg and used as a penicillin to treat infections.

Dose: adults and children over 5 years 250 mg every 4-6 hours.
Availability: NHS and private prescription.
Side effects: allergy, stomach disturbances.
Caution: in patients suffering from kidney disease.
Not to be used for: children over 5 years or for patients suffering from penicillin allergy.
Caution needed with: anticoagulants, the contraceptive pill.
Contains: PENICILLIN V POTASSIUM.
Other preparations: STABILLIN V-K (Boots), RIMAPEN (Rima), V-CIL-K, (Distaquaine V-K Syrup — now discontinued).

---

distigmine *see* Ubretid

---

disulfiram *see* Antabuse

---

dithranol *see* Anthranol, Antraderm, Dithrocream, Dithrolan, Exolan, Psoradrate, Psorin

---

Dithrocream
(Dermal)

A cream used as an antipsoriatic treatment for psoriasis.

Dose: apply to the affected area once a day and wash off after ½-1 hour or apply at night and wash off in the morning.
Availability: NHS, private prescription, over the counter.

Side effects: irritation, allergy.
Caution: stains skin and clothing.
Not to be used for: patients suffering from acute psoriasis.
Caution needed with:
Contains: DITHRANOL.
Other preparations: Dithrocream Forte, Dithrocream HP, Dithrocream 2%; ALPHODITH (Stafford-Miller), ANTHRANOL (Stiefel), EXOLAN (Dermal), PSORADRATE (Norwich Eaton). Some not available over the counter.

Dithrolan
(Dermal)

An ointment used as an antipsoriatic and skin softener to treat psoriasis.

Dose: before going to bed, bath and then apply the ointment to the affected area. Use once or twice a week.
Availability: NHS, private prescription, over the counter.
Side effects: irritation, allergy.
Caution: stains skin and clothing.
Not to be used for: patients suffering from acute psoriasis.
Caution needed with:
Contains: DITHRANOL, SALICYLIC ACID.
Other preparations: PSORIN (Thames).

Ditropan *see* Cystrin
(Smith and Nephew Pharm)

Diumide-K Continus
(ASTA)

A white/orange tablet used as a DIURETIC/potassium supplement combination to treat fluid retention including that associated with congestive heart failure, kidney and liver disease where a potassium supplement is needed.

Dose: 1 tablet a day in the morning.
Availability: NHS and private prescription.
Side effects: gout, bowel disturbances.
Caution: in pregnant women, nursing mothers, and in patients suffering from kidney or liver disease, diabetes, enlarged prostate, impaired urination, gout.
Not to be used for: children or for patients suffering from liver cirrhosis, raised potassium levels, Addison's disease.
Caution needed with: potassium-sparing DIURETICS, LITHIUM, DIGOXIN, some

antibiotics, NON-STEROID ANTI-INFLAMMATORY DRUGS, ANTIHYPERTENSIVES.
Contains: FRUSEMIDE, POTASSIUM CHLORIDE.
Other preparations: LASIKAL (Hoechst), LASIX + K (Hoechst).

Diuresal *see* **Lasix.** Product now discontinued.

---

diuretic

A drug which removes salt and water from the body, thus treating fluid
retention. Example FRUSEMIDE *see* Lasix.

Diurexan
(ASTA)

A white, scored tablet supplied at a strength of 20 mg and used as a
DIURETIC to treat high blood pressure, congestive heart failure, fluid retention.

Dose: high blood pressure 1 tablet a day in the morning increasing to 2
tablets a day if needed; fluid retention 2 tablets a day in the morning and
then 1-4 tablets a day as needed.
Availability: NHS and private prescription.
Side effects: low potassium levels, dizziness, stomach upset.
Caution: potassium supplements may be needed; care in pregnant
women, nursing mothers, and in patients suffering from gout, kidney or
liver disease, diabetes, enlarged prostate.
Not to be used for: children or for patients suffering from severe kidney
failure or cirrhosis of the liver.
Caution needed with: DIGOXIN, LITHIUM, ANTIHYPERTENSIVES.
Contains: XIPAMIDE.
Other preparations:

Dixarit
(Boehringer Ingelheim)

A blue tablet supplied at a strength of 25 micrograms and used as a blood
vessel antispasmodic drug to treat migraine, headache, menopausal
flushing.

Dose: 2-3 tablets morning and evening.
Availability: NHS and private prescription.

Side effects: sedation, dry mouth, dizziness, sleeplessness.
Caution: in nursing mothers or in patients suffering from depression.
Not to be used for: children.
Caution needed with: ANTIHYPERTENSIVES.
Contains: CLONIDINE hydrochloride.
Other preparations:

---

dl-methionine *see* Lipotriad

---

dl-threonine *see* Cicatrin

---

docosahexaenoic acid *see* Maxepa

---

docusate *see* Co-Danthrusate, Dioctyl, Dioctyl Ear Drops, Fletchers' Enemette, Normax, Waxsol

---

Dolmatil
(Squibb)

A white, scored tablet supplied at a strength of 200 mg and used as a sedative to treat schizophrenia.

Dose: over 14 years 2-4 tablets a day at first in 2 divided doses, the 1-6 tablets a day as needed.
Availability: NHS and private prescription.
Side effects: muscle spasms, restlessness, hands shaking, dry mouth, urine retention, palpitations, low blood pressure, weight gain, changes in libido, low body temperature, breast swelling, menstrual changes, jaundice, blood and skin changes, drowsiness, rarely fits.
Caution: in pregnant women or for patients suffering from hypomania, kidney disease, or epilepsy.
Not to be used for: for children under 14 years or for patients suffering from phaeochromocytoma (a disease of the adrenal glands).
Caution needed with: alcohol, tranquillizers, pain killers, ANTIHYPERTENSIVES, antidepressants, anticoagulants, antidiabetic drugs, LEVODOPA, ANTACIDS, SUCRALFATE.
Contains: SULPIRIDE.
Other preparations: SULPITIL (Farmitalia).

Dolobid
(Morson)

A peach tablet or an orange tablet according to strengths of 250 mg, 500 mg and used as an ANALGESIC to treat pain, rheumatoid arthritis, osteoarthritis.

Dose: 500 mg twice a day at first, then 250-500 mg twice a day. For arthritis 500-1000 mg a day adjusting according to response.
Availability: NHS and private prescription.
Side effects: stomach pain, dyspepsia, diarrhoea, rash, headache, dizziness, tinnitus.
Caution: in the elderly and in patients suffering from kidney, heart, or liver disease or with a history of stomach haemorrhage or ulcers.
Not to be used for: children, pregnant women, nursing mothers or for patients suffering from anti-inflammatory-induced allergy, asthma, or stomach ulcer.
Caution needed with: alcohol, INDOMETHACIN, anticoagulants.
Contains: DIFLUNISAL.
Other preparations:

Doloxene
(Eli Lilly)

An orange capsule supplied at a strength of 60 mg and used as an opiate to control pain.

Dose: 1 capsule 3-4 times a day.
Availability: controlled drug; NHS (when prescribed as a generic), private prescription.
Side effects: tolerance, dependence, drowsiness, constipation, rash, dizziness, nausea.
Caution: in pregnant women, the elderly, and in patients suffering from liver or kidney disease.
Not to be used for: children
Caution needed with: alcohol, sedatives, anticonvulsants, anticoagulants.
Contains: DEXTROPROPOXYPHENE.
Other preparations:

Doloxene Co.
(Eli Lilly)

A red/grey capsule used as an opiate to control pain.

Dose: 1 capsule 3-4 times a day.

D

Availability: private prescription only.
Side effects: tolerance, dependence, drowsiness, constipation, dizziness, nausea, rash.
Caution: in pregnant women, nursing mothers, the elderly, and in patients suffering from kidney, heart, or liver disease, anti-inflammatory induced allergy, or a history of bronchospasm.
Not to be used for: children or for patients suffering from stomach ulcer, haemophilia, and blood clotting disorders.
Caution needed with: alcohol, sedatives, anticoagulants, antidiabetics, uric acid-lowering drugs, anticonvulsants.
Contains: DEXTROPROPOXYPHENE NAPSYLATE, ASPIRIN, CAFFEINE.
Other preparations:

Dome-Acne — acne treatment. Product now discontinued.

Domical
(Berk)

A blue tablet, orange tablet, or brown tablet according to strengths of 10 mg, 25 mg, 50 mg and used as a TRICYCLIC antidepressant to treat depression.

Dose: adults 75 mg a day in divided doses at first increasing to up to 200 mg a day if needed, then usually 50-100 mg at night; elderly 10-50 mg a day at first.
Availability: NHS and private prescription.
Side effects: dry mouth, constipation, urine retention, blurred vision, palpitations, drowsiness, sleeplessness, dizziness, hands shaking, low blood presure, weight change, skin reactions, jaundice or blood changes, loss of libido may occur.
Caution: in nursing mothers or in patients suffering from heart disease, thyroid disease, epilepsy, diabetes, some other psychiatric conditions. Your doctor may advise regular blood tests.
Not to be used for: children, pregnant women, or for patients suffering from heart attacks, heart block, liver disease.
Caution needed with: alcohol, ANTICHOLINERGICS, adrenaline, MAOIS, BARBITURATES, other antidepressants, ANTIHYPERTENSIVES, CIMETIDINE, oestrogens.
Contains: AMITRIPTYLINE hydrochloride.
Other preparations: ELAVIL (DDSA), LENTIZOL (Parke-Davis), TRYPTIZOL (Morson).

---

domiphen *see* **Bradosol**

---

domperidone *see* **Evoxin, Motilium**

Dopamet *see* **Aldomet**
(Berk)

Doralese
(Bridge)

A yellow, triangular tablet supplied at a strength of 20 mg and used as an alpha-blocker to treat urine obstruction due to prostate disease.

Dose: 1 tablet twice a day (low dose in the elderly).
Availability: NHS and private prescription.
Side effects: dry mouth, nose blockage, weight gain, drowsiness, ejaculation failure.
Caution: in patients suffering from poor heart function, kidney or liver disease, Parkinson's disease, epilepsy, depression.
Not to be used for: patients suffering from heart failure.
Caution needed with: MAOIS, ANTIHYPERTENSIVES.
Contains: INDORAMIN.
Other preparations: BARATOL (Monmouth).

Dormonoct *see* **loprazolam.** Product now discontinued.

Dothapax *see* **Prothiaden**
(Ashbourne)

---

dothiepin *see* **Prothiaden**

Dovonex
(Leo)

An ointment used to treat mild to moderate psoriasis.

Dose: apply twice a day, not more than 100 g per week, for no more than

6 weeks.
Availability: NHS and private prescription.
Side effects: irritation, dermatitis.
Caution: in pregnant women and nursing mothers. Avoid the face.
Not to be used for: children, or for patients suffering from disorders of calcium metabolism.
Caution needed with:
Contains: CALCIPOTRIOL.
Other preparations:

D

doxazosin *see* **Cardura**

---

doxepin *see* **Sinequan**

---

doxycycline hydrochloride *see* **Vibramycin, Vibramycin 50**

---

doxylamine succinate *see* **Syndol**

Doxylar *see* **Vibramycin**
(Lagap)

Dozic
(R.P. Drugs)

A liquid used as a sedative to treat schizophrenia, mania, hypomania, organic psychoses, alcohol withdrawal symptoms, delirium tremens, behaviour problems among children.

Dose: elderly psychosis 0.5-2 mg 2-3 times a day at first then increase as needed to a maximum of 200 mg a day then decrease to 5-10 mg a day when control is achieved, anxiety 0.5 mg twice a day; adults 0.5 mg 2-3 times a day at first then as above, anxiety as above; children 0.05 mg per kg body weight a day in 2 divided doses.
Availability: NHS and private prescription.
Side effects: muscle spasms, restlessness, hands shaking, dry mouth, urine retention, palpitations, low blood pressure, weight gain, changes in libido, low body temperature, breast swelling, menstrual changes, jaun-

dice, blood and skin changes, drowsiness, rarely fits.
Caution: in pregnant women or in patients suffering from liver or kidney disease, epilepsy, severe cardiovascular disease, Parkinson's disease, or overactive thyroid gland.
Not to be used for: unconscious patients.
Caution needed with: alcohol, tranquillizers, pain killers, ANTIHYPERTENSIVES, antidepressants, anticonvulsants, antidiabetic drugs, LEVODOPA, RIFAMPICIN, LITHIUM.
Contains: HALOPERIDOL.
Other preparations: HALDOL (Janssen), SERENACE (Baker-Norton).

Dramamine
(Searle)

A white, scored tablet supplied at a strength of 50 mg and used as an ANTIHISTAMINE treatment for vertigo, nausea, vomiting, travel sickness.

Dose: adults 1-2 tablets 2-3 times a day; children 1-6 years ¼-½ tablet, 7-12 years ½-1 tablet 2-3 times a day.
Availability: NHS, over the counter, private prescription.
Side effects: drowsiness, reduced reactions, dry mouth, blurred vision, rarely skin eruptions.
Caution: in patients suffering from liver or kidney disease.
Not to be used for: infants under 1 year.
Caution needed with: alcohol, sedatives, some antidepressants (MAOIS).
Contains: DIMENHYDRENATE.
Other preparations:

Drapolene
(Wellcome)

A cream used as an antiseptic to treat nappy rash.

Dose: apply twice a day or each time the nappy is changed.
Availability: NHS, private prescription, over the counter.
Side effects:
Caution:
Not to be used for:
Caution needed with:
Contains: BENZALKONIUM CHLORIDE, CETRIMIDE.
Other preparations:

dried yeast *see* Tonivitan

Droleptan
(Janssen)

A yellow, scored tablet supplied at a strength of 10 mg and used as a sedative to treat manic agitation.

Dose: adults 5-20 mg every 4-8 hours; children 0.5-1 mg a day.
Availability: NHS and private prescription.
Side effects: muscle spasms, restlessness, hands shaking, dry mouth, urine retention, palpitations, low blood pressure, weight gain, changes in libido, low body temperature, breast swelling, menstrual changes, jaundice, blood and skin changes, drowsiness, rarely fits.
Caution: in pregnant women, nursing mothers and in patients suffering from severe liver disease, pyramidal or extrapyramidal symptoms (shaking and stiffness).
Not to be used for: patients suffering from severe clinical depression.
Caution needed with: alcohol, tranquillizers, pain killers, ANTIHYPERTENSIVES, antidepressants, anticonvulsants, antidiabetic drugs, LEVODOPA.
Contains: DROPERIDOL.
Other preparations: Droleptan Liquid.

Dromoran — opiate for severe pain. Product now discontinued.

---

droperidol *see* **Droleptan**

Droxalin — ANTACID. Product now discontinued.

Dryptal *see* Lasix
(Berk)

Dubam
(Norma)

An aerosol used as a topical ANALGESIC to relieve muscular pain.

Dose: spray on to the affected area for 2 seconds up to 4 times a day.
Availability: NHS, private prescription, over the counter.
Side effects: may be irritant.
Caution:

Not to be used for: areas near the eyes, or on broken or inflamed skin, or on membranes (such as the mouth).
Caution needed with:
Contains: GLYCOL SALICYLATE, METHYL SALICYLATE, ETHYL SALICYLATE, METHYL NICOTINATE.
Other preparations: Dubam Cream.

Dulcolax
(Windsor)

A yellow tablet supplied at a strength of 5 mg and used as a stimulant to treat constipation and for evacuation of the bowels before surgery.

Dose: adults 1-2 tablets at night; children under 10 years half adult dose.
Availability: NHS (when prescribed as a generic), private prescription, over the counter.
Side effects:
Caution:
Not to be used for:
Caution needed with:
Contains: BISACODYL.
Other preparations: Dulcolax Suppositories.

Duo-Autohaler —broncho-dilator aerosol. Product now discontinued.

Duofilm
(Stiefel)

A liquid used as a skin softener to treat warts.

Dose: apply the liquid to the wart once a day, allow to dry, and cover, rubbing down between applications.
Availability: NHS, private prescription, over the counter.
Side effects:
Caution: do not apply to healthy skin.
Not to be used for: warts on the face or anal and genital areas.
Caution needed with:
Contains: SALICYLIC ACID, LACTIC ACID.
Other preparations: CUPLEX (SNP), SALACTOL (Dermal), SALATAC (Dermal).

Duogastrone *see* Biogastrone. Product now discontinued.

Duovent
(Boehringer Ingelheim)

An aerosol used as a broncho-dilator to treat blocked airways.

Dose: adults 1-2 sprays 3-4 times a day; children over 6 years 1 spray 3 times a day.
Availability: NHS and private prescription.
Side effects: headache, dry mouth, dilation of the blood vessels.
Caution: in patients suffering from glaucoma, enlarged prostate, high blood pressure,overactive thyroid gland, heart muscle disease, angina, abnormal heart rhythms.
Not to be used for: children under 6 years.
Caution needed with: SYMPATHOMIMETICS.
Contains: FENOTEROL hydrobromide, IPRATROPIUM bromide.
Other preparations:

Duphalac
(Duphar)

A syrup used as a laxative to treat constipation, brain disease due to liver problems.

Dose: children 0-1 year 2.5 ml twice a day; 1-4 years 5 ml twice a day; 5-10 years 10 ml twice a day; adults15-50 ml 2-3 times a day until 2-3 soft stools are produced each day.
Availability: NHS (when prescribed as a generic), private prescription, over the counter.
Side effects: wind.
Caution:
Not to be used for: patients suffering from galactosaemia (an inherited disorder), blocked intestine.
Caution needed with: ANTACIDS, NEOMYCIN.
Contains: LACTULOSE.
Other preparations: LACTULOSE SOLUTION.

Duphaston
(Duphar)

A white, scored tablet supplied at a strength of 10 mg and used as a progestogen to treat period pain, habitual and threatened abortion, endometriosis (a womb disorder), infertility, premenstrual syndrome, and as an additional treatment to oestrogen in hormone replacement.

Dose: period pain 1 tablet twice a day from the fifth to the twenty-fifth day of the cycle; endometriosis 1 tablet 2-3 times a day from the fifth to the twenty-fifth day or continuously; premenstrual syndrome 1 tablet twice a day from the twelfth to the twenty-sixth day; hormone replacement 2 tablets a day for 12 days a month.

Availability: NHS and private prescription.
Side effects: irregular bleeding, breast discomfort, acne, headache.
Caution: in patients suffering from high blood pressure or tendency to thrombosis, migraine, liver abnormalities, ovarian cysts.
Not to be used for: children, pregnant women, women having suffered a previous ectopic pregnancy, or for patients suffering from severe heart or kidney disease, benign liver tumours, undiagnosed vaginal bleeding.
Caution needed with: BARBITURATES, PHENYTOIN, PYRIDONE, CARBAMAZEPINE, CHLORAL HYDRATE, DICHLORALPHENAZONE, ETHOSUXIMIDE, RIFAMPICIN, CHLORPHENESIN, MEPROBAMATE, GRISEOFULVIN.
Contains: DYDROGESTERONE.
Other preparations:

D

Duromine
(3M Healthcare)

A grey/green capsule or a grey/maroon capsule according to strengths of 15 mg, 30 mg and used as an appetite suppressant to treat obesity.

Dose: 15-30 mg once a day at breakfast.
Availability: controlled drug; NHS and private prescription.
Side effects: tolerance, addictions, mental disturbances, restlessness, nervousness, agitation, dry mouth, heart palpitations, raised blood pressure, fluid retention.
Caution: do not use for prolonged treatments. Care in patients suffering from high blood pressure, angina, abnormal heart rhythm.
Not to be used for: children, pregnant women, nursing mothers, or for patients suffering from hardening of the arteries, overactive thyroid gland, severe high blood pressure, or with a history of mental illness, alcoholism or drug addiction.
Caution needed with: MAOIS, SYMPATHOMIMETICS, METHYLDOPA, GUANETHIDINE, other appetite suppressants, antidepressants, tranquillizers.
Contains: PHENTERMINE.
Other preparations: IONAMIN (Lipha).

Dyazide
(Bridge)

A peach-coloured, scored tablet used as a DIURETIC to treat high blood pressure, fluid retention.

Dose: high blood pressure 1 tablet a day at first; fluid retention 1 tablet twice a day at first after meals and then 1 tablet a day or every other day. No more than 4 tablets a day.
Availability: NHS and private prescription.
Side effects: nausea, diarrhoea, cramps, weakness, headache, dry mouth, rash, blood changes.
Caution: in pregnant women, nursing mothers, and in patients suffering from liver or kidney disease, diabetes, electrolyte changes, gout, pancreatitis.
Not to be used for: patients suffering from severe or progressive kidney failure, raised potassium levels, Addison's disease (a disease of the adrenal glands).
Caution needed with: potassium supplements, potassium-sparing DIURETICS, LITHIUM, DIGOXIN, ANTIHYPERTENSIVES, INDOMETHACIN, ACE INHIBITORS.
Contains: TRIAMTERENE, HYDROCHLOROTHIAZIDE.
Other preparations: TRIAMAXCO (Ashbourne), TRIAMCO (Norton).

---

dydrogesterone *see* **Duphaston**

Dysman *see* **Ponstan**
(Ashbourne)

Dyspamet *see* **Tagamet**
(Bridge)

Dytac
(Bridge)

A maroon capsule supplied at a strength of 50 mg and used as a potassium-sparing DIURETIC to treat fluid retention especially when associated with congestive heart failure, liver or kidney disease.

Dose: 3-5 capsules a day in divided doses for 7 days, and then usually every other day.
Availability: NHS and private prescription.
Side effects: nausea, diarrhoea, cramps, weakness, headache, dry mouth, rash, blood changes.
Caution: in pregnant women, nursing mothers, and in patients suffering from kidney or liver disease, gout, electrolyte changes.
Not to be used for: children or for patients suffering from raised potas-

sium levels, or progressive kidney failure.
Caution needed with: potassium supplements, potassium-sparing DIURETICS, ANTIHYPERTENSIVES, INDOMETHACIN, ACE INHIBITORS.
Contains: TRIAMTERENE.
Other preparations:

Dytide
(Bridge)

A pale-yellow/maroon capsule used as a potassium-sparing DIURETIC to treat fluid retention.

Dose: 2 capsules after breakfast and 1 capsule after lunch at first, then 1 or 2 capsules every other day.
Availability: NHS and private prescription.
Side effects: nausea, diarrhoea, cramps, weakness, headache, dry mouth, rash, blood changes.
Caution: in pregnant women, nursing mothers, and in patients suffering from liver or kidney disease, diabetes, electrolyte changes, or gout.
Not to be used for: patients suffering from raised potassium levels, or progressive or severe kidney failure.
Caution needed with: potassium supplements, potassium-sparing DIURETICS, LITHIUM, DIGOXIN, ANTIHYPERTENSIVES, INDOMETHACIN, ACE INHIBITORS.
Contains: TRIAMTERENE, BENZTHIAZIDE.
Other preparations:

Ebufac *see* Brufen
(DDSA)

Econacort
(Princeton)

A cream used as a STEROID, antifungal, and antibacterial treatment for skin infections where there is also inflammation.

Dose: massage into the affected area night and morning.
Availability: NHS and private prescription.
Side effects: fluid retention, suppression of adrenal glands, thinning of the skin may occur.
Caution: use for short periods of time only.
Not to be used for: patients suffering from acne or any other skin infections caused by tuberculosis, ringworm, viruses, or fungi, or continuously especially in pregnant women.

Caution needed with:
Contains: ECONAZOLE nitrate, HYDROCORTISONE.
Other preparations:

---

econazole *see* **Econacort, Ecostatin, Ecostatin-1, Gyno-Pevaryl 1, Pevaryl**

Economycin *see* **tetracycline**
(DDSA)

Ecostatin
(Princeton)

A cream used as an antifungal treatment for fungal infections of the skin.

Dose: apply to the affected area night and morning.
Availability: NHS, private prescription, over the counter.
Side effects: irritation.
Caution: avoid the eyes.
Not to be used for:
Caution needed with:
Contains: ECONAZOLE nitrate.
Other preparations: Ecostatin Lotion, Ecostatin Powder, Ecostatin Spray, PEVARYL (Cilag).

Ecostatin-1
(Princeton)

A pessary plus applicator supplied at a strength of 150 mg and used as an antifungal and antibacterial treatment for thrush of the vulva or vagina.

Dose: 1 pessary inserted into the vagina at bed time.
Availability: NHS, private prescription, over the counter.
Side effects: mild burning or irritation.
Caution:
Not to be used for: children.
Caution needed with:
Contains: ECONAZOLE nitrate.
Other preparations: Ecostatin Pessaries, Ecostatin Cream, Ecostatin Twinpack, GYNO-PEVARYL (Cilag).

ecothiopate iodide *see* **Phospholine-Iodide**

Edecrin
(MSD)

A white, scored tablet supplied at a strength of 50 mg and used as a diuretic to treat fluid retention including that associated with congestive heart failure, or kidney or liver disease.

Dose: adults 1 tablet a day after breakfast at first, increasing by ½-1 tablet a day until the minimum effective dose usually of 1-3 tablets a day is found to a maximum of 8 in 2 divided doses; children 2-12 years ½ tablet a day after breakfast, then increasing by ½ tablet a day to the minimum effective dose.
Availability: NHS and private prescription.
Side effects: stomach upset, gout, jaundice, blood changes.
Caution: in pregnant women, and in patients suffering from liver disease, diabetes, enlarged prostate, impaired urination, or gout.
Not to be used for: infants, nursing mothers, or for patients suffering from cirrhosis of the liver, or severe kidney failure.
Caution needed with: LITHIUM, WARFARIN, DIGOXIN, ANTIHYPERTENSIVES, some antibiotics (eg aminoglycosides, cephalosporins).
Contains: ETHACRYNIC ACID.
Other preparations: Edecrin Injection.

Efalith
(Scotia)

An anti-inflammatory ointment used to treat seborrhoeic dermatitis.

Dose: apply thinly and evenly twice a day. Rub in gently.
Availability: NHS and private prescription.
Side effects: irritation.
Caution: in patients suffering from psoriasis. Avoid eyes and mucous membranes.
Not to be used for: children.
Caution needed with:
Contains: LITHIUM SUCCINATE, ZINC SULPHATE.
Other preparations:

Efamast
(Searle)

An oblong, soft capsule supplied at a strength of 40 mg and used to treat breast pain.

Dose: 3-4 capsules twice a day.
Availability: NHS and private prescription.
Side effects: nausea, diarrhoea, headache.
Caution: in patients suffering from epilepsy. Your doctor may suggest detailed breast examination before starting treatment.
Not to be used for: children.
Caution needed with:
Contains: GAMOLENIC ACID.
Other preparations:

Efcortelan *see* Hydrocortisone
(Glaxo)

Effercitrate
(Typharm)

A white, effervescent tablet used as an alkalizing agent to treat cystitis.

Dose: adults and children over 6 years 2 tablets dissolved in water up to 3 times a day with meals; children 1-6 years half adult dose.
Availability: NHS, private prescription, over the counter.
Side effects: raised potassium levels, stomach irritation, mild diuresis.
Caution: in patients suffering from kidney disease.
Not to be used for: infants under 1 year or for patients suffering from ulcerated or blocked small bowel.
Caution needed with: potassium-sparing DIURETICS.
Contains: CITRIC ACID, POTASSIUM BICARBONATE.
Other preparations: Potassium Citrate Mixture.

---

eicosapentaenoic acid *see* Maxepa

Elantan
(Schwarz)

A white, scored tablet supplied at strengths of 10 mg, 20 mg, 40 mg and used as a NITRATE treatment for the prevention of angina, and in addition to other treatments for congestive heart failure.

Dose: 10 mg twice a day at first increasing to 40-80 mg a day in 2 or 3

divided doses after meals to a maximum of 120 mg a day.
Availability: NHS and private prescription.
Side effects: headache, flushes, dizziness.
Caution:
Not to be used for: children.
Caution needed with:
Contains: ISOSORBIDE MONONITRATE.
Other preparations: Elantan LA, IMDUR (Astra), ISIB (Ashbourne) ISMO (Boehringer Mannheim), MCR-50 (Farmitalia), MONIT (Stuart), MONO-CEDOCARD (Farmitalia).

Elavil *see* Tryptizol
(DDSA)

Eldepryl
(Britannia)

A white, scored tablet supplied at strengths of 5 mg, 10 mg and used as an anti-parkinsonian treatment for Parkinson's disease.

Dose: 10 mg a day.
Availability: NHS and private prescription.
Side effects: low blood pressure on standing, involuntary movements, nausea, confusion, mental disorders.
Caution:
Not to be used for: children.
Caution needed with:
Contains: SELEGILINE HYDROCHLORIDE.
Other preparations:

Electrolade *see* Dioralyte
(Nicholas)

Eltroxin
(Evans)

A white, scored tablet or a white tablet according to strengths of 50 micrograms, 100 micrograms and used as a thyroid hormone to treat underactive thyroid gland in adults or children.

Dose: adults 50-100 micrograms a day at first increasing as needed by 50

micrograms a day every 3-4 weeks to a maximum of 100-200 micrograms a day; children 25 micrograms a day at first increasing if needed by 25 micrograms a day every 2-4 weeks and then reduce slightly.
Availability: NHS and private prescription.
Side effects: abnormal rhythms, chest pain, rapid heart rate, muscle cramp, headache, restlessness, excitability, flushing, sweating, diarrhoea, rapid weight loss.
Caution: in nursing mothers and in patients suffering from heart muscle or adrenal weakness.
Not to be used for:
Caution needed with: anticoagulants, TRICYCLICS, PHENYTOIN, CHOLESTYRAMINE.
Contains: anyhdrous SODIUM THYROXINE.
Other preparations:

E

Eludril
(Pierre Fabre)

A solution used as an antibacterial treatment for throat and mouth infections, gingivitis, ulcers.

Dose: dilute 10-15 ml with a-third of a glass of warm water and gargle or rinse the mouth 2-3 times a day.
Availability: NHS, private prescription, over the counter.
Side effects:
Caution:
Not to be used for: children under 6 years.
Caution needed with:
Contains: CHLORHEXIDINE DIGLUCONATE, CHLORBUTOL, CHLOROFORM.
Other preparations: Eludril Spray.

Emblon *see* Nolvadex-D
(Berk)

Emcor
(Merck)

An orange, heart-shaped tablet supplied at a strength of 10 mg and used as a ß-BLOCKER to treat angina, high blood pressure.

Dose: 10 mg once a day to a maximum of 20 mg a day.
Availability: NHS and private prescription.
Side effects: cold hands and feet, sleep disturbance, slow heart rate,

tiredness, wheezing, heart failure, stomach upset, dry eyes, rash.
Caution: in pregnant women, nursing mothers, and in patients suffering from diabetes, kidney or liver disorders, asthma. May need to be withdrawn before surgery. Withdraw gradually. Your doctor may advise additional treatment with DIURETICS or DIGOXIN.
Not to be used for: patients suffering from heart block or failure.
Caution needed with: VERAPAMIL, CLONIDINE withdrawal, some anti-arrhythmic drugs and anaesthetics, some ANTIHYPERTENSIVES, ERGOTAMINE, CIMETIDINE, sedatives, SYMPATHOMIMETICS, INDOMETHACIN, antidiabetics, RESERPINE.
Contains: BISOPROLOL FUMARATE.
Other preparations: Emcor LS, MONOCOR (Lederle).

Emeside
(L.A.B.)

An orange capsule supplied at a strength of 250 mg and used as an anticonvulsant to treat epilepsy.

Dose: adults up to 8 tablets a day; children under 6 years 1-4 tablets a day, 6-12 years as adult dose.
Availability: NHS and private prescription.
Side effects: stomach and brain disturbances, rash, blood changes, SLE (a multisystem disorder).
Caution: in pregnant women, nursing mothers, and in patients suffering from kidney or liver disease. Dose should be reduced gradually.
Not to be used for:
Caution needed with:
Contains: ETHOSUXIMIDE.
Other preparations: Emeside Syrup, ZARONTIN (Parke-Davis).

Emflex
(Merck)

An orange capsule supplied at a strength of 60 mg and used to treat rheumatoid arthritis, osteoarthritis, pain and inflammation after operation.

Dose: 2-3 capsules a day in divided doses, with food, milk, or ANTACID.
Availability: NHS and private prescription.
Side effects: stomach upset, headache, dizziness, fluid retention, chest pain, itching, blood changes, noises in the ears, blurred vision.
Caution: in patients suffering from psychiatric disorder, epilepsy, Parkinson's disease, liver or kidney disorder, congestive heart failure, some infections, body fluid imbalance, and in elderly patients. Your doctor

may advise regular examinations.

Not to be used for: children, pregnant women, nursing mothers, or for patients suffering from stomach ulcer, allergy to ASPIRIN or anti-inflammatory drugs, severe allergy, or with a history of a stomach/intestinal disorder.

Caution needed with: anticoagulants, some painkillers, PROBENECID, LITHIUM, TRIAMTERENE, ACE INHIBITORS, HALOPERIDOL, METHOTREXATE, ß-BLOCKERS, some DIURETICS, FRUSEMIDE.

Contains: ACEMETACIN.

Other preparations:

Emulsidern *see* Diprobath
(Dermal)

---

emulsifying ointment BP

An ointment used as an emollient to treat dry skin conditions.

Dose: apply as required, or use in place of soap.
Availability: NHS, private prescription, over the counter.
Side effects:
Caution:
Not to be used for:
Caution needed with:
Contains: emulsifying ointment BP.
Other preparations:

---

enalapril maleate *see* Innovace, Innozide

Enduron
(Abbott)

A square, pink, scored tablet supplied at a strength of 5 mg and used as a DIURETIC to treat fluid retention, high blood pressure.

Dose: adults ½-1 tablet a day to a maximum of 2 tablets a day; children in proportion to dose for adult of 70 kg bodyweight.
Availability: NHS and private prescription.
Side effects: low potassium levels, rash, sensitivity to light, blood changes, gout, tiredness.
Caution: in pregnant women, nursing mothers, and in patients suffering

from diabetes, gout, or liver or kidney disease. Potassium supplement may be necessary.
Not to be used for: patients suffering from severe kidney failure.
Caution needed with: LITHIUM, DIGOXIN, ANTIHYPERTENSIVES.
Contains: METHYCLOTHIAZIDE.
Other preparations:

---

enoxacin *see* **Comprecin**

Enteromide — sulphonamide to treat intestinal infections. Product now discontinued.

Epanutin
(Parke-Davis)

A white/purple capsule, a white/pink capsule, or a white/orange capsule according to strengths of 25 mg, 50 mg, 100 mg and used as an anticonvulsant to treat epilepsy, neuralgia.

Dose: adults usually 200-500 mg a day; children usually 4-8 mg per kg body weight a day, up to 300 mg a day.
Availability: NHS and private prescription.
Side effects: stomach upset, sleeplessness, unsteadiness, allergies, gum swelling, hairiness and motor activity in young people, blood changes, lymph gland swelling, nystagmus (abnormal eye movements).
Caution: in pregnant women, nursing mothers, and in patients suffering from liver disease. Dose should be reduced gradually. Maintain adequate levels of vitamin D.
Not to be used for:
Caution needed with: COUMARIN anticoagulants, ISONIAZID, CHLORAMPHENICOL, SULTHIAME, the contraceptive pill, DOXYCYCLINE.
Contains: PHENYTOIN sodium.
Other preparations: Epanutin Suspension, Epanutin Infatabs, Epanutin Parenteral.

---

ephedrine *see* **Auralgicin, CAM, Davenol, ephede nasal drops BP, Expurhin, Franol, Haymine**

---

ephedrine nasal drops BP

Drops used to treat congestion in the nose.

Dose: 1-2 drops in each nostril 3-4 times a day when required.
Availability: NHS, private prescription, over the counter.
Side effects: irritation, congestion, and less effect after excessive use.
Caution: in infants under 3 months. Avoid excessive use.
Not to be used for:
Caution needed with:
Contains: EPHEDRINE HYDROCHLORIDE.
Other preparations:

Ephynal
(Roche Nicholas)

A white tablet or a white, scored tablet according to strengths of 10 mg, 50 mg, 200 mg and used as a source of vitamin E to treat vitamin E deficiency, tropical vitamin E deficiency.

Dose: adults 10-15 mg a day; children 1-10 mg per kg body weight a day.
Availability: NHS, private prescription, over the counter.
Side effects:
Caution:
Not to be used for:
Caution needed with:
Contains: TOCOPHERYL ACETATE.
Other preparations: Ephynal Suspension, VITA-E (Bioglan).

Epifoam
(Stafford-Miller)

A foam supplied in an aerosol and used as a STEROID, local anaesthetic treatment for damage to the external genital area, skin disorders.

Dose: apply foam 3-4 times a day (2-3 times a day for skin disorders) with a sterile, non-absorbent pad.
Availability: NHS and private prescription.
Side effects: fluid retention, suppression of adrenal glands, thinning of skin may occur.
Caution: use for short periods of time only.
Not to be used for: patients suffering from infected wounds, or continuously especially in pregnant women.
Caution needed with:
Contains: HYDROCORTISONE acetate, PRAMOXINE hydrochloride.
Other preparations:

Epifrin *see* **Eppy.** Product now discontinued.

Epilim
(Sanofi Winthrop)

A lilac tablet supplied at strengths of 200 mg, 500 mg and used as an anticonvulsant to treat epilepsy.

Dose: adults 600 mg a day at first in 2 divided doses then increase by 200 mg every 3 days usually to 1-2 g a day and a maximum of 2.5 g a day; children under 20 kg body weight 20 mg per kg a day at first, over 20 kg 400 mg a day at first, increasing gradually to 40 mg per kg a day if needed.
Availability: NHS and private prescription.
Side effects: gain in weight, loss of hair, fluid retention, pancreatitis, liver failure, blood changes, neurological effects.
Caution: in pregnant women, in patients suffering from mental retardation, or who are undergoing major surgery.
Not to be used for: patients suffering from liver disease.
Caution needed with: antidepressants, other anticonvulsants, anticoagulants.
Contains: SODIUM VALPROATE.
Other preparations: Epilim Crushable, Epilim Syrup, Epilim Liquid, ORLEPT (CP Pharm).

Epinal — sympathomimetic/lubricant used to treat glaucoma. Product now discontinued.

Epogam
(Searle)

An oil-filled capsule supplied at a strength of 40 mg and used to relieve the symptoms of eczema.

Dose: adults 4-6 capsules twice a day; children over 1 year, 2-4 capsules twice a day.
Availability: NHS and private prescription.
Side effects: nausea, headache.
Caution: in patients suffering from epilepsy.
Not to be used for: children under 1 year.
Caution needed with:
Contains: GAMOLENIC ACID.
Other preparations: Epogam Paediatric.

227

Eppy
(SNP)

Drops used as a SYMPATHOMIMETIC to treat glaucoma.

Dose: 1 drop into the eye 1-2 times a day.
Availability: NHS, private prescription, over the counter.
Side effects: pain in the eye, headache, skin reactions, melanosis, red eye, rarely systemic effects.
Caution:
Not to be used for: patients suffering from absence of the lens, narrow-angle glaucoma.
Caution needed with: MAOIS, TRICYCLIC antidepressants
Contains: ADRENALINE.
Other preparations: SIMPLENE (SNP).

Equagesic
(Wyeth)

A pink/white/yellow tablet used as an opiate, ANALGESIC, and muscle relaxant to control pain in muscles or bones.

Dose: 2 tablets 3-4 times a day.
Availability: controlled drug; private prescription only.
Side effects: drowsiness, dizziness, nausea, unsteadiness, rash, blood changes.
Caution: in the elderly in patients with a history of epilepsy, or suffering from depression, suicidal behaviour, or liver disease.
Not to be used for: pregnant women, or for patients suffering from porphyria (a rare blood disorder), alcoholism, stomach ulcer, haemophilia, kidney disease, allergy to anti-inflammatory drugs or ASPIRIN.
Caution needed with: alcohol, sedatives, anticoagulants, antidiabetics, uric acid-lowering agents.
Contains: ETHOHEPTAZINE, MEPROBAMATE, ASPIRIN.
Other preparations:

Equanil
(Wyeth)

A white tablet or a white, scored tablet according to strengths of 200 mg, 400 mg and used as a tranquillizer for short-term treatment of anxiety, muscular tension.

Dose: elderly 200 mg 3 times a day; adults 400 mg 3 times a day and before going to bed.

Availability: controlled drug; NHS and private prescription.
Side effects: brain and stomach disturbances disturbances, low blood pressure, pins and needles, allergy, excitement, blood disorders.
Caution: in pregnant women, nursing mothers, and in patients with a history of epilepsy or depression, or patients suffering from liver or kidney disease. Patients should be warned that the drug is addictive
Not to be used for: alcoholics or for patients suffering from acute intermittent porphyria (a rare blood disorder).
Caution needed with: alcohol, sedatives, anticoagulants, PHENYTOIN, GRISEOFULVIN, RIFAMPICIN, STEROIDS taken by mouth, contraceptive pill, some antidepressants.
Contains: MEPROBAMATE.
Other preparations: MEPRATE (DDSA).

Eradacin
(Sanofi Winthrop)

A red/yellow capsule supplied at a strength of 150 mg and used as an antibiotic to treat acute gonorrhoea.

Dose: 2 capsules as a single dose.
Availability: NHS and private prescription.
Side effects: stomach upset, headache, dizziness, drowsiness.
Caution: in pregnant women and in patients suffering from liver or kidney disease.
Not to be used for: children.
Caution needed with:
Contains: ACROSOXACIN.
Other preparations:

---

ergotamine tartrate *see* **Cafergot, Lingraine, Medihaler-Ergotamine, Migril**

Erycen *see* **Erythrocin**
(Berk)

Erymax *see* **Erythrocin**
(Park-Davis)

Erythrocin
(Abbott)

A white, oblong tablet supplied at strengths of 250 mg, 500 mg and used as an antibiotic to treat infections, including acne.

Dose: 1-2 g a day.
Availability: NHS and private prescription.
Side effects: stomach disturbances, allergies.
Caution: in patients suffering from liver disease.
Not to be used for: children.
Caution needed with: THEOPHYLLINE, anticoagulants taken by mouth, CARBAMAZEPINE, DIGOXIN, TERFENADINE, ASTEMIZOLE.
Contains: ERYTHROMYCIN stearate.
Other preparations: Erythrocin IV Lactobionate, ARPIMYCIN, ERYCEN (Berk), ERYMAX (Parke-Davis), ERYTHROMID (Abbott), ERYTHROPED A (Abbott), ILOSONE (Dista), ILOTYCIN, RETCIN (DDSA), RONMIX (Ashbourne).

Erythromid *see* Erythrocin
(Abbott)

---

erythromycin *see* Erythrocin, Stiemycin, Stromba, Zineryt

Erythroped *see* Erythrocin

Esbatal *see* Bendogen. Product now discontinued.

Esidrex
(Ciba)

A white, scored tablet supplied at strengths of 25 mg, 50 mg, and used as a DIURETIC to treat fluid retention and high blood pressure.

Dose: adults, 25-100 mg once a day after breakfast, reducing to 25-50 mg on alternate days; children as advised by your doctor.
Availability: NHS and private prescription.
Side effects: low potassium levels, rash, sensitivity to light, blood changes, gout, tiredness.
Caution: in pregnant women, nursing mothers, and in patients suffering from gout, diabetes, liver or kidney damage. Potassium supplements may

be needed.
Not to be used for: patients suffering from severe kidney or liver disease, Addison's disease.
Caution needed with: LITHIUM, DIGOXIN, ANTIHYPERTENSIVES.
Contains: HYDROCHLOROTHIAZIDE.
Other preparations: HYDROSALURIC (MSD).

Esidrex K — DIURETIC and potassium supplement. Product now discontinued.

Eskamel
(S K B)

A cream used as a skin softener to treat acne.

Dose: apply a little to the affected area once a day.
Availability: NHS, private prescription, over the counter.
Side effects: irritation.
Caution: keep out of the eyes, nose, and mouth.
Not to be used for: patients suffering from acute local infection.
Caution needed with:
Contains: RESORCINOL, SULPHUR.
Other preparations:

Eskazole
(SKB)

A pale orange, rounded, oblong, scored tablet supplied at a strength of 400 mg and used to treat hydatid cysts.

Dose: 2 tablets a day in divided doses for 28 days, followed by 14 days without treatment.
Availability: NHS and private prescription.
Side effects: stomach upset, headache, dizziness, reversible hair loss, rash, fever, severe allergy, convulsions, brain irritation.
Caution: in patients under 60 kg body weight. Women of child-bearing age must use non-hormonal contraceptive measures during treatment and for 1 month afterwards. Your doctor may advise regular liver and blood tests.
Not to be used for: pregnant women, women who may become pregnant, children under 6 years.
Caution needed with:
Contains: ALBENDAZOLE

Other preparations:

Eskornade Spansule
(S K B)

A grey/clear capsule used as an ANTIHISTAMINE and SYMPATHOMIMETIC to treat congestion, running nose, and phlegm brought on by common cold, rhinitis, flu, sinusitis.

Dose: adults 1 capsule every 12 hours; children use syrup.
Availability: private prescription and over the counter.
Side effects: drowsiness.
Caution: in patients suffering from diabetes.
Not to be used for: patients suffering from cardiovascular problems, overactive thyroid gland.
Caution needed with: MAOIS, TRICYCLICS, sedatives, alcohol.
Contains: PHENYLPROPANOLAMINE HYDROCHLORIDE, DIPHENYLPYRALINE HYDROCHLORIDE.
Other preparations: Eskornade Syrup.

Estracombi *see* Estrapak

Estraderm
(Ciba)

A patch supplied at strengths of 25 micrograms, 50 micrograms, 100 micrograms and used as an oestrogen in oestrogen replacement therapy during the menopause. (Estraderm 50 used to prevent osteoporosis.)

Dose: apply a 50 microgram patch at first to a clean, hairless area of skin below the waist and replace with a new patch every 3-4 days on a different place. Adjust the dose as needed after 1 month to a maximum of 100 micrograms a day.
Availability: NHS and private prescription.
Side effects: headache, nausea, tender breasts, redness at the site of the patch, rashes, skin changes, liver function disorders, sodium retention.
Caution: in patients suffering from high blood pressure, kidney or heart disease, asthma, varicose veins, epilepsy, diabetes, thyroid disease, womb disease. Your doctor may advise that your blood pressure, breasts, pelvic organs should be checked regularly.
Not to be used for: pregnant women, nursing mothers, or for patients suffering from severe liver or kidney disease, breast, genital tract, or other oestrogen-dependent cancers, genital bleeding, some ear disorders, or a

history of or tendency towards thrombophlebitis, thromoboembolic diseases, cerebrovascular disease, sickle cell anaemia, porphyria, (a rare blood disorder).
Caution needed with: liver enzyme-inducing drugs (such as BARBITURATES, anti-epileptics), DIURETICS, ANTIHYPERTENSIVES.
Contains: OESTRADIOL.
Other preparations: CLIMAVAL (Sandoz), PROGYNOVA (Schering), ZUMENON (Duphar).

Estrapak
(Ciba)

A patch plus a red tablet supplied at strengths of 50 microgram and 1 mg respectively and used as oestrogen and progestogen in hormone replacement.

Dose: place patch on a clean, hairless are of skin below the waist and replace with a new patch every 3-4 days on a different area. 1 tablet a day from the fifteenth to the twenty-sixth days of each 28 days of oestrogen replacement. Start the treatment on the fifth day of the period if present.
Availability: NHS and private prescription.
Side effects: headache, nausea, tender breasts, redness at site of patch, rashes, skin changes, liver function disorders, sodium retention.
Caution: in patients with breast disease or a family history of breast cancer, high blood pressure, cholelithiasis (gallstones), kidney or heart disease, asthma, varicose veins, epilepsy, migraine, diabetes, thyroid disease, womb disease. Your doctor may advise that your blood pressure, breasts, pelvic organs should be checked regularly.
Not to be used for: children, pregnant women, nursing mothers or for patients suffering from severe liver or kidney disease, breast, genital tract, or other oestrogen-dependent cancers, genital bleeding, some ear disorders, or a history of or tendency towards thrombophlebitis, thromboembolic disorders, or cerebrovascular disease, sickle cell anaemia, porphyria (a rare blood disorder).
Caution needed with: liver enzyme-inducing drugs (such as BARBITURATES, anti-epileptics), DIURETICS, ANTIHYPERTENSIVES.
Contains: OESTRADIOL, NORETHISTERONE.
Other preparations: ESTRACOMBI, TRISEQUENS (Nova Nordisk).

---

ethacrynic acid *see* **Edecrin**

---

ethambutol *see* **Myambutol, Mynah**

E

ethamsylate see Dicynene

ethinyloestradiol *see* **BiNovum, Brevinor, Cilest, Conova 30, Controvlar, Dianette, ethinyloestradiol tablets, Eugynon 30, Femodene, Femodene ED, Loestrin 20, Logynon, Logynon ED, Marvelon, Mercilon, Microgynon 30, Minilyn, Minulet, Neocon 1/35, Norimin, Ovran, Ovranette, Ovysmen, PC4, Synphase, Tri-Minulet, Trinordiol, Trinovum, Trinovum-ED**

ethinyloestradiol tablets

White, round tablets supplied at strengths of 10 micrograms, 50 micrograms, and 1 mg, and used as an oestrogen treatment for menopausal symptoms, breast cancer.

Dose: for menopausal symptoms, 10-20 micrograms a day continuously or for 21 days, repeated after 7 days. Additional progestogen treatment may be necessary. For breast cancer, as advised by doctor.
Availability: NHS and private prescription.
Side effects: enlarged breasts, fluid retention, nausea, vaginal bleeding, weight gain, skin changes, liver disorders, jaundice, rashes, vomiting, headaches.
Caution: in patients suffering from high blood pressure, diabetes, heart disease, vascular disorders, asthma, kidney disease, epilepsy, womb diseases, thyroid disorder. Your doctor may advise you to have regular examinations.
Not to be used for: pregnant women, nursing mothers, or for patients suffering from sickle-cell anaemia, thrombosis, liver disorders, some cancers, undiagnosed vaginal bleeding, some ear, skin, and kidney disorders, jaundice, porphyria (a rare blood disorder), brain blood vessel disease.
Caution needed with: DIURETICS, ANTIHYPERTENSIVES, drugs which induce liver enzymes (eg BARBITURATES, CARBAMAZEPINE, PHENYTOIN, RIFAMPICIN).
Contains: ETHINYLOESTRADIOL.
Other preparations:

ethoheptazine *see* **Equagesic**

ethosuximide *see* **Emeside, Zarontin**

ethyl nicotinate *see* **Transvasin**

ethyl salicylate *see* **Dubam**

ethynodiol diacetate *see* **Conova 30**

etidronate disodium *see* **Didronel**

etodolac *see* **Lodine**

etretinate *see* **Tigason**

Eudemine — vasodilator/blood sugar elevator to treat high blood pressure. Product now discontinued.

Euglucon *see* **Daonil**
(Roussel)

Eugynon 30
(Schering)

A white tablet used as an oestrogen, progestogen contraceptive.

Dose: 1 tablet a day for 21 days starting on day 5 of the period.
Availability: NHS and private prescription.
Side effects: enlarged breasts, bloating and fluid retention, cramps, leg pains, mood change, reduction in sexual desire, headaches, nausea, vaginal erosion, discharge, and bleeding, weight gain, skin changes.
Caution: in patients suffering from high blood pressure, diabetes, vascular disorders, asthma, depression, kidney disease, multiple sclerosis, womb diseases. Your doctor may advise you not to smoke, to have regular examinations. You should stop treatment at the first sign of serious symptoms such as severe headache or jaundice. Treatment should be stopped before surgery.

Not to be used for: pregnant women, or for patients suffering from sickle-cell anaemia, history of heart disease or thrombosis, liver disorders, some cancers, undiagnosed vaginal bleeding, some ear, skin, and kidney disorders.

Caution needed with: RIFAMPICIN, TETRACYCLINES, GRISEOFULVIN, BARBITURATES, PHENYTOIN, PRIMIDONE, CARBAMAZEPINE, ETHOSUXIMIDE, CHLORAL HYDRATE, DICHLORALPHENAZONE.

Contains: ETHINYLOESTRADIOL, LEVONORGESTEROL.

Other preparations:

Euhypnos *see* Normison
(Farmitalia CE)

Eumovate Drops
(Glaxo)

Drops used as a STEROID treatment for inflammation of the eyes where there is no infection present.

Dose: 1-2 drops into the eye 4 times a day or every 1-2 hours for severe inflammation.
Availability: NHS and private prescription.
Side effects: rise in eye pressure, sensitization, resistance to NEOMYCIN, fungal infection, cataract, thinning cornea.
Caution: in pregnant women and infants — do not use for extended periods. Avoid using unnecessarily for any patients.
Not to be used for: patients suffering from glaucoma, dendritic ulcer, viral, fungal, tubercular, or weeping infections, or for patients who wear soft contact lenses.
Caution needed with:
Contains: CLOBETASONE BUTYRATE.
Other preparations: Eumovate-N (with NEOMYCIN for infected conditions).

Eumovate Cream
(Glaxo)

A cream used as a STEROID treatment for mild eczema and other skin disorders.

Dose: apply to the affected area 1-4 times a day.
Availability: NHS and private prescription.
Side effects: fluid retention, suppression of adrenal glands, thinning of the skin may occur.

Caution: use for short periods of time only.
Not to be used for: patients suffering from acne or any other skin infections caused by tuberculosis, ringworm, viruses, or fungi, or continuously especially in pregnant women.
Caution needed with:
Contains: CLOBETASONE BUTYRATE.
Other preparations: Eumovate Ointment.

Eurax
(Geigy)

A lotion used as a scabicide to treat scabies and itchy skin conditions.

Dose: scabies: apply to the body apart from the head and face after a hot bath; repeat after 24 hours and wash off the next day. Itching; apply when required.
Availability: NHS, private prescription, over the counter.
Side effects:
Caution: keep out of the eyes, and avoid areas of broken skin.
Not to be used for: patients suffering from acute exudative dermatitis.
Caution needed with:
Contains: CROTAMITON.
Other preparations: Eurax Cream.

Eurax-Hydrocortisone
(Zyma)

A cream used as a STEROID and anti-itch treatment for itching skin disorders.

Dose: apply to the affected area 2-3 times a day for 10-14 days (7 days if one face).
Availability: NHS and private prescription.
Side effects: fluid retention, suppression of adrenal glands, thinning of the skin may occur.
Caution: use for short periods of time only.
Not to be used for: patients suffering from acne or any other skin infections caused by tuberculosis, ringworm, viruses, ulcerated or weeping skin conditions, fungi, or continuously especially in pregnant women.
Caution needed with:
Contains: CROTAMITON, HYDROCORTISONE.
Other preparations:

Evacode *see* **Galcodine**
(Evans)

Evadyne
(Wyeth)

An orange tablet supplied at a strength of 25 mg and used as a TRICYCLIC antidepressant to treat depression.

Dose: 25 mg 3 times a day at first increasing if needed by 25 mg a day or every other day to a maximum of 100-150 mg a day, then 25 mg 3 times a day.
Availability: NHS and private prescription.
Side effects: dry mouth, constipation, urine retention, blurred vision, palpitations, drowsiness, sleeplessness, dizziness, hands shaking, low blood presure, weight change, skin reactions, jaundice or blood changes, loss of libido may occur.
Caution: in nursing mothers or in patients suffering from heart disease, thyroid disease, epilepsy, glaucoma, urinary retention, adrenal tumour, diabetes, some other psychiatric conditions. Your doctor may advise regular blood tests.
Not to be used for: children, pregnant women, or patients suffering from heart attacks, liver disease, heart block.
Caution needed with: alcohol, ANTICHOLINERGICS, adrenaline, MAOIS, BARBITURATES, other antidepressants, ANTIHYPERTENSIVES, CIMETIDINE, oestrogens.
Contains: BUTRYPTILINE HYDROCHLORIDE.
Other preparations:

Evaphol *see* **Galenphol**
(Evans)

Evoxin *see* **Motilium.** Product now discontinued.

Exelderm
(ICI)

A cream used as an antifungal treatment for fungal infections of the skin.

Dose: rub into the affected area twice a day for 2-3 weeks after the wounds have healed.

Availability: NHS and private prescription.
Side effects: irritation
Caution: keep out of the eyes; if the area becomes irritated, the treatment should be stopped.
Not to be used for:
Caution needed with:
Contains: SULCONAZOLE nitrate.
Other preparations:

Exirel
(3M Healthcare)

An olive green/turquoise-blue capsule or a beige/turquoise-blue capsule according to strengths of 10 mg, 15 mg and used as a broncho-dilator to treat bronchial spasm brought on by bronchial asthma, bronchitis, emphysema.

Dose: 10-15 mg 3-4 times a day up to a maximum of 60 mg a day.
Availability: NHS and private prescription.
Side effects: shaking of the hands, nervous tension, headache, dilation of the blood vessels.
Caution: in pregnant women and in patients suffering from high blood pressure, abnormal heart rhythms, angina, heart muscle disease, overactive thyroid.
Not to be used for: children.
Caution needed with: SYMPATHOMIMETICS.
Contains: PIRBUTEROL hydrochloride.
Other preparations: Exirel Inhaler. (Exirel Syrup — now discontinued.)

Exolan
(Dermal)

A cream used as an antipsoriatic treatment for psoriasis.

Dose: apply to the affected area 1-2 times a day.
Availability: NHS, private prescription, over the counter.
Side effects: irritation, allergy.
Caution:
Not to be used for: patients suffering from acute psoriasis.
Caution needed with:
Contains: DITHRANOL triacetate.
Other preparations: ALPHODITH (Stafford Miller), ANTHRANOL (Stiefel), DITHROCREAM (Dermal), PSORADRATE (Norwich Eaton) — some not available over the counter.

Expelix
(Cupal)

A liquid used to treat threadworms or roundworms.

Dose: adults, 15 ml a day for 7 days (threadworm), or 30 ml as a single dose (roundworm); children, 5-10 ml a day for 7 days (threadworm), or 10-25 ml as a single dose (roundworm) according to age. Treatment for roundworm should be repeated after 14 days.
Availability: NHS, private prescription, over the counter.
Side effects: nausea, vomiting, stomach pain, diarrhoea, allergy, breathing difficulty, ulceration of skin and eyes, dizziness, lack of co-ordination, drowsiness, confusion, muscle contractions.
Caution: in pregnant women and in patients suffering from epilepsy, liver or kidney disease, nervous diseases.
Not to be used for: children under 2 years (threadworm treatment), children under 1 year (roundworm treatment), or for patients with severe kidney disease.
Caution needed with: PYRANTEL.
Contains: PIPERAZINE HYDRATE.
Other preparations: PRIPSEN (Reckitt & Colman).

Expulin
(Galen)

A linctus used as an ANTIHISTAMINE, opiate, and SYMPATHOMIMETIC treatment for cough and congestion.

Dose: adults 10 ml 4 times a day; children 2-6 years 2.5-5 ml 4 times a day; 7-12 years 5-10 ml 4 times a day.
Availability: private prescription and over the counter.
Side effects: constipation, drowsiness, reduced reactions, anxiety, hands shaking, irregular or rapid heart rate, dry mouth, excitement, rarely skin eruptions.
Caution: in patients suffering from asthma, kidney disease, diabetes.
Not to be used for: children under 2 years or for patients suffering from liver disease, heart or thyroid isorders.
Caution needed with: MAOIS, alcohol, sedatives, TRICYCLICS.
Contains: PHOLCODINE, PSEUDOEPHEDRINE HYDROCHLORIDE, CHLORPHENIRAMINE HYDROCHLORIDE, CHLORPHENIRAMINE MALEATE.
Other preparations: Expulin Paediatric.

Expurhin
(Galen)

A linctus used as an ANTIHISTAMINE and SYMPATHOMIMETIC treatment for congestion, phlegm, and running nose in children.

Dose: 3 months-1 year 2.5-5 ml twice a day, 1-5 years 5-10 ml 3 times a day, 6-12 years 10-15 ml 3 times a day.
Availability: private prescription and over the counter.
Side effects: drowsiness, reduced reactions, anxiety, hands shaking, irregular or rapid heart rate, dry mouth, excitement, rarely skin eruptions.
Caution: in patients suffering from liver or kidney disease, diabetes.
Not to be used for: infants under 3 months, or for patients suffering from heart or thyroid disorders.
Caution needed with: alcohol, sedatives, some antidepressants (MAOIS), TRICYCLICS.
Contains: EPHEDRINE HYDROCHLORIDE, CHLORPHENIRAMINE MALEATE, MENTHOL.
Other preparations:

Exterol
(Dermal)

Drops used as a wax softener to remove ear wax.

Dose: hold 5-10 drops in the ear 1-2 times a day for 3-4 days.
Availability: NHS, private prescription, over the counter.
Side effects: slight fizzing.
Caution:
Not to be used for: patients suffering from perforated ear drum.
Caution needed with:
Contains: urea hydrogen peroxide, glycerin.
Other preparations:

F

Fabahistin
(Bayer)

An orange tablet supplied at a strength of 50 mg and used as an ANTIHISTAMINE to treat rhinitis, hay fever, other allergies.

Dose: 1-2 tablet 3 times a day.
Availability: NHS and private prescription.
Side effects: drowsiness, reduced reactions, rarely blood changes.
Caution:
Not to be used for: children.
Caution needed with: sedatives, MAOIS, alcohol.
Contains: MEBHYDROLIN.
Other preparations:

Fabrol
(Zyma)

A sachet of granules of 200 mg used as a protein to treat bronchitis, infections of the respiratory tract where phlegm is produced, complications in the abdomen associated with cystic fibrosis.

Dose: up to 6 sachets a day.
Availability: NHS in some circumstances (when prescribed as a generic), private prescription.
Side effects: nausea, heartburn, vomiting, headache, tinnitus, allergy, rarely bronchial spasm.
Caution: in patients suffering from diabetes.
Not to be used for:
Caution needed with:
Contains: ACETYLCYSTEINE.
Other preparations:

---

famotidine *see* Pepcid PM

Fansidar
(Roche)

A white, quarter-scored tablet used as a sulphonamide for the prevention and treatment of malaria.

Dose: prevention adults and children over 14 years 1 tablet a week, treatment 2-3 tablets as one dose or as advised by the physician; prevention children under 4 years quarter adult dose, treatment ½ tablet as one dose; prevention children 4-8 years half adult dose, treatment 1 tablet as one dose; prevention children 9-14 years three-quarters adult dose, treatment 2 tablets as one dose.
Availability: NHS and private prescription.
Side effects: rash, inflammation of the pharynx, itch, stomach upset, rare skin and blood changes.
Caution: patients should keep out of the sun. Your doctor may advise regular blood tests if the treatment is prolonged.
Not to be used for: new-born infants, pregnant women, nursing mothers or for patients suffering from severe kidney or liver disease, or sensitivity to sulphonamides.
Caution needed with: TRIMETHOPRIM.
Contains: SULFADOXINE, PYRIMETHAMINE.
Other preparations:

Farlutal *see* **Provera**
(Farmitalia CE)

Fasigyn
(Pfizer)

A white tablet supplied at a strength of 500 mg and used as an antibiotic for the treament and prevention of infection.

Dose: prevention 4 tablets as a single dose, treatment 4 tablets at first then 2 tablets a day for at least 5-6 days.
Availability: NHS and private prescription.
Side effects: stomach upset, furred tongue, unpleasant taste, swelling and brain disturbances, dark-coloured urine, rash.
Caution: in pregnant women and nursing mothers.
Not to be used for: children or for patients suffering from nervous disorders, blood changes. Your doctor may advise regular blood tests
Caution needed with: alcohol.
Contains: TINIDAZOLE.
Other preparations:

F

Faverin
(Duphar)

A yellow tablet supplied at a strength of 50 mg and used as an antidepressant to treat depression.

Dose: 2 tablets in the evening at first then usually 2-4 tablets a day in divided doses, up to a maximum of 6 tablets a day if needed.
Availability: NHS and private prescription.
Side effects: nausea, vomiting, sleepiness, diarrhoea, agitation, anorexia, tremor, convulsions
Caution: in patients suffering from liver or kidney disease.
Not to be used for: children, pregnant women, nursing mothers, or for patients with a history of epilepsy.
Caution needed with: PROPANOLOL, THEOPHYLLINE, PHENYTOIN, WARFARIN, MAOIS, alcohol, LITHIUM, TRYPTOPHAN.
Contains: FLUVOXAMINE MALEATE.
Other preparations:

Fectrim *see* **Septrin**
(DDSA)

Fefol Spansule
(S K B)

A clear/green capsule used for the prevention of iron and folic acid deficiency in pregnancy.

Dose: 1 capsule a day.
Availability: NHS, private prescription, over the counter.
Side effects: mild stomach upset.
Caution:
Not to be used for: children.
Caution needed with: TETRACYCLINES, LEVODOPA, PENICILLAMINE, ANTACIDS.
Contains: FERROUS SULPHATE, FOLIC ACID.
Other preparations: FERROGRAD FOLIC (Abott), SLOW FE FOLIC (Ciba)

Fefol Z Spansule
(S K B)

A clear/blue capsule used for the prevention of iron and folic acid deficiency in pregnancy where zinc supplement is also needed.

Dose: 1 capsule a day.
Availability: NHS, private prescription, over the counter.
Side effects: mild stomach upset.
Caution: in patients suffering from kidney disease.
Not to be used for: children.
Caution needed with: TETRACYCLINES, LEVODOPA, PENICILLAMINE, ANTACIDS.
Contains: FERROUS SULPHATE, FOLIC ACID, ZINC SULPHATE MONOHYDRATE.
Other preparations:

Fefol-Vit Spansule
(S K B)

A white/clear capsule used for the prevention of iron, folic acid, and vitamin deficiency in pregnancy.

Dose: 1 capsule a day.
Availability: private prescription and over the counter.
Side effects: mild stomach upset.
Caution:
Not to be used for: children.
Caution needed with: TETRACYCLINES, LEVODOPA, PENICILLAMINE, ANTACIDS.
Contains: FERROUS SULPHATE, FOLIC ACID, THIAMINE mononitrate, RIBOFLAVINE, PYRIDOXINE hydrochloride, NICOTINAMIDE, ASCORBIC ACID.
Other preparations: GIVITOL (Galen).

felbinac *see* **Traxam**

Feldene
(Pfizer)

A maroon/blue capsule or a maroon capsule according to strengths of 10 mg, 20 mg and used as a NON-STEROID ANTI-INFLAMMATORY DRUG to treat rheumatoid arthritis, osteoarthritis, ankylosing spondylitis, acute muscle or bone problems, acute gout, juvenile chronic arthritis.

Dose: adults 20 mg a day; for muscle or bone problems 40 mg a day for 2 days at first then 20 mg a day for 5-12 days; for gout 40 mg a day for 4-6 days. Children over 6 years and under 15 kg body weight 5 mg, 16-25 kg 10 mg, 26-45 kg 15 mg, over 46 kg 20 mg (all daily).
Availability: NHS and private prescription.
Side effects: stomach disturbances, swelling, brain disturbances, feeling of being unwell, tinnitus, skin reactions.
Caution: in pregnant women, nursing mothers, and in patients suffering from kidney or liver disease.
Not to be used for: patients suffering from anti-inflammatory- or ASPIRIN-induced allergy, stomach ulcer, history of recurring ulcers, recent anal inflammation.
Caution needed with: anticoagulants, other NON-STEROID ANTI-INFLAMMATORY DRUGS, antidiabetics, LITHIUM.
Contains: PIROXICAM.
Other preparations: Feldene Dispersible, Feldene Gel, Feldene Melt, Feldene Suppositories, Feldene Injection IM, PIROZIP (Ashbourne).

Felodipine *see* Plendil

Femerital — antispasmodic and ANALGESIC to relieve period pain. Product now discontinued.

Femodene
(Schering)

A white tablet used as an oestrogen, progestogen contraceptive.

Dose: 1 tablet a day for 21 days starting on day 1 of the period.
Availability: NHS and private prescription.
Side effects: enlarged breasts, bloating and fluid retention, cramps, leg

pains, mood change, reduction in sexual desire, headaches, nausea, vaginal erosion, discharge, and bleeding, weight gain, skin changes.
Caution: in patients suffering from high blood pressure, diabetes, vascular disorders, asthma, depression, kidney disease, multiple sclerosis, womb diseases. Your doctor may advise you not to smoke, to have regular examinations. You should stop treatment at the first sign of serious symptoms such as severe headache or jaundice. Treatment should be stopped before surgery.
Not to be used for: pregnant women, or for patients suffering from sickle-cell anaemia, history of heart disease or thrombosis, liver disorders, some cancers, undiagnosed vaginal bleeding, some ear, skin, and kidney disorders.
Caution needed with: RIFAMPICIN, TETRACYCLINES, GRISEOFULVIN, BARBITURATES, PHENYTOIN, PRIMIDONE, CARBAMAZEPINE, ETHOSUXIMIDE, CHLORAL HYDRATE, DICHLORALPHENAZONE.
Contains: ETHINYLOESTRADIOL, GESTODENE.
Other preparations: MINULET (Wyeth).

F Femodene ED
(Schering)

White tablets use as an oestrogen, progestogen contraceptive.

Dose: 1 tablet a day, starting on day 1 of period.
Availability: NHS and private prescription.
Side effects: enlarged breasts, bloating and fluid retention, cramps, leg pains, mood change, reduction in sexual desire, headaches, nausea, vaginal erosion, discharge and bleeding, weight gain, skin changes.
Caution: in patients suffering from high blood pressure, diabetes, vascular disorders, asthma, depression, kidney disease, multiple sclerosis, womb diseases. Your doctor may advise you not to smoke, and to have regular examinations. You should stop treatment at the first sign of serious symptoms such as severe headache or jaundice. Treatment should be stopped before surgery.
Not to be used for: pregnant women, or for patients suffering from sickle-cell anaemia, history of heart disease, or thombosis, liver disorders, some cancers, undiagnosed vaginal bleeding, some ear, skin, and kidney disorders.
Caution needed with: RIFAMPICIN, TETRACYCLINES, GRISEOFULVIN, BARBITURATES, PHENYTOIN, PRIMIDONE, CARBAMAZEPINE, ETHOSUXIMIDE, CHLORAL HYDRATE, DICHLORALPHENAZONE.
Contains: ETHINYLOESTRADIOL, GESTODENE, LACTOSE.
Other preparations:

Femulen
(Gold Cross)

A white tablet used as a progesterone contraceptive.

Dose: 1 tablet at the same time every day starting on day 1 of the period.
Availability: NHS and private prescription.
Side effects: irregular bleeding, breast discomfort, acne, headache, ovarian cyst.
Caution: in patients suffering from high blood pressure, tendency to thrombosis, migraine, liver abnormalities, ovarian cysts, some cancers. Your doctor may advise regular check-ups.
Not to be used for: pregnant women, or for patients suffering from severe heart or artery disease, benign liver tumours, vaginal bleeding, previous ectopic pregnancy.
Caution needed with: BARBITURATES, PHENYTOIN, PRIMIDONE, CARBAMAZEPINE, CHLORAL HYDRATE, DICHLORALPHENAZONE, ETHOSUXIMIDE, RIFAMPICIN, GLUTETHIMIDE, CHLORPROMAZINE, MEPROBAMATE, GRISEOFULVIN.
Contains: ETHYNODIOL DIACETATE.
Other preparations:

F

Fenbid Spansule
(S K B)

A pink/maroon capsule supplied at a strength of 300 mg and used as a NON-STEROID ANTI-INFLAMMATORY DRUG to treat pain, rheumatoid arthritis, osteoarthritis, ankylosing spondylitis, other joint diorders.

Dose: 2 capsules twice a day at first, then 3 capsules twice a day if needed, usually 1-2 capsules twice a day.
Availability: NHS and private prescription.
Side effects: dyspepsia, gastro-intestinal bleeding, rash, blood changes.
Caution: in pregnant women, and in patients suffering from heart failure, liver, kidney, or gastro-intestinal disease.
Not to be used for: children or patients suffering from asthma, stomach ulcer, or allergy to aspirin or anti-inflammatory drugs.
Caution needed with:
Contains: IBUPROFEN.
Other preparations: APSIFEN (APS), BRUFEN (Boots), EBUFAC (DDSA), IBUFHALAL (Halal), JUNIFEN (Boots), LIDIFEN (Berk), MOTRIN (Upjohn), PAXOFEN (Steinhard). Other brands are available over the counter (200 mg strength only).

fenbufen *see* **Lederfen**

fenchone *see* **Rowatinex**

---

fenfluramine *see* **Ponderax Pacaps**

---

fenofibrate *see* **Lipantil**

---

fenoprofen *see* **Fenopron**

Fenopron
(Dista)

An orange, oval tablet or orange, oblong, scored tablet according to strengths of 300 mg, 600 mg and used as a NON-STEROID ANTI-INFLAMMATORY DRUG to treat pain, rheumatoid arthritis, osteoarthritis, ankylosing spondylitis.

Dose: 300-600 mg 3-4 times a day to a maximum of 3 g a day.
Availability: NHS and private prescription.
Side effects: stomach intolerance, allergy, kidney and liver disorders, blood changes.
Caution: in the elderly, pregnant women, nursing mothers, and in patients with a history of stomach ulcer or stomach bleeding, or suffering from asthma, liver disease, or heart failure.
Not to be used for: children or for patients suffering from stomach ulcer, kidney disease, or allergy to ASPIRIN or anti-inflammatory drugs.
Caution needed with: anticoagulants, ASPIRIN, hydantoins, antidiabetics.
Contains: FENOPROFEN.
Other preparations: PROGESIC (Eli Lilly)

Fenostil Retard
(Zyma)

A white tablet supplied at a strength of 2.5 mg and used as an ANTIHISTAMINE treatment for rhinitis, urticaria, hay fever, other allergies.

Dose: 1 tablet night and morning.
Availability: NHS, private prescription, over the counter.
Side effects: drowsiness, reduced reactions.
Caution: in nursing mothers.
Not to be used for: children.

Caution needed with: sedatives, MAOIS, alcohol.
Contains: DIMETHINDENE maleate.
Other preparations:

---

fenoterol *see* Berotec, Duovent

Fentazin
(Evans)

A white tablet supplied at strengths of 2 mg, 4 mg and used as a sedative to treat anxiety, tension, chronic mental disorders, schizophrenia, vomiting, nausea, and other psychiatric problems.

Dose: usually 12 mg day in divided doses to a maximum of 24 mg day.
Availability: NHS and private prescription.
Side effects: muscle spasms, restlessness, hands shaking, blurred vision, dry mouth, urine retention, palpitations, low blood pressure, weight gain, changes in libido, low body temperature, breast swelling, menstrual changes, jaundice, blood and skin changes, drowsiness, rarely fits.
Caution: in pregnant women, nursing mothers, and in patients suffering from Parkinson's disease, liver disease, cardiovascular disease, kidney failure, epilepsy, glaucoma, myaesthenia gravis, adrenal tumour, enlarged prostate.
Not to be used for: children, unconscious patients, or those suffering from bone marrow depression.
Caution needed with: alcohol, tranquillizers, pain killers, ANTIHYPERTENSIVES, antidepressants, anticonvulsants, antidiabetic drugs, LEVODOPA.
Contains: PERPHENAZINE.
Other preparations: Fentazin Injection.

Feospan Spansule
(S K B)

A red/clear capsule supplied at a strength of 150 mg and used as a iron supplement to treat iron deficiency, anaemia

Dose: adults1-2 capsules a day; children 1-12 years 1 capsule a day.
Availability: NHS, private prescription, over the counter.
Side effects: mild stomach upset, allergy.
Caution:
Not to be used for: infants under 1 year.
Caution needed with: TETRACYCLINES, LEVODOPA, PENICILLAMINE, ANTACIDS.

Contains: FERROUS SULPHATE.
Other preparations: FERROGRAD (Abbott), SLOW-FE (Ciba).

Ferfolic SV
(Sinclair)

A pink tablet used as an iron supplement to treat iron and folic acid deficiencies.

Dose: 1 tablet 3 times a day.
Availability: NHS and private prescription.
Side effects: nausea, constipation
Caution:
Not to be used for: patients suffering from megaloblastic anaemia.
Caution needed with: TETRACYCLINES.
Contains: FOLIC ACID, FERROUS GLUCONATE.
Other preparations:

Fergon
(Sanofi Winthrop)

A red tablet supplied at a strength of 300 mg and used as an iron supplement to treat iron deficiency, anaemia.

Dose: adults treatment 4-6 tablets in divided doses 1 hour before food, prevention 2 tablets a day; children 6-12 years 1-3 tablets a day.
Availability: NHS, private prescription, over the counter.
Side effects: nausea, constipation.
Caution:
Not to be used for: children under 6 years.
Caution needed with: TETRACYCLINES, ANTACIDS.
Contains: FERROUS GLUCONATE.
Other preparations:

---

ferric ammonium citrate *see* Tonivitan A & D

Ferrocap *see* Fersamal
(Consolidated)

Ferrocap F *see* Folex 350
(Consolidated)

Ferrocontin Continus
(ASTA)

A red tablet supplied at a strength of 100 mg and used as an iron supplement to treat iron deficiency, anaemia.

Dose: 1 tablet a day.
Availability: NHS, private prescription, over the counter.
Side effects:
Caution:
Not to be used for: children under 10 years.
Caution needed with: TETRACYCLINES, PENICILLAMINE, ZINC.
Contains: FERROUS GLYCINE SULPHATE.
Other preparations: PLESMET (Napp).

Ferrocontin Folic
(ASTA)

A pale-orange tablet used as an iron supplement to prevent iron and FOLIC ACID deficiencies in pregnancy.

Dose: 1 tablet a day.
Availability: NHS, private prescription, over the counter.
Side effects:
Caution:
Not to be used for: children.
Caution needed with: TETRACYCLINES, PENICILLAMINE, ZINC.
Contains: FERROUS GLYCINE SULPHATE, FOLIC ACID.
Other preparations:

Ferrograd
(Abbott)

A red tablet supplied at a strength of 325 mg and used as an iron supplement to treat iron deficiency anaemia.

Dose: 1 tablet a day before food.
Availability: NHS, private prescription, and over the counter.
Side effects:
Caution: in patients suffering from slow bowel actions.
Not to be used for: children or for patients suffering from diverticular

disease, blocked intestine.
Caution needed with: TETRACYCLINES, LEVODOPA.
Contains: FERROUS SULPHATE.
Other preparations: FEOSPAN (SKB), SLOW FE (Ciba).

Ferrograd C
(Abbott)

A red, oblong tablet used as an iron supplement to treat iron deficiency anaemia where absorption is difficult.

Dose: 1 tablet a day before food.
Availability: private prescription and over the counter.
Side effects:
Caution: in patients suffering from slow bowel action.
Not to be used for: children or for patients suffering from diverticular disease, blocked intestine.
Caution needed with: TETRACYCLINES, LEVODOPA, Clinistix urine test.
Contains: FERROUS SULPHATE, ASCORBIC ACID.
Other preparations:

Ferrograd Folic
(Abbott)

A yellow/red tablet used as an iron supplement to treat anaemia in pregnancy.

Dose: 1 tablet a day before food.
Availability: NHS, private prescription, over the counter.
Side effects:
Caution: in patients suffering from slow bowel movements.
Not to be used for: children or for patients suffering from diverticular disease, intestinal blockage, vitamin B_{12} deficiency.
Caution needed with: TETRACYCLINES, LEVODOPA.
Contains: FERROUS SULPHATE, FOLIC ACID.
Other preparations:

Ferromyn
(Wellcome)

An elixir used as an iron supplement to treat iron deficiency anaemia.

Dose: adults and children over 10 years 5 ml 3 times a day; children up to 2 years up to 1 ml twice a day, 2-5 years 2.5 ml 3 times a day, 5-10 years

5 ml twice a day.
Availability: NHS, private prescription, over the counter.
Side effects: stomach upset.
Caution:
Not to be used for:
Caution needed with: TETRACYCLINES, ANTACIDS, LEVODOPA.
Contains: FERROUS SUCCINATE.
Other preparations:

---

ferrous fumarate *see* **BC 500 with Iron, Fersaday, Fersamal, Folex-350, Galfer, Galfervit, Givitol, Meterfolic, Pregaday, Unicap-M**

---

ferrous gluconate *see* **Ferfolic SV, Fergon**

---

ferrous glycine sulphate *see* **Ferrocontin Continus, Ferrocontin Continus Folic, Plesmet**

---

ferrous perchloride *see* **Glykola**

---

ferrous succinate *see* **Ferromyn**

---

ferrous sulphate *see* **Fefol Spansule, Fefol Z Spansule, Fefol-Vit Spansule, Feospan Spansule, Ferrograd, Ferrograd C, Ferrograd Folic, Fesovit Spansule, Fesovit Z Spansule, Octovit, Pregnavite Forte F, Slow-Fe,Slow-Fe Folic**

Fersaday
(Evans)

A brown tablet supplied at a strength of 100 mg and used as an iron supplement to treat iron deficiency.

Dose: 1 tablet 1-2 times a day.
Availability: NHS, private prescription, over the counter.
Side effects: stomach upset.

Caution: in patients with a history of stomach ulcer.
Not to be used for: children.
Caution needed with: TETRACYCLINES, ANTACIDS.
Contains: FERROUS FUMARATE.
Other preparations: FERROCAP (Consolidated), FERSAMAL (Evans), GALFER (Galen).

Fersamal
(Evans)

A brown tablet supplied at a strength of 65 mg and used as an iron supplement to treat iron deficiency.

Dose: adults 1 tablet 3 times a day; children use Fersamal Syrup.
Availability: NHS, private prescription, over the counter.
Side effects: stomach upset.
Caution: in patients with a history of stomach ulcer.
Not to be used for:
Caution needed with: TETRACYCLINES, ANTACIDS.
Contains: FERROUS FUMARATE.
Other preparations: Fersamal Syrup, FERROCAP (Consolidated), FERSADAY (Evans), GALFER (Galen).

Fesovit Spansule
(Wellcome)

A yellow/clear capsule used as an iron and vitamin supplement to treat iron deficiency anaemia needing vitamins B and C.

Dose: adults1 capsule 1-2 times a day; children 1-12 years 1 capsule a day.
Availability: private prescription and over the counter.
Side effects: mild stomach upset.
Caution:
Not to be used for: infants under 1 year.
Caution needed with: TETRACYCLINES, LEVODOPA.
Contains: FERROUS SULPHATE, ASCORBIC ACID, THIAMINE mononitrate, RIBOFLA-VINE, PYRIDOXINE hydrochloride, NICOTINAMIDE.
Other preparations:

Fesovit Z Spansule
(S K B)

An orange/clear capsule used as an iron, zinc, and vitamin supplement to treat iron defficiency anaemia where vitamins B and C and zinc are needed.

Dose: adults 1-2 capsules a day; children 1-12 years 1 capsule a day.
Availability: private prescription, over the counter.
Side effects: mild stomach upset.
Caution: in patients suffering from kidney failure.
Not to be used for: infants under 1 year.
Caution needed with: TETRACYCLINES, LEVODOPA, PENICILLAMINE, ANTACIDS.
Contains: FERROUS SULPHATE, ZINC SULPHATE MONOHYDRATE, ASCORBIC ACID, THIAMINE mononitrate, RIBOFLAVINE, PYRIDOXINE hydrochloride, NICOTINAMIDE.
Other preparations:

Finalgon — ointment to relieve muscular/skeletal pain. Product now discontinued.

---

finasteride *see* **Proscar**

F

Flagyl
(Rhone-Poulenc Rorer)

An off-white tablet or an off-white, capsule-shaped tablet according to strengths of 200 mg, 400 mg and used as an antibacterial treatment for trichomoniasis, non-specific vaginitis, other infections, dysentery, abscess of the liver, ulcerative gingivitis (gum disease).

Dose: adults up to 800 mg 2-3 times a day; children reduced doses according to age and condition.
Availability: NHS and private prescription.
Side effects: stomach upset, furred tongue, unpleasant taste, allergy, rash, swelling, brain disturbances, dark-coloured urine, nerve changes, seizures, white cell changes.
Caution: in patients with brain disorder caused by liver disease. Short-term high-dose treatment should not be used for pregnant women or nursing mothers.
Not to be used for:
Caution needed with: alcohol, PHENOBARBITONE, anticoagulants taken by mouth.
Contains: METRONIDAZOLE.
Other preparations: Flagyl-S Suspension, Flagyl Suppositories, Flagyl Injection, Flagyl Compak, METROLYL (Lagap), VAGINYL (DDSA), ZADSTAT (Lederle)

Flamazine
(SNP)

A cream used as an antibacterial treatment for wounds, burns, infected ulcers of the leg, bed sores, and where skin has been removed for grafting.

Dose: apply a layer up to 0.5 cm thick to the affected area; change dressing 3 times a week.
Availability: NHS and private prescription.
Side effects:
Caution: in patients suffering from kidney or liver disease.
Not to be used for: infants under 3 months or for pregnant women.
Caution needed with: PHENYTOIN, sulphonamide antibiotics, antidiabetics, enzyme wound treatments.
Contains: SILVER SULPHADIAZINE.
Other preparations:

---

flavoxate hydrochloride *see* Urispas

---

flecainide *see* Tambocor

Flemoxin Solutab *see* Amoxil
(Paines & Byrne)

Fletchers' Arachis Oil
(Pharmax)

A 130 ml, single-dose enema used as a faecal softener to treat faecal impaction.

Dose: 1 enema as required; children in proportion according to age and body weight.
Availability: NHS, private prescription, over the counter.
Side effects:
Caution: warm before use.
Not to be used for:
Caution needed with:
Contains: ARACHIS OIL.
Other preparations:

Fletchers' Enemette
(Pharmax)

A 5 ml, single-dose micro-enema supplied at a strength of 90 mg and used as a faecal softener to treat constipation, and for evacuation of bowels before surgery etc.

Dose: adults 1 as required; children over 3 years in proportion to age.
Availability: NHS, private prescription, over the counter.
Side effects:
Caution:
Not to be used for: children under 3 years.
Caution needed with:
Contains: DOCUSATE sodium.
Other preparations:

Fletchers' Phosphate
(Pharmax)

A 128 ml, single-dose enema used as a bowel evacuator to treat constipation, and for evacuation of the bowels before surgery etc.

Dose: adults 1 enema as required; children over 3 years in proportion to age.
Availability: NHS, private prescription, over the counter.
Side effects:
Caution: in patients with restricted sodium intake.
Not to be used for: children under 3 years, or for patients where the absorptive capacity of the colon is increased.
Caution needed with:
Contains: SODIUM ACID PHOSPHATE, SODIUM PHOSPHATE.
Other preparations:

Flexin Continus
(Napp)

A green, red, or yellow, scored tablet supplied at strengths of 25 mg, 50 mg, 75 mg and used as a NON-STEROID ANTI-INFLAMMATORY DRUG to treat acute rheumatoid arthritis, osteoarthritis, ankylosing spondylitis, degenerative joint disease of the hip, acute muscle or bone problems, lower back pain, other joint disorders, painful periods.

Dose: 1 tablet 1-2 times a day with food, milk, or an antacid.
Availability: NHS and private prescription.
Side effects: stomach bleeding, headache, corneal deposits, disturbances

of the retina, stomach intolerance, dizziness, brain effects, blood changes, kidney disorder, blood in the urine, noises in the ears, rash, inflammation of blood vessels.

Caution: in the elderly, and in patients suffering from liver or kidney disease, brain disorders, heart failure.

Not to be used for: children, pregnant women, nursing mothers, or for patients suffering from stomach ulcer, a history of stomach lesions, or allergy to ASPIRIN or anti-inflammatory drugs.

Caution needed with: anticoagulants, LITHIUM, STEROIDS, DIURETICS, ß-BLOCKERS, PROBENECID, METHOTREXATE, some ANALGESICS.

Contains: INDOMETHACIN.

Other preparations: ARTRACIN (DDSA), IMBRILON (Berk), INDOCID (Morson), INDOLAR (Lagap), INDOMAX (Ashbourne), INDOMID (Kabi Pharmacia), RIMACID ((Rima).

Flixonase
(A & H)

A nasal spray used as a STEROID to prevent and treat rhinitis, hay fever.

Dose: adults, 2 sprays in each nostril once a day in the morning, to a maximum of 4 sprays in each nostril a day; children over 4 years, 1-2 sprays in each nostril a day (for seasonal rhinitis only).

Availability: NHS and private prescription.

Side effects: irritation of the nose, nose bleed, taste and smell disturbances.

Caution: in pregnant women, nursing mothers, and in patients being transferred from STEROIDS taken orally.

Not to be used for: children under 4 years.

Caution needed with:

Contains: FLUTICASONE PROPIONATE.

Other preparations:

Florinef
(Squibb)

A pink, scored tablet supplied at a strength of 0.1 mg and used as a STEROID replacement treatment in Addison's disease, salt-losing adrenogenital syndrome (adrenal disorders).

Dose: adults ½-3 tablets a day; children in proportion to adult dose according to age, body weight, and severity of illness.

Availability: NHS and private prescription.

Side effects: high blood pressure, fluid retention, potassium loss, muscle

weakness, weight gain.
Caution: in pregnant women, in patients who have had recent bowel surgery, or who are suffering from inflamed veins, psychiatric disorders, virus infections, some cancers, some kidney diseases, thinning of the bones, ulcers, tuberculosis, other infections, high blood pressure, glaucoma, epilepsy, diabetes, underactive thyroid, liver disease, stress. Withdraw gradually.
Not to be used for:
Caution needed with: PHENYTOIN, PHENOBARBITONE, EPHEDRINE, RIFAMPICIN, DIURETICS, ANTICHOLINESTERASES, DIGOXIN, antidiabetic agents, anticoagulants, NON-STEROID ANTI-INFLAMMATORY DRUGS.
Contains: FLUDROCORTISONE acetate.
Other preparations:

---

flosequinan *see* **Manoplax**

Floxapen
(Beecham Research)

A black/caramel-coloured capsule supplied at strengths of 250 mg, 500 mg and used as a penicillin treatment for skin, soft tissue, ear, nose, and throat, and other infections.

Dose: adults and children over 10 years 1 capsule 4 times a day; children under 2 years quarter adult dose, 2-10 years half adult dose.
Availability: NHS and private prescription.
Side effects: allergy, stomach disturbances.
Caution:
Not to be used for: patients suffering from penicillin allergy.
Caution needed with:
Contains: FLUCLOXACILLIN sodium.
Other preparations: Floxapen Syrup, Floxapen Injection, FLUCOMIX (Ashbourne), LADROPEN (Berk), STAFOXIL (Brocades).

Fluanxol
(Lundbeck)

A red tablet supplied at strengths of 0.5 mg, 1 mg and used as a sedative for the short-term treatment of depression and anxiety.

Dose: adults 1-2 mg in the morning to a maximum of 3 mg a day in divided doses; elderly 0.5 mg in the morning to a maximum of 2 mg a day in divided doses.

Availability: NHS and private prescription.
Side effects: muscle spasms, restlessness, hands shaking, blurred vision, dry mouth, urine retention, palpitations, low blood pressure, weight gain, changes in libido, low body temperature, breast swelling, menstrual changes, jaundice, blood and skin changes, drowsiness, rarely fits.
Caution: in pregnant women, and in patients suffering from Parkinson's disease, severe hardening of the arteries, confusion in the elderly, severe kidney, liver, or heart disease.
Not to be used for: children or for excitable, overactive, or severely clinically depressed patients.
Caution needed with: alcohol, tranquillizers, pain killers, ANTIHYPERTENSIVES, antidepressants, anticonvulsants, antidiabetic drugs, LEVODOPA.
Contains: FLUPENTHIXOL dihydrochloride.
Other preparations: DEPIXOL (Lundbeck).

Fluclomix *see* **Floxapen**
(Ashbourne)

---

fluclorolone acetonide *see* **Topilar**

---

flucloxacillin *see* **Floxapen, Magnapen, Stafoxil, Staphlipen**

---

fluconazole *see* **Diflucan**

---

fludrocortisone *see* **Florinef**

---

flumethasone *see* **Locorten-Vioform**

---

flunisolide *see* **Syntaris**

---

flunitrazepam *see* **Rohypnol**

---

fluocinolone *see* **Synalar**

---

fluocinonide *see* **Metosyn**

---

fluocortolone hexanoate *see* **Ultradil, Ultralanum Plain Cream, Ultraproct**

---

fluocortolone pivalate *see* **Ultradil, Ultralanum Plain Cream, Ultraproct**

Fluorescein Minims
(SNP)

Drops used as a dye for staining purposes to enable abrasions or foreign bodies in the eye to be found.

Dose: 1 or more drops into the eye as needed.
Availability: NHS, private prescription, over the counter.
Side effects:
Caution:
Not to be used for:
Caution needed with: soft contact lenses.
Contains: SODIUM FLUORESCEIN.
Other preparations: Fluorescein and Lignocaine Minims.

---

fluorescein *see* **Fluorescein Minims**

---

fluorometholone *see* **FML, FML-Neo**

---

fluoxetine *see* **Prozac**

---

flupenthixol *see* **Depixol, Fluanxol**

---

fluphenazine *see* **Moditen, Motipress, Motival**

flurandrenolone *see* **Haelan**

flurazepam *see* **Dalmane**

flurbiprofen *see* **Froben**

fluticasone propionate *see* **Flixonase**

fluvoxamine *see* **Faverine**

FML
(Allergan)

Drops used as a STEROID treatment for inflammation of the eye where no infection is present.

Dose: 1-2 drops into the eye 2-4 times a day.
Availability: NHS and private prescription.
Side effects: rise in eye pressure, thinning cornea, fungal infection, cataract.
Caution: in pregnant women and infants — do not use for extended periods — or for patients suffering from glaucoma.
Not to be used for: infants under 2 years, or for patients suffering from viral, fungal, tubercular, or weeping infections, or who wear soft contact lenses.
Caution needed with:
Contains: FLUOROMETHOLONE.
Other preparations: FML-Neo (with NEOMYCIN for infected conditions).

Folex-350
(Rybar)

A pink tablet used as an iron supplement for the prevention of iron and FOLIC ACID deficiency in pregnancy.

Dose: 1 tablet a day.
Availability: NHS, private prescription, over the counter.
Side effects: nausea, constipation.
Caution:
Not to be used for: children or for patients suffering from megaloblastic anaemia.
Caution needed with: TETRACYCLINES.
Contains: FERROUS FUMARATE, FOLIC ACID.
Other preparations: GALFER FA (Galen), METERFOLIC (Sinclair), PREGADAY (Evans).

---

folic acid *see* **Fefol Spansule, Fefol Z Spansule, Fefol-Vit Spansule, Ferfolic SV, Ferrocontin Continus Folic, Ferrograd Folic, Folex-350, Folicin, Givitol, Irofol C, Ketovite, Lexpec, Meterfolic, Pregaday, Pregnavite Forte F, Slow-Fe Folic**

Folicin
(Paines & Byrne)

A white tablet used as an iron and mineral supplement for the prevention and treatment of anaemia in pregnancy.

Dose: 1-2 tablets a day.
Availability: NHS and private prescription.
Side effects: nausea, constipation.
Caution:
Not to be used for: children or patients suffering from megaloblastic anaemia.
Caution needed with: TETRACYCLINES, LEVODOPA.
Contains: FOLIC ACID, COPPER SULPHATE, MANGANESE SULPHATE, FERROUS SULPHATE.
Other preparations:

---

folinic acid *see* **Refolinon**

Forceval
(Unigreg)

A brown/red capsule used as a source of multivitamins and minerals to treat vitamin and mineral deficiencies.

F

Dose: adults 1 capsule a day; children over 5 years use Forceval Junior.
Availability: private prescription and over the counter.
Side effects:
Caution:
Not to be used for: children under 5 years, or for patients suffering from high calcium levels or iron absorption/storage disorders.
Caution needed with: PHENYTOIN, TETRACYCLINES, anticoagulants.
Contains: multivitamins and minerals.
Other preparations: Forceval Junior.

---

formaldehyde *see* **Veracur**

Fortagesic
(Sterling Research Laboratories)

A white tablet used as an ANALGESIC to relieve pain in the bones and muscles.

Dose: children 7-12 years 1 tablet up to 4 times a day; adults 2 tablets up to 4 times a day.
Availability: controlled drug; private prescription only.
Side effects: sedation, dizziness, nausea, psychological effects.
Caution: in pregnant women and in patients suffering from kidney, liver, or respiratory disease, or some blood disorders.
Not to be used for: children under 7 years, or for patients with respiratory depression, raised intracranial pressure, head injuries, or certain brain conditions, or for patients who depend on narcotics.
Caution needed with: MAOIS, narcotic ANALGESICS, alcohol.
Contains: PENTAZOCINE HYDROCHLORIDE, PARACETAMOL.
Other preparations:

Fortral
(Sanofi Winthrop)

A white tablet supplied at a strength of 25 mg and used as an ANALGESIC to relieve pain.

Dose: adults 1-4 tablets every 3-4 hours after meals; children 1-6 years by injection; children 6-12 years 1 tablet every 3-4 hours.
Availability: controlled drug; NHS (if prescribed as a generic) and private prescription.
Side effects: sedation, dizziness, nausea, psychological effects.
Caution: in pregnant women and in patients suffering from kidney, liver, or

respiratory disease.

Not to be used for: children under 1 year or for patients suffering from respiratory depression, raised intracranial pressure, head injury, certain brain conditions, some blood disorders, or dependence on narcotics.

Caution needed with: MAOIS, narcotic ANALGESICS, alcohol.

Contains: PENTAZOCINE HYDROCHLORIDE.

Other preparations: Fortral Capsules, Fortral Injection, Fortral Suppositories.

Fortunan *see* **Dozic.** Product now discontinued.

Fosfor
(Chancellor)

A syrup used as a food supplement.

Dose: adults 20 ml 3 times a day; children half adult dose.

Availability: private prescription and over the counter.

Side effects:

Caution:

Not to be used for:

Caution needed with:

Contains: PHOSPHORYLCOLAMINE.

Other preparations:

---

fosinopril sodium *see* **Staril**

---

framycetin *see* **Framycort, Framycort Ointment, Framygen, Framygen Ointment, Sofradex Drops, Sofradex Ointment, Soframycin, Soframycin Cream, Soframycin Eye Drops**

Framycort — antibiotic/STEROID drops/ointment for eye/ear infections and inflammation. Product now discontinued.

Framycort Ointment — antibacterial/STEROID ointment. Product now discontinued.

Framygen — antibiotic drops for outer ear inflammation. Product now discontinued.

Framygen Eye Ointment/Drops — antibiotic treatment for eye inflammation/infection. Product now discontinued.

---

frangula *see* **Roter**

Franol
(Sanofi Winthrop)

A white tablet used as a broncho-dilator to treat blocked airway brought on by chronic bronchitis or bronchial asthma.

Dose: 1 tablets 3 times a day and 1 tablet before going to bed if needed.
Availability: NHS and private prescription.
Side effects: nausea, stomach upset, headache, sleeplessness, rapid or abnormal heart rate, anxiety, tremor.
Caution: in the elderly, nursing mothers, and in patients suffering from kidney, heart or liver disease, stomach ulcer, agitation, overactive thyroid, glaucoma, enlarged prostate, adrenal tumour.
Not to be used for: children, pregnant women, or for patients suffering from coronary heart disease, high blood pressure, some blood disorders.
Caution needed with: CIMETIDINE, ERYTHROMYCIN, CIPROFLOXACIN, MAOIS, TRICYCLICS, SYMPATHOMIMETICS, INTERFERON, the contraceptive pill.
Contains: EPHEDRINE hydrochloride, THEOPHYLLINE.
Other preparations: Franol Plus.

Frisium
(Hoechst)

A blue capsule supplied at a strength of 10 mg and used as a sedative to treat anxiety, tension, agitation, and as an additional treatment for epilepsy.

Dose: elderly 1 tablet twice a day or 2 tablets at night; adults 1 tablet 2-3 times a day or 2-3 tablets at night. Maximum dose 6 tablets a day.
Availability: NHS (for epilepsy when prescribed as a generic) and private prescription.
Side effects: drowsiness, confusion, unsteadiness, low blood pressure, rash, changes in vision, changes in libido, retention of urine. Risk of

addiction increases with dose and length of treatment. May impair judgement.

Caution: in the elderly, pregnant women, nursing mothers, in women during labour, and in patients suffering from lung disorders, kidney or liver disorders. Avoid long-term use and withdraw gradually.

Not to be used for: children (except for epilepsy — use reduced doses), or for patients suffering from acute lung disorders, some chronic lung disorders, some obsessional and psychotic diseases.

Caution needed with: alcohol, other tranquillizers and anticonvulsants.

Contains: CLOBAZAM.

Other preparations:

Froben
(Boots)

A yellow tablet supplied at strengths of 50 mg, 100 mg and used as a NON-STEROID ANTI-INFLAMMATORY DRUG to treat rheumatoid disease, osteoarthritis, ankylosing spondylitis.

Dose: 150-200 mg a day in divided doses to a maximum of 300 mg a day.

Availability: NHS and private prescription.

Side effects: stomach intolerance, rash, rarely jaundice, blood changes, fluid retention.

Caution: in the elderly, pregnant women, nursing mothers, and in patients suffering from asthma, kidney, liver, or heart disease, allergy to ASPIRIN or anti-inflammatory drugs.

Not to be used for: children or for patients suffering from stomach ulcer or stomach bleeding.

Caution needed with: FRUSEMIDE, anticoagulants.

Contains: FLURBIPROFEN.

Other preparations: Froben Suppositories, Froben SR.

Frumax *see* Lasix
(Ashbourne)

Frumil
(Rhone-Poulenc Rorer)

An orange, scored tablet used as a potassium-sparing DIURETIC to treat fluid retention associated with heart failure, liver and kidney disease.

Dose: 1-2 tablets a day in the morning.

Availability: NHS and private prescription.

Side effects: feeling of being unwell, stomach upset, rash, blood changes.
Caution: in pregnant women, nursing mothers, and in patients suffering from liver or kidney disease, diabetes, electrolyte changes, enlarged prostate, gout, or impaired urination.
Not to be used for: children or for patients suffering from liver cirrhosis, progressive kidney failure, raised potassium levels.
Caution needed with: potassium supplements, potassium-sparing DIURETICS, LITHIUM, DIGOXIN, some antibiotics (aminoglycosides, cephalosporins), ANTIHYPERTENSIVES, NON-STEROID ANTI-INFLAMMATORY DRUGS, ACE INHIBITORS.
Contains: FRUSEMIDE, AMILORIDE hydrochloride.
Other preparations: Frumil Forte, Frumul LS, LASORIDE (Hoechst).

---

frusemide *see* Diumide-K Continus, Frumil, Frusene, Lasikal, Lasilactone, Lasipressin, Lasix, Lasíx + K, Lasoride

---

Frusene
(Fisons)

A yellow, scored tablet used as a potassium-sparing DIURETIC to treat fluid retention caused by heart or liver problems.

Dose: ½-2 tablets a day (occasionally up to 6 tablets a day).
Availability: NHS and private prescription.
Side effects: stomach upset, feeling of being unwell, rash, gout, blood changes.
Caution: in pregnant women, nursing mothers, and in patients suffering from kidney or liver disease, diabetes, electrolyte changes, enlarged prostate, impaired urination, gout.
Not to be used for: children or for patients suffering from cirrhosis of the liver, progressive kidney failure, or raised potassium levels.
Caution needed with: potassium supplements, potassium-sparing DIURETICS, LITHIUM, DIGOXIN, ANTIHYPERTENSIVES, some antibiotics (aminoglycosides, cephalosporin), NON-STEROID ANTI-INFLAMMATORY DRUGS, ACE INHIBITORS.
Contains: FRUSEMIDE, TRIAMTERENE.
Other preparations:

Frusid *see* Lasix
(DDSA)

Fucibet
(Leo)

A cream used as an antibacterial and STEROID treatment for eczema where there is also infection.

Dose: apply to the affected area 2-3 times a day at first and then reduce if possible.
Availability: NHS and private prescription.
Side effects: fluid retention, suppression of the adrenal glands, thinning of the skin may occur.
Caution: use for short periods of time only.
Not to be used for: patients suffering from acne or any other skin infections caused by tuberculosis, ringworm, viruses, or fungi, or continuously especially in pregnant women.
Caution needed with:
Contains: BETAMETHASONE valerate, FUSIDIC ACID.
Other preparations:

Fucidin
(Leo)

A white, oval tablet supplied at a strength of 250 mg and used as an antibiotic to treat infections.

Dose: 2 tablets 3 times a day; children use Fucidin Suspension.
Availability: NHS and private prescription.
Side effects: jaundice, stomach disturbances.
Caution: the liver should be checked regularly.
Not to be used for:
Caution needed with:
Contains: SODIUM FUSIDATE.
Other preparations: Fucidin Suspension.

Fucidin Cream
(Leo)

A cream used as an antibacterial treatment for skin infections.

Dose: apply to the affected area 3-4 times a day.
Availability: NHS and private prescription.
Side effects:
Caution:
Not to be used for:
Caution needed with:

Contains: FUSIDIC ACID.
Other preparations: Fucidin Gel, Fucidin Ointment.

Fucidin H
(Leo)

An ointment used as a STEROID and antibacterial treatment for skin disorders where there is inflammation and infection.

Dose: apply to the affected area 3-4 times a day.
Availability: NHS and private prescription.
Side effects: fluid retention, suppression of the adrenal glands, thinning of the skin may occur.
Caution: use for short periods of time only.
Not to be used for: patients suffering from acne or any other skin infections caused by tuberculosis, ringworm, viruses, or fungi, or continuously especially in pregnant women.
Caution needed with:
Contains: SODIUM FUSIDATE, HYDROCORTISONE acetate.
Other preparations: Fucidin H Cream, Fucidin H Gel.

Fucithalmic
(Leo)

Drops used as an antibacterial treatment for conjunctivitis.

Dose: 1 drop into the eye twice a day.
Availability: NHS and private prescription.
Side effects: temporary irritation, allergy.
Caution:
Not to be used for:
Caution needed with:
Contains: FUSIDIC ACID.
Other preparations:

Fulcin
(ICI)

A white, scored tablet or a white tablet according to strengths of 125 mg, 500 mg and used as an anti-fungal treatment for scalp, skin, and nail infections.

Dose: adults 125 mg 4 times a day or 500 mg once a day; children 10 mg per kg body weight in one or divided doses.

Availability: NHS and private prescription.
Side effects: stomach upset, headache, allergy, sensitivity to light, rarely a collagen disease, rash, blood changes.
Caution:
Not to be used for: pregnant women or for patients suffering from porphyria (a rare blood disorder), severe liver disease.
Caution needed with: COUMARIN anticoagulants, BARBITURATES, the contraceptive pill, alcohol.
Contains: GRISEOFULVIN.
Other preparations: Fulcin Suspension, GRISOVIN (Glaxo).

Full Marks
(Napp Consumer)

An alcohol-based lotion used to treat head and pubic lice.

Dose: rub into hair and leave to dry naturally. Shampoo after 2 hours and comb hair while still wet.
Availability: NHS, private prescription, over the counter.
Side effects:
Caution: in children under 6 months. Avoid the eyes.
Not to be used for:
Caution needed with:
Contains: PHENOTHRIN.
Other preparations: Full Marks Shampoo — now discontinued.

Fungilin
(Squibb)

A light-brown, scored tablet supplied at a strength of 100 mg and used as an antibiotic to treat intestinal thrush, and for the prevention of vaginal or skin thrush.

Dose: adults 1-2 tablets 4 times a day; children use Suspension.
Availability: NHS and private prescription.
Side effects: stomach upset.
Caution:
Not to be used for:
Caution needed with:
Contains: AMPHOTERICIN.
Other preparations: FUNGILIN LOZENGES, Fungilin Suspension.

Fungilin Cream/Ointment — antifungal treatment. Product now discontinued.

Fungilin Lozenges
(Squibb)

A yellow lozenge supplied at a strength of 10 mg and used as an antifungal treatment for thrush.

Dose: 1 lozenge allowed to dissolve slowly in the mouth 4-8 times a day.
Availability: NHS and private prescription.
Side effects:
Caution:
Not to be used for:
Caution needed with:
Contains: AMPHOTERICIN.
Other preparations: FUNGILIN, Fungilin Suspension

Furacin — antibacterial ointment. Product now discontinued.

Furadantin
(Norwich Eaton)

A yellow, pentagonal, scored tablet supplied at strengths of 50 mg, 100 mg and used as an antiseptic to treat infection of the urinary tract.

Dose: adults treatment 100 mg 4 times a day with food or milk, prevention 50-100 mg a day; children use suspension (reduced doses).
Availability: NHS and private prescription.
Side effects: stomach upset, allergy, jaundice, nerve inflammation, blood changes, possible liver damage.
Caution: in pregnant women, nursing mothers, and in patients suffering from anaemia, diabets, electrolyte imbalance, vitamin B deficiency, debilitation.
Not to be used for: infants under 1 month or for patients suffering from kidney problems resulting in reduced urine output.
Caution needed with: MAGNESIUM TRISILICATE, PROBENECID, SULPHINPYRAZONE, quinolone antibiotics.
Contains: NITROFURANTOIN.
Other preparations: Furadantin Suspension, MACROBID (Procter and Gamble) MACRODANTIN (Norwich Eaton), URANTOIN (DDSA).

fusafungine *see* **Locabiotal**

---

fusidic acid *see* **Fucibet, Fucidin Cream, Fucithalmic**

Fybogel
(Reckitt & Colman)

Plain or orange-flavoured, effervescent granules supplied in sachets of 3.5 g and used as a bulking agent in the treatment of diverticular disease, spastic and irritable colon, constipation.

Dose: adults 1 sachet in water evening and morning; children 2.5-5 ml in water evening and morning.
Availability: NHS, private prescription, over the counter.
Side effects:
Caution:
Not to be used for: patients suffering from intestinal obstruction.
Caution needed with:
Contains: ISPAGHULA husk.
Other preparations: Fybogel Orange, ISOGEL (Charwell), METAMUCIL (Procter and Gamble), REGULAN (Procter and Gamble).

G

Fybranta
(Norgine)

A mottled, pale-brown, chewable, 2 g tablet used as a bulking agent in the treatment of diverticular disease, irritable colon syndrome, constipation through a diet lacking in fibre.

Dose: adults 1-3 tablets with liquid 3-4 times a day; children in proportion.
Availability: private prescription and over the counter.
Side effects:
Caution:
Not to be used for:
Caution needed with:
Contains: BRAN.
Other preparations:

Galake *see* **co-dydramol**
(Galen)

Galcodine
(Galen)

A linctus supplied at a strength of 15 mg in 5 ml and used as an opiate to treat dry cough.

Dose: adults 5 ml 4 times a day; children 1-5 years use paediatric formula, 6-12 years 2.5-5 ml 3-4 times a day.
Availability: NHS, private prescription, over the counter.
Side effects: constipation.
Caution: in patients suffering from asthma.
Not to be used for: infants under 1 year, or for patients suffering from liver disease.
Caution needed with: MAOIS.
Contains: CODEINE PHOSPHATE.
Other preparations: Galcodine Paediatric, CODEINE LINCTUS.

Galenamox *see* Amoxil
(Galen)

Galenphol
(Galen)

A liquid supplied at a strength of 5 mg in 5 ml and used as an opiate to treat dry cough.

Dose: adults 5-10 ml 3-4 times a day; children 1-5 years 2.5-5 ml 3-4 times a day, 6-12 years 5 ml 3-4 times a day.
Availability: NHS, private prescription, over the counter.
Side effects: constipation.
Caution: in patients suffering from asthma.
Not to be used for: infants under 1 year, or for patients suffering from liver disease.
Caution needed with: MAOIS.
Contains: PHOLCODINE.
Other preparations: Galenphol Linctus Strong, Galenphol Linctus Paediatric, PAVACOL-D LINCTUS (Boehringer Ingelheim), PHOLCODINE LINCTUS, PHOLCOMED-D (Medo).

Galfer
(Galen)

A green/red capsule supplied at a strength of 290 mg and used as an iron supplement to treat iron-deficiency anaemia.

Dose: adults 1 capsule 1-2 times a day before food; children use syrup.
Availability: NHS, private prescription, over the counter.
Side effects: nausea, constipation.
Caution:
Not to be used for:
Caution needed with: TETRACYCLINES.
Contains: FERROUS FUMARATE.
Other preparations: Galfer Syrup, FERROCAP (Consolidated), FERSADAY
(Evans), FERSAMAL (Evans).

Galfer FA *see* **Folex 350**
(Galen)

Galfervit — iron and vitamin supplement. Product now discontinued.

Galpseud
(Galen)

A white tablet supplied at a strength of 60 mg and used as a
SYMPATHOMIMETIC to treat congestion of the nose, sinuses, and upper
respiratory tract.

Dose: adults 1 tablet 3 times a day; children use linctus.
Availability: NHS, private prescription, over the counter.
Side effects: anxiety, hands shaking, irregular or rapid heart rate, dry
mouth, excitement.
Caution: in patients suffering from diabetes.
Not to be used for: children under 2 years, or for patients suffering from
heart or thyroid disorders.
Caution needed with: MAOIS, TRICYCLICS.
Contains: PSEUDOEPHEDRINE hydrochloride.
Other preparations: Galpseud Linctus, SUDAFED (Wellcome).

G

Galpseud Plus
(Galen)

A linctus used as a SYMPATHOMIMETIC and ANTIHISTAMINE to treat allergic
rhinitis.

Dose: adults, 10 ml 3 times a day; children 2-6 years 2.5 ml 3 times a day,

children 6-12 years 5 ml 3 times a day.
Availability: NHS, private prescription, over the counter.
Side effects: drowsiness, impaired reactions.
Caution: in patients suffering from enlarged prostate, bladder disorder, severe kidney or liver disease.
Not to be used for: children under 2 years, or for patients suffering from epilepsy or high blood pressure.
Caution needed with: MAOIS, ANTIHYPERTENSIVES, other SYMPATHOMIMETICS, alcohol, sedatives.
Contains: PSEUDOEPHEDRINE HYDROCHLORIDE, CHLORPHENIRAMINE MALEATE.
Other preparations:

Gamanil
(Merck)

A maroon, scored tablet supplied at a strength of 70 mg and used as an antidepressant to treat depression.

Dose: 1 tablet in the morning and 1-2 tablets at night.
Availability: NHS and private prescription.
Side effects: dry mouth, constipation, urine retention, blurred vision, palpitations, drowsiness, sleeplessness, dizziness, hands shaking, low blood presure, weight change, skin reactions, jaundice or blood changes, loss of libido may occur.
Caution: in nursing mothers or in patients suffering from heart disease, thyroid disease, epilepsy, diabetes, glaucoma, adrenal tumour, urinary retention, some other psychiatric conditions. Your doctor may advise regular blood tests.
Not to be used for: children, pregnant women, or for patients suffering from heart attacks, heart block, liver disease.
Caution needed with: alcohol, ANTICHOLINERGICS, ADRENALINE, MAOIS, BARBITURATES, other antidepressants, ANTIHYPERTENSIVES, oestrogens, CIMETIDINE.
Contains: LOFEPRAMINE hydrochloride.
Other preparations:

---

gamolenic acid *see* Epogam, Efamast

Ganda
(SNP)

Drops used as a fluid channel drug to treat glaucoma.

Dose: 1 drop into the eye 1-2 times a day.

Availability: NHS and private prescription.
Side effects: pain in the eye, headache, redness, skin reactions, melanosis, rarely systemic effects, increase in eye pressure.
Caution: your doctor may advise that the conjunctiva and cornea should be checked every 6 months if you are undergoing prolonged treatment.
Not to be used for: patients suffering from narrow-angle glaucoma, absence of the lens.
Caution needed with: MAOIS.
Contains: GUANETHIDINE monosulphate, ADRENALINE.
Other preparations:

Garamycin *see* Cidomycin Drops
(Schering-Plough)

Gastrobid Continus *see* Maxolon
(Napp)

Gastrocote
(Boehringer Mannheim)

G

A white tablet used as an ANTACID and reflux suppressant to treat dyspepsia, hiatus hernia, oesophagitis

Dose: adults 1-2 tablets 4 times a day, children over 6 years as adult.
Availability: NHS, private prescription, over the counter.
Side effects: occasionally constipation.
Caution:
Not to be used for: children under 6 years.
Caution needed with: TETRACYCLINE antibiotics, tablets which are coated to protect the stomach.
Contains: ALGINIC ACID, ALUMINIUM HYDROXIDE, MAGNESIUM TRISILICATE, SODIUM BICARBONATE.
Other preparations: Gastrocote Liquid.

Gastroflux *see* Maxolon
(Ashbourne)

Gastromax *see* Maxolon
(Farmitalia CE)

Gastron
(Sanofi Winthrop)

A white tablet used as an ANTACID and reflux suppressant to treat reflux symptoms.

Dose: adults 1-2 tablets 3 times a day and 2 at bedtime.
Availability: NHS, private prescription, over the counter.
Side effects: occasionally constipation.
Caution: in pregnant women, and in patients suffering from high blood pressure, heart or kidney failure.
Not to be used for: children.
Caution needed with: tetracycline antibiotics, tablets which are coated to protect the stomach.
Contains: ALGINIC ACID, ALUMINIUM HYDROXIDE, SODIUM BICARBONATE, MAGNESIUM TRISILICATE.
Other preparations:

Gastrozepin
(Boots)

A white tablet used as an antispasm, ANTICHOLINERGIC treatment for gastric and duodenal ulcers.

Dose: adults 1 tablet twice a day before meals for 4-6 weeks.
Availability: NHS and private prescription.
Side effects: blurred vision, confusion, dry mouth.
Caution:
Not to be used for: children, or for patients with glaucoma, inflammatory bowel disease, intestinal obstruction, or enlarged prostate.
Caution needed with:
Contains: PIRENZEPINE.
Other preparations:

Gaviscon
(Reckitt & Colman)

A white tablet or pink liquid used as an ANTACID and reflux suppressant to treat reflux symptoms.

Dose: children use sachets; adults 1-2 tablets or 10-20 ml after meals and at night.
Availability: NHS, private prescription, over the counter.
Side effects: occasionally constipation.
Caution: in pregnant women, and in patients suffering from high blood

G

pressure, heart or kidney failure.
Not to be used for:
Caution needed with: TETRACYCLINE antibiotics, tablets which are coated to protect the stomach.
Contains: SODIUM ALGINATE, SODIUM BICARBONATE, CALCIUM CARBONATE.
Other preparations: Gaviscon Infant Sachets.

Geangin *see* Cordilox
(Cusi)

---

gelatin *see* Orabase

Gelcosal
(Quinoderm)

A gel used as an antipsoriatic and skin softener to treat psoriasis, dermatitis, when the condition is scaling.

Dose: massage into the affected area twice a day.
Availability: NHS, private prescription, over the counter.
Side effects:
Caution:
Not to be used for:
Caution needed with:
Contains: COAL TAR SOLUTION, TAR, SALICYLIC ACID.
Other preparations: CAPASAL (Dermal), IONIL-T (Galderma).

Gelcotar
(Quinoderm)

A gel used as an antipsoriatic treatment for psoriasis, dermatitis.

Dose: massage into the affected area twice a day.
Availability: NHS, private prescription, over the counter.
Side effects: irritation, sensitivity to light.
Caution:
Not to be used for: patients suffering from acute psoriasis.
Caution needed with:
Contains: COAL TAR SOLUTION, TAR.
Other preparations: Gelcotar Liquid, CARBO-DOME (Lagap), CLINITAR (Shire), PSORIDERM (Dermal), PSORIGEL (Galderma).

gemfibrozil *see* Lopid

Genisol
(Fisons)

A liquid used as an antipsoriatic and anti-dandruff treatment for psoriasis, dandruff, seborrhoeic inflammation of the scalp.

Dose: shampoo once a week or as needed.
Availability: NHS, private prescription, over the counter.
Side effects:
Caution: avoid eyes.
Not to be used for:
Caution needed with:
Contains: COAL TAR, SODIUM SULPHOSUCCINATED UNDECYLENIC MONOALKYOLAMIDE.
Other preparations:

Gentamicin Minims
(SNP)

Drops used as an aminoglycoside antibiotic to treat bacterial infections of the eye.

Dose: 1 drop into the eye as needed.
Availability: NHS and private prescription.
Side effects:
Caution:
Not to be used for:
Caution needed with:
Contains: GENTAMICIN sulphate.
Other preparations: CIDOMYCIN DROPS (Roussel), GARAMYCIN (Schering-Plough), GENTICIN (Nicholas).

---

gentamicin *see* Cidomycin Cream, Cidomycin Drops, Gentamicin Minims, Genticin Cream, Gentisone HC, Gentisone HC Drops

---

gentian mixture, acid

A tonic used to to improve appetite.

Dose: 10-20 ml ½ hour before a meal.

Availability: NHS, private prescription, over the counter.
Side effects:
Caution:
Not to be used for: children.
Caution needed with:
Contains:
Other preparations: gentian mixture, alkaline.

---

gentian violet *see* **crystal violet paint**

Genticin Cream
(Nicholas)

A cream used as an aminoglycoside antibiotic to treat skin infections such as ulcers, burns, wounds, impetigo, inflammation of the follicles.

Dose: apply to the affected area 3-4 times a day.
Availability: NHS and private prescription.
Side effects: sensitization.
Caution: in patients with large areas of affected skin.
Not to be used for:
Caution needed with:
Contains: GENTAMICIN.
Other preparations: Genticin Ointment — now discontinued, CIDOMYCIN CREAM (Roussel).

G

Genticin Drops *see* Cidomycin Drops
(Nicholas)

Gentisone HC Cream
(Nicholas)

A cream used as a STEROID and antibacterial treatment for allergic or other skin disorders where there is also infection and inflammation.

Dose: apply to the affected area 3-4 times a day.
Availability: NHS and private prescription.
Side effects: fluid retention, suppression of adrenal glands, thinning of the skin.
Caution: use for short periods of time only.
Not to be used for: continuously especially for pregnant women, or for

patients suffering from tubercular, fungal, viral, or ringworm infections.
Caution needed with:
Contains: GENTAMICIN sulphate, HYDROCORTISONE acetate.
Other preparations: Gentisone HC Ointment.

Gentisone HC Drops
(Nicholas)

Drops used as an antibiotic, STEROID treatment for inflammation of the outer ear, acute weeping inflammation of the middle ear.

Dose: 2-4 drops into the ear 3-4 times a day and at night.
Availability: NHS and private prescription.
Side effects: additional infection.
Caution: in pregnant women, infants, and in patients suffering from perforated ear drum. Use for short periods of time only.
Not to be used for:
Caution needed with:
Contains: GENTAMICIN sulphate, HYDROCORTISONE acetate.
Other preparations:

G

Gestanin
(Organon)

A white tablet supplied at a strength of 5 mg and used as a progestogen treatment for threatened or habitual abortion, threatened labour.

Dose: up to 8 tablets a day depending on condition.
Availability: NHS and private prescription.
Side effects: nausea.
Caution: in nursing mothers, and in patients suffering from diabetes, migraine, epilepsy, high blood pressure, and liver, kidney, or heart disease.
Not to be used for: children or for patients with a history of thromboembolic disorders, breast or genital cancer, liver disease, abnormal vaginal bleeding, porphyria (a rare blood disorder).
Caution needed with:
Contains: ALLYLOESTRENOL.
Other preparations:

---

gestodene *see* **Femodene, Femodene ED, Minulet, Tri-Minulet**

---

gestrinone *see* **Dimetriose**

Gevral
(Lederle)

A brown capsule used as a source of multivitamins and minerals to treat vitamin and mineral deficiencies.

Dose: 1 capsule a day.
Availability: private prescription and over the counter.
Side effects:
Caution:
Not to be used for:
Caution needed with: LEVODOPA.
Contains: multivitamins and minerals.
Other preparations:

Givitol
(Galen)

A maroon/red capsule used as an iron, folic acid, and vitamin supplement to treat iron and folic acid deficiencies in pregnancy where vitamin supplements are also needed.

Dose: 1 capsule a day before food.
Availability: private prescription and over the counter.
Side effects: nausea, constipation.
Caution:
Not to be used for: children.
Caution needed with: TETRACYCLINES, LEVADOPA.
Contains: FERROUS FUMARATE, ASCORBIC ACID, RIBOFLAVINE, PYRIDOXINE hydrochloride, NICOTINAMIDE, FOLIC ACID.
Other preparations:

Glandosane
(Fresenius)

An aerosol used to provide artificial saliva for dry mouth and throat.

Dose: spray into the mouth and throat for 1-2 seconds as needed.
Availability: NHS, private prescription, over the counter.
Side effects:
Caution:
Not to be used for:

G

Caution needed with:
Contains: CARBOXYMETHYLCELLULOSE SODIUM, SORBITOL, POTASSIUM CHLORIDE, SODIUM CHLORIDE, MAGNESIUM CHLORIDE, CALCIUM CHLORIDE, DIPOTASSIUM HYDROGEN PHOSPHATE.
Other preparations:

Glauline — ß-BLOCKER drops to treat glaucoma. Product now discontinued.

---

glibenclamide *see* **Daonil**

Glibenese
(Pfizer)

A white, oblong, scored tablet supplied at a strength of 5 mg and used as a sulphonylurea to treat diabetes.

Dose: ½-1 tablet a day with breakfast or lunch at first increasing if needed by ½-1 tablet a day every 3-5 days to a maximum of 6 tablets a day in divided doses.
Availability: NHS and private prescription.
Side effects: allergy including skin rash.
Caution: in the elderly and in patients suffering from kidney failure.
Not to be used for: children, pregnant women, nursing mothers, during surgery, or for patients suffering from juvenile diabetes, liver or kidney impairment, hormone disorders, stress, infections.
Caution needed with: ß-BLOCKERS, MAOIS, STEROIDS, DIURETICS, alcohol, anticoagulants, lipid-lowering agents, ASPIRIN, some antibiotics (RIFAMPICIN, sulphonamides, CHLORAMPHENICOL), GLUCAGON, CYCLOPHOSPHAMIDE, the contraceptive pill.
Contains: GLIPIZIDE.
Other preparations: MINODIAB (Farmitalia CE).

---

gliclazide *see* **Diamicron**

---

glipizide *see* **Glibenese, Minodiab**

Gluco-lyte *see* Dioralyte
(Cupal)

Glucagon
(Lilly, Novo)

An injection administered by the subcutaneous, intramuscular, or intravenous route to treat severe low blood glucose levels (eg in diabetics when too much insulin has been used). A similar effect can be achieved by giving the patient sugar by mouth, if conscious.

Dose: adults and children 0.5-1 mg immediately.
Availability: NHS and private prescription.
Side effects: nausea, vomiting, diarrhoea, low blood potassium levels, allergy.
Caution: in pregnant women and nursing mothers. If a suitable response is not seen within 20 mintues of the dose, further treatment is needed urgently.
Not to be used for: patients suffering from adrenal tumour, pancreatic tumour.
Caution needed with: WARFARIN.
Contains: GLUCAGON HYDROCHLORIDE.
Other preparations:

G

Glucophage
(Lipha)

A white tablet supplied at strengths of 500 mg, 850 mg and used as an antidiabetic to treat diabetes.

Dose: 500-850 mg twice a day with meals at first increasing gradually if needed to a maximum of 3 g a day, and then reduce to 2 x 850 mg or 3 x 500 mg a day in divided doses.
Availability: NHS and private prescription.
Side effects: allergy including skin rash, rarely acidosis (a metabolic disorder).
Caution: in the elderly and in patients suffering from kidney failure.
Not to be used for: children, pregnant women, nursing mothers, during pregnancy, or for patients suffering from juvenile diabetes, liver or kidney impairment, hormone disorders, stress, infections.
Caution needed with: ß-BLOCKERS, MAOIS, STEROIDS, DIURETICS, alcohol, anticoagulants, lipid-lowering agents, ASPIRIN, some antibiotics (RIFAMPICIN, sulphonamides, CHLORAMPHENICOL), GLUCAGON, CYCLOPHOSPHAMIDE, the contraceptive pill.

Contains: METFORMIN HYDROCHLORIDE.
Other preparations: ORABET (Lagap).

---

glucose *see* Dioralyte, Rehidrat

Glucotard — bulking agent to treat diabetes. Product now discontinued.

Glurenorm
(Sanofi Winthrop)

A white, scored tablet supplied at a strength of 30 mg and used as an antidiabetic to treat diabetes.

Dose: 1½-2 tablets a day in divided doses before food to a maximum of 6 tablets a day.
Availability: NHS and private prescription.
Side effects: allergy including skin rash.
Caution: in the elderly and in patients suffering from kidney failure.
Not to be used for: children, pregnant women, nursing mothers, during surgery, or for patients suffering from juvenile diabetes, liver or kidney impairment, hormone disorders, stress, infections.
Caution needed with: ß-BLOCKERS, MAOIS, STEROIDS, DIURETICS, alcohol, anticoagulants, lipid-lowering agents, ASPIRIN, some antibiotics (RIFAMPICIN, sulphonamides, CHLORAMPHENICOL), GLUCAGON, CYCLOPHOSPHAMIDE, the contraceptive pill.
Contains: GLIQUIDONE.
Other preparations:

---

glutamic acid hydrochloride *see* Muripsin

---

glutaraldehyde *see* Glutarol, Verucasep

Glutarol
(Dermal)

A solution used as a virucidal, skin-drying agent to treat warts.

Dose: apply the solution to the wart twice a day and rub down hard skin.

Availability: NHS, private prescription, over the counter.
Side effects: staining of the skin.
Caution: do not apply to healthy skin.
Not to be used for: warts on the face or anal and genital areas.
Caution needed with:
Contains: GLUTARALDEHYDE.
Other preparations: VERUCASEP (Galen).

---

glycerin/glycerol *see* Exterol, glycerol suppositories, magnesium sulphate paste, Micolette, Relaxit, sodium bicarbonate ear drops, Ung Merck

---

glycerol suppositories

Suppositories supplied at strengths of 1 g, 2 g, 4 g and used as a lubricant to treat constipation.

Dose: adults 4 g suppository as necessary; children 2 g suppository, infants 1 g suppository.
Availability: NHS, private prescription, over the counter.
Side effects:
Caution:
Not to be used for:
Caution needed with:
Contains: GLYCEROL (glycerin)
Other preparations:

---

glyceryl trinitrate *see* Coro-Nitro, Deponit, Nitrocontin Continus, Nitrolingual, Percutol, Suscard Buccal, Sustac, Transiderm-Nitro

---

glycine *see* Cicatrin, Paynocil, Titralac

---

glycol salicylate *see* Bayolin, Cremalgin, Dubam, Salonair

Glyconon *see* Rastinon
(DDSA)

G

Glykola — liquid tonic. Product now discontinued.

Glymese *see* **Diabinese**
(DDSA)

Glytrin *see* **Nitrolingual**
(Sanofi Winthrop)

---

grain fibre *see* **Proctofibe**

---

gramicidin *see* **Graneodin, Neosporin, Sofradex Drops, Sofradex Eye Ointment, Tri-Adcortyl, Tri-Adcortyl Otic,**

Graneodin
(Squibb)

An ointment used as an aminoglycoside and protein to treat skin infections such as impetigo and beard infections.

Dose: apply 2-4 times a day.
Availability: NHS and private prescription.
Side effects: hearing damage, sensitization.
Caution: in patients with large areas of affected skin; do not use with dressings.
Not to be used for: fungal, viral, or deep infections.
Caution needed with:
Contains: NEOMYCIN sulphate, GRAMICIDIN.
Other preparations:

Gregoderm
(Unigreg)

An ointment used as a STEROID, antibacterial treatment for psoriasis, itch of the anal and genital area, and other skin disorders where there is also inflammation and infection.

Dose: apply to the affected area 2-3 times a day.
Availability: NHS and private prescription.

Side effects: fluid retention, suppression of the adrenal glands, thinning of the skin may occur.
Caution: use for short periods of time only.
Not to be used for: continuously especially for pregnant women, or for patients suffering from acne or any other tubercular, fungal, viral, or ringworm infections.
Caution needed with:
Contains: NEOMYCIN sulphate, NYSTATIN, POLYMYXIN B SULPHATE.
Other preparations:

---

griseofulvin *see* Fulcin, Grisovin

Grisovin
(Glaxo)

A white tablet supplied at strengths of 125 mg, 500 mg and used as an antifungal treatment for infections of the nails, skin, and scalp.

Dose: adults 500 mg-1 g a day in divided doses after meals; children 10 mg per kg body weight a day in divided doses.
Availability: NHS and private prescription.
Side effects: drowsiness, gastric upset, headache, allergies, sensitivity to light, rarely precipitation of SLE (a rare collagen disease).
Caution: in pregnant women and in patients on prolonged treatment.
Not to be used for: patients suffering from porphyria (a rare blood disease), liver disease, SLE (a rare collagen disease).
Caution needed with: BARBITURATES, COUMARIN anticoagulants, alcohol, the contraceptive pill.
Contains: GRISEOFULVIN.
Other preparations: FULCIN (ICI).

---

guaiphenesin *see* Bricanyl Expectorant, Dimotane Expectorant, Noradran

---

guanethidine *see* Ganda, Ismelin, Ismelin Eye Drops

Guanor
(R P Drugs)

G

A liquid used as an expectorant, ANTIHISTAMINE, mucus softener to treat cough, bronchial congestion.

Dose: adults 5-10 ml every 2-3 hours; children 1-5 years 2.5 ml every 3-4 hours, 6-12 years 5 ml every 3-4 hours.
Availability: private prescription and over the counter.
Side effects: drowsiness, reduced reactions.
Caution:
Not to be used for: infants under 1 year.
Caution needed with: sedatives, alcohol.
Contains: AMMONIUM CHLORIDE, DIPHENHYDRAMINE hydrochloride, SODIUM CITRATE, MENTHOL.
Other preparations: BENYLIN EXPECTORANT (Warner-Lambert).

---

guar gum *see* **Glucotard, Guarem**

Guarem
(Rybar)

Dispersible granules in a 5 g sachet used as a bulking agent to treat diabetes and dumping syndrome.

Dose: ½-1 sachet dispersed in 100 ml of liquid immediately before each meal or stirred into food and eaten with 100 ml liquid.
Availability: NHS, private prescription, over the counter.
Side effects: wind, swollen abdomen.
Caution: glucose levels should be checked in diabetics.
Not to be used for: children or for patients suffering from a blocked intestine or oesophageal disease.
Caution needed with:
Contains: GUAR GUM.
Other preparations: GUARINA (Norgine).

Guarina *see* **Guarem**
(Norgine)

Gyno-Daktarin 1
(Janssen)

A white vaginal capsule supplied at a strength of 1200 mg and used as an antifungal treatment for thrush of the vulva or vagina.

Dose: 1 capsule inserted high into the vagina as a single dose.
Availability: NHS, private prescription, over the counter.
Side effects: mild burning or irritation.
Caution:
Not to be used for: children.
Caution needed with:
Contains: MICONAZOLE nitrate.
Other preparations: Gyno-Daktarin Pessaries, Gyno-Daktarin CombiPack, Gyno-Daktarin Tampons — now discontinued, GynoDaktarin Cream.

Gyno-Pevaryl 1
(Cilag)

A pessary supplied at a strength of 150 mg and used as an antifungal treatment for vaginal thrush.

Dose: 1 pessary inserted into the vagina at night as a single dose.
Availability: NHS, private prescription, over the counter.
Side effects: mild burning or irritation.
Caution:
Not to be used for: children.
Caution needed with:
Contains: ECONAZOLE nitrate.
Other preparations: Gyno-Pevaryl 1CP, Gyno-Pevaryl Cream, Gyno-Pevaryl Pessaries, Gyno-Pevaryl Combipack.

H

H₂ antagonist (blocker)

A drug which works on the stomach to reduce acid production by blocking the histamine pathway. Example RANITIDINE *see* Zantac.

Haelan
(Dista)

A cream used as a STEROID treatment for skin disorders.

Dose: apply to the affected area 2-3 times a day.
Availability: NHS and private prescription.
Side effects: fluid retention, suppression of the adrenal glands, thinning of the skin may occur.
Caution: use for short periods of time only.
Not to be used for: continuously especially for pregnant women, or for

patients suffering from acne, or any other tubercular, viral, fungal, or ringworm skin infections.
Caution needed with:
Contains: FLURANDRENOLONE.
Other preparations: Haelan Ointment, Haelan Tape (not available on NHS), Haelan-X — now discontinued, Haelan-C (with CLIOQUINOL for infected conditions).

Halciderm
(Squibb)

A cream used as a STEROID treatment for acute skin disorders.

Dose: apply to the affected area 2-3 times a day.
Availability: NHS and private prescription.
Side effects: fluid retention, suppression of the adrenal glands, thinning of the skin may occur.
Caution: do not dilute the cream. Use for short periods of time only.
Not to be used for: continuously especially for pregnant women, or for patients suffering from other tubercular, fungal, viral, or ringworm infections.
Caution needed with:
Contains: HALCINONIDE.
Other preparations:

H

halcinonide *see* Halciderm

Halcion — sleeping tablet for occasional use. Product now discontinued.

Haldol
(Janssen)

A blue tablet or a yellow tablet according to strengths of 5 mg, 10 mg and used as a sedative to treat schizophrenia, mental or behavioural disorders, mania, hypomania, alcohol withdrawal symptoms, delirium tremens, behavioural disorders in children, nausea, vomiting, medication before an anaesthetic.

Dose: adults 0.5-5 mg 2-3 times a day at first increasing gradually to a maximum of 200 mg a day if needed; children 0.05 mg per kg body weight a day in 2 divided doses.

Availability: NHS and private prescription.
Side effects: muscle spasms, restlessness, hands shaking, blurred vision, dry mouth, urine retention, palpitations, low blood pressure, weight gain, changes in libido, low body temperature, breast swelling, menstrual changes, jaundice, blood and skin changes, drowsiness, rarely fits.
Caution: in pregnant women, nursing mothers, and in patients suffering from liver or kidney failure, severe cardiovascular disease, Parkinson's disease, overactive thyroid gland, epilepsy.
Not to be used for: unconscious patients.
Caution needed with: alcohol, tranquillizers, pain killers, ANTIHYPERTENSIVES, antidepressants, anticonvulsants, antidiabetics, LEVODOPA.
Contains: HALOPERIDOL DECANOATE.
Other preparations: Haldol Oral Liquid, DOZIC (R.P. Drugs), SERENACE (Baker Norton).

Half-Betadur CR *see* Inderal LA
(Monmouth)

Half-Inderal LA *see* Inderal LA
(ICI)

Half-Securon SR *see* Securon SR
(Knoll)

Halfan
(SKF)

A white, scored, capsule-shaped tablet used to treat malaria.

Dose: adults and children over 37 kg in weight, 6 tablets taken in 3 divided doses at 6-hourly intervals. Repeat the dose one week later.
Availability: NHS and private prescription.
Side effects: stomach upset, abdominal pain, blood changes.
Caution: in women of child-bearing age, and in patients suffering from complicated malarial conditions, or malaria involving the brain.
Not to be used for: children under 37 kg body weight, pregnant women, nursing mothers, or for preventing malaria.
Caution needed with:
Contains: HALOFANTRINE.
Other preparations:

H

halofantrine *see* **Halfan**

---

haloperidol decanoate *see* **Haldol**

---

haloperidol *see* **Dozic, Serenace**

Halycitrol
(LAB)

An emulsion used as a multivitamin preparation to treat VITAMIN A and VITAMIN D deficiencies.

Dose: adults and children over 6 months 5 ml a day; infants under 6 months 2.5 ml a day.
Availability: private prescription and over the counter.
Side effects: vitamin poisoning.
Caution: in patients suffering from kidney disease, sarcoidosis (a chest disease that affects calcium levels), and in pregnant women.
Not to be used for:
Caution needed with:
Contains: VITAMIN A, VITAMIN D.
Other preparations:

Hamarin *see* Zyloric
(Nicholas)

Harmogen
(Abbott)

An orange, oval, scored tablet supplied at a strength of 1.5 mg and used as an oestrogen to treat menopausal oestrogen deficiency.

Dose: 1-3 tablets a day for 3-4 weeks then 5-7 days without tablets.
Availability: NHS and private prescription.
Side effects: enlarged breasts, fluid retention, nausea, vaginal bleeding, weight gain, skin changes, liver disorders, jaundice, rashes, vomiting, headaches.
Caution: in patients suffering from high blood pressure, diabetes, heart disease, vascular disorders, asthma, kidney disease, epilepsy, migraine, womb diseases, thyroid disorder. Your doctor may advise you to have

regular examinations.

Not to be used for: pregnant women, nursing mothers, or for patients suffering from sickle-cell anaemia, thrombosis, liver disorders, some cancers, undiagnosed vaginal bleeding, some ear, skin, and kidney disorders, jaundice, porphyria (a rare blood disorder), brain blood vessel disease.

Caution needed with: DIURETICS, ANTIHYPERTENSIVES, drugs which induce liver enzymes (eg BARBITURATES, CARBAMAZEPINE, PHENYTOIN, RIFAMPICIM).

Contains: PIPERAZINE OESTRONE SULPHATE.

Other preparations:

Haymine
(Pharmax)

A yellow tablet used as an ANTIHISTAMINE and SYMPATHOMIMETIC treatment for allergies.

Dose: 1 tablet in the morning and 1 tablet at night if needed.
Availability: NHS, private prescription, over the counter.
Side effects: drowsiness, reduced reactions, dizziness.
Caution:
Not to be used for: children or for patients suffering from overactive thyroid gland, high blood pressure, coronary thrombosis.
Caution needed with: sedatives, MAOIS, alcohol.
Contains: CHLORPHENIRAMINE maleate, EPHEDRINE hydrochloride.
Other preparations:

H

Heminevrin
(Astra)

A syrup used as a sedative for the short-term treatment of sleeplessness in the elderly, agitated states, tension and anxiety, daytime sedation in senile mental disorder, confusion, alcohol withdrawal symptoms, pre-eclamptic toxaemia, severe epilepsy.

Dose: 10 ml in water or fruit juice before going to bed. For sedation 5-10 ml 3 times a day. (Different doses for alcohol withdrawal. Injection used for toxaemia and epilepsy.)
Availability: NHS and private prescription.
Side effects: blocked and irritating nose, irritating eyes, stomach disturbances, severe allergy, sedation, excitement, confusion.
Caution: in patients suffering from long-term lung weakness, kidney or liver disease. Patients should be warned of impaired ability.
Not to be used for: children, nursing mothers, or patients suffering from

acute lung weakness.
Caution needed with: alcohol and sedatives.
Contains: CHLORMETHIAZOLE EDISYLATE.
Other preparations: Heminevrin Capsules, Heminevrin IV, Heminevrin Solution.

heparinoid *see* **Anacal, Bayolin, Hirudoid, Lasonil,**

Herpid
(Boehringer Ingelheim)

A solution used as an anti-viral treatment for herpes-type skin infections.

Dose: apply locally 4 times a day for 4 days.
Availability: NHS and private prescription.
Side effects:
Caution:
Not to be used for: children, pregnant women, nursing mothers.
Caution needed with:
Contains: IDOXURIDINE, DIMETHYL SULPHOXIDE.
Other preparations: IDURIDIN (Ferring), VIRUDOX (Bioglan).

hexachlorophane *see* **Dermalex, Ster-Zac DC, Ster-Zac Powder, Torbetol**

hexamine hippurate *see* **Hiprex**

hexetidine *see* **Oraldene**

Hexopal
(Sanofi Winthrop)

A white, scored tablet supplied at a strength of 500 mg and used as a vasodilator to treat Raynaud's phenomenon (a condition caused by spasm of the blood vessels), intermittent claudication (difficulty walking caused by circulation disorders).

Dose: 2 tablets 3-4 times a day.

Availability: NHS and private prescription.
Side effects:
Caution: in pregnant women.
Not to be used for: children.
Caution needed with:
Contains: INOSITOL NICOTINATE.
Other preparations: Hexopal Forte, Hexopal Suspension.

---

hexyl nicotinate *see* **Transvasin**

Hibiscrub
(ICI)

A solution used as a disinfectant for cleansing and disinfecting skin and hands.

Dose: use as a liquid soap.
Availability: NHS, private prescription, over the counter.
Side effects:
Caution:
Not to be used for:
Caution needed with:
Contains: CHLORHEXIDINE gluconate.
Other preparations: HIBISOL (ICI), HIBITANE (ICI), PHISOMED (Sterling), UNISEPT (Seton Healthcare).

H

Hibisol
(ICI)

A solution used as a disinfectant for cleansing and disinfecting skin and hands.

Dose: rub vigorously on to the skin until dry.
Availability: NHS, private prescription, over the counter.
Side effects:
Caution:
Not to be used for:
Caution needed with:
Contains: CHLORHEXIDINE gluconate, ISOPROPYL ALCOHOL.
Other preparations: HIBISCRUB (ICI), HIBITANE (ICI), PHISOMED (Sterling), UNISEPT (Seton Healthcare).

Hibitane
(ICI)

A cream used as a disinfectant for cleansing and disinfecting hands and skin before surgery, and for prevention of infections in wounds and after surgery.

Dose: apply freely to the affected area as needed.
Availability: NHS, private prescription, over the counter.
Side effects:
Caution:
Not to be used for:
Caution needed with:
Contains: CHLORHEXIDINE gluconate.
Other preparations: Hibitane Obstetric Cream, Hibitane Concentrate, Hibitane 20% Gluconate, HIBISCRUB (ICI), HIBISOL (ICI), PHISOMED (Sterling), UNISEPT (Seton Healthcare)..

Hioxyl
(Quinoderm)

A cream used as a disinfectant to treat minor wounds, infections, bed sores, leg ulcers.

Dose: apply freely as needed and cover with a dressing.
Availability: NHS, private prescription, over the counter.
Side effects:
Caution:
Not to be used for:
Caution needed with:
Contains: HYDROGEN PEROXIDE.
Other preparations:

Hiprex
(3M Healthcare)

A white, oblong, scored tablet supplied at a strength of 1 g and used as an antibacterial treatment for infections of the urinary tract.

Dose: adults 1 g twice a day; children 6-12 years half adult dose.
Availability: NHS, private prescription, over the counter.
Side effects: stomach upset, rash, bladder irritation.
Caution:
Not to be used for: children under 6 years, or for patients suffering from severe dehydration, severe kidney failure, or electrolyte changes.

Caution needed with: sulphonamide antibiotics, SODIUM BICARBONATE, SODIUM CITRATE, POTASSIUM CITRATE.
Contains: HEXAMINE HIPPURATE.
Other preparations:

Hirudoid
(Panpharma)

A cream used as an anti-inflammatory agent to treat superficial thrombophlebitis and bruising.

Dose: apply liberally up to 4 times a day.
Availability: NHS, private prescription, over the counter.
Side effects:
Caution:
Not to be used for: children under 5 years, or on open wounds or mucous membranes.
Caution needed with:
Contains: HEPARINOID.
Other preparations: Hirudoid Gel.

Hismanal
(Janssen)

A white, scored tablet supplied at a strength of 10 mg and used as an ANTIHISTAMINE treatment for hay fever, allergic rhinitis, skin allergies.

Dose: adults 1 tablet a day 1 hour before food; children 6-12 years half adult dose.
Availability: NHS, private prescription, over the counter.
Side effects: rarely drowsiness or gain in weight, heart rhythm disturbance.
Caution: women of child-bearing age should take steps to avoid conception during and for some weeks after the treatment.
Not to be used for: children under 6 years, pregnant women.
Caution needed with: KETOCONAZOLE, ERYTHROMYCIN, ITRACONAZOLE.
Contains: ASTEMIZOLE.
Other preparations: Hismanal Suspension, Pollon-eze (Janssen).

Histalix
(Wallace)

A syrup used as an ANTIHISTAMINE, expectorant, and sputum softener to

H

treat bronchial and nasal congestion.

Dose: adults 5-10 ml every 3 hours; children half adult dose.
Availability: private prescription and over the counter.
Side effects: drowsiness, reduced reactions, rarely skin eruptions.
Caution:
Not to be used for:
Caution needed with: alcohol, sedatives.
Contains: DIPHENHYDRAMINE HYDROCHLORIDE, AMMONIUM CHLORIDE, SODIUM CITRATE, MENTHOL.
Other preparations: BENYLIN EXPECTORANT (Warner Lambert), GUANOR (R.P. Drugs).

Histryl Spansule
(Wellcome)

A pink/clear capsule supplied at a strength of 5 mg and used as an ANTIHISTAMINE treatment for rhinitis, severe allergic conditions, insect bites and stings, allergies to food or other drugs.

Dose: 1-2 capsules night and morning.
Availability: NHS, private prescription, over the counter.
Side effects: drowsiness, reduced reactions, dry mouth, blurred vision, dizziness.
Caution: in nursing mothers.
Not to be used for: children.
Caution needed with: sedatives, alcohol.
Contains: DIPHENYLPYRALINE HYDROCHLORIDE.
Other preparations: Histryl Paediatric.

Homatropine Minims
(SNP)

Drops used as an ANTICHOLINERGIC preparation for pupil dilation.

Dose: 1 or more drops into the eye as needed.
Availability: NHS and private prescription.
Side effects:
Caution:
Not to be used for: patients suffering from narrow-angle glaucoma.
Caution needed with:
Contains: HOMATROPINE HYDROBROMIDE.
Other preparations: Homatropine Eye Drops.

homatropine hydrobromide *see* **Homatropine**

---

homatropine *see* **APP**

Hormofemin *see* **Ortho Dienoestrol**. Product now discontinued.

Hormonin
(Shire)

A pink, scored tablet used as an oestrogen treatment for symptoms associate with the menopause.

Dose: 1-2 tablets a day.
Availability: NHS and private prescription.
Side effects: enlarged breasts, fluid retention, headaches, nausea, vaginal bleeding, weight gain, skin changes, rashes, liver disorders, jaundice, vomiting.
Caution: in patients suffering from high blood pressure, diabetes, heart disease, vascular disorders, asthma, kidney disease, epilepsy, womb diseases, migraine, thyroid disorder. Your doctor may advise you to have regular examinations.
Not to be used for: pregnant women, nursing mothers, or for patients suffering from sickle-cell anaemia, thrombosis, liver disorders, some cancers, undiagnosed vaginal bleeding, some ear, skin, and kidney disorders, jaundice, porphyria (a rare blood disorder), brain blood vessel disease.
Caution needed with: DIURETICS, ANTIHYPERTENSIVES, drugs which induce liver enzymes (eg BARBITURATES, PHENYTOIN, CARBAMAZEPINE, RIFAMPICIN).
Contains: OESTRIOL, OESTRONE, OESTRADIOL.
Other preparations:

Humulin see Insulin
(Lilly)

Hydergine
(Sandoz)

A white tablet supplied at strengths of 1.5 mg, 4.5 mg and used as a vasodilator as an additional treatment for elderly patients suffering from dementia.

Dose: 4.5 mg a day.
Availability: NHS and private prescription.
Side effects: stomach upset, flushes, rash, blocked nose, cramps, headache, dizziness, low blood pressure when standing.
Caution: in patients suffering from slow heart rate.
Not to be used for: children
Caution needed with:
Contains: CODERGOCRINE MESYLATE.
Other preparations:

---

hydralazine *see* Apresoline

Hydrenox
(Boots)

A white, scored tablet supplied at a strength of 50 mg and used as a DIURETIC to treat fluid retention, high blood pressure.

Dose: adults fluid retention 1-4 tablets a day as a single dose in the morning, then ½-1 tablet a day every other day, high blood pressure ½-1 tablet a day; children 1 mg per kg bodyweight a day.
Availability: NHS and private prescription.
Side effects: low potassium levels, rash, sensitivity to light, blood changes, gout, tiredness.
Caution: in the elderly, in pregnant women, nursing mothers, and in patients suffering from diabetes, liver or kidney disease, or gout; your doctor may advise that a potassium supplement is needed.
Not to be used for: patients suffering from severe kidney failure.
Caution needed with: LITHIUM, DIGOXIN, ANTIHYPERTENSIVES.
Contains: HYDROFLUMETHIAZIDE.
Other preparations:

Hydrocal *see* hydrocortisone cream

---

hydrochlorothiazide *see* Capozide, Carace Plus, Co-Betaloc, Dyazide, Esidrex, Hydromet, Hydrosaluric, Hypertane, Kalten, Innozide, Moducren, Moduret 25, Moduretic, Normetic, Secadrex, Serpasil Esidrex, Sotazide, Tolerzide

hydrocortisone cream

A cream used as a STEROID treatment for eczema, itch, and other skin disorders.

Dose: apply to the affected area 1-4 times a day.
Availability: NHS and private prescription.
Side effects: fluid retention, suppression of adrenal glands, thinning of the skin may occur.
Caution: use for short periods of time only.
Not to be used for: continuously especially for pregnant women, or for patients suffering from acne or any other tubercular, viral, fungal, or ringworm skin infections.
Caution needed with:
Contains: hydrocortisone.
Other preparations: Hydrocortisone Ointment, DIODERM (Dermal), EFCORTELAN (Glaxo), HYDROCAL (Bioglan), HYDROCORTISTAB (Boots), HYDROCORTISYL (Roussel), LOCOID (Brocades), MILDISON LIPOCREAM (Brocades). Some other brands available over the counter for certain conditions only..

---

hydrocortisone *see* **Actinac, Alphaderm, Alphosyl HC, Anugesic-HC, Anusol HC, Barquinol HC, Calmurid HC, Canesten-HC, Carbo-Cort, Chloromycetin Hydrocortisone, Cobadex, Colifoam, Corlan, Cortenema, Cortucid, Daktacort, Econacort, Epifoam, Eurax-Hydrocortisone, Framycort, Fucidin H, Gentisone HC, Gregoderm, Hydrocortistab, Hydroderm, Mildison Lipocream, Neo-Cortef, Nystaform-HC, Otosporin, Proctofoam HC, Proctosedyl, Quinocort, Sential, Tarcortin, Terra-Cortril, Timodine, Tri-Cicatrin, Uniroid, Vioform-Hydrocortisone, Xyloproct**

---

hydrocortisone suppositories *see* **Colifoam**

Hydrocortistab Tablets
(Boots)

A white, scored tablet supplied at a strength of 20 mg and used as a STEROID for replacement treatment in adrenocortical deficiency, inflammation in allergies, and rheumatic and collagen diseases.

Dose: adults and children as advised by the physician.
Availability: NHS and private prescription.
Side effects: high blood sugar, thin bones, mood changes, ulcers, high

H

blood pressure, fluid retention, potassium loss, muscle weakness.
Caution: in pregnant women, in patients who have had recent bowel surgery, or who are suffering from inflamed veins, psychiatric disorders, virus infections, some cancers, some kidney diseases, thinning of the bones, ulcers, tuberculosis, other infections, high blood pressure, glaucoma, epilepsy, diabetes, underactive thyroid, liver disease, stress. Withdraw gradually.
Not to be used for:
Caution needed with: PHENYTOIN, PHENOBARBITONE, EPHEDRINE, RIFAMPICIN, DIURETICS, ANTICHOLINESTERASES, DIGOXIN, antidiabetic agents, anticoagulants, NON-STEROID ANTI-INFLAMMATORY DRUGS.
Contains: HYDROCORTISONE.
Other preparations: Hydrocortistab Injection, HYDROCORTONE (MSD).

Hydrocortistab Cream/Ointment *see* hydrocortisone cream
(Boots)

Hydrocortisyl *see* hydrocortisone cream
(Roussel)

Hydrocortone
(MSD)

A white, quarter-scored tablet or a white, scored, oval tablet according to strengths of 10 mg, 20 mg and used as a STEROID replacement treatment in adrenocortical deficiency.

Dose: as advised by the physician.
Availability: NHS and private prescription.
Side effects: high blood sugar, thin bones, mood changes, ulcers, high blood pressure, fluid retention, potassium loss, muscle weakness.
Caution: in pregnant women, in patients who have had recent bowel surgery, or who are suffering from inflamed veins, psychiatric disorders, virus infections, some cancers, some kidney diseases, thinning of the bones, ulcers, tuberculosis, other infections, high blood pressure, glaucoma, epilepsy, diabetes, underactive thyroid, liver disease, stress. Withdraw gradually.
Not to be used for:
Caution needed with: PHENYTOIN, PHENOBARBITONE, EPHEDRINE, RIFAMPICIN, DIURETICS, ANTICHOLINESTERASES, DIGOXIN, antidiabetic agents, anticoagulants, NON-STEROID ANTI-INFLAMMATORY DRUGS.
Contains: HYDROCORTISONE.

Other preparations: HYDROCORTISTAB (Boots).

Hydroderm — antibacterial/steroid ointment. Product now discontinued.

---

hydroflumethiazide *see* **Hydrenox**

---

hydrogen peroxide *see* **Hioxyl**

Hydromet
(MSD)

A pink tablet used as an ANTIHYPERTENSIVE treatment for high blood pressure.

Dose: adults 1 tablet twice a day at first increasing at 2-day intervals to a maximum of 12 tablets a day; children as advised by physician.
Availability: NHS and private prescription.
Side effects: sedation, headache, weakness, depression, slow heart rate, blocked nose, dry mouth, stomach upset, blood changes.
Caution: in pregnant women, nursing mothers, and in patients with a history of liver disease, or in patients suffering from some blood disorders, gout, diabetes, liver or kidney disease. Your doctor may advise that potassium supplements may be needed.
Not to be used for: patients suffering from depression, liver disease, severe kidney failure, phaeochromocytoma (a disease of the adrenal glands).
Caution needed with: TRICYCLICS, MAOIS, ANTIHYPERTENSIVES, HYDRALAZINE, DIGOXIN, LITHIUM.
Contains: METHYLDOPA, HYDROCHLOROTHIAZIDE.
Other preparations:

Hydromol *see* Diprobath
(Quinoderm)

Hydrosaluric
(MSD)

A white, scored tablet supplied at strengths of 25 mg, 50 mg and used as a DIURETIC to treat fluid retention, high blood pressure.

Dose: adults as a diuretic 25-100 mg once or twice a day, high blood pressure 25-50 mg a day at first, then up to not more than 100 mg a day; infants under 6 months up to 3.5 mg per kg bodyweight a day, 6 months-2 years 12.5-37.5 mg a day, 2-12 years 37.5-100 mg a day all in 2 divided doses.
Availability: NHS and private prescription.
Side effects: low potassium levels, rash, sensitivity to light, blood changes, gout, tiredness.
Caution: in pregnant women and in patients suffering from diabetes, liver or kidney disease, electrolyte imbalance, or gout. Your doctor may advise that a potassium supplement is needed.
Not to be used for: nursing mothers or for patients suffering from severe kidney or liver failure.
Caution needed with: LITHIUM, DIGOXIN, ANTIHYPERTENSIVES, sedatives, ACE INHIBITORS, STEROIDS, antidiabetics, muscle relaxants, anti-inflammatories.
Contains: HYDROCHLOROTHIAZIDE.
Other preparations: ESIDREX (Ciba).

---

hydrotalcite *see* Altacite Plus

---

hydrous ointment BP

A cream used as an emollient to treat dry skin conditions.

Dose: apply as required
Availability: NHS, private prescription, over the counter.
Side effects:
Caution:
Not to be used for:
Caution needed with:
Contains: hydrous ointment BP (oily cream).
Other preparations:

---

hydroxocobalamin *see* Lipoflavonoid, Lipotriad

---

hydroxyapatite compound *see* Ossopan

---

hydroxychloroquine *see* Plaquenil
306

hydroxyzine *see* **Atarax**

Hygroton
(Ciba-Geigy)

A pale-yellow, scored tablet supplied at a strength of 50 mg and used as a DIURETIC to treat high blood pressure, fluid retention.

Dose: adults fluid retention 50 mg a day or 100-200 mg every other day at first, then 50-100 mg 3 times a week as a single dose after breakfast, high blood pressure 25-50 mg a day as a single dose after breakfast; children 2 mg per kg a day.
Availability: NHS and private prescription.
Side effects: abnormal heart rhythm, stomach disturbances, rash, sensitivity to light, blood changes, gout, tiredness, electrolyte distrubances, visual disturbances, impotence, low blood pressure when standing, dizziness, rarely liver disturbances.
Caution: in the elderly, pregnant women, nursing mothers, and in patients suffering from diabetes, kidney or liver disease, high blood lipids, severe thickening of the arteries or gout. Your doctor may advise that a potassium supplement is needed.
Not to be used for: patients suffering from Addison's disease, severe kidney or liver failure, low sodium or potassium levels, high calcium or uric acid levels.
Caution needed with: LITHIUM, DIGOXIN, ANTIHYPERTENSIVES, NON-STEROID ANTI-INFLAMMATORY DRUGS, INSULIN, antidiabetics.
Contains: CHLORTHALIDONE.
Other preparations:

H

Hygroton K
(Geigy)

A pink tablet used as a DIURETIC with potassium supplement to treat high blood pressure, fluid retention.

Dose: high blood pressure 1 tablet 1-2 times a day; fluid retention 1-2 tablets a day or 2-4 tablets 3 times a week.
Availability: NHS and private prescription.
Side effects: abnormal heart rhythm, stomach disturbances, rash, sensitivity to light, blood changes, gout, tiredness, electrolyte disturbances, rarely liver changes.
Caution: in the elderly, and in patients suffering from diabetes, gout, liver or kidney disease, high blood lipids.
Not to be used for: pregnant women, nursing mothers, or for patients

suffering from severe kidney or liver failure, Addison's disease, raised potassium levels, low sodium or potassium levels, high calcium or uric acid levels, gastro-intestinal inflammation or obstruction.
Caution needed with: LITHIUM, DIGOXIN, ANTIHYPERTENSIVES, potassium-sparing DIURETICS, ACE INHIBITORS, NON-STEROID ANTI-INFLAMMATORY DRUGS.
Contains: CHLORTHALIDONE, POTASSIUM CHLORIDE.
Other preparations:

hyoscine *see* Buscopan, hyoscine eye drops, Scopoderm

hyoscine eye drops

Drops usually supplied at a strength of 0.25% and used to dilate the eye pupil.

Dose: as directed by the doctor.
Availability: NHS and private prescription.
Side effects:
Caution: in very young and very old patients.
Not to be used for: patients with some types of glaucoma.
Caution needed with:
Contains: HYOSCINE HYDROBROMIDE.
Other preparations:

hyoscyamine sulphate *see* Peptard

Hypertane
(Schwarz)

A white, scored tablet used as a DIURETIC and potassium-sparing diuretic to treat congestive heart failure, high blood pressure, cirrhosis of the liver with ascites especially where the potassium balance must be controlled.

Dose: adults usually 1-2 tablets a day up to a maximum of 4 tablets; elderly according to kidney function and response.
Availability: NHS and private prescription.
Side effects: rash, sensitivity to light, blood changes, gout.
Caution: in patients suffering from diabetes, electrolyte changes, gout, kidney or liver disease.
Not to be used for: children, pregnant women, nursing mothers, or for patients suffering from raised potassium levels, progressive or severe

kidney failure.
Caution needed with: potassium supplements and potassium-sparing DIURETICS, DIGOXIN, LITHIUM, ANTIHYPERTENSIVES, ACE INHIBITORS.
Contains: HYDROCHLOROTHIAZIDE, AMILORIDE hydrochloride.
Other preparations: AMILCO (Baker Norton), AMILMAXCO (Ashbourne), CO-AMILOZIDE, MODURETIC (MSD).

Hypon
(Calmic)

A yellow tablet used as an ANALGESIC for the relief of headache, rheumatism, neuralgia, period pain, colds.

Dose: 1-2 tablets every 4 hours.
Availability: private prescription and over the counter.
Side effects: stomach upset, allergy, asthma.
Caution: in the elderly, pregnant women, and in patients with a history of allergy to aspirin or asthma, impaired liver or kidney function, indigestion.
Not to be used for: children, nursing mothers, or for patients suffering from haemophilia, ulcers.
Caution needed with: anticoagulants, some antidiabetic drugs, anti-inflammatory agents, METHOTREXATE, SPIRONOLACTONE, some uric acid-lowering drugs, STEROIDS.
Contains: ASPIRIN, CAFFEINE, CODEINE PHOSPHATE.
Other preparations:

Hypotears
(Iolab)

Drops used to moisten dry eyes.

Dose: 1-2 drops every 3-4 hours or as needed.
Availability: NHS, private prescription, over the counter.
Side effects:
Caution:
Not to be used for: patients who wear soft contact lenses.
Caution needed with:
Contains: POLYETHYLENE GLYCOL, POLYVINYL ALCOHOL.
Other preparations: LIQUIFILM TEARS (Allergan), SNO TEARS (S&N).

Hypovase
(Invicta)

A white tablet, orange, scored tablet, or white, scored tablet according to strengths of 500 micrograms, 1 mg, 2 mg, 5 mg and used as a vasodilator to treat congestive heart failure, high blood pressure, Raynaud's phenomenon, additional treatment in urinary obstruction caused by prostate enlargement.

Dose: for heart failure 500 micrograms 3-4 times a day at first, increasing to 1 mg 3-4 times a day, followed by 4-20 mg a day in divided doses to maintain treatment. For high blood pressure 500 micrograms on first evening, then 500 micrograms 2-3 times a day for 3-7 days increasing as needed to a maximum of 20 mg a day. For Raynaud's phenomenon or prostate enlargement 500 micrograms twice a day at first then 1-2 mg twice a day.
Availability: NHS and private prescription.
Side effects: loss of consciousness, dizziness, lassitude, dry mouth, blurred vision, rash.
Caution: in patients suffering from fainting when they urinate.
Not to be used for: children.
Caution needed with: ANTIHYPERTENSIVES.
Contains: PRAZOSIN HYDROCHLORIDE.
Other preparations: ALPHAVASE (Ashbourne).

---

hypromellose *see* Epinal, hypromellose eye drops, Ilube, Isopto Alkaline, Isopto Atropine, Isopto Carbachol, Isopto Carpine, Isopto Plain, Maxidex, Maxitrol, Tears Naturale

H

---

hypromellose eye drops

Drops used to treat tear defiency.

Dose: 1-2 drops 3 times a day or as required.
Availability: NHS, private prescription, over the counter.
Side effects:
Caution:
Not to be used for:
Caution needed with:
Contains: HYPROMELLOSE.
Other preparations BJ6 (Martindale, Thornton & Ross), ISOPTO ALKALINE (Alcon), ISOPTO PLAIN (Alcon), TEARS NATURALE (Alcon).

Hypurin *see* Insulin
(CP Pharmaceuticals)

Hytrin
(Abbott)

A white, yellow, brown, or blue tablet according to strengths of 1 mg, 2 mg, 5 mg, 10 mg and used as an ANTIHYPERTENSIVE to treat high blood pressure.

Dose: 1 mg at bed time at first, then increase dose at weekly intervals to a usual dose of 2-10 mg once a day.
Availability: NHS and private prescription.
Side effects: fainting with first dose, dizziness, lowered blood pressure on standing, lassitude, swelling of the limbs.
Caution: in patients with a history of liver disease or suffering from fainting.
Not to be used for: children.
Caution needed with:
Contains: TERAZOSIN HYDROCHLORIDE.
Other preparations:

Ibrufhalal *see* Brufen
(Halal)

Ibufac *see* Brufen
(DDSA)

Ibugel *see* Proflex
(Dermal)

Ibumed *see* Brufen
(Medipharma Labs)

---

ibuprofen *see* Brufen, Codafen, Junifen, Proflex

Idoxene
(Spodefell)

An ointment used as an anti-viral treatment for herpetic keratitis (viral infection of the cornea).

Dose: Apply 4 times a day and at night until 3-5 days after symptoms have gone but for no more than 3 weeks.
Availability: NHS and private prescription.
Side effects: local irritation, swelling, pain.
Caution: in pregnant women.
Not to be used for:
Caution needed with: STEROIDS, BORIC ACID.
Contains: IDOXURIDINE.
Other preparations:

---

idoxuridine *see* **Herpid, Idoxene, Kerecid, Virudox**

Iduridin *see* **Herpid**
(Ferring)

Ilosone *see* **Erythrocin**
(Dista)

Ilotycin *see* **Erythrocin.** Product now discontinued

Ilube
(Cusi)

Drops used to moisten dry eyes.

Dose: 1-2 drops into the eye 3-4 times a day.
Availability: NHS and private prescription.
Side effects:
Caution:
Not to be used for: patients who wear soft contact lenses.
Caution needed with:
Contains: ACETYLCYSTEINE, HYPROMELLOSE.
Other preparations:

Imbrilon see Indocid
(Berk)

Imdur *see* Elantan
(Astra)

Imigran
(Glaxo)

A white, capsule-shaped tablet supplied at a strength of 100 mg and used to treat migraine.

Dose: 1 tablet soon after onset of attack. If migraine responds but then recurs, repeat the dose, to a maximum of 3 tablets in 24 hours.Repeat doses should not be used if migraine did not respond initially.
Availability: NHS and private prescription.
Side effects: tiredness, dizziness, feelings of heaviness and weakness, throat symptoms, chest pain, raised blood pressure, liver disorder.
Caution: in pregnant women, nursing mothers, and in patients suffering from liver or kidney disorder.
Not to be used for: children, the elderly, or for patients suffering from heart disease or disorder, or uncontrolled high blood pressure.
Caution needed with: MAOIS, LITHIUM, ERGOTAMINE, some antidepressants.
Contains: SUMATRIPTAN.
Other preparations: Imigran Injection (also used to treat cluster headache).

---

imipramine *see* Tofranil

Imodium
(Janssen)

A dark green/grey capsule supplied at a strength of 2 mg and used to treat diarrhoea.

Dose: acute diarrhoea, 2 capsules initially then 1 after each loose bowel motion, to a maximum of 8 capsules a day. Chronic diarrhoea, 2-4 capsules a day in divided doses. Children use syrup.
Availability: NHS, private prescription, over the counter.
Side effects: rash.
Caution: in patients suffering from severe ulcerative colitis.
Not to be used for: children under 4 years.
Caution needed with:
Contains: LOPERAMIDE.
Other preparations: Imodium Syrup (only available on prescription), ARRET (Janssen), diocalm ultra (SKB).

I

Imperacin *see* **Tetracycline**
(ICI)

Imtack
(Astra)

An aerosol used as a NITRATE to treat and prevent angina.

Dose: 1-3 doses sprayed under the tongue (while holding breath) at start of an attack or before exertion.
Availability: NHS, private prescription, over the counter.
Side effects: flushes, headache, dizziness.
Caution: do not inhale the spray.
Not to be used for: for children.
Caution needed with:
Contains: ISOSORBIDE DINITRATE.
Other preparations: CEDOCARD (Famitalia), ISOKET RETARD (Schwarz), ISORDIL (Monmouth), SONI-SLO (Lipha), SORBICHEW (Stuart), SORBID-SA (Stuart), SORBITRATE (Stuart), VASCARDIN (Nicholas).

Imunovir
(Leo)

A white tablet supplied at a strength of 500 mg and used as an anti-viral treatment for genital herpes, warts, and other herpes-type infections.

Dose: herpes 8 tablets a day for 7-14 days; warts 6 tablets a day for 14-28 days.
Availability: NHS and private prescription.
Side effects: increased levels of uric acid.
Caution: in patients suffering from kidney disease, gout, raised uric acid levels.
Not to be used for: children.
Not to be used with:
Contains: INOSINE PRANOBEX.
Other preparations:

---

indapamide hemihydrate *see* **Natrilix**

Inderal
(ICI)

A pink tablet supplied at strengths of 10 mg, 40 mg, 80 mg and used as a ß-BLOCKER to treat angina, migraine, high blood pressure, anxiety, abnormal heart rhythm, other heart conditions, and as an additional treatment for thyrotoxicosis.

Dose: adults high blood pressure 80 mg twice a day at first, then adjust each week according to response, thyrotoxicosis 10-40 mg 3-4 times a day, migraine 40 mg 2-3 times a day, angina 40 mg 2-3 times a day up to 480 mg a day; children thyrotoxicosis 0.25-0.5 mg per kg bodyweight 3-4 times a day, migraine half adult dose. Other conditions as advised by doctor.
Availability: NHS and private prescription.
Side effects: cold hands and feet, sleep disturbance, slow heart rate, tiredness, wheezing, heart failure, stomach upset.
Caution: in pregnant women, nursing mothers, and in patients suffering from diabetes, kidney or liver disorders, asthma. May need to be withdrawn before surgery. Withdraw gradually. Your doctor may advise additional treatment with DIURETICS or DIGOXIN.
Not to be used for: patients suffering from heart block or failure.
Caution needed with: VERAPAMIL, CLONIDINE withdrawal, some anti-arrhythmic drugs and anaesthetics, RESERPINE, CIMETIDINE, sedatives, SYMPATHOMIMETICS, INDOMETHACIN, antidiabetics, ERGOTAMINE, some ANTIHYPERTENSIVES.
Contains: PROPRANOLOL HYDROCHLORIDE.
Other preparations: ANGILOL (DDSA), APSOLOL (APS), BEDRANOL SR (Lagap), BERKOLOL (Berk), BETA-PROGRANE (Tillomed), BETADUR CR (Monmouth), CARDINOL (CP Pharm), HALF BETADUR CR (Monmouth), HALF INDERAL LA (ICI), INDERAL LA (ICI), PROPANIX (Ashbourne).

Inderal LA
(ICI)

A lavender/pink capsule supplied at a strength of 160 mg and used as a ß-BLOCKER to treat angina, high blood pressure, anxiety, migraine, and as an additional treatment for thyrotoxicosis.

Dose: 80 or 160 mg a day to a maximum of 240 mg a day. High blood pressure 160 mg a day at first increasing by 80 mg at a time until there is an effective response. Thyrotoxicosis 80 or 160 mg a day to a maximum of 240 mg a day.
Availability: NHS and private prescription.
Side effects: cold hands and feet, sleep disturbance, slow heart rate, tiredness, wheezing, heart failure, stomach upset, dry eyes, rash.
Caution: in pregnant women, nursing mothers, and in patients suffering from diabetes, kidney or liver disorders, asthma. May need to be with-

drawn before surgery. Withdraw gradually. Your doctor may advise additional treatment with DIURETICS or DIGOXIN. Potassium supplements may be needed.

Not to be used for: children or for patients suffering from heart block or failure.

Caution needed with: VERAPAMIL, CLONIDINE withdrawal, some ANTIHYPERTENSIVES, anaesthetics, RESERPINE, CIMETIDINE, sedatives, SYMPATHOMIMETICS, INDOMETHACIN, antidiabetics, ERGOTAMINE.

Contains: PROPRANOLOL HYDROCHLORIDE, BENDROFLUAZIDE.

Other preparations: ANGILOL (DDSA), APSOLOL (APS), BEDRANOL SR (Lagap), BERKOLOL (Berk), BETA-PROGRANE (Tillomed), BETADUR CR (Monmouth), CARDINOL (CP Pharm), HALF BETADUR CR (Monmouth), HALF INDERAL LA (ICI), INDERAL (ICI) PROPANIX (Ashbourne).

Inderetic
(ICI)

A white capsule used as a ß-BLOCKER to treat high blood pressure.

Dose: 1 capsule twice a day.
Availability: NHS and private prescription.
Side effects: cold hands and feet, sleep disturbance, slow heart rate, tiredness, wheezing, heart failure, stomach upset, low blood potassium, rash, sensitivity to light, blood changes, gout, dry eyes.
Caution: in pregnant women, nursing mothers, and in patients suffering from diabetes, kidney or liver disorders, asthma, gout. May need to be withdrawn before surgery. Withdraw gradually. Your doctor may advise additional treatment with DIURETICS or DIGOXIN, blood tests.
Not to be used for: children or for patients suffering from heart block or failure, severe kidney failure.
Caution needed with: VERAPAMIL, CLONIDINE withdrawal, some anti-arrhythmic drugs, some ANTIHYPERTENSIVES, anaesthetics, RESERPINE, CIMETIDINE, sedatives, SYMPATHOMIMETICS, INDOMETHACIN, other DIURETICS, antidiabetics, ERGOTAMINE.
Contains: PROPANOLOL HYDROCHLORIDE.
Other preparations: INDEREX (double strength).

Inderex *see* Inderetic
(ICI)

Indocid
(Morson)

316

An ivory capsule supplied at strengths of 25 mg, 50 mg and used as a NON-STEROID ANTI-INFLAMMATORY DRUG to treat rheumatoid arthritis, osteoarthritis, degenerative disease of the hip joint, ankylosing spondylitis, acute gout, lumbago, acute joint disorders, orthopaedic procedures, period pain.

Dose: 50-200 mg a day in divided doses.
Availability: NHS and private prescription.
Side effects: gastro-intestinal bleeding, headache, corneal deposits, disturbances of the retina, gastro-intestinal intolerance, dizziness, brain disturbances, blood changes.
Caution: in the elderly, and in patients suffering from kidney or liver disease, brain disorders.
Not to be used for: children, pregnant women, nursing mothers, or for patients suffering from stomach ulcer, history of stomach lesions, aspirin/anti-inflammatory drug allergy, recent proctitis, severe allergic swelling.
Caution needed with: anticoagulants, LITHIUM, DIURETICS, ß-BLOCKERS, PROBENECID, aminoglycoside antibiotics, METHOTREXATE, STEROIDS, some ANALGESICS.
Contains: INDOMETHACIN.
Other preparations: Indocid Suspension, Indocid Suppositories, Indocid-R. ARTRACIN (DDSA), FLEXIN (Napp), IMBRILON (Berk), INDOLAR SR (Lagap), INDOMAX (Ashbourne), INDOMOD (Pharmacia), RIMACID (Rima).

Indolar SR *see* **Indocid**
(Lagap)

Indomax *see* **Indocid**
(Ashbourne)

---

indomethacin *see* **Flexin Continus, Indocid**

Indomod *see* **Indocid**
(Kabi Pharmacia)

---

indoramin *see* **Baratol, Doralese**

Infacol *see* **Asilone**
(Pharmax)

Initard *see* **insulin**
(Novo Nordisk)

Innovace
(MSD)

A round white tablet, a white scored, or red or peach, triangular tablet according to strengths of 2.5 mg, 5 mg, 10 mg, 20 mg and used as an ACE INHIBITOR to treat congestive heart failure, high blood pressure.

Dose: heart failure adults 2.5 mg at first in hospital, 10-20 mg thereafter. High blood pressure 5 mg a day at first, then 10-20 mg to a maximum of 40 mg once a day; elderly or patients suffering from kidney disease start with 2.5 mg a day.
Availability: NHS and private prescription.
Side effects: low blood pressure, kidney failure, swelling, rash, headache, tiredness, dizziness, stomach upset, and rarely a cough.
Caution: fluid depletion may cause a marked drop in blood pressure. Dose of diuretic given may need to be reduced. Care in patients suffering from some kidney diseases, severe heart failure, and in nursing mothers and patients being anaesthetized.
Not to be used for: children, pregnant women, or for patients suffering from some heart defects..
Caution needed with: other ANTIHYPERTENSIVES, LITHIUM, potassium supplements, potassium-sparing DIURETICS.
Contains: ENALAPRIL MALEATE.
Other preparations:

Innozide
(MSD)

A yellow, scored tablet used as an ACE INHIBITOR and DIURETIC to treat mild to moderate high blood pressure.

Dose: 1-2 tablets once a day.
Availability: NHS and private prescription.
Side effects: dizziness, tiredness, headache, cramp, weakness, low blood pressure, cough, impotence, chest pain, rash, kidney failure, severe allergy.
Caution: in nursing mothers, and in patients suffering from body fluid

imbalance, blood vessel disease in the heart or brain, diabetes, gout, liver or kidney disease, and during anaesthesia.
Not to be used for: children, pregnant women, or for patients suffering from inability to produce urine, or with a history of severe allergy to ACE INHIBITORS.
Caution needed with: LITHIUM, NON-STEROID ANTI-INFLAMMATORY drugs, some DIURETICS, potassium supplements, sedatives, antidiabetics, STEROIDS.
Contains: ENALPRIL MALEATE, HYDROCHLOROTHIAZIDE.
Other preparations:

---

inosine pranobex *see* Imunovir

---

inositol *see* Hexopal, Ketovite, Lipoflavonoid, Lipotriad

Insulatard *see* insulin
(Novo Nordisk)

---

insulin

An injectable liquid used to treat diabetes.

Dose: usually by subcutaneous injection (occasionally intramuscular or intravenous, depending on type of insulin), according to patient's requirements.
Availability: NHS, private prescription; over the counter.
Side effects: allergy at injection site, alteration in fat at injection site. Low blood sugar if too much insulin given.
Caution: in patients transferring from other types of insulin, in pregnant women, and in patients suffering from infection, emotional distress, or liver or kidney disease.
Not to be used for:
Caution needed with: ß-BLOCKERS, MAOIS, STEROIDS, DIURETICS, the contraceptive pill, alcohol.
Contains: (*see* table below)
Other preparations: (*see* table below)

Human Actraphane
(Novo Nordisk)

Ingredients: human neutral insulin, human isophane insulin.
Duration of action: biphasic (mixed effect).

Human Actrapid
(Novo Nordisk)

Ingredients: human neutral insulin.
Duration of action: short-acting.

Human Initard 50/50
(Novo Nordisk)

Ingredients: human neutral insulin, human isophane insulin.
Duration of action: biphasic (mixed effect).

Human Insulatard
(Novo Nordisk)

Ingredients: human isophane insulin.
Duration of action: intermediate-acting.

Human Mixtard
(Novo Nordisk)

Ingredients: human neutral insulin, human isophane insulin.
Duration of action: biphasic (mixed effect).

Human Monotard
(Novo Nordisk)

Ingredients: human insulin zinc suspension (mixed).
Duration of action: intermediate-acting.

Human Protaphane
(Novo Nordisk)

Ingredients: human isophane insulin.
Duration of action: intermediate-acting.

Human Ultratard
(Novo Nordisk)

Ingredients: human insulin zinc suspension (crystalline).
Duration of action: long-acting.

Human Velosulin
(Novo Nordisk)

Ingredients: human neutral insulin.
Duration of action: short-acting.

Humulin I
(Lilly)

Ingredients: human isophane insulin.
Duration of action: intermediate-acting.

Humulin Lente
(Lilly)

Ingredients: human insulin zinc suspension (mixed).
Duration of action: intermediate-acting.

Humulin M1, M2, M3, M4
(Lilly)

Ingredients: human neutral insulin, human isophane insulin.
Duration of action: biphasic (mixed effect).

Humulin S
(Lilly)

Ingredients: human neutral insulin.
Duration of action: short-acting.

Humulin Zn
(Lilly)

I

Ingredients: human insulin zinc suspension (crystalline).
Duration of action: intermediate-acting.

Hypurin Isophane
(CP Pharmaceuticals)

Ingredients: beef isophane insulin.
Duration of action: intermediate-acting.

Hypurin Lente
(CP Pharmaceuticals)

Ingredients: beef insulin zinc suspension.
Duration of action: long-acting.

Hypurin Neutral
(CP Pharmaceuticals)

Ingredients: beef neutral insulin.
Duration of action: short-acting.

Hypurin Protamine Zinc
(CP Pharmaceuticals)

Ingredients: beef protamine zinc insulin.
Duration of action: long-acting.

Initard 50/50
(Novo Nordisk)

Ingredients: pork neutral insulin, pork isophane insulin.
Duration of action: biphasic (mixed effect).

Insulatard
(Novo Nordisk)

Ingredients: pork isophane insulin.
Duration of action: intermediate-acting.

Isophane
(Evans)

Ingredients: beef isophane insulin.
Duration of action: intermediate-acting.

Lentard MC
(Novo Nordisk)

Ingredients: beef and pork insulin zinc suspensions (mixed).
Duration of action: intermediate-acting.

Lente
(Evans)

Ingredients: beef insulin zinc suspension (mixed).
Duration of action: long-acting.

Mixtard
(Novo Nordisk)

Ingredients: pork neutral insulin, pork isophane insulin.
Duration of action: biphasic (mixed effect).

Neutral
(Evans)

Ingredients: beef neutral insulin.
Duration of action: short-acting.

Penmix 10/90, 20/80, 30/70, 40/60, 50/50
(Novo Nordisk)

Ingredients: human neutral insulin, human isophane insulin.
Duration of action: biphasic (mixed effect).

Pur-in Isophane
(CP Pharmaceuticals)

I

Ingredients: human isophane insulin.
Duration of action: intermediate-acting.

Pur-in Mix 15/85, 25/75, 50/50
(CP Pharmaceuticals)

Ingredients: human neutral insulin, human isophane insulin.
Duration of action: biphasic (mixed effect).

Pur-in Neutral
(CP Pharmaceuticals)

Ingredients: human neutral insulin.
Duration of action: short-acting.

Rapitard MC
(Novo Nordisk)

Ingredients: pork neutral insulin, beef crystalline insulin.
Duration of action: Biphasic (mixed effect).

Semitard MC
(Novo Nordisk)

Ingredients: pork insulin zinc suspension (amorphous).
Duration of action: intermediate-acting

Velosulin
(Novo Nordisk)

Ingredients: pork neutral insulin.
Duration of action: short-acting.

Intal
(Fisons)

A yellow/clear spincap (delivery capsule) supplied at a strength of 20 mg and used as an anti-asthmatic drug for the prevention of bronchial asthma.

Dose: 4 a day at regular intervals in Spinhaler (delivery system) increasing

if needed to 6-8 a day. Treatment should be continuous.
Availability: NHS and private prescription.
Side effects: passing cough, irritated throat, rarely bronchial spasm.
Caution:
Not to be used for:
Caution needed with:
Contains: SODIUM CROMOGLYCATE.
Other preparations: Intal Inhaler, Intal Nebuliser Solution, CROMOGEN (Baker Norton). (Intal 5 Inhaler — now discontinued.)

Intal Compound
(Fisons)

An orange/clear Spincap (delivery capsule) used as an anti-asthmatic drug for the prevention of bronchial asthma.

Dose: 4 a day at regular intervals in Spinhaler (delivery system) up to 6-8 a day if needed. Treatment should be continuous.
Availability: NHS and private prescription.
Side effects: passing cough, irritated throat, headache, abnormal heart rhythms, rapid heart rate, dilation of the blood vessels, rarely bronchial spasm.
Caution: in patients suffering from diabetes, high blood pressure.
Not to be used for: patients suffering from heart disease, overactive thyroid, cardiac asthma.
Not to be used with: MAOIS, SYMPATHOMIMETICS, TRICYCLICS.
Contains: SODIUM CROMOGLYCATE, ISOPRENALINE SULPHATE.
Other preparations:

Integrin
(Sanofi Winthrop)

A white capsule or a white, scored tablet according to strengths of 10 mg, 40 mg and used as a sedative to treat anxiety, schizophrenia, mental disorders, delirium.

Dose: anxiety 10 mg 3-4 times a day to a maximum of 60 mg a day; others 40 mg 2-3 times a day to a maximum of 300 mg a day.
Availability: NHS and private prescription.
Side effects: tremor, ANTI-CHOLERGENIC effects, low blood pressure episodes, sedation, agitation, changes in some blood tests.
Caution: in the elderly, pregnant women, nursing mothers, and in patients suffering from kidney or liver damage, heart or lung disease, epilepsy, parkinsonism, or underactive thyroid. Your doctor may advise that blood

and liver tests should be made regularly, and that your judgement and abilities may be reduced.
Not to be used for: children, or for patients suffering from glaucoma or bone marrow depression.
Caution needed with: MAOIS, alcohol, sedatives, ANTIHYPERTENSIVES.
Contains: OXYPERTINE.
Other preparations:

Intralgin
(3M Healthcare)

A gel used as an ANALGESIC rub to treat muscle strains, sprains.

Dose: massage gently into the affected area as needed.
Availability: NHS, private prescription, and over the counter.
Side effects: may be irritant.
Caution:
Not to be used for: areas near the eyes or on broken or inflamed skin or on membranes (such as the mouth).
Caution needed with:
Contains: SALICYLAMIDE, BENZOCAINE.
Other preparations:

Iodosorb
(Perstorp)

Powder in a sachet used as an absorbant, antibacterial treatment for leg ulcers and moist wounds.

Dose: apply a 3 mm coating and cover with a dressing; repeat the treatment before the dressing is saturated.
Availability: NHS and private prescription.
Side effects:
Caution: in patients having thyroid investigation.
Not to be used for: pregnant women or nursing mothers.
Caution needed with:
Contains: CADEXOMER IODINE.
Other preparations: Iodosorb Ointment.

Ionamin
(Lipha)

A yellow/grey capsule or a yellow capsule according to strengths of 15 mg,

30 mg and used as an appetite suppressant to treat obesity.

Dose: adults 15-30 mg once a day at breakfast time.
Availability: controlled drug; NHS and private prescription.
Side effects: tolerance, addiction, mental disturbances, restlessness, nervousness, agitation, dry mouth, heart palpitations, raised blood pressure.
Caution: in patients suffering from angina, abnormal heart rhythms, high blood pressure.
Not to be used for: children, pregnant women, nursing mothers, or for patients suffering from hardening of the arteries, overactive thyroid gland, severe high blood pressure, or with a history of mental illness, alcoholism, or drug addiction.
Caution needed with: MAOIS, SYMPATHOMIMETICS, METHYLDOPA, GUANETHIDINE, sedatives.
Contains: PHENTERMINE.
Other preparations: DUROMINE (3M Healthcare).

Ionax
(Galderma)

An gel used as an abrasive, antibacterial preparation to clean the skin in the treatment of acne.

Dose: wet the face, then rub in once or twice a day, and rinse.
Availability: NHS, private prescription, over the counter.
Side effects:
Caution:
Not to be used for: for children under 12 years.
Caution needed with:
Contains: POLYETHYLENE GRANULES, BENZALKONIUM CHLORIDE.
Other preparations:

Ionil T
(Galderma)

A shampoo used as an antipsoriatic treatment for seborrhoeic inflammation of the scalp.

Dose: shampoo once or twice a week.
Availability: NHS, private prescription, over the counter.
Side effects: irritation, sensitivity to light.
Caution:
Not to be used for: patients suffering from acute psoriasis.
Caution needed with:

Contains: SALICYLIC ACID, BENZALKONIUM CHLORIDE, COAL TAR SOLUTION.
Other preparations: CAPASAL (Dermal), GELCOSAL (Quinoderm).

---

ipecacuanha *see* **Alophen**

Ipral *see* **Monotrim**
(Squibb)

---

ipratropium *see* **Atrovent, Duovent, Rinatec**

---

iprindole *see* **Prondol**

Irofol C *see* **Fefol.** Product now discontinued.

Isib *see* **Elantan**
(Ashbourne)

Isisfen *see* **Brufen**
(Isis)

Ismelin Tablets
(Ciba)

A white tablet or a pink tablet according to strengths of 10 mg, 25 mg and used as an ANTIHYPERTENSIVE treatment for high blood pressure.

Dose: adults 10 mg a day at first increasing by 10 mg at a time at weekly intervals if needed; children as advised by physician.
Availability: NHS and private prescription.
Side effects: low blood pressure on standing up, diarrhoea, failure of ejaculation, fluid retention, blood changes, slow heartbeat.
Caution: in pregnant women and in patients undergoing anaesthesia or suffering from kidney disease, stomach ulcer, or hardening of the arteries.
Not to be used for: patients suffering from phaeochromocytoma (a

disease of the adrenal glands), kidney or heart failure.
Caution needed with: TRICYCLIC antidepressants, SYMPATHOMIMETICS, MAOIS, DIURETICS, RESERPINE-like drugs, anti-arrhythmics, DIGOXIN, sedatives, ANTIHYPERTENSIVES, the contraceptive pill, antidiabetics.
Contains: GUANETHIDINE.
Other preparations:

Ismelin Eye Drops
(Zyma)

Drops used as a fluid balance altering drug to treat glaucoma and lid retraction.

Dose: 1 drop into the eye 1-2 times a day.
Availability: NHS and private prescription.
Side effects: swelling, redness, or inflammation of the eye.
Caution:
Not to be used for: children or patients suffering from narrow angle glaucoma or who wear soft contact lenses.
Caution needed with: MAOIS.
Contains: GUANETHIDINE monosulphate.
Other preparations:

ISMO
(Boehringer Mannheim)

A white tablet or white, scored tablet according to strengths of 10 mg, 20 mg, 40 mg and used as a NITRATE treatment for angina, and in addition to other treatment for congestive heart failure etc.

Dose: 10 mg a day for 2 days, then 10 mg twice a day for 3 days, followed by 20 mg 2-3 times a day; no more than 120 mg a day.
Availability: NHS and private prescription. (Some strengths available over the counter.)
Side effects: headache, flushes, dizziness.
Caution:
Not to be used for: children.
Caution needed with:
Contains: ISOSORBIDE MONONITRATE.
Other preparations: Ismo-retard, ELANTAN (Schwartz), IMDUR (Astra), ISIB (Ashbourne), MCR-50 (Farmitalia), MONIT (Stuart), MONO-CEDOCARD (Farmitalia).

I

Iso-Autohaler *see* **Medihaler-Iso.** Product now discontinued.

---

isoaminile linctus

A linctus supplied at a strength of 40 mg in 5 ml and used as an anti-tussive agent to treat cough.

Dose: adults 5 ml 3-5 times a day; children 2.5-5 ml 3-5 times a day.
Availability: NHS and private prescription.
Side effects: constipation, dizziness, nausea.
Caution:
Not to be used for:
Caution needed with:
Contains: ISOAMINILE CITRATE.
Other preparations: Dimyril (not available on NHS).

---

isocarboxazid *see* **Marplan**

---

isoconazole nitrate *see* **Travogyn**

---

isoetharine hydrochloride *see* **Numotac**

---

isoetharine mesylate *see* **Bronchilator**

Isogel
(A & H)

Granules used as a bulking agent to treat constipation, diarrhoea, irritable colon, and for colostomy control.

Dose: adults 10 ml in water once or twice a day with meals, children half adult dose.
Availability: NHS, private prescription, over the counter.
Side effects:
Caution:
Not to be used for:
Caution needed with:
Contains: ISPAGHULA husk.

Other preparations: FYBOGEL (Reckitt and Coleman), METAMUCIL (Procter and Gamble), REGULAN (Procter and Gamble).

Isoket Retard
(Schwarz)

A yellow, scored tablet or an orange, scored tablet according to strengths of 20 mg, 40 mg and used as a NITRATE for the prevention of angina.

Dose: 20-40 mg every 12 hours to a maximum of 160 mg a day.
Availability: NHS, private prescription, over the counter.
Side effects: headache, flushes, dizziness.
Caution:
Not to be used for: children or for patients suffering from uncompensated heart shock, severe low blood pressure, anaemia, brain haemorrhage.
Caution needed with:
Contains: ISOSORBIDE DINITRATE.
Other preparations: Isoket 0.1%, CEDOCARD RETARD (Farmitalia), IMTACK (Astra), ISORDIL (Monmouth), SONI-SLO (Lipha), SORBICHEW (Stuart), SORBID-SA (Stuart), SORBITRATE (Stuart), VASCARDIN (Nicholas).

---

isometheptene mucate *see* Midrid

---

isomide *see* Dirythmin SA
(Monmouth)

---

isoniazid *see* isoniazid tablets, Mynah, Rifater, Rifinah

---

isoniazid tablets

Tablets supplied at strengths of 50 mg, 100 mg, and used in combination with other drugs to treat and prevent tuberculosis.

Dose: usually adults, 300 mg a day; children, 10 mg/kg body weight per day.
Availability: NHS and private prescription.
Side effects: nausea, vomiting, allergy including rashes, nerve inflammation, convulsions, mental disturbances, blood changes, liver disorder.
Caution: in nursing mothers, or in patients suffering from kidney or liver damage, alcoholism, epilepsy, or a history of mental disorder.

Not to be used for: patients suffering from drug-induced liver disease, or porphyria (a rare blood disorder).
Caution needed with: ANTACIDS, anti-epileptics, DIAZEPAM, THEOPHYLLINE.
Contains: ISONIAZID.
Other preparations: isoniazid elixir.

Isophane *see* Insulin
(Evans)

---

isoprenaline *see* Duo-Autohaler, Intal Compound, Iso-Autohaler, Medihaler-Duo, Medihaler-Iso, Saventrine

---

isopropyl alcohol *see* Hibisol, Manusept

---

isopropyl myristate *see* Diprobath, Hydromol

Isopto Alkaline
(Alcon)

Drops used to lubricate the eyes.

Dose: 1-2 drops into the eye 3 times a day.
Availability: NHS, private prescription, over the counter.
Side effects:
Caution:
Not to be used for: patients who wear soft contact lenses.
Caution needed with:
Contains: HYPROMELLOSE.
Other preparations: HYPROMELLOSE EYE DROPS, ISOPTO PLAIN (Alcon).

Isopto Atropine
(Alcon)

Eye drops used as an ANTICHOLINERGIC and lubricant to treat uveitis (inflammation in the eye) and used to prepare the eye for examination.

Dose: for uveitis, 1 drop 3 times a day. For examination, adults, 1-2 drops 1 hour before examination; children 1 drop twice a day for 1-2 days before

examination.
Availability: NHS and private prescription.
Side effects: stinging, dry mouth, blurred vision, intolerance to light, rapid heart rate, headache, mental or behavioural changes.
Caution: in infants.
Not to be used for: patients suffering from some types of glaucoma, or who wear soft contact lenses.
Caution needed with:
Contains: ATROPINE SULPHATE, HYPROMELLOSE.
Other preparations: ATROPINE MINIMS, atropine eye drops.

Isopto Carbachol
(Alcon)

Drops used as a cholinergic and lubricant treatment for glaucoma.

Dose: 2 drops into the eye 3 times a day.
Availability: NHS and private prescription.
Side effects:
Caution:
Not to be used for: children or for patients suffering from damaged cornea, acute iritis, or who wear soft contact lenses.
Caution needed with:
Contains: CARBACHOL, HYPROMELLOSE.
Other preparations:

Isopto Carpine
(Alcon)

Drops used as a cholinergic, lubricant treatment for glaucoma.

Dose: 2 drops into the eye 3 times a day.
Availability: NHS and private prescription.
Side effects:
Caution:
Not to be used for: patients suffering from acute iritis or who wear soft contact lenses.
Caution needed with:
Contains: PILOCARPINE, HYPROMELLOSE.
Other preparations: PILOCARPINE MINIMS (SNP), SNO PILO (S & N), OCUSERT PILO (SNP), OPULETS PILOCARPINE (Alcon).

Isopto Frin
(Alcon)

Drops to relieve redness of the eye caused by minor irritations.

Dose: 1-2 drops into the eye up to 4 times a day.
Availability: NHS, private prescription, over the counter.
Side effects:
Caution: in infants and patients suffering from narrow angle glaucoma.
Not to be used for: patients who wear soft contact lenses.
Caution needed with:
Contains: PHENYLEPHRINE hydrochloride, HYPROMELLOSE.
Other preparations:

Isopto Plain
(Alcon)

Drops used to moisten dry eyes.

Dose: 1-2 drops into the eye 3 times a day.
Availability: NHS, private prescription, over the counter.
Side effects:
Caution:
Not to be used for: patients who wear soft contact lenses.
Caution needed with:
Contains: HYPROMELLOSE.
Other preparations: HYPROMELLOSE EYE DROPS, ISOPTO ALKALINE (Alcon).

Isordil
(Monmouth)

A white, scored tablet supplied at strengths of 10 mg, 30 mg and used as a NITRATE for the prevention of angina, acute congestive heart failure.

Dose: 5-15 mg under the tongue every 2-3 hours at first, then 10-60 mg swallowed 4 times a day. 40-120 mg a day for the prevention of angina.
Availability: NHS, private prescription, over the counter.
Side effects: headache, flushes, dizziness, may make chest pain worse.
Caution: heart function should be checked in the case of heart failure.
Not to be used for: children.
Caution needed with:
Contains: ISOSORBIDE DINITRATE.
Other preparations: Isordil Sublingual, Isordil Tembids, CEDOCARD (Farmitalia), CEDOCARD RETARD (Farmitalia), IMTACK (Astra), ISOKET RETARD (Schwarz), SONI-SLO (Lipha), SORBICHEW (Stuart) SORBID-SA (Stuart),

SORBITRATE (Stuart), VASCARDIN (Nicholas).

---

isosorbide dinitrate *see* **Cedocard, Cedocard Retard, Imtack, Isoket Retard, Isordil, Soni-Slo, Sorbichew, Sorbid SA, Sorbitrate, Vascardin**

---

isosorbide mononitrate *see* **Elantan, ISMO, Monit, Mono-Cedocard**

---

isotretinoin *see* **Roaccutane, Isotrex**

Isotrex
(Stiefel)

A gel used to treat acne.

Dose: apply once or twice a day, sparingly, for a minimum of 6-8 weeks. Do not apply to angles of the nose.
Availability: NHS and private prescription.
Side effects: irritation.
Caution: avoid mouth, eyes, mucous membranes, damaged skin. Avoid ultraviolet light.
Not to be used for: pregnant women, nursing mothers, children, or patients with a history of skin cancer.
Caution needed with: skin-softening agents (eg BENZOYL PEROXIDE).
Contains: ISOTRETINOIN.
Other preparations: ROACCUTANE (Roche).

---

ispaghula *see* **Colven, Fybogel, Isogel, Manevac, Regulan**

---

isradipine *see* **Prescal**

Istin
(Pfizer)

White tablets supplied at strengths of 5 mg, 10 mg, and used to treat high blood pressure and poor blood supply to the heart (when associated with angina).

Dose: 5-10 mg once a day.
Availability: NHS and private prescription.
Side effects: headache, fluid retention, tiredness, nausea, flushing, dizziness.
Caution: in pregnant women, nursing mothers, and in patients suffering from liver disorder.
Not to be used for: children.
Caution needed with:
Contains: AMLODIPINE BESYLATE.
Other preparations:

---

itraconazole *see* **Sporanox**

Junifen
(Boots)

An orange-flavoured suspension used as a NON-STEROID ANTI-INFLAMMATORY DRUG to treat pain and fever in children.

Dose: 1-2 years 2.5 ml, 3-7 years 5 ml, 8-12 years 10 ml, all 3-4 times a day.
Availability: NHS and private prescription.
Side effects: stomach upset or bleeding, rash, blood changes.
Caution: in patients suffering from asthma, allergy to ASPIRIN or anti-inflammatory drugs, heart failure, liver or kidney disorder.
Not to be used for: children under 1 year, or weighing less than 7 kg, or suffering from stomach ulcer.
Caution needed with:
Contains: IBUPROFEN.
Other preparations:

K

Kalspare
(Cusi)

An orange, scored tablet used as a DIURETIC combination to treat high blood pressure, fluid retention.

Dose: high blood pressure 1 tablet a day in the morning increasing to 2 tablets if needed, fluid retention 1 tablet a day in the morning increasing to 2 a day after 7 days if the condition fails to respond.

Availability: NHS and private prescription.
Side effects: rash, sensitivity to light, blood changes, gout, cramps
Caution: in pregnant women, nursing mothers, and in patients suffering
from diabetes, electrolyte changes, gout, kidney or liver disease.
Not to be used for: children, and for patients suffering from progressive
or severe kidney failure, raised potassium levels.
Caution needed with: potassium supplements, potassium-sparing
DIURETICS, LITHIUM, DIGOXIN, ANTIHYPERTENSIVES, ACE INHIBITORS.
Contains: CHLORTHALIDONE, TRIAMTERENE.
Other preparations: Kalspare LS.

Kalten
(Stuart)

A red and cream capsule used as a ß-BLOCKER and DIURETIC combination to
treat high blood pressure.

Dose: 1 capsule a day
Availability: NHS and private prescription.
Side effects: cold hands and feet, sleep disturbance, slow heart rate,
tiredness, wheezing, heart failure, stomach upset, rash, sensitivity to light,
blood changes, gout, cramps, dry eyes.
Caution: in pregnant women, nursing mothers, and in patients suffering
from diabetes, electrolyte changes, gout, kidney or liver disease, asthma.
Not to be used for: children, and for patients suffering from progressive
or severe kidney or liver failure, raised potassium levels, heart block or
failure.
Caution needed with: potassium supplements, potassium-sparing
DIURETICS, LITHIUM, DIGOXIN, ANTIHYPERTENSIVES, ACE INHIBITORS, VERAPAMIL,
CLONIDINE withdrawal, some anti-arrhythmic drugs and anaesthetics,
RESERPINE, ERGOTAMINE, CIMETIDINE, sedatives, SYMPATHOMIMETICS, INDOMETHACIN.
Contains: ATENOLOL, HYDROCHLOROTHIAZIDE, AMILORIDE hydrochloride
Other preparations:

K

Kamillosan
(Norgine)

An ointment used as a wetting agent to treat chapped skin, sore nipples,
nappy rash.

Dose: apply twice a day or after breastfeeding. For nappy rash, apply at
each nappy change.
Availability: NHS and private prescription.
Side effects:

Caution:
Not to be used for:
Caution needed with:
Contains: CHAMOMILE OIL, CHAMOMILE EXTRACT.
Other preparations: Kamillosan Baby Cream.

Kay-Cee-L
(Geistlich)

A syrup used as a potassium supplement to treat potassium deficiency.

Dose: adults, 10-50 ml a day in divided doses after food; children as advised by doctor.
Availability: NHS, private prescription, over the counter.
Side effects:
Caution:
Not to be used for: patients suffering from kidney damage or dehydration.
Caution needed with:
Contains: POTASSIUM CHLORIDE.
Other preparations: LEO K (Leo), SLOW-K (Ciba).

Keflex
(Eli Lilly)

A dark green/white capsule or dark green/light green capsule supplied at strengths of 250 mg, 500 mg and used as a cephalosporin antibiotic to treat respiratory, soft tissue, urine, and skin infections.

Dose: adults 1-4 g a day in divided doses; children 25-50 mg per kg body weight a day in divided doses.
Availability: NHS and private prescription.
Side effects: allergic reactions, stomach disturbances.
Caution: in patients suffering from kidney disease or who are very sensitive to penicillin.
Not to be used for:
Caution needed with: loop DIURETICS.
Contains: CEPHALEXIN.
Other preparations: Keflex Tablets, Keflex Chewable, Keflex Suspension, CEPOREX (Glaxo).

Kelfizine W
(Farmitalia CE)

A white tablet supplied at a strength of 2 g and used as a sulphonamide to treat bronchitis, urine infections.

Dose: 1 tablet a week.
Availability: NHS and private prescription.
Side effects: anaemia, stomach disturbances, sore tongue, rash, blood changes when used for an extended period of treatment.
Caution: in patients suffering from liver or kidney disease, blood disorders. Your doctor may advise that blood should be checked regularly for patients on extended periods of treatment.
Not to be used for: children, pregnant women, nursing mothers.
Caution needed with: TRIMETHOPRIM, antidiabetics taken by mouth.
Contains: SULFAMETOPYRAZINE.
Other preparations:

Kemadrin
(Wellcome)

A white, scored tablet supplied at a strength of 5 mg and used as an ANTICHOLINERGIC to treat Parkinson's disease.

Dose: ½ tablet 3 times a day after meals at first, increasing every 2-3 days by ½-1 tablet to a maximum of 6 tablets a day.
Availability: NHS and private prescription.
Side effects: ANTICHOLINERGIC effects, confusion at high doses.
Caution: in patients suffering from heart problems, stomach obstruction, glaucoma, enlarged prostate. Reduce dose slowly.
Not to be used for: children or patients suffering from movement disorders.
Caution needed with: phenothiazines, ANTIHISTAMINES, antidepressants, some tranquillizers.
Contains: PROCYCLIDINE hydrochloride
Other preparations: ARPICOLIN (RP Drugs).

K

Keralyt — skin softener for thickened skin. Product now discontinued.

Kerecid — antiviral drops/ointment for herpes eye infections. Product now discontinued.

Kerlone
(Lorex)

A white, scored tablet supplied at a strength of 20 mg and used as a ß-BLOCKER to treat high blood pressure.

Dose: 1 tablet a day; elderly ½ tablet a day at first.
Availability: NHS and private prescription.
Side effects: cold hands and feet, sleep disturbance, slow heart rate, tiredness, wheezing, heart failure, stomach upset, dry eyes, rash.
Caution: in pregnant women, nursing mothers, and in patients suffering from diabetes, kidney or liver disorders, asthma. May need to be withdrawn before surgery. Withdraw gradually. Your doctor may advise additional treatment with DIURETICS or DIGOXIN.
Not to be used for: children or for patients suffering from heart block or failure.
Caution needed with: VERAPAMIL, CLONIDINE withdrawal, some anti-arrhythmic drugs and anaesthetics, RESERPINE, some ANTIHYPERTENSIVES, ERGOTAMINE, CIMETIDINE, sedatives, SYMPATHOMIMETICS, INDOMETHACIN, antidiabetics.
Contains: BETAXOLOL hydrochloride.
Other preparations:

Kest
(Torbet)

A white tablet used as a stimulant to treat constipation.

Dose: adults 1-2 tablets at night.
Availability: private prescription and over the counter.
Side effects: allergic reactions to PHENOLPHTHALEIN, blood changes.
Caution: in patients suffering from kidney problems.
Not to be used for: children
Caution needed with:
Contains: MAGNESIUM SULPHATE, PHENOLPHTHALEIN.
Other preparations:

ketazolam *see* **Anxon**

keterolac trometamol *see* **Toradol**

ketoconazole *see* **Nizoral, Nizoral Cream**

ketoprofen *see* **Orudis**

---

ketotifen *see* **Zaditen**

Ketovite
(Paines & Byrne)

A yellow tablet used as a multivitamin supplement in artificial diets.

Dose: 1 tablet 3 times a day plus 5 ml of Ketovite Liquid a day.
Availability: NHS, private prescription, over the counter.
Side effects:
Caution:
Not to be used for:
Caution needed with: LEVODOPA.
Contains: tablet: ACETOMENAPHTHONE, THIAMINE, RIBOFLAVINE, PYRIDOXINE, NICOTINAMIDE, CALCIUM PANTOTHENATE, ACSORBIC ACID, TOCOPHERYL ACETATE, INOSITOL, BIOTIN, FOLIC ACID; liquid: VITAMIN A, VITAMIN D, CHOLINE, CYANOCOBALAMIN.
Other preparations: Ketovite Liquid.

Kiditard *see* **Kinidin Durules**
(Delandale)

Kinidin Durules
(Astra)

A white tablet supplied at a strength of 250 mg and used as an anti-arrhythmic drug to treat abnormal heart rhythm.

Dose: 1 tablet at first, then 2-5 tablets twice a day.
Availability: NHS and private prescription.
Side effects: allergies, liver disease, quinine excess, heart muscle toxicity.
Caution: in patients with congestive heart failure, low blood pressure, rapid heart rate, low potassium levels.
Not to be used for: children, pregnant women, or for patients suffering from acute infection, myasthenia gravis (a muscle disorder), severe heart disease.
Caution needed with: DIGOXIN, anticoagulants, ANTIHYPERTENSIVES, CIMETIDINE.

K

Contains: QUINIDINE bisulphate
Other preparations: KIDITARD (Delandale).

Klaricid
(Abbott)

A yellow, oval tablet supplied at a strength of 250 mg and used as an antibiotic to treat infections of the respiratory tract, skin, and soft tissues.

Dose: 1-2 tablets twice a day for 7-14 days.
Availability: NHS and private prescription.
Side effects: nausea, vomiting, diarrhoea, abdominal pain, headache, rash.
Caution: in pregnant women, nursing mothers, and in patients suffering from kidney or liver damage.
Not to be used for: children.
Caution needed with: THEOPHYLLINE, anticoagulants, DIGOXIN, CARBAMAZEPINE.
Contains: CLARITHROMYCIN.
Other preparations:

Kloref
(Cox)

A white, effervescent tablet used as a potassium supplement to treat potassium deficiency.

Dose: adults 1-2 tablets in water 3 times a day; children as advised by the physician.
Availability: NHS, private prescription, and over the counter.
Side effects:
Caution: in patients suffering from kidney disease.
Not to be used for: patients suffering from increased chloride levels or other rare metabolic disorders.
Caution needed with:
Contains: BETAINE HYDROCHLORIDE, POTASSIUM BENZOATE, POTASSIUM BICARBONATE, POTASSIUM CHLORIDE.
Other preparations: Kloref-S

---

kola liquid extract *see* Glykola

---

kola nut dried extract *see* Labiton

342

Kolanticon
(Marion Merrell Dow)

A gel used as an ANTACID, antispasm, and ANTICHOLINERGIC treatment for bowel/stomach spasm, acidity, wind, ulcers.

Dose: adults 10-20 ml every 4 hours.
Availability: NHS, over the counter, private prescription.
Side effects: occasionally constipation, blurred vision, confusion, dry mouth.
Caution:
Not to be used for: children or for patients suffering from glaucoma, inflammatory bowel disease, intestinal obstruction, or enlarged prostate.
Caution needed with: TETRACYCLINE antibiotics and tablets which are coated to protect the stomach.
Contains: ALUMINIUM HYDROXIDE, MAGNESIUM OXIDE, DICYCLOMINE HYDROCHLORIDE, DIMETHICONE.
Other preparations:

Konakion
(Roche)

A white tablet supplied at a strength of 10 mg and used as a vitamin K derivative to treat blood disorders which result in bleeding tendency.

Dose: up to 40 mg in 24 hours; children use injectable form.
Availability: NHS, private prescription, over the counter.
Side effects: flushing, sweating, poor oxygen supply (resulting in bluish colour to skin and mucous membranes).
Caution:
Not to be used for:
Caution needed with:
Contains: PHYTOMENADIONE.
Other preparations: Konakion Injection (available only on prescription).

l-cysteine *see* Cicatrin

L

labetalol *see* Trandate

Labiton
(LAB)

A liquid used as a tonic.

Dose: 10-20 ml twice a day.
Availability: private prescription and over the counter.
Side effects:
Caution:
Not to be used for: children, or for patients suffering from hepatitis or who are taking sedatives.
Caution needed with: sedatives.
Contains: THIAMINE hydrochloride, P-AMINOBENZOIC ACID, KOLA NUT DRIED EXTRACT, alcohol, CAFFEINE.
Other preparations:

Labosept
(LAB)

A red hexagonal-shaped pastille supplied at a strength of 0.25 mg and used as an antiseptic treatment for throat and mouth infections.

Dose: suck 1 pastille every 4 hours.
Availability: NHS, private prescription, over the counter.
Side effects:
Caution:
Not to be used for:
Caution needed with:
Contains: DEQUALINIUM CHLORIDE.
Other preparations:

Labrocol *see* Trandate
(Lagap)

Lacri-Lube
(Allergan)

An ointment used for lubricating the eyes and protecting the cornea.

Dose: apply into the eye as needed.
Availability: NHS, private prescription, over the counter.
Side effects:
Caution:
Not to be used for:
Caution needed with:
Contains: LIQUID PARAFFIN, WOOL FAT.

---

lactic acid *see* **Calmurid HC, Cuplex, Duofilm, Salactol, Tampovagan, Variclene**

Lactitol
(Zyma)

Powder supplied in 10 g sachets and used as a laxative to treat constipation, brain disease due to liver problems.

Dose: constipation adults, 2 sachets a day initially, then 1 sachet a day; children ¼-2 sachets a day according to age, adjusted according to response. Other conditions 0.5-0.7 g/kg body weight a day in 3 divided doses with meals.
Availability: NHS and private prescription.
Side effects: stomach discomfort, wind, bloating, itching around the anus.
Caution: in pregnant women, the elderly, or debilitated patients. Adequate fluid intake must be maintained.
Not to be used for: patients suffering from galactosaemia (an inherited disorder), or blocked intestine.
Caution needed with: ANTACIDS, NEOMYCIN.
Contains: LACTITOL.
Other preparations:

---

lactose *see* **Logynon ED, Femodene ED, Trinovum ED**

---

lactulose *see* **Duphalac**

Ladropen *see* **Floxapen**
(Berk)

L

---

laevulose *see* **Rehidrat**

Lamictal
(Wellcome)

A yellow tablet supplied at strengths of 25 mg, 50 mg, 100 mg, and used as an anticonvulsant to treat epilepsy.

Dose: 50 mg twice a day, increasing to 100-200 mg twice a day. Dose may need adjustment if other anticonvulsants are also taken.
Availability: NHS and private prescription.
Side effects: rash, severe allergy, double or blurred vision, dizziness, drowsiness, headache, stomach upset.
Caution: in pregnant women, nursing mothers, and in patients suffering from rash, fever, influenza, drowsiness, or worsening of symptoms. Must be withdrawn gradually.
Not to be used for: children, the elderly, or for patients suffering from liver or kidney damage.
Caution needed with: PHENYTOIN, CARBAMAZEPINE, PHENOBARBITONE, PRIMIDONE, SODIUM VALPROATE.
Contains: LAMOTRIGINE.
Other preparations:

Lamisil
(Sandoz)

A white, scored tablet supplied at a strength of 250 mg and used as an antifungal treatment for fungal infections of skin and nails.

Dose: athlete's foot, 1 tablet a day for 2-6 weeks. Groin infection, 1 tablet a day for 2-4 weeks. Body infection, 1 tablet a day for 4 weeks. Nail infection, 1 tablet a day for 6 weeks-3 months.
Availability: NHS and private prescription.
Side effects: upset stomach, nausea, allergic skin reactions.
Caution: in pregnant women, nursing mothers, and in patients suffering from severe liver disorder, kidney damage.
Not to be used for: children.
Caution needed with: drugs affecting liver enzymes (eg BARBITURATES, CARBAMAZEPINE, DICHLORALPHENAZONE, PHENYTOIN, PRIMIDONE, RIFAMPICIN, ALLOPURINOL, CIMETIDINE, CIPROFLOXACIN, ERYTHROMYCIN).
Contains: TERBINAFINE.
Other preparations: Lamisil Cream.

---

lamotrigine *see* Lamictal

Lamprene
(Ciba-Geigy)

A brown capsule supplied at a strength of 100 mg and used as an anti-leprotic drug to treat leprosy.

Dose: as advised by the physician.
Availability: NHS and private prescription.
Side effects: skin, hair, faeces and urine discoloration, dry skin, itch, stomach disturbance.
Caution: in pregnant women, nursing mothers, or in patients suffering from stomach pain, diarrhoea, kidney or liver disease.
Not to be used for:
Caution needed with:
Contains: CLOFAZIMINE.
Other preparations:

---

lanatoside C *see* Cedilanid

---

lanolin oil *see* Alpha Keri

Lanoxin
(Wellcome)

A white, scored tablet supplied at a strength of 0.25 mg used as a heart muscle stimulant for digitalis treatment especially heart failure.

Dose: adults 1-2 tablets a day; elderly ½-1 tablet a day; children 10-20 micrograms a day in single or divided doses.
Availability: NHS and private prescription.
Side effects: stomach upset, visual changes, and heart rhythm changes.
Caution: the elderly and in patients suffering from heart block, potassium deficiency, lung disease, kidney and thyroid disorders.
Not to be used for: raised calcium levels, rapid heart rate, some heart muscle disorders.
Caution needed with: calcium injections and tablets, some DIURETICS, QUINIDINE, LITHIUM, ANTACIDS, antibiotics, other heart muscle stimulants.
Contains: DIGOXIN.
Other preparations: Lanoxin 125, Lanoxin-PG, Lanoxin-PG Elixir, Lanoxin Injection.

L

Laractone *see* Aldactone. Product now discontinued.

Laraflex *see* **Naprosyn**
(Lagap)

Larapam *see* **Feldene**. Product now discontinued.

Laratrim *see* **Septrin**
(Lagap)

Largactil
(Rhone-Poulenc Rorer)

A white tablet supplied at strengths of 10 mg, 25 mg, 50 mg, 100 mg and used as a sedative to treat brain disturbances needing sedation, premedication, inducing hypothermia, nausea, vomiting, schizophrenia, mood change.

Dose: adults 25 mg 3 times a day at first increasing if needed by 25 mg a day to 75-300 mg a day; children as advised by physician.
Availability: NHS and private prescription.
Side effects: muscle spasms, restlessness, hands shaking, dry mouth, urine retention, palpitations, low blood pressure, weight gain, blurred vision, changes in libido, low body temperature, breast swelling, menstrual changes, jaundice, blood and skin changes, drowsiness, rarely fits.
Caution: in pregnant women and nursing mothers.
Not to be used for: unconscious patients, the elderly, or for patients suffering from bone marrow depression, liver or kidney disease, heart failure, epilepsy, parkinsonism, underactive thyroid, enlarged prostate, glaucoma.
Caution needed with: alcohol, tranquillizers, pain killers, ANTIHYPERTENSIVES, antidepressants, anticonvulsants, antidiabetic drugs, LEVODOPA.
Contains: CHLORPROMAZINE hydrochloride.
Other preparations: Largactil Syrup, Largactil Forte Suspension, Largactil Injection, CHLORACTIL (DDSA).

Lariam
(Roche)

A white, quarter-scored tablet supplied at a strength of 250 mg, and used to treat and prevent malaria.

Dose: for prevention adults, 1 tablet a week; children, 1 tablet a week according to age. Start one week before departure and continue for 4 weeks after return. Maximum use 3 months. For treatment, as advised by doctor.
Availability: NHS and private prescription.
Side effects: dizziness, nausea, vomiting, stomach upset, loss of appetite, headache, slow pulse rate, skin changes, psychological changes.
Caution: in patients suffering from heart conduction disorders. Women must use reliable contraception during treatment and for 3 months afterwards.
Not to be used for: pregnant women, nursing mothers, or for patients suffering from liver or kidney damage, or history of psychiatric disorder or convulsions.
Caution needed with: QUININE, SODIUM VALPROATE, typhoid vaccination.
Contains: MEFLOQUINE HYDROCHLORIDE.
Other preparations:

Larodopa
(Cambridge)

A white, quarter-scored tablet supplied at a strength of 500 mg and used as an anti-parkinsonian drug to treat Parkinson's disease.

Dose: ¼ tablet twice a day after meals at first increasing after 7 days to ¼ tablet 4-5 times a day, then increasing every 7 days by ¾ tablet a day to 5-16 tablets a day in 4-5 divided doses.
Availability: NHS and private prescription.
Side effects: nausea, vomiting anorexia, low blood pressure on standing up, involuntary movments, heart and brain disturbances, discoloration of urine.
Caution: in pregnant women and in patients suffering from heart, liver, kidney, lung, or endocrine disease, stomach ulcer, and glaucoma.Your doctor may advise that blood and liver, kidney, and cardiovascular systems should be checked regularly.
Not to be used for: children, adults aged under 25, or for patients suffering from severe mental disorder, glaucoma, or a history of malignant melanoma.
Caution needed with: MAOIS, PYRIDOXINE, ANTIHYPERTENSIVES, SYMPATHOMIMETICS, FERROUS SULPHATE, some other similar drugs.
Contains: LEVODOPA.
Other preparations: BROCADOPA (Brocades)

L

Lasikal
(Hoechst)

A white/yellow, double-layered tablet used as a DIURETIC and potassium supplement to treat fluid retention where a potassium supplement is needed.

Dose: 2 tablets a day as a single dose in the morning, then either 4 tablets a day in 2 doses if needed, or 1 tablet a day.
Availability: NHS and private prescription.
Side effects: stomach upset, rash, gout.
Caution: in pregnant women, nursing mothers, or in patients suffering from liver or kidney disease, enlarged prostate, diabetes, or impaired urination.
Not to be used for: children, or for patients suffering from cirrhosis of the liver, raised potassium levels, or Addison's disease.
Caution needed with: potassium-sparing DIURETICS, DIGOXIN, LITHIUM, some antibiotics, NON-STEROID ANTI-INFLAMMATORY DRUGS, ANTIHYPERTENSIVES.
Contains: FRUSEMIDE, POTASSIUM CHLORIDE.
Other preparations: DIUMIDE-K (ASTA), LASIX + K (Hoechst).

Lasilactone
(Hoechst)

A blue/white capsule used as a DIURETIC combination to treat fluid retention, some types of high blood pressure.

Dose: 1-4 capsules a day.
Availability: NHS and private prescription.
Side effects: stomach upset, gout, rash, blood changes, breast swelling.
Caution: in pregnant women, nursing mothers, young patients, or in patients suffering from enlarged prostate, impaired urination, diabetes, kidney or liver disease.
Not to be used for: children, or for patients suffering from severe or progressive kidney failure, liver cirrhosis, raised potassium levels, Addison's disease.
Caution needed with: potassium supplements, potassium-sparing DIURETICS, ANTIHYPERTENSIVES, DIGOXIN, LITHIUM, aminoglycoside and cephalosporin antibiotics, NON-STEROID ANTI-INFLAMMATORY DRUGS, ACE INHIBITORS.
Contains: FRUSEMIDE, SPIRONOLACTONE.
Other preparations:

Lasipressin
(Hoechst)

A white, oblong, scored tablet used as a ß-BLOCKER and DIURETIC to treat high blood pressure.

Dose: 1 tablet in the morning at first increasing to 2 tablets a day if needed.
Availability: NHS and private prescription.
Side effects: cold hands and feet, sleep disturbance, slow heart rate, tiredness, wheezing, heart failure, stomach upset, rash, gout, sensitivity to light, weakness, blood changes, dry eyes.
Caution: pregnant women, nursing mothers, and in patients suffering from asthma, diabetes, kidney or liver disorders, gout, enlarged prostate, impaired urination.
Not to be used for: for patients suffering from heart block or failure, liver cirrhosis, or severe kidney failure.
Caution needed with: VERAPAMIL, CLONIDINE withdrawal, some anti-arrhythmic drugs and anaesthetics, RESERPINE, ANTIHYPERTENSIVES, ERGOTAMINE, CIMETIDINE, sedatives, SYMPATHOMIMETICS, INDOMETHACIN, DIGOXIN, LITHIUM, aminoglycoside and cephalosporin antibiotics, NON-STEROID ANTI-INFLAMMATORY DRUGS.
Contains: FRUSEMIDE, PENBUTOLOL sulphate
Other preparations:

Lasix
(Hoechst)

A white, scored tablet supplied at strengths of 20 mg, 40 mg and used as a DIURETIC to treat fluid retention, high blood pressure.

Dose: 20-80 mg a day or every other day as one dose.
Availability: NHS and private prescription.
Side effects: stomach upset, rash, gout.
Caution: in pregnant women, nursing mothers, and in patients suffering from liver or kidney disease, gout, diabetes, enlarged prostate, impaired urination.
Not to be used for: patients suffering from liver cirrhosis.
Caution needed with: DIGOXIN, LITHIUM, aminoglycoside and cephalosporin antibiotics, ANTIHYPERTENSIVES, NON-STEROID ANTI-INFLAMMATORY DRUGS.
Contains: FRUSEMIDE.
Other preparations: Lasix 500, Lasix Paediatric Liquid, Lasix Injection, DRYPTAL (Berk), FRUMAX (Ashbourne), FRUSID (DDSA), RUSYDE (CP Pharm).

L

Lasix + K
(Hoechst)

Ten white, scored tablets plus 20 pale-yellow tablets supplied at strengths of 40 mg plus 750 mg and used as a DIURETIC and potassium supplement.

Dose: 1 white tablet a day in the morning and 2 pale-yellow tablets a day at noon and in the evening.
Availability: NHS and private prescription.
Side effects: stomach upset, rash, gout.
Caution: in pregnant women, nursing mothers, and in patients suffering from liver or kidney disease, enlarged prostate, diabetes, gout, impaired urination.
Not to be used for: patients suffering from liver cirrhosis, raised potassium levels, Addison's disease.
Caution needed with: potassium-sparing DIURETICS, DIGOXIN, LITHIUM, aminoglycoside and cephalosporin antibiotics, NON-STEROID ANTI-INFLAMMATORY DRUGS, ANTIHYPERTENSIVES.
Contains: FRUSEMIDE plus POTASSIUM CHLORIDE.
Other preparations: DIUMIDE-K (ASTA), LASIKAL (Hoechst).

Lasma
(Pharmax)

A white, elongated, scored tablet supplied at a strength of 300 mg and used as a broncho-dilator to treat brochial spasm brought on by asthma, bronchitis, emphysema.

Dose: 1 tablet every 12 hours increasing by ½ tablet if needed.
Availability: NHS, private prescription, over the counter.
Side effects: rapid heart rate, nausea, stomach upset, headache, abnormal heart rhythms.
Caution: in pregnant women, nursing mothers, and in patients suffering from heart or liver disease, or stomach ulcer.
Not to be used for: children.
Caution needed with: CIMETIDINE, ERYTHROMYCIN, CIPROFLOXACIN, interferon, STEROIDS, DIURETICS, other broncho-dilators.
Contains: THEOPHYLLINE.
Other preparations: BIOPHYLLINE (Delandale), NUELIN SA (3M Healthcare), PRO-VENT (Wellcome), SABIDAL SR, SLO-PHYLLIN (Lipha), TEDRAL, THEO-DUR (Astra), UNIPHYLLIN-CONTINUS (Napp).

Lasonil
(Bayer)

An ointment used as an anti-inflammatory preparation to treat bruises, sprains, soft tissue injuries.

Dose: apply 2-3 times a day.
Availability: NHS, private prescription, over the counter.
Side effects:
Caution:
Not to be used for: if there are open or infected wounds.
Caution needed with:
Contains: HEPARINOID.
Other preparations:

Lasoride
(Hoechst)

A yellow tablet used as a potassium-sparing DIURETIC combination used for fast diuretic treatment where maintaining potassium is important.

Dose: adults 1-2 tablets a day in the morning; elderly according to kidney function, response to treatment and potassium level.
Availability: NHS and private prescription.
Side effects: general feeling of being unwell, stomach upset, itch, blood changes, reduced alertness, calcium loss, rarely minor mental disturbances, altered liver function, ototoxicity, pancreatitis.
Caution: in the elderly, pregnant women, nursing mothers, and in patients suffering from enlarged prostate, impaired urination, diabetes, and gout.
Not to be used for: patients suffering from liver cirrhosis, severe or progressive kidney failure, raised potassium levels, Addison's disease (a disease of the adrenal glands), electrolyte imbalance.
Caution needed with: potassium supplements and potassium-sparing DIURETICS, LITHIUM, aminoglycoside or cephalosporin antibiotics, NON-STEROID ANTI-INFLAMMATORY DRUGS, DIGOXIN, ANTIHYPERTENSIVES, antidiabetic drugs
Contains: FRUSEMIDE, AMILORIDE hydrochloride.
Other preparations: FRUMIL (Rhone-Poulenc Rorer).

---

laureth *see* **Alcos-Anal**

---

lauromacrogol *see* **Anacal, Balneum Plus**

L

Laxoberal
(Windsor)

A liquid used as a stimulant to treat constipation, and for evacuation of the bowels before surgery etc.

Dose: adults 5-15 ml at night, children under 5 years 2.5 ml at night, 5-10 years 2.5-5 ml at night.
Availability: NHS (when prescribed as a generic), private prescription, over the counter.
Side effects:
Caution: in patients suffering from inflammatory bowel disease.
Not to be used for:
Caution needed with: antibiotics.
Contains: SODIUM PICOSULPHATE.
Other preparations: PICOLAX (Ferring), SODIUM PICOSULPHATE.

Ledercort
(Lederle)

A blue, oblong, scored tablet or a white, oblong, scored tablet according to strengths of 2 mg, 4 mg and used as a STEROID treatment for rheumatoid arthritis, allergies.

Dose: as advised by physician.
Availability: NHS and private prescription.
Side effects: raised blood sugar levels, thinning of the bones, mood changes, stomach ulcer.
Caution: in pregnant women, in patients who have had recent bowel surgery or who are suffering from inflamed veins, psychiatric disorders, virus infections, some cancers, some kidney diseases, thinning of the bones, ulcers, tuberculosis, other infections, high blood pressure, glaucoma, epilepsy, diabetes, underactive thyroid, liver disease, stress. Withdraw gradually.
Not to be used for:
Caution needed with: PHENYTOIN, PHENOBARBITONE, EPHEDRINE, RIFAMPICIN, DIURETICS, ANTICHOLINESTERASES, DIGOXIN, antidiabetics, anticoagulants, NON-STEROID ANTI-INFLAMMATORY DRUGS.
Contains: TRIAMCINOLONE.
Other preparations:

Ledercort Cream
(Lederle)

A cream used as a STEROID treatment for skin disorders where there is inflammation.

Dose: apply a small quantity to the affected area 3-4 times a day.
Availability: NHS and private prescription.
Side effects: fluid retention, suppression of adrenal glands, thinning of the skin may occur.
Caution: use for short periods of time only.
Not to be used for: patients suffering from acne or any other skin infections caused by tuberculosis, ringworm, viruses, or fungi, or continuously especially in pregnant women.
Caution needed with:
Contains: TRIAMCINOLONE acetonide.
Other preparations: (Ledercort Ointment — now discontinued.)

Lederfen
(Lederle)

A blue, oblong tablet or a blue, oblong, scored tablet according to strengths of 300 mg, 450 mg and used as a NON-STEROID ANTI-INFLAMMATORY DRUG to treat rheumatoid arthritis, osteoarthritis, ankylosing spondylitis, and acute muscle or bone problems.

Dose: either 300 mg in the morning and 600 mg at night or 450 mg twice a day.
Availability: NHS and private prescription.
Side effects: rash, stomach intolerance.
Caution: in the elderly, pregnant women, nursing mothers, and in patients suffering from heart failure, kidney or liver disorders.
Not to be used for: children or for patients suffering from anti-inflammatory drug/ASPIRIN allergy, stomach ulcer, or history of gastro-intestinal disease.
Caution needed with: some ANALGESICS, anticoagulants.
Contains: FENBUFEN.
Other preparations: Lederfen Capsules, Lederfen F

Ledermycin
(Lederle)

L

A dark-red/pale-red capsule supplied at a strength of 150 mg and used as a TETRACYCLINE to treat respiratory and soft tissue infections.

Dose: 2 capsules twice a day or 1 capsule 4 times a day.
Availability: NHS and private prescription.
Side effects: stomach disturbances, sensitivity to light, additional infections.

Caution: in patients suffering from liver or kidney disease.
Not to be used for: children, nursing mothers, or women in the last half of pregnancy.
Caution needed with: milk, ANTACIDS, mineral supplements, contraceptive pill.
Contains: DEMECLOCYCLINE.
Other preparations: (Ledermycin Tablets — now discontinued.)

Lejfibre — bulking agent to treat constipation. Product now discontinued.

---

lemon bioflavonoid complex *see* **Lipoflavonoid**

Lenium
(Janssen)

An anti-dandruff preparation.

Dose: twice a week for the first two weeks, once a week for two further weeks, then once every 3-6 weeks.
Availability: NHS, private prescription, over the counter.
Side effects:
Caution: keep out of the eyes and any areas of broken skin; do not use within 48 hours of waving or colouring substances.
Not to be used for:
Caution needed with:
Contains: SELENIUM SULPHIDE.
Other preparations: SELSUN (Abbott).

Lentard *see* **insulin**
(Novo Nordisk)

Lente *see* **insulin**
(Evans)

Lentizol
(Parke-Davis)

A pink capsule or pink/red capsule according to strengths of 25 mg, 50 mg and used as a TRICYCLIC antidepressant to treat depression especially where sedation is needed.

Dose: adults usually 50 mg before going to bed, up to a maximum of 100 mg; elderly 25-75 mg a day at first.
Availability: NHS and private prescription.
Side effects: dry mouth, constipation, urine retention, blurred vision, palpitations, drowsiness, sleeplessness, dizziness, hands shaking, low blood presure, weight change, skin reactions, jaundice or blood changes, loss of libido may occur.
Caution: in nursing mothers or in patients suffering from heart disease, thyroid disease, epilepsy, diabetes, glaucoma, adrenal tumour, urinary retention, some other psychiatric conditions. Your doctor may advise regular blood tests.
Not to be used for: children, pregnant women, or for patients suffering from heart attacks, liver disease, heart block.
Caution needed with: alcohol, ANTICHOLINERGICS, ADRENALINE, MAOIS, BARBITURATES, other antidepressants, CIMETEDINE, oestrogens, ANTIHYPERTENSIVES.
Contains: AMITRIPTYLINE hydrochloride.
Other preparations: DOMICAL (Berk), ELAVIL (DDSA), TRYPTIZOL (Morson).

Leo K
(Leo)

A white, oval tablet used as a potassium supplement to treat potassium deficiency.

Dose: adults 3-5 tablets a day in divided doses; children as advised by the physician.
Availability: NHS, private prescription, over the counter.
Side effects: ulcers or blockage in the small bowel.
Caution: in patients suffering from kidney disease.
Not to be used for:
Caution needed with:
Contains: POTASSIUM CHLORIDE.
Other preparations: KAY-CEE-L (Geistlich), SLOW-K (Ciba).

Lergoban *see* **Histryl**. Product now discontinued.

---

levobunolol *see* **Betagan**

---

levodopa *see* **Larodopa, Madopar, Sinemet**

levonorgestrel *see* **Cyclo-Progynova 1mg, Eugynon 30, Logynon, Logynon ED, Microgynon 30, Microval, Norgeston, Ovran, Ovranette, Nuvelle**

levorphanol *see* **Dromoran**

Lexotan
(Roche)

A lilac, hexagonal, scored tablet or a pink, hexagonal, scored tablet according to strengths of 1.5 mg, 3 mg and used for the short-term treatment of anxiety.

Dose: elderly 1.5-9 mg a day in divided doses, adults 3-18 mg a day in divided doses.
Availability: private prescription only.
Side effects: drowsiness, confusion, unsteadiness, low blood pressure, rash, changes in vision, changes in libido, retention of urine. Risk of addiction increases with dose and length of treatment. May impair judgement.
Caution: in the elderly, pregnant women, nursing mothers, in women during labour, and in patients suffering from lung disorders, kidney or liver disorders. Avoid long-term use and withdraw gradually.
Not to be used for: children or for patients suffering from acute lung diseases, some chronic lung diseases, some obsessional and psychotic diseases.
Caution needed with: alcohol and other tranquillizers and anticonvulsants.
Contains: BROMAZEPAM.
Other preparations:

L

Lexpec
(RP Drugs)

A syrup used as a folic acid supplement to treat megaloblastic anaemia (anaemia with large red blood cells).

Dose: adults 20-40 ml a day for 14 days then 5-20 ml a day; children 10-

30 ml a day.
Availability: NHS and private prescription.
Side effects: nausea, constipation, mottled teeth.
Caution: mottled teeth can be minimized by drinking syrup through a straw.
Not to be used for: megaloblastic anaemia caused by vitamin B_{12} deficiency.
Caution needed with: TETRACYCLINES.
Contains: FOLIC ACID.
Other preparations: Lexpec with Iron, Lexpec with Iron-M, folic acid tablets.

Li-liquid *see* Litarex
(RP DRugs)

Libanil *see* Daonil
(APS)

Librium
(Roche)

A yellow-green, light blue-green, or dark blue-green tablet according to strengths of 5 mg, 10, mg, 25 mg and used as a tranquillizer to treat anxiety, symptoms of acute alcohol withdrawal, short-term treatment of sleeplessness where sedation during the day does not cause difficulty.

Dose: elderly 5 mg a day at first; adults 30 mg a day at first; 40-100 mg a day in severe cases.
Availability: NHS (when prescribed as a generic) and private prescription.
Side effects: drowsiness, confusion, unsteadiness, low blood pressure, rash, changes in vision, changes in libido, retention of urine. Risk of addiction increases with dose and length of treatment. May impair judgement.
Caution: in the elderly, pregnant women, nursing mothers, in women during labour, and in patients suffering from lung disorders, kidney or liver disorders. Avoid long-term use and withdraw gradually.
Not to be used for: children or for patients suffering from acute lung diseases, some chronic lung diseases, some obsessional and psychotic diseases.
Caution needed with: alcohol and other tranquillizers and anticonvulsants.
Contains: CHLORDIAZEPOXIDE.

L

Other preparations: Librium Capsules, CHLORDIAZEPOXIDE, TROPIUM (DDSA)

Lidifen *see* Brufen
(Berk)

---

lidoflazine *see* Clinium

Lignocaine and Fluorescein
(SNP)

Drops used as a local anaesthetic and dye for carrying out procedures on the eye.

Dose: 1 or more drops into the eye as needed. Protect eye.
Availability: NHS and private prescription.
Side effects:
Caution:
Not to be used for:
Caution needed with:
Contains: LIGNOCAINE HYDROCHLORIDE, SODIUM FLUORESCEIN.
Other preparations:

---

lignocaine *see* Betnovate Rectal, Lignocaine and Fluorescein, Xylocaine, Xyloproct

---

Limbitrol 5
(Roche)

A pink/green capsule used as a TRICYCLIC antidepressant to treat depression and anxiety.

Dose: 1 tablet 3 times a day.
Availability: private prescription only.
Side effects: dry mouth, constipation, palpitations, sleeplessness, shaking hands, weight change, skin reactions, jaundice or blood changes, drowsiness, confusion, unsteadiness, low blood pressure, rash, changes in vision, changes in libido, retention of urine. Risk of addiction increases with dose and length of treatment. May impair judgement.
Caution: in nursing mothers, in women during labour, and in patients suffering from lung disorders, kidney or liver disorders, overactive thyroid,

L

adrenal tumour, epilepsy, urinary retention, glaucoma, diabetes. Avoid long-term use and withdraw gradually.
Not to be used for: children, the elderly, pregnant women, or for patients suffering from acute lung diseases, some chronic lung diseases, some obsessional and psychotic diseases, heart disease, liver disease, epilepsy.
Caution needed with: alcohol and other tranquillizers and anticonvulsants, ANTICHOLINERGICS, ADRENALINE, MAOIS, BARBITURATES, other antidepressants, ANTIHYPERTENSIVES, CIMETEDINE, oestrogens.
Contains: AMITRIPTYLINE hydrochloride, CHLORDIAZEPOXIDE.
Other preparations: Limbitrol 10.

Lincocin — antibiotic preparation. Product now discontinued.

---

lincomycin *see* **Lincocin**

---

lindane *see* **Lorexane, Quellada**

Lingraine
(Sanofi Winthrop)

A green tablet supplied at a strength of 2 mg and used as an ergot preparation to treat migraine, headache.

Dose: 1 tablet under the tongue at the beginning of a migraine attack, and repeat if needed ½-1 hour later to a maximum of 3 tablets in 24 hours or 6 tablets in a week.
Availability: NHS and private prescription.
Side effects: nausea, stomach pain, leg cramps.
Caution:
Not to be used for: children, pregnant women, nursing mothers, or for patients suffering from coronary, peripheral, or occlusive vascular disease, severe high blood pressure, kidney or liver disease, sepsis, overactive thyroid, porphyria (a rare blood disorder).
Caution needed with: ERYTHROMYCIN, ß-BLOCKERS.
Contains: ERGOTAMINE tartrate.
Other preparations: CAFERGOT (Sandoz), MEDIHALER ERGOTAMINE (3M Healthcare), MIGRIL (Wellcome).

L

Lioresal
(Ciba)

A white, scored tablet supplied at a strength of 10 mg and used as a muscle relaxant to treat voluntary muscle spasticity caused by cerebrovascular accidents, cerebral palsy, meningitis, multiple sclerosis, spinal lesions.

Dose: adults ½ tablet 3 times a day at first increasing as needed by ½ tablet 3 times a day every 3 days to a maximum of 10 tablets a day; children as advised by doctor.
Availability: NHS and private prescription.
Side effects: nausea, sedation, confusion, muscle tiredness, reduced alertness, low blood pressure, heart, lung, and circulation disorder, problems with urination. Rarely visual disturbance, rash, or liver disorder.
Caution: in the elderly, pregnant women, and in patients suffering from epilepsy, stroke, liver/kidney disorder, diabetes, or mental disorders. Withdraw treatment gradually.
Not to be used for: patients suffering from stomach ulcer.
Caution needed with: ANTIHYPERTENSIVES, LITHIUM, TRICYCLIC antidepressants, IBUPROFEN, LEVODOPA, CARBIDOPA.
Contains: BACLOFEN.
Other preparations: Lioresal Liquid, BACLOSPAS (Ashbourne).

Liothyronine see Tertroxin

Lipantil
(Distriphar UK)

A white capsule supplied at a strength of 100 mg and used as a lipid-lowering agent to lower cholesterol or triglycerides.

Dose: 2-4 capsules a day.
Availability: NHS and private prescription.
Side effects: stomach upset, dizziness, headache, tiredness, rashes.
Caution: in patients suffering from kidney impairment.
Not to be used for: pregnant women, nursing mothers, or for patients suffering from severe kidney or liver problems, gall bladder disease.
Caution needed with: anticoagulants, PHENYLBUTAZONE, antidiabetic drugs taken by mouth.
Contains: FENOFIBRATE.
Other preparations:

L

Lipobase *see* Diprobase
(Brocades)

Lipoflavonoid
(Lipomed)

A black/pink capsule used as a multivitamin treatment for vitamin B deficiency.

Dose: 3 capsules 3 times a day for 2-3 months reducing to 2 capsules 3 times a day.
Availability: private prescription and over the counter.
Side effects:
Caution:
Not to be used for: children.
Caution needed with:
Contains: CHOLINE BITARTRATE, INOSITOL, METHIONINE, ASCORBIC ACID, LEMON BIOFLAVONOID COMPLEX, THIAMINE, RIBOFLAVINE, NICOTINAMIDE, PYRIDOXINE, PANTHENOL, HYDROXOCOBALAMIN.
Other preparations:

Lipostat
(Squibb)

A pink, oblong tablet supplied at a strength of 10 mg, 20 mg, and used as a lipid-lowering agent to treat raised cholesterol.

Dose: 10 mg at night initially, increasing to 10-40 mg at night.
Availability: NHS and private prescription.
Side effects: rash, muscle pain, headache, chest pain, nausea, vomiting, diarrhoea, tiredness.
Caution: in patients with a history of liver disease. Your doctor may advise regular tests during treatment.
Not to be used for: children, pregnant women, nursing mothers, or for patients suffering from liver disease.
Caution needed with: CHOLESTYRAMINE, COLESTIPOL.
Contains: PRAVASTATIN.
Other preparations:

L

Lipotriad
(Lipomed)

A clear pink capsule used as a multivitamin treatment for vitamin B deficiency.

Dose: 3 capsules 3 times a day for 2-3 months then reducing to 2 capsules 3 times a day.
Availability: private prescription and over the counter.
Side effects:
Caution:
Not to be used for: children.
Caution needed with: LEVODOPA.
Contains: CHOLINE BITARTRATE, INOSITOL, DL-METHIONINE, HYDROXOCOBALAMIN, THIAMINE, RIBOFLAVINE, NICOTINAMIDE, PYRIDOXINE, PANTHENOL.
Other preparations: (Lipotriad Liquid — now discontinued.)

---

liquid paraffin *see* **Alpha Keri, Balmandol, Coal tar and salicylic acid ointment, Diprobase, Diprobath, Hydromol, Lipobase, liquid paraffin and magnesium hydroxide emulsion, Lubrifilm, Oilatum, Petrolagar No 1, Polytar Emollient, simple eye ointment, Unguentum Merck**

---

liquid paraffin and magnesium hydroxide emulsion

An emulsion used as a laxative to treat constipation.

Dose: 5-20 ml when required.
Availability: NHS, private prescription, over the counter.
Side effects: colic,
Caution: in the elderly, and in patients who are weak or suffering from kidney or liver damage.
Not to be used for: sudden, severe symptoms.
Caution needed with:
Contains: LIQUID PARAFFIN, MAGNESIUM HYDROXIDE.
Other preparations:

Liquifilm Tears
(Allergan)

Drops used to lubricate dry eyes.

Dose: 1 drop into the eye as needed.
Availability: NHS, private prescription, over the counter.
Side effects:
Caution:
Not to be used for: patients who wear soft contact lenses.

Caution needed with:
Contains: POLYVINYL ALCOHOL.
Other preparations: SNO TEARS (S&N).

---

liquorice *see* Caved-S

---

lisinopril *see* Carace, Carace Plus, Zestril

Liskonum
(S K B)

A white, scored, oblong tablet supplied at a strength of 450 mg and used as a sedative to treat mania, hypomania, manic depression.

Dose: as judged by blood tests to keep a constant level.
Availability: NHS and private prescription.
Side effects: nausea, diarrhoea, hand tremor, muscular weakness, brain and heart disturbances, weight gain, fluid retention, underactive or over active thyroid gland, thirst and frequent urination, kidney changes, skin reactions, intoxication.
Caution: treatment should be started in hospital and a careful check on the functioning of the kidneys and thyroid should be made, as well as ensuring that there is an adequate consumption of salt and fluid. Your doctor may advise blood tests to gauge dose.
Not to be used for: children, for pregnant women, nursing mothers, or for patients suffering from disturbed sodium balance, Addison's disease, kidney or heart disease, or underactive thyroid.
Caution needed with: DIURETICS, NON-STEROID ANTI-INFLAMMATORY DRUGS, CARBAMAZEPINE, PHENYTOIN, HALOPERIDOL, FLUPENTHIXOL, METHYLDOPA, PHENYTOIN, FLUOXAMINE.
Contains: LITHIUM CARBONATE.
Other preparations: CAMCOLIT (Norgine), PHASAL (Lagap), PRIADEL (Delandale).

---

lisuride *see* Revanil

Litarex
(CP Pharmaceuticals)

A white, oval tablet supplied at a strength of 564 mg and used as a sedative to treat acute mania, and for the prevention of recurring mood changes.

Dose: 1 tablet morning and evening at first and then as advised by the physician.
Availability: NHS and private prescription.
Side effects: nausea, diarrhoea, hand tremor, muscular weakness, brain and heart disturbances, weight gain, fluid retention, underactive or overactive thyroid gland, thirst and frequent urination, skin reactions.
Caution: treatment should be started in hospital, thyroid function should be checked regularly, and there should be an adequate consumption of salt and fluid. Your doctor may advise frequent blood tests to gauge dose.
Not to be used for: children, pregnant women, nursing mothers, or for patients suffering from Addison's disease, kidney or cardiovascular disease, underactive thyroid, in cases where there is a disturbed sodium balance.
Caution needed with: DIURETICS, NON-STEROID ANTI-INFLAMMATORY DRUGS, CARBAMAZEPINE, FLUPENTHIXOL, METHYLDOPA, PHENYTOIN, HALOPERIDOL, antidepressants.
Contains: LITHIUM CITRATE.
Other preparations: LI-LIQUID (RP Drugs).

---

lithium carbonate *see* **Camcolit, Liskonum, Phasal, Priadel**

---

lithium citrate *see* **Litarex**

---

lithium succinate *see* **Efalith**

Lithofalk
(Thames)

A scored tablet used as a bile acid to dissolve gallstones.

Dose: 2 tablets (patients over 80 kg, 3 tablets) a day at bedtime for 6-24 months.
Availability: NHS and private prescription.
Side effects: diarrhoea, itching, minor liver abnormalities, blood changes.
Caution:
Not to be used for: children, pregnant women, or for patients suffering from chronic liver disease, or inflammatory disease of the intestine.

Caution needed with: the contraceptive pill.
Contains: CHENODEOXYCHOLIC ACID, URSODEOXYCHOLIC ACID.
Other preparations:

Livial
(Organon)

A white tablet supplied at a strength of 2.5 mg, and used to treat symptoms associated with the menopause.

Dose: 1 tablet a day for a minimum of 3 months.
Availability: NHS and private prescription.
Side effects: changes in body weight, dizziness, headache, seborrhoeic dermatitis, vaginal bleeding, stomach upset, liver disorder, hair growth, fluid retention.
Caution: in patients who have transferred from a similar drug, or who suffer from kidney disorder, epilepsy, migraine, diabetes, or high cholesterol levels.
Not to be used for: children, pregnant women, nursing mothers, or for patients suffering from some tumours, undiagnosed vaginal bleeding, blood vessel disorder of the brain or heart, severe liver disorders.
Caution needed with: ANTICOAGULANTS, PHENYTOIN, CARBAMAZEPINE, RIFAMPICIN.
Contains: TIBOLONE.
Other preparations:

Loasid *see* **Unigest.** Product now discontinued.

Lobak
(Sanofi Winthrop)

A white, scored tablet used as a muscle relaxant and ANALGESIC to relieve painful muscle spasm

Dose: adults 1-2 tablets 3 times a day to a maximum of 8 tablets a day; elderly half normal adult dose.
Availability: private prescription only.
Side effects: reduced alertness, drowsiness, dizziness, rash, dry mouth, jaundice.
Caution: in pregnant women, nursing mothers, and in patients suffering from kidney or liver disease.
Not to be used for: children.
Caution needed with: alcohol, sedatives MAOIS.
Contains: CHLORMEZANONE, PARACETAMOL.

L

Locabiotal
(Servier)

An aerosol supplied at a strength of 125 micrograms and used as an anti-inflammatory, antibiotic treatment for infection, inflammation, of the nose, mouth, and throat.

Dose: adults 5 sprays into the mouth or 3 sprays into each nostril 5 times a day; children 3-5 years 2 sprays into the mouth 3 times a day or 1 spray into each nostril 5 times a day, 6-12 years 3 sprays into the mouth 3 times a day or 2 sprays in each nostril 5 times a day, over 12 years 4 sprays into the mouth 3 times a day or 3 sprays in each nostril 5 times a day.
Availability: NHS and private prescription.
Side effects:
Caution:
Not to be used for: children under 3 years.
Caution needed with:
Contains: FUSAFUNGINE.
Other preparations:

Loceryl
(Roche)

A cream used as an antifungal treatment for fungal skin infection.

Dose: apply once a day in the evening, until 3-5 days after apparent cure.
Availability: NHS and private prescription.
Side effects: itching, burning.
Caution: avoid contact with eyes, ears, mucous membranes.
Not to be used for: children, pregnant women, nursing mothers.
Caution needed with:
Contains: AMOROLFINE.
Other preparations: Loceryl Lacquer (for nail infections).

L

Locoid *see* **hydrocortisone cream**
(Brocades)

Locoid-C
(Brocades)

A cream/ointment used as an antibacterial and STEROID to treat eczema, psoriasis, and other skin conditions which are also infected with bacteria or fungi.

Dose: apply 2-4 times a day.
Availability: NHS and private prescription.
Side effects: fluid retention, suppression of adrenal glands, thinning of the skin may occur.
Caution: use for short periods of time only.
Not to be used for: continuous use, especially on pregnant women, or for patients suffering from acne or any other tubercular or viral infection of the skin.
Caution needed with:
Contains: HYDROCORTISONE 17-BUTYRATE, CHLORQUINALDOL.
Other preparations:

Locorten-Vioform
(Zyma)

Drops used as an antibacterial, STEROID treatment for inflammation of the outer ear where secondary infections may be present.

Dose: 2-3 drops into the ear twice a day for 7-10 days.
Availability: NHS and private prescription.
Side effects: irritation, hair discoloration.
Caution: in nursing mothers.
Not to be used for: patients suffering from perforated ear drum or primary infections of the outer ear.
Caution needed with:
Contains: CLIOQUINOL, FLUMETHASONE PIVALATE.
Other preparations:

Lodine
(Wyeth)

A dark-grey/light-grey capsule or light grey capsule, marked with 2 red bands tablet supplied at strengths of 200 mg, 300 mg and used as a NON-STEROID ANTI-INFLAMMATORY DRUG to treat rheumatoid arthritis and osteoarthritis.

Dose: 200-300 mg twice a day to a maximum of 600 mg a day.
Availability: NHS and private prescription.
Side effects: nausea, stomach pain, headache, dizziness, tinnitus, rash, swelling.
Caution: in the elderly on long-term treatment and in patients suffering

L

from kidney or liver disease, heart failure.
Not to be used for: children, pregnant women, nursing mothers, or for patients suffering from stomach ulcer, a history of stomach ulcer or gastro-intestinal bleeding, allergy to anti-inflammatory drugs/aspirin.
Caution needed with: anticoagulants, antidiabetic drugs.
Contains: ETODOLAC.
Other preparations: Lodine Tablets.

Iodoxamide *see* Alomide

Loestrin 20
(Parke-Davis)

A blue tablet used as an oestrogen, progestogen contraceptive.

Dose: 1 tablet a day for 21 days starting on day 5 of the period.
Availability: NHS and private prescription.
Side effects: enlarged breasts, bloating and fluid retention, cramps, leg pains, mood change, reduction in sexual desire, headaches, nausea, vaginal erosion, discharge, and bleeding, weight gain, skin changes.
Caution: in patients suffering from high blood pressure, diabetes, vascular disorders, asthma, depression, kidney disease, multiple sclerosis, womb diseases. Your doctor may advise you not to smoke, to have regular examinations. You should stop treatment at the first sign of serious symptoms such as severe headache or jaundice. Treatment should be stopped before surgery.
Not to be used for: pregnant women, or for patients suffering from sickle-cell anaemia, history of heart disease or thrombosis, liver disorders, some cancers, undiagnosed vaginal bleeding, some ear, skin, and kidney disorders.
Caution needed with: RIFAMPICIN, TETRACYCLINES, GRISEOFULVIN, BARBITURATES, PHENYTOIN, PRIMIDONE, CARBAMAZEPINE, ETHOSUXIMIDE, CHLORAL HYDRATE, DICHLORALPHENAZONE.
Contains: ETHINYLOESTRADIOL, NORETHISTERONE acetate.
Other preparations: Loestrin 30.

---

lofepramine *see* Gamanil

Logynon
(Schering)

A brown tablet, or a white tablet and an ochre tablet used as an oestrogen, progestogen contraceptive.

Dose: 1 tablet a day for 21 days starting on day 1 of the period.
Availability: NHS and private prescription.
Side effects: enlarged breasts, bloating and fluid retention, cramps, leg pains, mood change, reduction in sexual desire, headaches, nausea, vaginal erosion, discharge, and bleeding, weight gain, skin changes.
Caution: in patients suffering from high blood pressure, diabetes, vascular disorders, asthma, depression, kidney disease, multiple sclerosis, womb diseases. Your doctor may advise you not to smoke, to have regular examinations. You should stop treatment at the first sign of serious symptoms such as severe headache or jaundice. Treatment should be stopped before surgery.
Not to be used for: pregnant women, or for patients suffering from sickle-cell anaemia, history of heart disease or thrombosis, liver disorders, some cancers, undiagnosed vaginal bleeding, some ear, skin, and kidney disorders.
Caution needed with: RIFAMPICIN, TETRACYCLINES, GRISEOFULVIN, BARBITURATES, PHENYTOIN, PRIMIDONE, CARBAMAZEPINE, ETHOSUXIMIDE, CHLORAL HYDRATE, DICHLORALPHENAZONE.
Contains: ETHINYLOESTRADIOL, LEVONORGESTREL.
Other preparations: TRINORDIOL (Wyeth).

Logynon ED
(Schering)

A brown tablet, white tablet, and ochre tablet, or white and ochre tablet and white tablet used as an oestrogen, progestogen contraceptive.

Dose: 1 tablet a day for 28 days starting on day 1 of the period.
Availability: NHS and private prescription.
Side effects: enlarged breasts, bloating and fluid retention, cramps, leg pains, mood change, reduction in sexual desire, headaches, nausea, vaginal erosion, discharge, and bleeding, weight gain, skin changes.
Caution: in patients suffering from high blood pressure, diabetes, vascular disorders, asthma, depression, kidney disease, multiple sclerosis, womb diseases. Your doctor may advise you not to smoke, to have regular examinations. You should stop treatment at the first sign of serious symptoms such as severe headache or jaundice. Treatment should be stopped before surgery.
Not to be used for: pregnant women, or for patients suffering from sickle-cell anaemia, history of heart disease or thrombosis, liver disorders, some cancers, undiagnosed vaginal bleeding, some ear, skin, and kidney disorders.

L

Caution needed with: RIFAMPICIN, TETRACYCLINES, GRISEOFULVIN, BARBITURATES, PHENYTOIN, PRIMIDONE, CARBAMAZEPINE, ETHOSUXIMIDE, CHLORAL HYDRATE, DICHLORALPHENAZONE.
Contains: ETHINYLOESTRADIOL, LEVONORGESTREL, LACTOSE.
Other preparations:

Lomotil
(Gold Cross)

A white tablet used to slow down intestinal contents and as an ANTICHOLINERGIC to treat diarrhoea.

Dose: adults, 4 tablets initially, then 2 every 6 hours; children 4-8 years, 1 tablet 3 times a day, 9-12 years, 1 tablet 4 times a day, 13-16 years, 2 tablets 3 times a day.
Availability: NHS and private prescription.
Side effects: allergy, stomach upset, ANTICHOLINERGIC effects, disturbance of brain and spinal cord.
Caution: in pregnant women, nursing mothers, or in patients suffering from liver disorder, dehydration, body fluid imbalance.
Not to be used for: children under 4 years, or for patients suffering from blockage in the intestine, jaundice, colitis.
Caution needed with: MAOIS, sedatives
Contains: DIPHENOXYLATE HYDROCHLORIDE, ATROPINE SULPHATE (CO-PHENOTROPE).
Other preparations: Lomotil Liquid.

Loniten
(Upjohn)

A white tablet supplied at strengths of 2.5 mg, 5 mg, 10 mg and used as a vasodilator to treat high blood pressure.

Dose: adults 5 mg a day at first increasing at 3-day intervals to up to 10 mg a day and then by 10 mg at a time to a maximum of 50 mg a day; children 0.2 mg per kg of bodyweight a day at first, increasing at 3-day intervals by 0.1-0.2 mg per kg bodyweight to a maximum of 1 mg per kg bodyweight a day.
Availability: NHS and private prescription.
Side effects: hair growth, swelling, rapid heart rate.
Caution: angina or heart attack patients need to be monitored carefully. Other antihypertensives need to be withdrawn (apart from ß-BLOCKERS and DIURETICS). Needs to be given in conjunction with some other ANTIHYPERTENSIVE drugs.
Not to be used for: patients suffering from phaeochromocytoma (a

disease of the adrenal glands).
Caution needed with:
Contains: MINOXIDIL.
Other preparations: REGAINE (Upjohn) — local application for the treatment of male pattern baldness.

---

loperamide *see* Imodium

Lopid
(Parke-Davis)

A white/maroon capsule and white oval tablet supplied at strengths of 300 mg, 600 mg and used as a lipid-lowering agent to treat raised lipid levels.

Dose: usually 600 mg twice a day to a maximum of 1500 mg a day.
Availability: NHS and private prescription.
Side effects: stomach upset, rashes, impotence, headache, dizziness, painful extremities, muscle aches, blurred vision.
Caution: your doctor may advise a lipid check; blood count, and liver function should be checked before treatment; eyes, blood, and serum should be checked regularly.
Not to be used for: pregnant women, nursing mothers, alcoholics, or patients suffering from gallstones or liver disease.
Caution needed with: anticoagulants.
Contains: GEMFIBROZIL.
Other preparations:

---

loprazolam tablets

A tablet supplied at a strength of 1 mg and used as a sleeping tablet for the short-term treatment of sleeplessness or waking at night.

Dose: elderly up to 1 tablet before going to bed; adults 1-2 tablets before going to bed.
Availability: NHS and private prescription.
Side effects: drowsiness, confusion, unsteadiness, low blood pressure, rash, changes in vision, changes in libido, retention of urine. Risk of addiction increases with dose and length of treatment. May impair judgement.
Caution: in the elderly, pregnant women, nursing mothers, in women during labour, and in patients suffering from lung disorders, kidney or liver disorders. Avoid long-term use and withdraw gradually.
Not to be used for: children, or for patients suffering from acute lung

L

diseases, some chronic lung diseases, some obsessional and psychotic diseases.

Caution needed with: alcohol, other tranquillizers, anticonvulsants.
Contains: LOPRAZOLAM mesylate.
Other preparations: Dormonoct (now discontinued).

Lopresor
(Ciba-Geigy)

A pink, scored tablet or a pale-blue, scored tablet according to strengths of 50 mg, 100 mg and used as a ß-BLOCKER to treat angina, for the prevention of heart muscle damage, high blood pressure, and as an additional treatment in thyrotoxicosis, migraine.

Dose: angina 50-100 mg 2-3 times a day. High blood pressure 100 mg a day at first increasing to 200 mg a day if needed. Thyrotoxicosis 50 mg 4 times a day. Migraine 100-200 mg a day in divided doses.
Availability: NHS and private prescription.
Side effects: cold hands and feet, sleep disturbance, slow heart rate, tiredness, wheezing, heart failure, stomach upset, dry eyes, rash.
Caution: in pregnant women, nursing mothers, and in patients suffering from diabetes, kidney or liver disorders, asthma. May need to be withdrawn before surgery. Withdraw gradually. Your doctor may advise additional treatment with DIURETICS or DIGOXIN.
Not to be used for: children, or for patients suffering from heart block or failure.
Caution needed with: VERAPAMIL, CLONIDINE withdrawal, some anti-arrhythmic drugs and anaesthetics, RESERPINE, some ANTIHYPERTENSIVES, ERGOTAMINE, CIMETIDINE, sedatives, antidiabetics, SYMPATHOMIMETICS, INDOMETHACIN.
Contains: METOPROLOL tartrate
Other preparations: Lopresor SR, ARBRALENE (Berk), BETALOC (Astra), MEPRANIX (Ashbourne).

Lopresoretic
(Ciba-Geigy)

An off-white, scored tablet used as a ß-BLOCKER/thiazide DIURETIC combination to treat high blood pressure.

Dose: 1 tablet a day in the morning at first, increasing to 3-4 tablets a day as needed.
Availability: NHS and private prescription.
Side effects: cold hands and feet, sleep disturbance, slow heart rate,

tiredness, wheezing, heart failure, stomach upset, low blood potassium, rash, sensitivity to light, blood changes, gout, dry eyes, rash.
Caution: in pregnant women, nursing mothers, and in patients suffering from diabetes, kidney or liver disorders, gout, asthma. May need to be withdrawn before surgery. Withdraw gradually. Your doctor may advise potassium supplements, blood tests.
Not to be used for: children, or for patients suffering from heart block or failure, severe kidney failure.
Caution needed with: VERAPAMIL, CLONIDINE withdrawal, some anti-arrhythmic drugs and anaesthetics, RESERPINE, some ANTIHYPERTENSIVES, ERGOTAMINE, CIMETIDINE, sedatives, SYMPATHOMIMETICS, INDOMETHACIN, LITHIUM, DIGOXIN, other DIURETICS.
Contains: METOPROLOL tartrate, CHLORTHALIDONE.
Other preparations:

---

loratidine *see* Clarityn

---

lorazepam

A tablet supplied at strengths of 1 mg, 2.5 mg and used as a sedative to treat anxiety.

Dose: elderly 0.5-2 mg a day in divided doses; adults 1-4 mg a day in divided doses.
Availability: NHS and private prescription.
Side effects: drowsiness, confusion, unsteadiness, low blood pressure, rash, changes in vision, changes in libido, retention of urine. Risk of addiction increases with dose and length of treatment. May impair judgement.
Caution: in the elderly, pregnant women, nursing mothers, in women during labour, and in patients suffering from lung disorders, kidney or liver disorders. Avoid long-term use and withdraw gradually.
Not to be used for: children, or for patients suffering from acute lung diseases, some chronic lung diseases, some obsessional and psychotic diseases.
Caution needed with: alcohol, other tranquillizers, anticonvulsants.
Contains: lorazepam.
Other preparations: ATIVAN (Wyeth) — available on NHS only if prescribed as a generic.

L

Lorexane *see* **Quellada.** Product now discontinued.

lormetazepam

A tablet supplied at strengths of 0.5 mg, 1 mg and used as a sedative to treat sleeplessness.

Dose: elderly 0.5 mg before going to bed; adults 1 mg before going to bed.
Availability: NHS and private prescription.
Side effects: drowsiness, confusion, unsteadiness, low blood pressure, rash, changes in vision, changes in libido, retention of urine. Risk of addiction increases with dose and length of treatment. May impair judgement.
Caution: in the elderly, pregnant women, nursing mothers, in women during labour, and in patients suffering from lung disorders, kidney or liver disorders. Avoid long-term use and withdraw gradually.
Not to be used for: children, or for patients suffering from acute lung diseases, some chronic lung diseases, some obsessional and psychotic diseases.
Caution needed with: alcohol, other tranquillizers, anticonvulsants.
Contains: lormetazepam.
Other preparations:

Losec
(Astra)

A pink/brown capsule tablet supplied at a strength of 20 mg and used as an anti-ulcer drug for ulcers which are difficult to treat, and as a treatment for reflux oesophagitis.

Dose: usually 1-2 capsules a day for up to 8 weeks; rarely up to 6 capsules a day.
Availability: NHS and private prescription.
Side effects: constipation, diarrhoea, headache, nausea, rashes.
Caution: your doctor may advise endoscopic checks of the stomach.
Not to be used for: pregnant women or nursing mothers.
Caution needed with: DIAZEPAM, PHENYTOIN, WARFARIN.
Contains: OMEPRAZOLE.
Other preparations:

Lotriderm *see* Betnovate
(Schering-Plough)

Lotussin — ANTIHISTAMINE/antitussive cough linctus. Product now discontinued.

Loxapac
(Novex)

A yellow/green capsule, light-green/dark-green capsule, or blue/dark-green capsule according to strengths 10 mg, 25 mg, 50 mg, and used to treat mental disorders.

Dose: 20-50 mg a day in 2 divided doses, increasing to a maximum of 250 mg a day.
Availability: NHS and private prescription.
Side effects: drowsiness, dizziness, faintness, muscle twitching, weakness, confusion, rapid heart beat, low or high blood pressure, changes in heart activity, skin reactions, ANTICHOLINERGIC effects, nausea, vomiting, breathing difficulty, changes in the eye.
Caution: in pregnant women, nursing mothers, and in patients suffering from epilepsy, cardiovascular disease, glaucoma, urine retention.
Not to be used for: children, or for patients in a coma or depressed state because of drugs.
Caution needed with: sedatives, ANTICHOLINERGICS.
Contains: LOXAPINE SUCCINATE.
Other preparations:

---

loxapine *see* **Loxapac**

Lubrifilm
(Cusi)

An eye ointment used to lubricate and protect the eye in various eye disorders.

Dose: apply as required.
Availability: NHS, private prescription, over the counter.
Side effects: vision may be blurred.
Caution:
Not to be used for: patients allergic to any of the ingredients.
Caution needed with:
Contains: WOOL FAT, YELLOW SOFT PARAFFIN, LIQUID PARAFFIN.
Other preparations: SIMPLE EYE OINTMENT.

L

Ludiomil
(Ciba)

A peach tablet, greyish red tablet, pale-orange tablet, or brownish orange tablet according to strengths of 10 mg, 25 mg, 50 mg, 75 mg and used as a tetracyclic antidepressant to treat depression.

Dose: adults 25-75 mg a day at first usually at night or in 3 divided doses, then adjusted as needed after 1-2 weeks; elderly 30 mg a day at first at night or in 3 divided doses.
Availability: NHS and private prescription.
Side effects: convulsions, rash, reduced reactions, ANTICHOLINERGIC effects.
Caution: in the elderly, in pregnant women, nursing mothers, and in patients suffering from cardiovascular disease, overactive thyroid, schizophrenia.
Not to be used for: children or for patients suffering from mania, severe kidney or liver disease, history of epilepsy, narrow-angle glaucoma, recent heart attack, retention of urine.
Caution needed with: MAOIS, ANTIHYPERTENSIVES, SYMPATHOMIMETICS, BARBITURATES, PHENYTOIN, tranquillizers, CIMETEDINE, alcohol, anaesthetics.
Contains: MAPROTILINE hydrochloride.
Other preparations:

Luminal — a BARBITURATE. Product now discontinued.

Lurselle
(Marion Merrell Dow)

A white, scored tablet supplied at a strength of 250 mg and used as a lipid-lowering agent to treat elevated lipids.

Dose: 2 tablets twice a day with morning and evening meals.
Availability: NHS and private prescription.
Side effects: diarrhoea, stomach upset.
Caution: in patients suffering from heart disorders. Cease treatment 6 months before a planned pregnancy.
Not to be used for: children, pregnant women, or nursing mothers.
Caution needed with:
Contains: PROBUCOL.
Other preparations:

Lustral
(Invicta)

White, capsule-shaped tablets supplied at strengths of 50 mg, 100 mg, and used to treat the symptoms of depression, and to prevent relapse and further depressive episodes.

Dose: 50 mg once a day after food, increasing if necessary to a maximum of 100 mg a day, or up to 150 mg for 8 weeks.
Availability: NHS and private prescription.
Side effects: dry mouth, nausea, diarrhoea, shaking, sweating, stomach discomfort, sexual disturbances.
Caution: in pregnant women, nursing mothers, patients undergoing electroconvulsive therapy, or suffering from unstable epilepsy.
Not to be used for: children, or for patients suffering from kidney or liver disorder.
Caution needed with: MAOIS, LITHIUM, TRYPTOPHAN.
Contains: SERTRALINE.
Other preparations:

Lyclear
(Wellcome)

A conditioning lotion applied to the head to treat head lice.

Dose: shampoo hair as usual, then apply enough to saturate hair and scalp. Leave for 10 minutes, then rinse and dry.
Availability: NHS, private prescription, over the counter.
Side effects:
Caution: in children under 2 years, pregnant women, and nursing mothers. Avoid eyes.
Not to be used for: infants under 6 months.
Caution needed with:
Contains: PERMETHRIN.
Other preparations: Lyclear Cream (used to treat scabies).

---

lymecycline *see* **Tetralysal 300**

---

lynoestrenol *see* **Minilyn**

---

lypressin *see* **Syntopressin**

---

lysuride *see* **Revanil**

L

Maalox
(Rhone-Poulenc Rorer)

A white tablet used as an ANTACID to treat gastric and duodenal ulcer, gastritis, heartburn, acidity.

Dose: adults 1-2 tablets after meals and at bedtime.
Availability: NHS, private prescription, over the counter.
Side effects: occasionally constipation.
Caution:
Not to be used for: children.
Caution needed with: TETRACYCLINE antibiotics, tablets which are coated to protect the stomach.
Contains: ALUMINIUM HYDROXIDE, MAGNESIUM HYDROXIDE.
Other preparations: Maalox suspension, Maalox TC. MUCOGEL (Pharmax).

Maalox Plus *see* Asilone
(Rhone-Poulenc Rorer)

Macrobid *see* Furandantin
(Procter and Gamble)

Macrodantin
(Norwich Eaton)

A yellow/white capsule or a yellow capsule according to strengths of 50 mg, 100 mg and used as an antiseptic to treat infection of the urinary tract.

Dose: adults treatment 50-100 mg 4 times a day with food or milk, prevention 50-100 mg a day; children treatment 3 mg per kg a day, prevention 1 mg per kg.
Availability: NHS and private prescription.
Side effects: stomach upset, allergy, blood disorders, nerve damage, jaundice, possible liver damage.
Caution: in the elderly, pregnant women, nursing mothers, and in patients suffering from anaemia, diabetes, electrolyte imbalance, vitamin B deficiency, debilitation.
Not to be used for: infants under 1 month or for patients suffering from kidney failure.
Caution needed with: MAGNESIUM TRISILICATE, PROBENECID, SULPHINPYRAZONE, quinolone antibiotics.
Contains: NITROFURANTOIN.

M

Madopar
(Roche)

A blue/grey capsule, blue/pink capsule, or blue/caramel capsule according to strengths of 62.5 mg, 125 mg, 250 mg and used as an anti-parkinsonian combination to treat Parkinson's disease.

Dose: adults over 25 years 1 low-dose capsule 3-4 times a day after meals at first increasing by 2 low-dose capsules a day 1-2 times a week up to 8-16 low-dose capsules a day in divided doses or as advised by the physician; elderly 1 low-dose capsule twice a day at first increasing by 1 low-dose capsule every 3-4 days.
Availability: NHS and private prescription.
Side effects: nausea, vomiting, anorexia, low blood pressure on standing, involuntary movements, heart and brain disturbances, discoloration of urine, rarely haemolytic anaemia.
Caution: in patients suffering from cardiovascular, liver, lung, endocrine or kidney disease, stomach ulcer, mental disturbance, glaucoma, bone changes. Your doctor may advise that blood, liver, kidney, and cardiovascular systems should be checked regularly.
Not to be used for: children, adults under 25 years, pregnant women, nursing mothers, or for patients suffering from severe mental disorders, glaucoma, history of malignant melanoma.
Caution needed with: MAOIS, ANTIHYPERTENSIVES, SYMPATHOMIMETICS, FERROUS SULPHATE, other similar drugs.
Contains: LEVODOPA, BENSERAZIDE HYDROCHLORIDE (CO-BENELDOPA).
Other preparations: Madopar Dispersible Tablets, Madopar CR.

Magnapen
(Beecham)

A turquoise/black capsule used as a penicillin to treat serious infections.

Dose: adults 1 capsule 4 times a day ½-1 hour before food; children use syrup.
Availability: NHS and private prescription.
Side effects: allergies, stomach disturbances.
Caution: in patients suffering from glandular fever.
Not to be used for: for patients suffering from penicillin allergy.
Caution needed with:
Contains: AMPICILLIN, FLUCLOXACILLIN (CO-FLUAMPICIL).

M

Other preparations: Magnapen Syrup.

magnesium alginate *see* Algicon

magnesium carbonate *see* Algicon, APP, Bellocarb, Caved-S, magnesium carbonate aromatic mixture, Nulacin, Roter, Topal

magnesium carbonate aromatic mixture

A mixture used as an ANTACID to treat stomach discomfort.

Dose: 10 ml 3 times a day in water.
Availability: NHS, private prescription, over the counter.
Side effects: diarrhoea, belching.
Caution: in patients suffering from kidney damage.
Not to be used for: patients with low phosphate levels in the blood.
Caution needed with: ASPIRIN, DIFLUNISAL, QUINIDINE, some antibiotics (especially TETRACYCLINES) PHENYTOIN, ITRACONAZOLE, KETOCONAZOLE, FOSINOPRIL, DIPYRIDAMOLE, CHLOROQUINE, HYDROXYCHLOROQUINE, some sedatives, PENICILLAMINE.
Contains: MAGNESIUM CARBONATE, SODIUM BICARBONATE, aromatic cardamon tincture.
Other preparations:

magnesium chloride *see* Glandosane

magnesium citrate *see* Picolax

magnesium hydroxide *see* Actonorm, Andursil, Carbellon, Diovol, liquid paraffin and magnesium hydroxide emulsion, Maalox, Maalox Plus, magnesium hydroxide mixture, Mucaine, Octovit

magnesium hydroxide mixture

A mixture used as a laxative to treat constipation.

M

Dose: 25-50 ml when required.
Availability: NHS, private prescription, over the counter.
Side effects: colic.
Caution: in the elderly, and in patients who are weak or suffering from kidney or liver damage.
Not to be used for: sudden, severe symptoms.
Caution needed with:
Contains: MAGNESIUM HYDROXIDE.
Other preparations:

---

magnesium oxide *see* Asilone, Kolanticon, Nulacin, Polyalk

---

magnesium sulphate (Epsom salts)

An osmotic laxative used to evacuate the bowels quickly.

Dose: adults 5-10 g in water on an empty stomach.
Availability: NHS, private prescription, over the counter.
Side effects:
Caution: in patients suffering from kidney disease.
Not to be used for:
Caution needed with:
Contains:
Other preparations:

---

magnesium sulphate *see* Kest, magnesium sulphate (Epsom Salts), magnesium sulphate paste

---

magnesium sulphate paste

A paste used to treat boils.

Dose: apply under a dressing.
Availability: NHS, private prescription, over the counter.
Side effects:
Caution: stir before use.
Not to be used for:
Caution needed with:
Contains: MAGNESIUM SULPHATE, GLYCEROL, PHENOL.
Other preparations:

M

---

magnesium trisilicate mixture

A white liquid used as an ANTACID to treat acidity, dyspepsia.

Dose: 10 ml 3 times a day in water.
Availability: NHS, private prescription, over the counter.
Side effects: diarrhoea.
Caution: in patients suffering from kidney impairment.
Not to be used for: children.
Caution needed with: tablets which are coated to protect the stomach
Contains: MAGNESIUM TRISILICATE.
Other preparations: magnesium trisilicate tablets co., magnesium trisilicate powder.

---

magnesium trisilicate *see* Aluhyde, Bellocarb, Droxalin, Gastrocote, Gastron, Genusil, magnesium trisilicate mixture, Nulacin

---

Malatex — anti-inflammatory solution to treat skin ulcers, sores, and burns. Product now discontinued.

---

malathion *see* Derbac-M, Prioderm, Suleo-M

---

malic acid *see* Aserbine, Malatex

Malinal — ANTACID tablets/suspension. Product now discontinued.

Maloprim
(Wellcome)

A white, scored tablet used as a sulphone preparation for the prevention of malaria.

Dose: adults and children over 10 years 1 tablet a week; children 5-10 years half adult dose. Continue for 4 weeks after leaving area.
Availability: NHS and private prescription.
Side effects: blood disorders, sensitive skin.
Caution: in pregnant women, nursing mothers, and in patients suffering

from liver or kidney disease.
Not to be used for:
Caution needed with: TRIMETHOPRIM.
Contains: DAPSONE, PYRIMETHAMINE.
Other preparations:

---

maltose *see* **Nulacin**

Manevac
(Galen)

Granules used as a stimulant and bulking agent to treat constipation.

Dose: adults 5-10 ml at night and before breakfast if needed; children over 5 years 5 ml daily.
Availability: NHS, private prescription, over the counter.
Side effects: wind, distension, diarrhoea.
Caution:
Not to be used for: children under 5 years, or for patients suffering from obstruction of the intestine, coeliac disease.
Caution needed with:
Contains: ISPAGHULA, SENNOSIDES.
Other preparations:

---

manganese glycerophosphate *see* **Tonivitan A & D, Tonivitan B, Verdiviton**

---

manganese *see* **Metatone**

---

manganese sulphate *see* **Folicin**

Manoplax
(Boots)

A white hexagonal tablet supplied at strengths of 50 mg, 100 mg, and used as an additional treatment for congestive heart failure.

Dose: initially 50 mg once a day for 4 weeks, then increasing if necessary

M

to a maximum of 150 mg a day.
Availability: NHS and private prescription.
Side effects: headache, dizziness, heart beat or rhythm disturbance, low blood pressure, stomach upset, taste disturbance, anaemia, joint pains, body fluid changes, sensitivity to light, feeling of being unwell, rash, vertigo.
Caution: in nursing mothers, and in patients suffering from low blood pressure, severe liver of kidney disorder, rapid heart rate.
Not to be used for: children, pregnant women, or for patients suffering from obstructed outflow from the heart.
Caution needed with: anticoagulants, cimetidine, other drugs affecting blood vessels (vasodilators).
Contains: FLOSEQUINAN.
Other preparations:

Manusept
(Hough, Hoseason)

A solution used as a disinfectant for cleansing and disinfecting skin and hands before surgery.

Dose: rub into the skin until dry.
Availability: NHS, private prescription, over the counter.
Side effects:
Caution: keep out of the eyes.
Not to be used for:
Caution needed with:
Contains: TRICLOSAN, ISOPROPYL ALCOHOL.
Other preparations:

MAOI (mono-amine oxidase inhibitor)

An antidepressant agent which may interact with some foods and other drugs. Example ISOCARBOXAZID *see* Marplan.

maprotiline *see* Ludiomil

M

Marevan
(Evans)

A brown tablet, blue tablet, or pink tablet according to strengths of 1 mg, 3 mg, 5 mg and used as an anticoagulant to thin the blood.

Dose: 10-15 mg a day initially, then as directed.
Availability: NHS and private prescription.
Side effects: rash, diarrhoea, blood changes, hair loss.
Caution: in the elderly or very ill patients, and for patients suffering from high blood pressure, weight changes, kidney disease, or vitamin K deficiency.
Not to be used for: children, pregnant women, within 24 hours of surgery or labour, or for patients suffering from kidney or liver disease, or haemorrhagic conditions.
Caution needed with: NON-STEROID ANTI-INFLAMMATORY DRUGS, oral antidiabetics, QUINIDINE, antibiotics, PHENFORMIN, CIMETIDINE, drugs affecting liver chemistry, STEROIDS, IMIDAZOLE antifungal drugs,
Contains: sodium WARFARIN.
Other preparations:

Marplan
(Cambridge)

A pink, scored tablet supplied at a strength of 10 mg and used as an MAOI to treat depression.

Dose: adults 3 tablets a day at first, then 1-2 tablets a day; elderly half adult dose.
Availability: NHS and private prescription.
Side effects: severe high blood pressure reactions with certain foods, sleeplessness, low blood pressure, dizziness, drowsiness, weakness, dry mouth, constipation, stomach upset, blurred vision, urinary difficulties, ankle swelling, rash, jaundice, weight gain, confusion, sexual desire changes.
Caution: in the elderly and in patients suffering from epilepsy.
Not to be used for: children, or for patients suffering from liver disease, blood changes, heart disease, phaeochromocytoma, overactive thyroid, brain artery disease.
Caution needed with: amphetamines or similar SYMPATHOMIMETIC drugs, TRICYCLIC antidepressants, PETHIDINE and other narcotics, some cough mixtures and appetite suppressants containing sympathomimetics. BARBITURATES, sedatives, alcohol, and antidiabetics may be enhanced. ANTICHOLINERGIC side effects are increased. Cheese, Bovril, Oxo, meat extracts, broad beans, banana, Marmite, yeast extracts, wine, beer, other alcohol, pickled herrings, vegetable proteins. (Up to 14 days after cessation.)
Contains: ISOCARBOXAZID.
Other preparations:

M

Marvelon
(Organon)

A white tablet used as an oestrogen, progestogen contraceptive.

Dose: 1 tablet a day for 21 days starting on day 1 or day 5 of the period.
Availability: NHS and private prescription.
Side effects: enlarged breasts, bloating and fluid retention, cramps, leg pains, mood change, reduction in sexual desire, headaches, nausea, vaginal erosion, discharge, and bleeding, weight gain, skin changes.
Caution: in patients suffering from high blood pressure, diabetes, vascular disorders, asthma, depression, kidney disease, multiple sclerosis, womb diseases. Your doctor may advise you not to smoke, to have regular examinations. You should stop treatment at the first sign of serious symptoms such as severe headache or jaundice. Treatment should be stopped before surgery.
Not to be used for: pregnant women, or for patients suffering from sickle-cell anaemia, history of heart disease or thrombosis, liver disorders, some cancers, undiagnosed vaginal bleeding, some ear, skin, and kidney disorders.
Caution needed with: RIFAMPICIN, TETRACYCLINES, GRISEOFULVIN, BARBITURATES, PHENYTOIN, PRIMIDONE, CARBAMAZEPINE, ETHOSUXIMIDE, CHLORAL HYDRATE, DICHLORALPHENAZONE.
Contains: ETHINYLOESTRADIOL, DESOGESTREL.
Other preparations:

Maxepa
(Innovex)

A clear, soft capsule used as a lipid-lowering agent to treat elevated lipids.

Dose: 5 capsules twice a day with food.
Availability: NHS, private prescription, over the counter.
Side effects: nausea, belching
Caution: in patients suffering from bleeding disorders.
Not to be used for: children.
Caution needed with: anticoagulants
Contains: EICOSAPENTAENOIC ACID, DOCOSAHEXAENOIC ACID.
Other preparations: Maxepa Liquid.

M

Maxidex
(Alcon)

Drops used as a STEROID, lubricant treatment for inflammation of the front of the eye.

Dose: 1-2 drops every hour, reducing as inflammation subsides. (Mild disease 4-6 times a day.)
Availability: NHS and private prescription.
Side effects: cataract, thinning cornea, fungal infection, rise in eye pressure.
Caution: in pregnant women and infants — do not use for extended periods.
Not to be used for: patients suffering from viral, fungal, tubercular, or weeping infections, glaucoma, or for patients who wear soft contact lenses.
Caution needed with:
Contains: DEXAMETHASONE, HYPROMELLOSE.
Other preparations:

Maxitrol
(Alcon)

Drops used as a STEROID, aminoglycoside antibiotic, lubricant, and protein treatment for infected inflammation of the eye.

Dose: 1-2 drops into the eye 4-6 times a day.
Availability: NHS and private prescription.
Side effects: rise in eye pressure, fungal infection, thinning cornea, cataract.
Caution: in pregnant women and infants— do not use for extended periods.
Not to be used for: patients suffering from glaucoma, viral, fungal, tubercular, or weeping infections, or for patients who wear soft contact lenses.
Caution needed with:
Contains: DEXAMETHASONE, NEOMYCIN sulphate, HYPROMELLOSE, POLYMYXIN B SULPHATE.
Other preparations: Maxitrol Ointment.

Maxivent *see* Ventolin
(Ashbourne)

Maxolon
(Beecham)

A white tablet supplied at a strength of 10 mg and used as an anti-sickness (anti-dopaminergic), antispasm drug to treat nausea, vomiting,

M

dyspepsia, wind, heartburn, and other symptoms related to stomach and bowels, intolerance to cytotoxic drugs, congestive heart failure, after operations, deep X-ray or cobalt treatment.

Dose: adults over 20 years10 mg 3 times a day; children and young adults use only for special circumstances such as in sickness caused by cancer treatment (reduced doses).
Availability: NHS and private prescription.
Side effects: occasionally parkinsonian-type symptoms, extra-pyramidal reactions (tremor, rigidity).
Caution: in pregnant women, nursing mothers, and in patients suffering from liver and kidney problems or epilepsy.
Not to be used for: where recent gastric or bowel surgery has occurred. Some rare tumours such as phaeochromocytoma (a disease of the adrenal glands) or prolactin-dependent breast cancers.
Caution needed with: ANTICHOLINERGICS, some sedatives, tranquillizers and antidepressants.
Contains: METOCLOPRAMIDE.
Other preparations: Maxolon Syrup, Maxolon Paediatric Liquid, Maxolon SR. GASTROBID CONTINUS (Napp), GASTROFLUX (Ashbourne), GASTROMAX (Farmitalia CE), METOX, METRAMID, MYGDALON (DDSA), PARMID (Lagap), PRIMPERAN (Berk).

Maxtrex
(Farmitalia)

A yellow tablet or a yellow, scored tablet according to strengths of 2.5 mg, 10 mg, and used to treat severe psoriasis. Also used to treat some cancer conditions.

Dose: as advised by your doctor.
Availability: NHS and private prescription.
Side effects: stomach pain, liver and bone marrow disorder, rash.
Caution: in the elderly and the young, and in patients suffering from blood or gastro-intestinal disorders, mental illness, liver or kidney damage. Your doctor may advise regular tests.
Not to be used for: pregnant women, nursing mothers, or for patients suffering from severe kidney or liver damage, serious blood disorders.
Caution needed with: alcohol, some vaccines, FOLIC ACID, ETRETINATE, anticonvulsants, NON-STEROID ANTI-INFLAMMATORY DRUGS, some other drugs.
Contains: METHOTREXATE.
Other preparations:

M

mazindol *see* **Teronac**

MCR-50 *see* **ISMO**
(Farmitalia CE)

---

mebendazole *see* **Vermox**

---

mebeverine *see* **Colofac, Colven**

---

mebhydrolin *see* **Fabahistin**

---

medazepam *see* **Nobrium**

Medicoal
(Torbet)

Effervescent granules used as an adsorbent to treat poisoning and overdosing with drugs.

Dose: 5-10 g in 100 ml of water, repeat up to a maximum of 50 g.
Availability: NHS, private prescription, over the counter.
Side effects:
Caution:
Not to be used for: poisoning where there is a known antidote or for poisoning by acids, alkalis, iron salts, cyanides, MALATHION, DDT, some antidiabetics.
Caution needed with: drugs taken by mouth.
Contains: activated CHARCOAL.
Other preparations:

Medihaler-Duo — broncho-dilator aerosol to treat bronchial spasm. Product now discontinued.

Medihaler-EPI
(3M-Healthcare)

An aerosol supplied at a strength of 0.28 mg and used as a SYMPATHOMIMETIC additional treatment for sensitivity to drugs or stings due to

M

previous exposure.

Dose: adults at least 20 sprays; children 10-15 sprays.
Availability: NHS and private prescription.
Side effects: nervousness, shaking hands, dry mouth, stomach pain.
Caution: in patients suffering from diabetes.
Not to be used for: patients suffering from heart disease, high blood pressure, overactive thyroid, abnormal heart rhythm.
Caution needed with: MAOIS, TRICYCLICS, other SYMPATHOMIMETICS.
Contains: ADRENALINE ACID TARTRATE.
Other preparations:

Medihaler-Ergotamine
(3M Healthcare)

An aerosol used to treat migraine.

Dose: 1 dose repeated if needed after 5 minutes up to a maximum of 6 doses in 24 hours or 15 doses in a week.
Availability: NHS and private prescription.
Side effects: nausea, muscular pain.
Caution:
Not to be used for: children under 10 years, pregnant women, nursing mothers, or for patients suffering from coronary, peripheral, or occlusive vascular disease, severe high blood pressure, kidney or liver disease, or sepsis.
Caution needed with: ERYTHROMYCIN, ß-BLOCKERS.
Contains: ERGOTAMINE TARTRATE.
Other preparations: CAFERGOT (Sandoz), LINGRAINE (Sanofi-Winthrop), MIGRIL (Wellcome).

Medihaler-Iso
(3M Healthcare)

An aerosol supplied at a strength of 0.08 mg and used as a ß-agonist to treat bronchial asthma, chronic bronchitis.

Dose: 1-3 sprays and again after 30 minutes if needed, to a maximum of 24 sprays in 24 hours.
Availability: NHS and private prescriptions.
Side effects: rapid or abnormal heart rate, dry mouth, nervousness.
Caution: in pregnant women, and in patients suffering from diabetes, high blood pressure.
Not to be used for: patients suffering from heart disease, overactive thyroid.

M

Caution needed with: MAOIS, SYMPATHOMIMETICS, TRICYCLICS.
Contains: ISOPRENALINE sulphate.
Other preparations: Medihaler Iso Forte. SAVENTRINE (Pharmax).

Medilave
(Martindale)

A gel used as an antiseptic and local anaesthetic to treat abrasions or ulcers in the mouth, teething.

Dose: apply to the affected area without rubbing in 3-4 times a day.
Availability: NHS, private prescription, over the counter.
Side effects:
Caution:
Not to be used for: infants under 6 months.
Caution needed with:
Contains: BENZOCAINE, CETYLPYRIDINIUM.
Other preparations:

Medised Suspension
(Panpharma)

A suspension used as an ANALGESIC, ANTIHISTAMINE treatment to relieve pain and fever associated with congestion, chicken pox.

Dose: children 3 months-1 year 5 ml up to 4 times a day, 1-6 years 10 ml up to 4 times a day, 6-12 years 20 ml up to 4 times a day.
Availability: private prescription, and over the counter.
Side effects: drowsiness.
Caution: in patients with liver or kidney disease.
Not to be used for: infants under 3 months.
Caution needed with: alcohol, sedatives, other medicines containing PARACETAMOL.
Contains: PARACETAMOL, PROMETHAZINE hydrochloride.
Other preparations: (Medised Tablets — now discontinued.)

Meditar — treatment stick for psoriasis/eczema. Product now discontinued.

M

Medocodene *see* **Co-codamol.** Product now discontinued.

Medomet *see* **Aldomet**
(DDSA)

Medrone
(Upjohn)

A pink, quarter-scored, oval tablet, a white, quarter-scored, oval tablet, a white, quarter-scored tablet, or a light-blue scored tablet according to strengths of 2 mg, 4 mg, 16 mg, 100 mg and used as a STEROID treatment for rheumatoid arthritis, inflammatory conditions, allergies.

Dose: as advised by the physician.
Availability: NHS and private prescription.
Side effects: high blood sugar, thin bones, mood changes, ulcers.
Caution: pregnant women,or for patients who have had recent bowel surgery, or who are suffering from inflamed veins, psychiatric disorders, virus infections, some cancers, some kidney diseases, thinning of the bones, ulcers, tuberculosis, other infections, high blood pressure, glaucoma, epilepsy, diabetes, underactive thyroid, liver disease, stress. Withdraw gradually.
Not to be used for:
Caution needed with: PHENYTOIN, PHENOBARBITONE, EPHEDRINE, RIFAMPICIN, DIURETICS, ANTI-CHOLINESTERASES, DIGOXIN, antidiabetic agents, anticoagulants, NON-STEROID ANTI-INFLAMMATORY DRUGS.
Contains: METHYLPREDNISOLONE.
Other preparations:

Medrone Lotion — STEROID/skin softener to treat acne/dermatitis. Product now discontinued.

---

medroxyprogesterone *see* **Provera**

---

mefenamic acid *see* **Ponstan, Ponstan Forte**

---

mefloquine *see* **Lariam**

---

mefruside *see* **Baycaron**

394

Megace
(Bristol-Myers Squibb)

A white, scored tablet or an off-white, oval, scored tablet according to strengths of 40 mg, 160 mg and used as a progestogen treatment for breast cancer or endometrial cancer.

Dose: breast cancer 160 mg a day for at least 2 months; endometrial cancer 40-320 mg a day.
Availability: NHS and private prescription.
Side effects: gain in weight, skin allergies, nausea.
Caution: in patients suffering from thrombophlebitis.
Not to be used for: children or pregnant women.
Caution needed with:
Contains: MEGESTROL ACETATE.
Other preparations:

Megaclor *see* **tetracycline.** Product now discontinued.

---

megestrol *see* **Megace**

Melleril
(Sandoz)

A white tablet supplied at strengths of 10 mg, 25 mg, 50 mg, 100 mg and used as a sedative to treat schizophrenia, manic mental disorders, senile confusion, behavioural disorders, epilepsy in children.

Dose: adults 30-100 mg a day at first increasing to 600 mg a day if needed; children under 5 years 1 mg per kg body weight a day, 5-12 years 75-150 mg a day, to a maximum of 300 mg a day.
Availability: NHS and private prescription.
Side effects: muscle spasms, restlessness, blurred vision, hands shaking, constipation, dry mouth, urine retention, palpitations, low blood pressure, weight gain, changes in libido, low body temperature, breast swelling, menstrual changes, jaundice, blood and skin changes, drowsiness, rarely fits.
Caution: in patients suffering from liver disease, kidney disease, cardio-vascular disease, epilepsy, glaucoma, myaesthenia gravis, enlarged prostate, severe lung disease, parkinsonism, adrenal tumour.
Not to be used for: pregnant women, nursing mothers, severely depressed or unconscious patients or for patients suffering from blood disorders, severe heart disease.

M

Caution needed with: alcohol, tranquillizers, pain killers, ANTIHYPERTENSIVES, antidepressants, anticonvulsants, antidiabetic drugs, LEVODOPA.
Contains: THIORIDAZINE hydrochloride.
Other preparations: Melleril Suspension, Melleril Syrup.

---

menadiol diphosphate *see* Synkavit

Menophase
(Syntex)

Five pink tablets, 8 orange tablets, 2 yellow tablets, 3 green tablets, 6 blue tablets, and 4 lavender tablets used as an oestrogen, progestogen treatment for symptoms associated with the menopause, and prevention of thinning of the bones after menopause.

Dose: 1 tablet a day.
Availability: NHS and private prescription.
Side effects: enlarged breasts, bloating and fluid retention, cramps, leg pains, mood change, reduction in sexual desire, headaches, nausea, vaginal erosion, discharge, and bleeding, weight gain, skin changes.
Caution: in patients suffering from high blood pressure, diabetes, vascular disorders, asthma, depression, kidney disease, multiple sclerosis, womb diseases. Your doctor may advise you not to smoke, to have regular check-ups.
Not to be used for: children, pregnant women, or for patients suffering from sickle-cell anaemia, history of heart disease or thrombosis, liver disorders, some cancers, undiagnosed vaginal bleeding, some ear, skin, and kidney disorders.
Caution needed with: DIURETICS, ANTIHYPERTENSIVES, and drugs that change liver enzymes, RIFAMPICIN, TETRACYCLINES, GRISEOFULVIN, BARBITURATES, PHENYTOIN, PRIMIDONE, CARBAMAZEPINE, ETHOSUXIMIDE, CHLORAL HYDRATE, DICHLORALPHENAZONE.
Contains: MESTRANOL, NORETHISTERONE,
Other preparations:

---

menthol *see* **Aradolene, Aspellin, Balmosa, Benylin Expectorant, Copholco, Copholcoids, Expurhin, Guanor, Histalix, Phytocil, Rowachol, Salonair, Tercoda, Terpoin**

---

menthone *see* **Rowachol**

Menzol *see* **Primolut-N**
(Schwarz)

---

mepacrine hydrochloride *see* **mepacrine tablets**

---

mepacrine tablets

Tablets supplied at a strength of 100 mg and used to treat giardiasis (an intestinal infection).

Dose: adults, 1 tablet every 8 hours; children, 2 mg/kg body weight every 8 hours.
Availability: NHS and private prescription.
Side effects: stomach upset, dizziness, headache, nausea, vomiting, mental disorder, excitation, yellow discoloration of skin and urine, skin disorders, liver disorders, blood changes, changes in vision, discoloured palate and nails.
Caution: in the elderly, and in patients suffering from liver disorder or a history of mental disorder.
Not to be used for: patients suffering from psoriasis.
Caution needed with: PRIMAQUIN.
Contains: MEPACRINE HYDROCHLORIDE.
Other preparations:

---

mepenzolate *see* **Cantil**

Mepranix *see* **Betaloc**
(Ashbourne)

Meprate *see* **Equanil**

---

meprobamate *see* **Equagesic, Equanil, Tenavoid**

---

meptazinol *see* **Meptid**

M

Meptid
(Wyeth)

An orange, oval tablet tablet supplied at a strength of 200 mg and used as an ANALGESIC to relieve pain.

Dose: 1 tablet every 3-6 hours as needed.
Availability: NHS and private prescription.
Side effects: dizziness, nausea.
Caution: in patients with liver or kidney disease or respiratory depression.
Not to be used for: children.
Caution needed with:
Contains: MEPTAZINOL.
Other preparations:

---

mequitazine *see* **Primalan**

Merbentyl
(Marion Merrell Dow)

A white tablet supplied at strengths of 10 mg, 20 mg and used as an antispasm, ANTICHOLINERGIC treatment for bowel and stomach spasm.

Dose: children 6 months-2 years 5-10 mg 3-4 times a day before feeds, over 2 years 10 mg 3 times a day, adults 10-20 mg 3 times a day between meals.
Availability: NHS and private prescription.
Side effects: dry mouth, thirst, dizziness.
Caution: in patients suffering from glaucoma, enlarged prostate, hiatus hernia with reflux oesophagitis.
Not to be used for:
Caution needed with:
Contains: DICYCLOMINE.
Other preparations: Merbentyl syrup.

Mercilon
(Organon)

A white tablet used as an oestrogen, progestogen contraceptive.

Dose: 1 tablet a day for 21 days starting on day 1 or day 5 of the period.
Availability: NHS and private prescription.
Side effects: enlarged breasts, bloating and fluid retention, cramps, leg pains, mood change, reduction in sexual desire, headaches, nausea,

vaginal erosion, discharge, and bleeding, weight gain, skin changes.
Caution: in patients suffering from high blood pressure, diabetes, vascular disorders, asthma, depression, kidney disease, multiple sclerosis, womb diseases. Your doctor may advise you not to smoke, to have regular examinations. You should stop treatment at the first sign of serious symptoms such as severe headache or jaundice. Treatment should be stopped before surgery.
Not to be used for: pregnant women, or for patients suffering from sickle-cell anaemia, history of heart disease or thrombosis, liver disorders, some cancers, undiagnosed vaginal bleeding, some ear, skin, and kidney disorders.
Caution needed with: RIFAMPICIN, TETRACYCLINES, GRISEOFULVIN, BARBITURATES, PHENYTOIN, PRIMIDONE, CARBAMAZEPINE, ETHOSUXIMIDE, CHLORAL HYDRATE, DICHLORALPHENAZONE.
Contains: ETHINYLOESTRADIOL, DESOGESTREL.
Other preparations:

Merocaine
(Marion Merrell Dow)

A green lozenge used as an antiseptic and local anaesthetic to treat painful infections of the throat and mouth, and as an additional treatment for tonsillitis and pharyngitis.

Dose: 1 lozenge allowed to dissolve in the mouth every 2 hours up to a maximum of 8 lozenges in 24 hours.
Availability: NHS, private prescription, over the counter.
Side effects:
Caution:
Not to be used for: children.
Caution needed with:
Contains: CETYLPYRIDINIUM CHLORIDE, BENZOCAINE.
Other preparations:

Merocet
(Marion Merrell Dow)

A solution used as an antiseptic to treat infections of the throat and mouth.

Dose: rinse the mouth or gargle with the solution diluted or undiluted every 3 hours or as needed.
Availability: NHS, private prescription, over the counter.
Side effects:
Caution:

M

Not to be used for: children under 6 years.
Caution needed with:
Contains: CETYLPYRIDINIUM CHLORIDE.
Other preparations: Merocets Lozenge

---

mesalazine *see* **Asacol**

---

mesterolone *see* **Pro-Viron**

Mestinon
(Roche)

A white tablet tablet supplied at a strength of 60 mg and used as a nerve conduction enhancer to treat paralytic ileus, myasthenia gravis (muscular disorders).

Dose: paralytic ileus adults 1-4 tablets as required; children ¼ -1 tablet as required. For myasthenia gravis adults 5-20 tablets a day in divided doses; infants 5-10 mg every 4 hours, under 6 years ½ tablet initially, 6-12 years 1 tablet intitially.
Availability: NHS and private prescription.
Side effects: nausea, salivation, diarrhoea, colic.
Caution: in patients suffering from bronchial asthma, heart disease, epilepsy, Parkinson's disease.
Not to be used for: patients with bowel or urinary obstruction.
Caution needed with: some drugs used in anaesthesia.
Contains: PYRIDOSTIGMINE BROMIDE.
Other preparations:

---

mestranol *see* **Menophase, Norinyl-1, Ortho-Novin 1/50**

Metalpha *see* **Aldomet**
(Ashbourne)

M

Metamucil *see* **Fybogel**
(Procter and Gamble)

Metatone
(Warner-Lambert)

A liquid used as a source of vitamin B$_1$ and minerals and used as a tonic.

Dose: adults 5-10 ml 2-3 times a day; children 6-12 years half adult dose.
Availability: private prescription and over the counter.
Side effects:
Caution:
Not to be used for: children under 6 years.
Caution needed with:
Contains: THIAMINE hydrochloride, CALCIUM GLYCEROPHOSPHATE, MANGANESE, POTASSIUM, SODIUM.
Other preparations:

Metenix
(Hoechst)

A blue tablet tablet supplied at a strength of 5 mg and used as a DIURETIC to treat high blood pressure, fluid retention, swollen abdomen, or toxaemia of pregnancy.

Dose: high blood pressure 5 mg a day at first, then reduce to 5 mg every other day after 3-4 weeks; fluid retention 5-10 mg as a single dose; no more than 80 mg in 24 hours.
Availability: NHS and private prescription.
Side effects: low potassium levels, headache, stomach upset, cramps, rash.
Caution: in pregnant women, nursing mothers, and in patients suffering from liver disease, gout, or diabetes. Potassium supplements may be needed.
Not to be used for: patients suffering from liver cirrhosis or kidney failure.
Caution needed with: DIGOXIN, LITHIUM, ANTIHYPERTENSIVES.
Contains: METOLAZONE.
Other preparations: XURET (Galen).

Meterfolic
(Sinclair)

A grey tablet used as an iron and folic acid supplement in the prevention of iron and folic acid deficiencies in pregnancy.

Dose: 1 tablet 1-2 times a day.
Availability: NHS and private prescription.
Side effects: nausea, constipation.

M

Caution: in patients suffering from haemolytic anaemia, or with a history of stomach ulcer.
Not to be used for: children or for patients suffering from vitamin B$_{12}$ deficiency.
Caution needed with: TETRACYCLINES.
Contains: FERROUS FUMARATE, FOLIC ACID.
Other preparations: FOLEX-350 (Rybar), GALFER FA (Galen).

---

metformin *see* **Glucophage**

---

methadone *see* **Physeptone**

---

methionine *see* **Lipoflavonoid, Pameton**

---

methixene hydrochloride *see* **Tremonil**

---

methocarbamol *see* **Robaxin, Robaxisal**

---

methoserpidine *see* **Decaserpyl, Decaserpyl Plus**

---

methotrexate *see* **Maxtrex**

---

methotrimeprazine *see* **Nozinan, Veractil**

---

methyclothiazide *see* **Enduron**

M

methyl nicotinate *see* **Cremalgin, Dubam**

methyl salicylate *see* **Aspellin, Balmosa, Dubam, Monphytol, Phytex**

---

methyl undecoanate *see* **Monphytol**

---

methylcellulose granules *see* **Celevac.** Product now discontinued.

---

methylcellulose *see* **Celevac, Cologel, methylcellulose granules, Nilstim**

---

methylcysteine hydrochloride *see* **Visclair**

---

methyldopa *see* **Aldomet, Hydromet**

---

methylphenobarbitone *see* **Prominal**

---

methylprednisolone *see* **Medrone, Medrone Lotion, Neo-Medrone Cream, Neo-Medrone Lotion**

---

methyprylone *see* **Noludar**

---

methysergide *see* **Deseril**

Metipranolol Minims
(SNP)

Drops used as a ß-BLOCKER to treat high eye pressure.

Dose: 1 drop into the eye twice a day.
Availability: NHS and private prescription.
Side effects: slight smarting, temporary headache.

M

Caution: in pregnant women, and in patients suffering from heart block.
Not to be used for: children, or for patients suffering from heart failure, blocked airways disease, or abnormal heart rhythm.
Caution needed with: VERAPAMIL, other ß-BLOCKERS.
Contains: METIPRANOLOL.
Other preparations:

---

metipranolol *see* **Metipranolol Minims**

---

metoclopramide *see* **Maxolon, Migravess Forte, Paramax**

---

metolazone *see* **Metenix**

---

metoprolol *see* **Betaloc**

Metopirone
(Ciba)

A cream capsule tablet supplied at a strength of 250 mg and used as a hormone blocker to treat Cushing's syndrome, and with glucocorticoids to treat resistant oedema caused by increased aldosterone secretion (adrenal gland disorder).

Dose: Cushing's syndrome 1-24 tablets a day; oedema 10-18 tablets a day.
Availability: NHS and private prescription.
Side effects: nausea, vomiting, low blood pressure, allergies.
Caution: in patients suffering from underactive pituitary gland.
Not to be used for: children, pregnant women, or nursing mothers.
Caution needed with:
Contains: METYRAPONE.
Other preparations:

M

metoprolol *see* **Betaloc, Co-Betaloc, Lopresor, Lopresoretic, Metoros**

Metoros *see* **Betaloc.** Product now discontinued.

Metosyn
(Stuart)

A cream used as a STEROID treatment for allergic and other skin conditions where there is also inflammation.

Dose: massage into the affected area morning and night at first and then reduce to once a day as soon as possible.
Availability: NHS and private prescription.
Side effects: fluid retention, suppression of adrenal glands, thinning of the skin may occur.
Caution: use for short periods of time only.
Not to be used for: patients suffering from acne or any other skin infections caused by tuberculosis, ringworm, viruses, or fungi, or continuously especially in pregnant women.
Caution needed with:
Contains: FLUOCINONIDE.
Other preparations: Metosyn Ointment, Metosyn Scalp Lotion.

Metox *see* **Maxolon.** Product now discontinued.

Metramid *see* **Maxolon.** Product now discontinued.

Metrogel
(Sandoz)

A gel used to treat rosacea (a skin disorder of the face).

Dose: apply twice a day for 8-9 weeks.
Availability: NHS and private prescription.
Side effects: irritation.
Caution:
Not to be used for: children or for pregnant women
Caution needed with:
Contains: METRONIDAZOLE.
Other preparations:

M

Metrolyl *see* **Flagyl**
(Lagap)

---

metronidazole *see* **Flagyl, Metrogel**

---

metyrapone *see* **Metopirone**

---

mexiletine *see* **Mexitil**

Mexitil
(Boehringer Ingelheim)

A red/purple capsule or a red capsule according to strengths of 50 mg, 200 mg and used as an anti-arrhythmic treatment for abnormal heart rhythm.

Dose: 400-600 mg at first, then 2 hours later and thereafter 200-250 mg 3-4 times a day.
Availability: NHS and private prescription.
Side effects: stomach and brain disorders, low blood pressure.
Caution: in patients suffering from nerve conduction defects in the heart, low blood pressure, heart, liver, or kidney failure, Parkinson's disease.
Not to be used for: children.
Caution needed with:
Contains: MEXILETENE hydrochloride.
Other preparations: Mexitil Perlongets, Mexitil Injection

---

mianserin *see* **Bolvidon, Norval**

Micolette
(Cusi)

A micro-enema used as a faecal softener and lubricant to treat constipation, and for the evacuation of bowels before surgery.

Dose: adults and children over 3 years 1-2 enemas.
Availability: NHS, private prescription, over the counter.
Side effects:

---

miconazole *see* **Acnidazil, Daktacort, Daktarin, Daktarin Cream, Daktarin Oral Gel, Gyno-Daktarin 1**

Micralax
(Evans)

A disposable enema used as a faecal softener and lubricant to treat constipation, and for evacuation of bowels

Dose: adults and children over 3 years 1 enema.
Availability: NHS, private prescription, over the counter.
Side effects:
Caution:
Not to be used for: for children or patients suffering from inflammatory bowel disease.
Caution needed with:
Contains: SODIUM CITRATE, SODIUM ALKYLSULPHOACETATE, SORBIC ACID.
Other preparations:

Microgynon 30
(Schering)

A beige tablet used as an oestrogen, progestogen contraceptive.

Dose: 1 tablet a day for 21 days starting on day 5 of the period.
Availability: NHS and private prescription.
Side effects: enlarged breasts, bloating and fluid retention, cramps, leg pains, mood change, reduction in sexual desire, headaches, nausea, vaginal erosion, discharge, and bleeding, weight gain, skin changes.
Caution: in patients suffering from high blood pressure, diabetes, vascular disorders, asthma, depression, kidney disease, multiple sclerosis, womb diseases. Your doctor may advise you not to smoke, to have regular examinations. You should stop treatment at the first sign of serious symptoms such as severe headache or jaundice. Treatment should be stopped before surgery.

M

Not to be used for: pregnant women, or for patients suffering from sickle-cell anaemia, history of heart disease or thrombosis, liver disorders, some cancers, undiagnosed vaginal bleeding, some ear, skin, and kidney disorders.

Caution needed with: RIFAMPICIN, TETRACYCLINES, GRISEOFULVIN, BARBITURATES, PHENYTOIN, PRIMIDONE, CARBAMAZEPINE, ETHOSUXIMIDE, CHLORAL HYDRATE, DICHLORALPHENAZONE.

Contains: ETHINYLOESTRADIOL, LEVONORGESTREL.

Other preparations: OVRANETTE (Wyeth).

Micronor
(Cilag)

A white tablet used as a progesterone contraceptive.

Dose: 1 tablet at the same time every day starting on day 1 of the period.

Availability: NHS and private prescription.

Side effects: irregular bleeding, breast discomfort, acne, headache.

Caution: in patients suffering from high blood pressure, tendency to thrombosis, migraine, liver abnormalities, ovarian cysts. Your doctor may advise regular check-ups.

Not to be used for: pregnant women, or for patients suffering from severe heart or artery disease, benign liver tumours, vaginal bleeding, previous ectopic pregnancy.

Caution needed with: BARBITURATES, PHENYTOIN, PRIMIDONE, CARBAMAZEPINE, CHLORAL HYDRATE, DICHLORALPHENAZONE, ETHOSUXIMIDE, RIFAMPICIN, GLUTETHIMIDE, CHLORPROMAZINE, MEPROBAMATE, GRISEOFULVIN.

Contains: NORETHISTERONE.

Other preparations: NORIDAY (Syntex).

Microval
(Wyeth)

A white tablet used as a progesterone contraceptive.

Dose: 1 tablet at the same time every day starting on day 1 of the period.

Availability: NHS and private prescription.

Side effects: irregular bleeding, breast discomfort, acne, headache.

Caution: in patients suffering from high blood pressure, tendency to thrombosis, migraine, liver abnormalities, ovarian cysts. Your doctor may advise regular check-ups.

Not to be used for: pregnant women, or for patients suffering from severe heart or artery disease, benign liver tumours, vaginal bleeding, previous ectopic pregnancy.

M

Caution needed with: BARBITURATES, PHENYTOIN, PRIMIDONE, CARBAMAZEPINE, CHLORAL HYDRATE, DICHLORALPHENAZONE, ETHOSUXIMIDE, RIFAMPICIN, GLUTETHIMIDE, CHLORPROMAZINE, MEPROBAMATE, GRISEOFULVIN.
Contains: LEVONORGESTREL.
Other preparations: NORGESTON (Schering).

Mictral
(Sanofi Winthrop)

Granules in a sachet used as an antiseptic to treat cystitis and some infections of the urinary tract.

Dose: the contents of 1 sachet dissolved in water 3 times a day for 3 days.
Availability: NHS and private prescription.
Side effects: stomach problems, disturbed vision, rash, seizures, anaemia, blood changes, sensitivity to light.
Caution: in pregnant women, nursing mothers, and in patients suffering from liver disease. Keep out of sunlight.
Not to be used for: children or patients suffering from kidney disease, with a history of convulsions, or porphyria (a rare blood disorder).
Caution needed with: anticoagulants, antibacterials.
Contains: NALIDIXIC ACID, SODIUM CITRATE, CITRIC ACID, SODIUM BICARBONATE.
Other preparations: NEGRAM (Sanofi Winthrop), URIBEN (RP Drugs).

Micturin — ANTIHISTAMINE-type treatment for frequent/urgent urination. Product now discontinued.

Midamor *see* Amiloride
(Morson)

Midrid
(Shire)

A red capsule used as an ANALGESIC to treat migraine.

Dose: 2 capsules at the beginning of the migraine attack, then 1 capsule every hour to a maximum of 5 capsules in 12 hours.
Availability: NHS, private prescription, over the counter.
Side effects: dizziness.
Caution: in pregnant women and nursing mothers.
Not to be used for: children, or for patients suffering from severe kidney,

M

liver, or heart disease, gastritis, severe high blood pressure, or glaucoma.
Caution needed with: MAOIS, other medicines containing PARACETAMOL.
Contains: ISOMETHEPTENE MUCATE, PARACETAMOL.
Other preparations:

Migraleve
(Charwell)

A pink tablet and a yellow tablet according to strength and contents and used as an ANALGESIC, ANTIHISTAMINE treatment for migraine.

Dose: adults 2 pink tablets at the beginning of the attack, and then 2 yellow tablets every 4 hours if needed to a maximum of 2 pink tablets and 6 yellow tablets in 24 hours; children 10-14 years half adult dose.
Availability: NHS, private prescription, over the counter.
Side effects: drowsiness.
Caution: in patients suffering from kidney or liver disease.
Not to be used for: children under 10 years.
Caution needed with: other medicines containg PARACETAMOL.
Contains: pink: BUCLIZINE hydrochloride, PARACETAMOL, CODEINE phosphate; yellow: PARACETAMOL, CODEINE phosphate.
Other preparations:

Migravess
(Bayer)

A white, scored, effervescent tablet used as an anti-emetic and ANALGESIC to treat migraine.

Dose: adults 2 tablets dissolved in water at the beginning of the attack, then up to a maximum of 6 tablets in 24 hours; children 12-15 years half adult dose.
Availability: NHS and private prescription.
Side effects: extrapyramidal reactions (shaking and rigidity), drowsiness, diarrhoea.
Caution: in pregnant women or in patients suffering from kidney or liver disease, asthma.
Not to be used for: children under 12 years or for patients suffering from stomach ulcer, haemophilia, or allergy to ASPIRIN or anti-inflammatory drugs.
Caution needed with: ANTI-CHOLINERGICS, some sedatives, anticoagulants, antidiabetics and uric acid-lowering agents.
Contains: METOCLOPRAMIDE HYDROCHLORIDE, ASPIRIN.
Other preparations: Migravess Forte.

M

Migril

(Wellcome)

A white, scored tablet used as an ergot preparation to treat migraine.

Dose: 1 tablet at the beginning of an attack, then ½-1 tablet every ½ hour if needed to a maximum of 4 tablets for any 1 attack and 6 tablets in any 1 week.
Availability: NHS and private prescription.
Side effects: rebound headache, poor circulation, abdominal pain, drowsiness, dry mouth.
Caution: in patients suffering from sepsis, anaemia, overactive thyroid.
Not to be used for: children, pregnant women, nursing mothers, or for patients suffering from coronary, peripheral, or occlusive vascular disease, severe high blood pressure, kidney or liver disease.
Caution needed with: ERYTHROMYCIN, ß-BLOCKERS, sedatives.
Contains: ERGOTAMINE tartrate, CYCLIZINE hydrochloride, CAFFEINE hydrate.
Other preparations: CAFERGOT (Sandoz), LINGRAINE (Sanofi Withrop), MEDIHALER ERGOTAMINE (3M Healthcare).

Mildison Lipocream

(Brocades)

A cream used as a STEROID treatment for eczema and other skin disorders.

Dose: apply a small quantity to the affected area 2-3 times a day.
Availability: NHS and private prescription.
Side effects: fluid retention, suppression of adrenal glands, thinning of the skin may occur.
Caution: do not use for children or for facial conditions for longer than 5 days.
Not to be used for: with covering dressings or for patients suffering from bacterial, fungal, or viral infections, or for extended treatments in pregnant women.
Caution needed with:
Contains: HYDROCORTISONE.
Other preparations: DIODERM (Dermal), EFCORTELAN (Glaxo), HYDROCAL (Bioglan), HYDROCORTISONE CREAM, HYDROCORTISYL (Roussel), LOCOID (Brocades). Some other brands available over the counter for certain conditions only.

M

Minamino — vitamin and mineral supplement. Product now discontinued.

Min-i-jet adrenaline
(IMS)

A ready-to-use injection for emergency treatment of severe allergy. (Also used by trained medical personnel to treat heart attack.)

Dose: for severe allergy, 0.05 ml-1 ml injected by the intramuscular route (according to age), and repeated if necessary every 10 minutes.
Availability: NHS and private prescription.
Side effects: anxiety, shaking, rapid heart beat, heart beat irregularity, dry mouth, cold hands and feet.
Caution: in the elderly, and in patients suffering from overactive thyroid, diabetes, heart disease, high blood pressure.
Not to be used for:
Caution needed with: anaesthetics, antidepressants, ANTIHYPERTENSIVES, ß-BLOCKERS, breathing stimulants, other SYMPATHOMIMETICS.
Contains: ADRENALINE.
Other preparations: Adrenaline Injection, MEDIHALER-EPI (3M Healthcare).

Minilyn — oral contraceptive. Product now discontinued.

Minocin 50
(Lederle)

A beige tablet supplied at a strength of 50 mg and used as an antibiotic treatment for acne.

Dose: 1 tablet twice a day for at least 6 weeks.
Availability: NHS and private prescription.
Side effects: stomach disturbances, allergies, ear disorder, additional infections.
Caution: in patients suffering from liver disease.
Not to be used for: children, nursing mothers, women in the last half of pregnancy, or for patients suffering from kidney failure.
Caution needed with: ANTACIDS, mineral supplements.
Contains: MINOCYCLINE hydrochloride.
Other preparations: MINOCIN MR.

M

Minocin *see* **Tetracycline**

---

minocycline *see* **Minocin, Minocin 50**

412

Minodiab
(Farmitalia CE)

A white tablet supplied at strengths of 2.5 mg, 5 mg and used as an antidiabetic treatment for diabetes.

Dose: 2.5-5 mg a day in divided doses at first titrating by 2.5 or 5 mg a day every 7 days, then usually 2.5-30 mg a day to a maximum of 40 mg a day, taken in divided doses 15-20 minutes before food.
Availability: NHS and private prescription.
Side effects: allergy, including skin rash.
Caution: in the elderly and in patients suffering from kidney failure.
Not to be used for: children, pregnant women, nursing mothers, during surgery, or for patients suffering from juvenile diabetes, liver or kidney disorders, stress, infections.
Caution needed with: ß-BLOCKERS, MAOIS, STEROIDS, DIURETICS, alcohol, anticoagulants, lipid-lowering agents, ASPIRIN, some antibiotics (RIFAMPICIN, sulphonamides, CHLORAMPHENICOL), GLUCAGON, CYCLOPHOSPHAMIDE, the contraceptive pill.
Contains: GLIPIZIDE.
Other preparations: GLIBENESE (Pfizer).

---

minoxidil *see* Loniten, Regaine

Mintec
(Innovex)

A green/ivory capsule used as an anti-spasm treatment for irritable bowel syndrome, spastic colon.

Dose: adults 1-2 tablets 3 times a day before meals.
Availability: NHS, over the counter, private prescription.
Side effects:
Caution:
Not to be used for: children.
Caution needed with:
Contains: PEPPERMINT OIL.
Other preparations: COLPERMIN (Farmitalia CE).

Mintezol
(MSD)

An orange, scored, chewable tablet supplied at a strength of 500 mg and used to treat worms and other associated conditions and infections.

Dose: under 60 kg body weight 25 mg per kg twice a day with food; over 60 kg body weight 1.5 g twice a day with food.
Availability: NHS and private prescription.
Side effects: reduced alertness, stomach and brain disturbances, allergy, liver damage, changes to sight and hearing, low blood pressure, bed wetting.
Caution: in patients suffering from liver or kidney disease.
Not to be used for: pregnant women or nursing mothers.
Caution needed with: xanthine derivatives (such as THEOPHYLLINE).
Contains: THIABENDAZOLE.
Other preparations:

Minulet
(Wyeth)

A white tablet used as an oestrogen, progestogen contraceptive.

Dose: 1 tablet a day for 21 days starting on day 1 of the period.
Availability: NHS and private prescription.
Side effects: enlarged breasts, bloating and fluid retention, cramps, leg pains, mood change, reduction in sexual desire, headaches, nausea, vaginal erosion, discharge, and bleeding, weight gain, skin changes.
Caution: in patients suffering from high blood pressure, diabetes, vascular disorders, asthma, depression, kidney disease, multiple sclerosis, womb diseases. Your doctor may advise you not to smoke, to have regular examinations. You should stop treatment at the first sign of serious symptoms such as severe headache or jaundice. Treatment should be stopped before surgery.
Not to be used for: pregnant women, or for patients suffering from sickle-cell anaemia, history of heart disease or thrombosis, liver disorders, some cancers, undiagnosed vaginal bleeding, some ear, skin, and kidney disorders.
Caution needed with: RIFAMPICIN, TETRACYCLINES, GRISEOFULVIN, BARBITURATES, PHENYTOIN, PRIMIDONE, CARBAMAZEPINE, ETHOSUXIMIDE, CHLORAL HYDRATE, DICHLORALPHENAZONE.
Contains: ETHINYLOESTRADIOL, GESTODENE.
Other preparations: FEMODENE (Schering).

M

Miraxid
(Fisons)

A white tablet used as a penicillin treatment for respiratory, ear, and urinary infections.

Dose: 2-4 tablets twice a day with food or drink. (Reduced doses for children.)
Availability: NHS and private prescription.
Side effects: allergy, stomach disturbances.
Caution: in patients suffering from lymphatic leukaemia. Your doctor may advise regular liver and kidney checks.
Not to be used for: patients suffering from glandular fever or penicillin allergy.
Caution needed with:
Contains: PIVAMPICILLIN, PIVMECILLINAM HYDROCHLORIDE.
Other preparations: Miraxid Paediatric Syrup, Miraxid 450.

---

misoprostol *see* **Cytotec, Napratec**

Mixtard *see* **insulin**
(Novo Nordisk)

Mobiflex
(Roche)

A brown, five-sided tablet supplied at a strength of 20 mg and used as a NON-STEROID ANTI-INFLAMMATORY DRUG to treat osteoarthritis, rheumatoid arthritis.

Dose: 1 tablet a day.
Availability: NHS and private prescription.
Side effects: stomach disturbances, swelling, headache, rash, blood changes, liver changes, disturbances of the eyesight.
Caution: in the elderly or in patients suffering from liver or kidney disease, heart failure.
Not to be used for: children, pregnant women, patients with a history of or suffering from stomach ulcer, gastro-intestinal bleeding, gastritis, allergy to ASPIRIN or anti-inflammatory drugs.
Caution needed with: anticoagulants, antidiabetics taken by mouth, other NON-STEROID ANTI-INFLAMMATORY DRUGS, LITHIUM.
Contains: TENOXICAM.
Other preparations:

M

Modalim
(Sanofi Winthrop)

A white, capsule-shaped tablet supplied at a strength of 100 mg and used to treat high blood lipid levels which cannot be controlled by diet alone.

Dose: 1-2 tablets a day as a single dose.
Availability: NHS and private prescription.
Side effects: headache, vertigo, rash, stomach upset, muscle pain, impotence, hair loss, dizziness, drowsiness.
Caution: in patients suffering from liver or kidney disease.
Not to be used for: children, pregnant women, nursing mothers, or for patients suffering from severe liver or kidney disease.
Caution needed with: anticoagulants, antidiabetics, the contraceptive pill.
Contains: CIPROFIBRATE.
Other preparations:

Moditen
(Squibb)

A pink tablet, yellow tablet, or white tablet according to strengths of 1 mg, 2.5 mg, 5 mg and used as a sedative to treat schizophrenia, behavioural problems, anxiety, tension, senile disorders.

Dose: adults 1-2 mg a day at first up to 2-4 mg a day if needed (Maximum 20 mg a day); senile elderly use lower doses.
Availability: NHS and private prescription.
Side effects: muscle spasms, restlessness, constipation, blurred vision, hands shaking, dry mouth, urine retention, palpitations, low blood pressure, weight gain, changes in libido, low body temperature, breast swelling, menstrual changes, jaundice, blood and skin changes, drowsiness, rarely fits.
Caution: in the elderly, pregnant women, nursing mothers, and in patients suffering from tremor or rigidity, liver, lung, or heart disorder, thyroid disorder, epilepsy, glaucoma, myaesthenia gravis, or enlarged prostate.
Not to be used for: children or for patients suffering from phaeochromocytoma, kidney or liver failure, poor brain circulation, severe heart weakness, severe depression or coma.
Caution needed with: alcohol, tranquillizers, pain killers, ANTIHYPERTENSIVES, antidepressants, anticonvulsants, antidiabetic drugs, LEVODOPA.
Contains: FLUPHENAZINE hydrochloride.
Other preparations:

M

Modrasone
(Schering Plough)

A cream used as a STEROID treatment for skin disorders.

Dose: apply to the affected area 2-3 times a day.
Availability: NHS and private prescription.
Side effects: fluid retention, suppression of adrenal glands, thinning of the skin may occur.
Caution: use for short periods of time only.
Not to be used for: patients suffering from acne or any other skin infections caused by tuberculosis, ringworm, viruses, or fungi, or continuously especially in pregnant women.
Caution needed with:
Contains: ALCLOMETASONE DIPROPRIONATE.
Other preparations: Modrasone Ointment.

Modrenal
(Fusillon)

Capsules supplied at strengths of 60 mg, 120 mg and used as an adrenal inhibitor and hormone blocker.

Dose: 60 mg 4 times a day for the first 3 days, then adjust as needed up to a maximum of 960 mg a day.
Availability: NHS and private prescription.
Side effects: flushing, nausea, running nose, diarrhoea.
Caution: in patients suffering from kidney or liver disease, stress. Your doctor may wish to ensure there is no tumour of the adrenal glands.
Not to be used for: children, pregnant women, or for patients suffering from severe kidney or liver disease.
Caution needed with: ALDOSTERONE antagonists (another hormone blocker), AMILORIDE, TRIAMTERENE.
Contains: TRILOSTANE.
Other preparations:

Moducren
(Morson)

A blue, scored, square tablet used as a ß-BLOCKER/DIURETIC/ potassium-sparing DIURETIC combination to treat high blood pressure.

Dose: 1-2 tablets a day.
Availability: NHS and private prescription.
Side effects: cold hands and feet, sleep disturbance, slow heart rate,

M

tiredness, wheezing, heart failure, stomach upset, rash, sensitivity to light, blood changes, gout, cramps, dry eyes.

Caution: in pregnant women, nursing mothers, and in patients suffering from diabetes, electrolyte changes, gout, kidney or liver disease.

Not to be used for: children, and for patients suffering from progressive or severe kidney failure, raised potassium levels, heart block or failure, asthma.

Caution needed with: potassium supplements, potassium-sparing DIURETICS, LITHIUM, DIGOXIN, ANTIHYPERTENSIVES, ACE INHIBITORS, VERAPAMIL, CLONIDINE withdrawal, some anti-arrhythmic drugs and anaesthetics, RESERPINE, ERGOTAMINE, CIMETIDINE, sedatives, SYMPATHOMIMETICS, INDOMETHACIN, antidiabetics.

Contains: HYDROCHLOROTHIAZIDE, AMILORIDE hydrochloride, TIMOLOL maleate.

Other preparations:

Moduret 25
(Du Pont)

A near-white, diamond-shaped tablet used as a potassium-sparing DIURETIC to treat high blood pressure.

Dose: 1-4 tablets a day in divided doses.

Availability: NHS and private prescription.

Side effects: rash, sensitivity to light, blood changes, gout.

Caution: in patients suffering from diabetes, electrolyte changes, gout, liver or kidney disease.

Not to be used for: children, pregnant women, nursing mothers, or for patients suffering from raised potassium levels, progressive or severe kidney failure.

Caution needed with: potassium supplements, potassium-sparing DIURETICS, DIGOXIN, LITHIUM, ANTIHYPERTENSIVES, ACE INHIBITORS.

Contains: AMILORIDE hydrochloride, HYDROCHLOROTHIAZIDE.

Other preparations: AMILCO (Baker Norton), CO-AMILOZIDE, MODURETIC (Du Pont).

Moduretic
(Du Pont)

A peach-coloured, diamond-shaped, scored tablet used as a potassium-sparing DIURETIC to treat high blood pressure, congestive heart failure, liver cirrhosis with fluid retention.

Dose: 1-2 tablets a day increasing to up to 4 tablets a day if needed.

Availability: NHS and private prescription.

M

Side effects: rash, sensitivity to light, blood changes, gout.
Caution: in patients suffering from diabetes, electrolyte changes, gout, kidney or liver damage
Not to be used for: children, pregnant women, nursing mothers, or for patients suffering from raised potassium levels, progressive or severe kidney failure.
Caution needed with: potassium supplements, potassium-sparing DIURETICS, DIGOXIN, LITHIUM, ANTIHYPERTENSIVES, ACE INHIBITORS.
Contains: AMILORIDE hydrochloride, HYDROCHLOROTHIAZIDE (CO-AMILOZIDE).
Other preparations: Moduretic Solution, AMILCO (Baker Norton), AMILMAXCO (Ashbourne), CO-AMILOZIDE, MODURET-25 (Du Pont).

Mogadon
(Roche)

A white, scored tablet supplied at a strength of 5 mg and used as a sleeping tablet for the short-term treatment of sleeplessness where sedation during the day does not cause difficulty.

Dose: elderly ½-1 tablet before going to bed; adults 1-2 tablets before going to bed.
Availability: NHS (when prescribed as a generic) and private prescription.
Side effects: drowsiness, confusion, unsteadiness, low blood pressure, rash, changes in vision, changes in libido, retention of urine. Risk of addiction increases with dose and length of treatment. May impair judgement.
Caution: in the elderly, pregnant women, nursing mothers, in women during labour, and in patients suffering from lung disorders, kidney or liver disorders. Avoid long-term use and withdraw gradually.
Not to be used for: children, or for patients suffering from acute lung diseases, some chronic lung diseases, some obsessional and psychotic diseases.
Caution needed with: alcohol, other tranquillizers, anticonvulsants.
Contains: NITRAZEPAM.
Other preparations: Mogadon Capsules (not available on NHS), nitrazepam tablets, REMNOS (DDSA), SOMNITE (Norgine), SUREM, UNISOMNIA.

Molcer
(Wallace)

Drops as a wax softener to soften ear wax.

Dose: fill ear with the drops and plug with cotton wool; leave for 2 nights and then clean out.

M

Availability: NHS, private prescription, over the counter.
Side effects:
Caution:
Not to be used for: patients suffering from perforated ear drum.
Caution needed with:
Contains: sodium DOCUSATE.
Other preparations: DIOCTYL EAR DROPS (Medo), WAXSOL (Norgine).

Molipaxin
(Roussel)

A pink, scored tablet supplied at a strength of 150 mg and used as a sedative to treat depression and anxiety.

Dose: adults 1 tablet a night at first or as divided doses daily after meals, then increase to 2 tablets a day after 1 week if needed, up to a maximum of 4 tablets a day; elderly ⅔ tablet at night at first or as divided doses daily after meals up to a maximum of 2 tablets a day.
Availability: NHS and private prescription.
Side effects: drowsiness, dizziness, headache, penile erection.
Caution: in patients suffering from epilepsy, severe kidney or liver disease.
Not to be used for: children.
Caution needed with: muscle relaxants, anaesthetics, alcohol, sedatives, MAOIS, CLONIDINE.
Contains: TRAZODONE hydrochloride.
Other preparations: Molipaxin Capsules, Molipaxin CR, Molipaxin Liquid.

Monistat *see* **Gyno-Daktarin.** Product now discontinued.

Monit
(Stuart)

A white, scored tablet supplied at a strength of 20 mg and used as a NITRATE for the prevention of angina.

Dose: 10 mg twice a day at first, then usually 20 mg 2-3 times a day.
Availability: NHS, private prescription, over the counter.
Side effects: headache, flushes, dizziness.
Caution:
Not to be used for: children.
Caution needed with:
Contains: ISOSORBIDE MONONITRATE.

M

Other preparations: Monit LS, Monit SR, ELANTAN (Schwarz), IMDUR (Astra), ISIB (Ashbourne), ISMO (Boehringer Mannheim), MCR-50 (Farmitalia), MONO-CEDOCARD (Farmitalia).

Mono-Cedocard
(Farmitalia)

An orange, scored tablet or a white, scored tablet according to strengths of 10 mg, 20 mg, 40 mg and used as a NITRATE for the prevention of angina.

Dose: 20-120 mg a day in divided doses.
Availability: NHS, private prescription, over the counter.
Side effects: headache, flushes, dizziness.
Caution:
Not to be used for: children.
Caution needed with:
Contains: ISOSORBIDE MONONITRATE.
Other preparations: ELANTAN (Schwarz), IMDUR (Astra), ISIB (Ashbourne), ISMO (Boehringer Mannheim), MCR-50 (Farmitalia), MONIT (Stuart).

Monocor
(Lederle)

A pink tablet or a white tablet according to strengths of 5 mg, 10 mg and used as a ß-BLOCKER to treat angina, high blood pressure.

Dose: 10 mg once a day to a maximum of 20 mg a day.
Availability: NHS and private prescription.
Side effects: cold hands and feet, sleep disturbance, slow heart rate, tiredness, wheezing, heart failure, stomach upset, dry eyes, rash.
Caution: in pregnant women, nursing mothers, and in patients suffering from diabetes, kidney or liver disorders, asthma. May need to be withdrawn before surgery. Withdraw gradually. Your doctor may advise additional treatment with DIURETICS or DIGOXIN.
Not to be used for: children or for patients suffering from heart block or failure..
Caution needed with: VERAPAMIL, CLONIDINE withdrawal, some anti-arrhythmic drugs and anaesthetics, RESERPINE, some ANTIHYPERTENSIVES, ERGOTAMINE, CIMETIDINE, sedatives, antidiabetics, SYMPATHOMIMETICS, INDOMETHACIN.
Contains: BISOPROLOL fumarate.
Other preparations: EMCOR (Merck).

M

monosulfiram *see* **Tetmosol**

Monotard *see* **insulin**
(Novo Nordisk)

Monotrim
(Duphar)

A white, scored tablet supplied at strengths of 100 mg, 200 mg and used as an antibiotic to treat infections, urine infections.

Dose: adults 200 mg twice a day, children 6 weeks-5 months 25 mg twice a day, 6 months-5 years 50 mg twice a day, 6-12 years 100 mg twice a day.
Availability: NHS and private prescription.
Side effects: stomach disturbances, skin reactions.
Caution: in the elderly and in patients suffering from kidney disease from folate deficiency (vitamin deficiency). Your doctor may advise regular blood tests.
Not to be used for: infants under 6 weeks, pregnant women, or for patients suffering from severe kidney disease where regular blood tests cannot be made.
Caution needed with:
Contains: TRIMETHOPRIM.
Other preparations: Monotrim Suspension, Monotrim Injection, IPRAL (Squibb), TIEMPE (DDSA), TRIMOGAL (Lagap), TRIMOPAN (Berk).

Monovent
(Lagap)

A syrup used as a broncho-dilator to treat bronchial spasm brought on by asthma, bronchitis, or emphysema.

Dose: adults 10-15 mg twice a day or every 8 hours; children reduced doses.
Availability: NHS and private prescription.
Side effects: shaking of the hands, dilation of the blood vessels, tension, headache.
Caution: in pregnant women and in diabetics, or in patients suffering from high blood pressure, abnormal heart rhythms, heart muscle disorders, overactive thyroid gland, angina.
Not to be used for:
Caution needed with: SYMPATHOMIMETICS.

M

Contains: TERBUTALINE sulphate.
Other preparations: BRICANYL (Astra). (Monovent/Monovent SA tablets —
now discontinued.)

Monphytol
(LAB)

A paint used as an anti-fungal treatment for athlete's foot.

Dose: paint on to the affected area twice a day at first then once a week.
Availability: NHS, private prescription, over the counter.
Side effects:
Caution:
Not to be used for: children or pregnant women.
Caution needed with:
Contains: CHLORBUTOL, METHYL UNDECOANATE, SALICYLIC ACID, METHYL SALICYLATE,
PROPYL SALICYLATE, PROPYL UNDECOANATE.
Other preparations:

---

morphine *see* MST Continus, Nepenthe, Oramorph

Motilium
(Sanofi Winthrop)

A white tablet supplied at a strength of 10 mg and used as an anti-emetic
drug to treat acute nausea and vomiting.

Dose: adults 10-20 mg every 4-8 hours; children use in rare situations in
reduced doses.
Availability: NHS and private prescription.
Side effects: blood changes.
Caution:
Not to be used for: pregnant women.
Caution needed with:
Contains: DOMPERIDONE.
Other preparations: Motilium Suspension, Motilium Suppositories.

Motipress
(Squibb)

A yellow, triangular tablet used as a sedative to treat anxiety/depression.

M

Dose: 1 tablet a day at bedtime for up to 3 months.
Availability: NHS and private prescription.
Side effects: muscle spasms, restlessness, sleeplessness, dizziness, hands shaking, dry mouth, constipation, blurred vision, urine retention, palpitations, low blood pressure, weight change, changes in libido, low body temperature, breast swelling, menstrual changes, jaundice, blood and skin changes, drowsiness, rarely fits.
Caution: in patients with a history of epilepsy or brain damage, nursing mothers, and in patients suffering from heart disease, glaucoma, adrenal tumour, urinary retention, thyroid disease, epilepsy, diabetes, some other psychiatric conditions. Your doctor may advise regular blood and liver tests.
Not to be used for: children, pregnant women or for patients suffering from Parkinson's disease, heart attacks, liver disease, heart block.
Caution needed with: alcohol, ANTICHOLINERGICS, ADRENALINE, MAOIS, BARBITU-RATES tranquillizers, pain killers, ANTIHYPERTENSIVES, antidepressants, anticonvulsants, antidiabetic drugs, LEVODOPA, CIMETIDINE, oestrogen.
Contains: FLUPHENAZINE hydrochloride, NORTRIPTYLINE
Other preparations: MOTIVAL (Squibb).

Motival
(Squibb)

A triangular, pink tablet used as a sedative to treat anxiety/depression

Dose: 1 tablet 2-3 times a day for up to 3 months.
Availability: NHS and private prescription.
Side effects: muscle spasms, restlessness, sleeplessness, dizziness, hands shaking, dry mouth, constipation, blurred vision, urine retention, palpitations, low blood pressure, weight change, changes in libido, low body temperature, breast swelling, menstrual changes, jaundice, blood and skin changes, drowsiness, rarely fits.
Caution: in patients with a history of epilepsy or brain damage, nursing mothers, and in patients suffering from heart disease, urinary retention, adrenal tumour, glaucoma, thyroid disease, epilepsy, diabetes, some other psychiatric conditions. Your doctor may advise regular blood and liver tests.
Not to be used for: children, pregnant women or for patients suffering from Parkinson's disease, heart attacks, liver disease, heart block.
Caution needed with: alcohol, ANTICHOLINERGICS, ADRENALINE, MAOIS, BARBITU-RATES, CIMETIDINE, tranquillizers, pain killers, ANTIHYPERTENSIVES, antidepressants, anticonvulsants, antidiabetic drugs, LEVODOPA.
Contains: FLUPHENAZINE hydrochloride, NORTRIPTYLINE hydrochloride.
Other preparations: MOTIPRESS (Squibb).

M

Motrin *see* **Brufen**
(Upjohn)

Movelat
(Panpharma)

A cream and a gel used as an anti-inflammatory rub to relieve arthritis, fibrositis, soft tissue pain.

Dose: massage gently into the affected area up to 4 times a day.
Availability: NHS, private prescription, over the counter.
Side effects:
Caution:
Not to be used for:
Caution needed with:
Contains: SALICYLIC ACID, MUCOPOLYSACCHARIDE POLYSULPHATE.
Other preparations:

MST Continus
(Napp)

A brown tablet, light-green tablet, purple tablet, orange tablet, or grey tablet according to strengths of 10 mg, 15 mg, 30 mg, 60 mg, 100 mg, 200 mg and used as an opiate for the prolonged relief of severe pain.

Dose: 10-20 mg twice a day at first, then as advised by physician.
Availability: controlled drug; NHS and private prescription.
Side effects: tolerance, addiction, constipation, nausea, vomiting.
Caution: in the elderly and in patients suffering from kidney or liver disease and underactive thyroid.
Not to be used for: children, pregnant women, or patients suffering from respiratory depression or blocked airways, acute liver disease.
Caution needed with: MAOIS, sedatives, alcohol.
Contains: MORPHINE sulphate.
Other preparations: MST Continus Suspension, NEPENTHE (Evans), ORAMORPH (Boehringer Ingelheim), SEVREDOL (Napp), SRM-RHOTARD (Farmitalia CE).

Mucaine
(Wyeth)

A white liquid used as an ANTACID plus local anaesthetic to treat oesophagitis and hiatus hernia.

M

Dose: adults 5-10 ml 3-4 times a day before meals.
Availability: NHS and private prescription.
Side effects: occasional constipation.
Caution:
Not to be used for: children.
Caution needed with: TETRACYCLINE antibiotics.
Contains: OXETHAZAINE, ALUMINIUM HYDROXIDE, MAGNESIUM HYDROXIDE.
Other preparations:

Mucodyne
(Rorer)

A syrup supplied at a strength of 250 mg and used as a mucus softener to clear phlegm, running nose, glue ear in children.

Dose: adults 15 ml 3 times a day reducing to 10 ml; children over 2 years use paediatric syrup.
Availability: NHS (only if for a child with tracheostomy), private prescription.
Side effects: stomach disturbance, nausea, rash.
Caution: in pregnant women and in patients with a history of stomach ulcer.
Not to be used for: children under 2 years or for patients suffering from stomach ulcer.
Caution needed with:
Contains: CARBOCISTEINE.
Other preparations: Mucodyne Capsules, Mucodyne Paediatric.

Mucogel *see* Maalox
(Pharmax)

Multilind *see* Nystan Cream. Product now discontinued.

Multivite *see* Vitamins Capsules BPC. Product now discontinued.

M

mupirocin *see* Bactroban Nasal

Muripsin
(Norgine)

An oblong, orange tablet used as a source of hydrochloric acid/proteolytic enzyme to treat low stomach acid.

Dose: adults 1-2 with meals; children as advised.
Availability: NHS, private prescription, over the counter.
Side effects:
Caution:
Not to be used for:
Caution needed with:
Contains: GLUTAMIC ACID HYDROCHLORIDE, PEPSIN.
Other preparations:

Myambutol
(Lederle)

A yellow tablet or a grey tablet according to strengths of 100 mg, 400 mg and used as an anti-tubercular, additional treatment and preventive drug for tuberculosis.

Dose: adults 15 mg per kg body weight once a day; children treatment 25 mg per kg body weight once a day for 60 days, then 15 mg per kg body weight once a day; prevention 15 mg per kg body weight once a day.
Availability: NHS and private prescription.
Side effects: visual changes, eye inflammation.
Caution: in nursing mothers and in patients suffering from kidney disease. Eyes should be checked regularly.
Not to be used for: patients suffering from inflamation of the optic nerve.
Caution needed with:
Contains: ETHAMBUTOL.
Other preparations:

Mycardol
(Sanofi Winthrop)

A white, scored tablet supplied at a strength of 30 mg and used as a NITRATE in addition to glyceryl trintrate in the treatment of angina.

Dose: 2 tablets 3-4 times a day.
Availability: NHS, private prescription, over the counter.
Side effects: headache, flushes, dizziness, rapid heart rate, nausea, vomiting.
Caution: in pregnant women and in patients suffering from glaucoma.

M

427

Not to be used for: children or for patients suffering from coronary thrombosis, bleeding in the brain, anaemia.
Caution needed with:
Contains: PENTAERYTHRITOL TETRANITRATE.
Other preparations:

Mycifradin
(Upjohn)

A tablet supplied at a strength of 500 mg and used as an aminoglycoside antibiotic to treat skin and mucous membrane infections, and to sterilize the bowel before surgery.

Dose: as advised by the physician.
Availability: NHS and private prescription.
Side effects: hearing damage, sensitization.
Caution: in patients with large areas of affected skin, and in patients suffering from kidney failure.
Not to be used for:
Caution needed with:
Contains: NEOMYCIN sulphate.
Other preparations: NEOMYCIN ELIXIR, NIVEMYCIN (Boots).

Myciguent *see* **Neomycin.** Product now discontinued.

Mydriacyl
(Alcon)

Drops used as an ANTICHOLINERGIC pupil dilator.

Dose: 1-2 drops into the eye with 1-5 minutes between each drop, then a further drop into the eye after 30 minutes if needed.
Availability: NHS and private prescription.
Side effects: temporary smarting, dry mouth, blurred vision, aversion to light, rapid heart rate, headache, mental and behavioural changes, stinging.
Caution: in infants and in patients where the eye pressure is not known.
Not to be used for: patients suffering from narrow angle glaucoma or who wear soft contact lenses.
Caution needed with:
Contains: TROPICAMIDE.
Other preparations:

M

Mydrilate
(Boehringer Ingelheim)

Drops used as an ANTICHOLINERGIC pupil dilator

Dose: adults 1 drop into the eye; children reduced dose.
Availability: NHS and private prescription.
Side effects: systemic anticholinergic effects.
Caution: in patients suffering from inflamed eye.
Not to be used for: patients suffering from glaucoma.
Caution needed with:
Contains: CYCLOPENTOLATE HYDROCHLORIDE.
Other preparations: ALNIDE (Cusi).

Mygdalon *see* Maxolon
(DDSA)

Mynah
(Lederle)

A yellow tablet or orange tablet according to different strengths and used as an anti-tuberculous drug combination for the prevention and treatment of tuberculosis.

Dose: 15 mg per kg body weight of ETHAMBUTOL plus 300 mg ISONIAZID once a day.
Availability: NHS and private prescription.
Side effects: visual changes, eye inflammation, hepatitis, sleeplessness, restlessness, rheumatic disorders.
Caution: in nursing mothers, in patients with a history of epilepsy, or patients suffering kidney or liver disease, chronic alcoholism. Eyes should be tested regularly.
Not to be used for: children or or patients suffering from inflammation of the optic nerve.
Caution needed with: alcohol.
Contains: ETHAMBUTOL, ISONIAZID.
Other preparations:

Myotonine
(Glenwood)

A white tablet supplied at strengths of 10 mg, 25 mg and used as a cholinergic drug to treat bowel paralysis or partial paralysis, urinary

M

retention, reflux oesophagitis.

Dose: adults 10-25 mg 3-4 times a day; children in proportion to a 70 kg adult.
Availability: NHS and private prescription.
Side effects: nausea, vomiting, urination, abdominal cramps, blurred vision, sweating.
Caution:
Not to be used for: pregnant women or for patients suffering from asthma, overactive thyroid, urinary or gastro-intestinal blockage, marked vagotonia, slow heart rate, recent heart attacks, epilepsy, Parkinson's disease, low blood pressure.
Caution needed with:
Contains: BETHANECHOL CHLORIDE.
Other preparations:

Mysoline
(ICI)

A white, scored tablet supplied at a strength of 250 mg and used as an anticonvulsant to treat epilepsy

Dose: ½ a tablet at night at first, increasing every 3 days by ½ a tablet to 2 tablets a day, then increase by 1 tablet at a time to 6 tablets a day; children same as adults at first increasing by ½ tablet a day. Lower maximum doses for children.
Availability: NHS and private prescription.
Side effects: drowsiness, hangover, dizziness, allergies, headache, confusion, excitement, anaemia.
Caution: in patients suffering from kidney, liver, or lung disease. Dependence (addiction) may develop.
Not to be used for: children, young adults, pregnant women, nursing mothers, the elderly, patients with a history of drug or alcohol abuse, or suffering from porphyria (a rare blood disorder), or in the management of pain.
Caution needed with: anticoagulants (blood-thinning drugs), alcohol, other tranquillizers, STEROIDS, the contraceptive pill, GRISEOFULVIN, RIFAMPICIN, PHENYTOIN, METRONIDAZOLE, CHLORAMPHENICOL.
Contains: PRIMIDONE.
Other preparations: Mysoline Suspension.

M

Mysteclin *see* Tetracycline
(Squibb)

nabilone *see* **Cesamet**

---

nabumetone *see* **Relifex**

Nacton Forte
(Bencard)

An orange tablet supplied at a strength of 4 mg and used as an anti-spasm, ANTICHOLINERGIC treatment for spasm, acidity, ulcers.

Dose: 4 mg 3 times a day and at bedtime.
Availability: NHS and private prescription.
Side effects: blurred vision, confusion, dry mouth.
Caution: in patients suffering from rapid heart rate, glaucoma, or difficulty in passing urine.
Not to be used for: children.
Caution needed with:
Contains: POLDINE METHYLSULPHATE.
Other preparations: Nacton 2 mg.

---

nadolol *see* **Corgard, Corgaretic 40**

---

nafarelin *see* **Synarel**

---

naftidrofuryl oxalate *see* **Praxilene**

Nalcrom
(Fisons)

A clear capsule supplied at a strength of 100 mg and used as an anti-allergy drug to treat allergies to foods.

Dose: adults 2 capsules 4 times a day before meals; children over 2 years 1 capsule 4 times a day before meals.
Availability: NHS and private prescription.
Side effects: rash, pain in the joints, nausea.
Caution:
Not to be used for: infants under 2 years.

N

nalidixic acid *see* **Mictral, Negram**

Nalorex
(Du Pont)

A mottled, orange, scored tablet supplied at a strength of 50 mg and used as a narcotic antagonist as a treatment for patients who have been detoxified from opioid dependency.

Dose: ½ tablet a day at first, then 1 tablet a day for 3 months.
Availability: NHS and private prescription.
Side effects: vomiting, drowsiness, dizziness, stomach cramps, joint and muscle pain.
Caution: in patients suffering from liver or kidney disease.
Not to be used for: patients suffering from acute liver disease, liver failure, or current dependence on opiates.
Caution needed with:
Contains: NALTREXONE HYDROCHLORIDE.
Other preparations:

naltrexone hydrochloride *see* **Nalorex**

naphazoline hydrochloride *see* **Vasocon-A**

Napratec
(Searle)

Yellow, oblong, scored tablets and white, hexagonal scored tablets supplied together in one pack to treat rheumatoid arthritis, osteoarthritis, and ankylosing spondylitis where the stomach also needs protecting against the effects of the medication.

Dose: 1 of each tablet twice a day with food.
Availability: NHS and private prescription.
Side effects: stomach upset, diarrhoea, abdominal pain, vaginal bleeding, heavy periods, rash, itching, severe allergy, headache, dizziness, noise in

N

the ears, vertigo, blood changes.

Caution: in the elderly, and in patients suffering from asthma, liver or kidney damage, disorders affecting blood vessels. Women of child-bearing age must use effective contraception.

Not to be used for: children, pregnant women, nursing mothers, or for patients suffering from allergy to ASPIRIN or anti-inflammatory drugs, or stomach ulcer.

Caution needed with: anticoagulants, PHENYTOIN, some antidiabetics, sulphonamide antibiotics, DIURETICS, LITHIUM, ß-BLOCKERS, PROBENECID, METHOTREXATE.

Contains: NAPROXEN (yellow tablets), MISOPROSTOL (white tablets).
Other preparations:

Naprosyn
(Syntex)

A yellow, scored tablet or a yellow, oblong, scored tablet according to strengths of 250 mg, 500 mg and used as a non-steroid anti-inflammatory drug to treat rheumatoid arthritis, osteoarthritis, ankylosing spondylitis, acute gout.

Dose: adults 250-500 mg twice a day at first; for gout 750 mg at first then 250 mg every 8 hours. Children 5-16 years 10 mg per kg body weight a day in 2 divided doses.

Availability: NHS and private prescription.

Side effects: rash, stomach intolerance, headache, tinnitus, vertigo, blood changes.

Caution: in the elderly, pregnant women, nursing mothers, and in patients suffering from kidney or liver disease, heart failure, asthma, or a history of gastro-intestinal lesions.

Not to be used for: children under 5 years, or for patients suffering from stomach ulcer or allergy to aspirin or NON-STEROID ANTI-INFLAMMATORY DRUGS.

Caution needed with: anticoagulants, hydantoins, some antidiabetics, LITHIUM, ß-BLOCKERS, METHOTREXATE, PROBENECID, FRUSEMIDE.

Contains: NAPROXEN.

Other preparations: Naprosyn Suspension, Naprosyn EC Tablets, Naprosyn Granules, Naprosyn Suppositories, ARTHROSIN (Ashbourne), ARTHROXEN (CP Pharm), LARAFLEX (Lagap), NAPRATEC (Searle), NYCOPREN (Lundbeck), PRANOXEN (Napp), PROSAID (BHR), RHEUFLEX (Goldcrest), RIMOXYN (Rima), SYNFLEX (Syntex), VALROX (Shire).

---

naproxen *see* **Napratec, Naprosyn, Synflex**

N

Nardil
(Warner)

An orange tablet supplied at a strength of 15 mg and used as an MAOI to treat depression, phobias.

Dose: 1 tablet 3 times a day at first reducing gradually according to response.
Availability: NHS and private prescription.
Side effects: severe high blood pressure reactions with certain foods, sleeplessness, low blood pressure, dizziness, drowsiness, weakness, dry mouth, constipation, stomach upset, blurred vision, urinary difficulties, ankle swelling, rash, jaundice, weight gain, confusion, sexual desire changes.
Caution: in the elderly and in patients suffering from epilepsy.
Not to be used for: children, or for patients suffering from liver disease, blood changes, heart disease, phaeochromocytoma, overactive thyroid, brain artery disease.
Caution needed with: amphetamines or similar SYMPATHOMIMETIC drugs, TRICYCLIC antidepressants, PETHIDINE and other similar ANALGESICS, some cough mixtures and appetite supressants containing SYMPATHOMIMETICS. BARBITURATES, sedatives, alcohol, and antidiabetics may be enhanced. ANTICHOLINERGIC side effects are increased. Cheese, Bovril, Oxo, meat extracts, broad beans, banana, Marmite, yeast extracts, wine, beer, other alcohol, pickled herrings, vegetable proteins. (Up to 14 days after cessation.)
Contains: PHENELZINE SULPHATE.
Other preparations:

Narphen
(Napp)

A white, scored tablet supplied at a strength of 5 mg and used as an opiate to control severe, prolonged pain including biliary and pancreatic pain.

Dose: 1 tablet every 4-6 hours either swallowed or under the tongue. No single dose should exceed 4 tablets.
Availability: controlled drug; NHS and private prescription.
Side effects: tolerance, addiction, nausea, dizziness, constipation.
Caution: in the elderly, pregnant women, women in labour, or patients suffering from underactive thyroid, or liver or kidney disease.
Not to be used for: children or for patients in coma, or suffering from breathing difficulty, blocked airways, acute alcoholism, epilepsy.
Caution needed with: MAOIS, sedatives, alcohol.

N

434

Contains: PHENAZOCINE HYDROBROMIDE.
Other preparations:

Naseptin
(ICI)

A cream used as an antibacterial treatment for infections of the nose.

Dose: apply into each nostril 2-4 times a day.
Availability: NHS and private prescription.
Side effects: sensitive skin.
Caution: avoid prolonged use.
Not to be used for:
Caution needed with:
Contains: CHLORHEXIDINE HYDROCHLORIDE, NEOMYCIN sulphate.
Other preparations:

---

natamycin *see* **Pimafucin, Pimafucin 2½%, Pimafucin Cream**

Natrilix
(Servier)

A pink tablet supplied at a strength of 2.5 mg and used as a vasorelaxant to treat high blood pressure.

Dose: 1 tablet in the morning.
Availability: NHS and private prescription.
Side effects: low potassium level, nausea, headache.
Caution: in pregnant women and in patients suffering from severe kidney or liver disease.
Not to be used for: children, nursing mothers, or for patients suffering from severe liver failure or who have recently suffered a stroke.
Caution needed with: DIURETICS, anti-arrhythmics, DIGOXIN, STEROIDS, laxatives, LITHIUM.
Contains: INDAPAMIDE HEMIHYDRATE.
Other preparations:

Navidrex
(Ciba)

A white, scored tablet supplied at a strength of 0.5 mg and used as a DIURETIC to treat heart failure, fluid retention, high blood pressure.

N

Dose: adults ½-2 tablets a day, up to 3 tablets a day if needed; children as advised by physician.
Availability: NHS and private prescription.
Side effects: rash, sensitivity to light, blood changes, stomach upset, pancreatitis, headache, dizziness, tingling sensation, electrolyte and metabolic disturbances, lung and liver changes.
Caution: the elderly, and in patients suffering from diabetes, kidney or liver disease, gout, high blood lipid levels. Potassium supplements may be needed.
Not to be used for: pregnant women, nursing mothers, or for patients suffering from inability to produce urine or severe kidney failure, low sodium or potassium levels, Addison's disease, high calcium or uric acid levels.
Caution needed with: DIGOXIN, LITHIUM, ANTIHYPERTENSIVES, NON-STEROID ANTI-INFLAMMATORY DRUGS.
Contains: CYCLOPENTHIAZIDE.
Other preparations:

Navidrex-K — DIURETIC with potassium supplement. Product now discontinued.

Navispare
(Ciba)

A yellow tablet used as a DIURETIC to treat high blood pressure.

Dose: 1-2 tablets once a day in the morning.
Availability: NHS and private prescription.
Side effects: rash, sensitivity to light, blood changes, gout, tiredness, stomach upset.
Caution: in pregnant women, nursing mothers, and in patients suffering from diabetes, liver or kidney damage, gout, high acidity in the blood, high blood lipid levels.
Not to be used for: children, or for patients suffering from severe kidney or liver failure, high potassium levels, Addison's disease, diabetic kidney disorders, persistent low potassium or sodium levels or high calcium levels.
Caution needed with: DIGOXIN, LITHIUM, some other DIURETICS, ACE-INHIBITORS, potassium supplements.
Contains: CYCLOPENTHIAZIDE, AMILORIDE.
Other preparations:

N

Naxogin 500 — antiprotozoal tablet. Product now discontinued.

---

nefopam hydrochloride *see* **Acupan**

Negram
(Sanofi Winthrop)

A pale-brown tablet supplied at a strength of 500 mg and used as an antiseptic to treat urinary and stomach infections.

Dose: adults acute infections 2 tablets 4 times a day for at least 7 days, chronic infections 1 tablet 4 times a day; children 3 months-12 years up to 50 mg per kg body weight a day.
Availability: NHS and private prescription.
Side effects: stomach upset, disturbed vision, rash, blood changes, seizures, sensitivity to light.
Caution: in pregnant women, nursing mothers and in patients suffering from liver or kidney disease. Keep out of the sunlight.
Not to be used for: infants under 3 months or for patients with a history of convulsions, porphyria (a rare blood disorder).
Caution needed with: anticoagulants, PROBENECID, antibacterials.
Contains: NALIDIXIC ACID.
Other preparations: Negram Suspension, URIBEN (RP Drugs).

Neo-Cortef
(Upjohn)

Drops used as an antibiotic, STEROID, and aminoglycoside antibiotic treatment for inflammation of the outer ear or infected inflammation of the eye.

Dose: 1-2 drops into the eye up to 6 times a day or 2-3 drops into the ear 3-4 times a day.
Availability: NHS and private prescription.
Side effects: additional infection, sensitization, fungal infection, thinning cornea, cataract, rise in eye pressure.
Caution: in pregnant women and infants — avoid using over extended periods.
Not to be used for: patients suffering from perforated ear drum, or viral, tubercular, fungal, or acute weeping infections, glaucoma.
Caution needed with:
Contains: NEOMYCIN sulphate, HYDROCORTISONE acetate.
Other preparations: Neo-Cortef Ointment.

N

Neo-Medrone Cream
(Upjohn)

A cream used as an antibacterial, STEROID treatment for allergic and other skin disorders where there is also inflammation and infection.

Dose: apply to the affected area 1-3 times a day.
Availability: NHS and private prescription.
Side effects: fluid retention, suppression of adrenal glands, thinning of the skin may occur.
Caution: use for short periods of time only.
Not to be used for: patients suffering from acne or any other skin infections caused by tuberculosis, ringworm, viruses, or fungi, or continuously especially in pregnant women.
Caution needed with:
Contains: METHYLPREDNISOLONE acetate, NEOMYCIN sulphate.
Other preparations:

Neo-Medrone Lotion — STEROID/antibacterial treatment for acne/dermatitis. Product now discontinued.

Neo-Mercazole
(Nicholas)

A pink tablet supplied at strengths of 5 mg, 20 mg and used as an antithyroid treatment for thyrotoxicosis.

Dose: adults 20-60 mg a day at first in 2-3 divided doses, then 5-15 mg a day for 6-18 months, or continue with 20-60 mg a day with thyroxine; children 5-15 mg a day at first in divided doses.
Availability: NHS and private prescription.
Side effects: rash, headache, nausea, joint pain, bone marrow depression; inform the physician of sore throat, mouth ulcer.
Caution: in pregnant women. Your doctor may advise regular blood tests.
Not to be used for: nursing mothers or patients with a blocked trachea.
Caution needed with:
Contains: CARBIMAZOLE.
Other preparations:

Neo-Naclex
(Evans)

A white, scored tablet supplied at a strength of 5 mg and used as a

N

diuretic to treat fluid retention, high blood pressure, congestive heart failure, nephrotic syndrome (a kidney disease).

Dose: adults fluid retention 1-2 tablets once a day at first then ½-1 tablet from time to time, high blood pressure ½-2 tablets a day; children fluid retention in proportion to the dose for a 70 kg adult.
Availability: NHS and private prescription.
Side effects: low potassium levels, rash, sensitivity to light, blood changes, gout, impotence.
Caution: in pregnant women, nursing mothers, and in patients suffering from diabetes, kidney or liver disease, gout. Potassium supplements may be needed.
Not to be used for: patients suffering from severe kidney failure, raised calcium levels.
Caution needed with: DIGOXIN, LITHIUM, ANTIHYPERTENSIVES.
Contains: BENDROFLUAZIDE.
Other preparations: APRINOX (Boots), BENDROFLUAZIDE TABLETS, BERKOZIDE (Berk), CENTYL (Leo).

Neo-Naclex-K
(Goldcrest)

A double-layered pink/white tablet used as a DIURETIC with potassium supplement to treat high blood pressure, chronic fluid retention.

Dose: adults high blood pressure 1-4 tablets a day, fluid retention 2 tablets a day increasing to 4 tablets a day if needed then 1-2 tablets from time to time. Children, fluid retention proportion to dose for 70 kg adult.
Availability: NHS and private prescription.
Side effects: rash, sensitivity to light, blood changes, gout, impotence.
Caution: in pregnant women, nursing mothers, and in patients suffering from diabetes, liver or kidney disease, gout.
Not to be used for: patients suffering from severe kidney failure, raised calcium or potassium levels, Addison's disease.
Caution needed with: DIGOXIN, LITHIUM, potassium-sparing DIURETICS, ANTIHYPERTENSIVES, some antidiabetic drugs.
Contains: BENDROFLUAZIDE, POTASSIUM CHLORIDE.
Other preparations: CENTYL-K (Leo).

Neocon 1/35
(Cilag)

A peach-coloured tablet used as an oestrogen, progestogen contraceptive.

N

Dose: 1 tablet a day for 21 days starting on day 5 of the period.
Availability: NHS and private prescription.
Side effects: enlarged breasts, bloating and fluid retention, cramps, leg pains, mood change, reduction in sexual desire, headaches, nausea, vaginal erosion, discharge, and bleeding, weight gain, skin changes.
Caution: in patients suffering from high blood pressure, diabetes, vascular disorders, asthma, depression, kidney disease, multiple sclerosis, womb diseases. Your doctor may advise you not to smoke, to have regular examinations. You should stop treatment at the first sign of serious symptoms such as severe headache or jaundice. Treatment should be stopped before surgery.
Not to be used for: pregnant women, or for patients suffering from sickle-cell anaemia, history of heart disease or thrombosis, liver disorders, some cancers, undiagnosed vaginal bleeding, some ear, skin, and kidney disorders.
Caution needed with: RIFAMPICIN, TETRACYCLINES, GRISEOFULVIN, BARBITURATES, PHENYTOIN, PRIMIDONE, CARBAMAZEPINE, ETHOSUXIMIDE, CHLORAL HYDRATE, DICHLORALPHENAZONE.
Contains: ETHINYLOESTRADIOL, NORETHISTERONE.
Other preparations: NORIMIN (Syntex).

Neogest
(Schering)

A brown tablet used as a progesterone contraceptive.

Dose: 1 tablet at the same time every day starting on day 1 of the period.
Availability: NHS and private prescription.
Side effects: irregular bleeding, breast discomfort, acne, headache.
Caution: in patients suffering from high blood pressure, tendency to thrombosis, migraine, liver abnormalities, ovarian cysts. Your doctor may advise regular check-ups.
Not to be used for: pregnant women, or for patients suffering from severe heart or artery disease, benign liver tumours, vaginal bleeding, previous ectopic pregnancy.
Caution needed with: BARBITURATES, PHENYTOIN, PRIMIDONE, CARBAMAZEPINE, CHLORAL HYDRATE, DICHLORALPHENAZONE, ETHOSUXIMIDE, RIFAMPICIN, GLUTETHIMIDE, CHLORPROMAZINE, MEPROBAMATE, GRISEOFULVIN.
Contains: NORGESTREL.
Other preparations:

---

neomycin eye drops

Drops used as an aminoglycoside antibiotic to treat bacterial infections of the eye.

Dose: adults 1 or more drops into the eye as needed; children 1 drop into the eye as needed.
Availability: NHS and private prescription.
Side effects:
Caution:
Not to be used for:
Caution needed with:
Contains: NEOMYCIN sulphate.
Other preparations: MYCIGUENT (Upjohn), Neomycin Minims (SNP).

---

neomycin *see* **Audicort, Betnovate-N, Cicatrin, Dexa-Rhinaspray, Eumovate-N, Gregoderm, Graneodin, Hydroderm, Maxitrol, Mycifradin, Myciguent, Naseptin, Neo-Cortef, Neo-Medrone Cream, Neo-Medrone Lotion, neomycin cream BPC, neomycin eye drops, Neosporin, Nivemycin, Otomize, Otosporin, Polybactrin, Tri-Adcortyl, Tri-Adcortyl Otic, Tricicatrin, Tribiotic, Uniroid, Vibrocil**

---

neomycin cream BPC

A cream used as an antibacterial preparation to treat skin infection.

Dose: apply up to 3 times a day, up to a maximum of 60 g a day for 3 weeks. Do not repeat within 3 months.
Availability: NHS and private private prescription.
Side effects: allergy.
Caution: with large open wounds, and in patients allergic to other similar antibiotics.
Not to be used for:
Caution needed with:
Contains: neomycin cream BPC.
Other preparations:

Neophryn — SYMPATHOMIMETIC nasal spray/drops to clear nasal congestion. Product now discontinued.

Neosporin
(Cusi)

Drops used as a peptide and aminoglycoside antibiotic to treat eye infections, prevention of eye infections before and after eye operations, removal of foreign bodies from the eye.

Dose: 1-2 drops 2-4 times a day or more often if needed.
Availability: NHS and private prescription.
Side effects:
Caution: in patients suffering from existing eye defect.
Not to be used for:
Caution needed with:
Contains: POLYMYXIN B SULPHATE, NEOMYCIN sulphate, GRAMICIDIN.
Other preparations:

---

neostigmine *see* Prostigimin

Neotigason
(Roche)

A brown/white capsule or brown/yellow capsule according to strengths of 10 mg, 25 mg, and used to treat severe extensive psoriasis.

Dose: initially 25-30 mg once a day, increasing to a maximum of 75 mg a day if needed.
Availability: NHS and private prescription.
Side effects: dryness, erosion of mucous membranes, hair loss, liver disorder, blood changes, nausea, headache, drowsiness, sweating, loss of appetite, mood changes, thickening of bones.
Caution: women of child-bearing age must use effective contraception during treatment and for 2 years afterwards. Blood must not be donated during treatment or for 1 year afterwards. Your doctor may advise regular tests and examinations.
Not to be used for: children, pregnant women, or for patients suffering from kidney or liver damage.
Caution needed with: high doses of VITAMIN A, METHOTREXATE.
Contains: ACITRETIN.
Other preparations:

Nepenthe
(Evans)

An opiate solution used as an additional treatment for the relief of severe pain.

N

Dose: adults 1-2 ml not more often than every 4 hours; children 1-5 years 0.25-0.5 ml, 6-12 years 0.5-1 ml not more often than every 4 hours.
Availability: controlled drug; NHS and private prescription.
Side effects: tolerance, addiction, nausea, vomiting, constipation.
Caution: in the elderly,pregnant women, women in labour, and in patients suffering from liver disease or underactive thyroid. The solution should be stored in a tightly sealed container in a cool place.
Not to be used for: children under 1 year, or for patients suffering from respiratory depression or blocked airways.
Caution needed with: other opiates, MAOIS, sedatives, alcohol.
Contains: anhydrous MORPHINE in solution.
Other preparations: Nepenthe Injection (now discontinued).

Nephril
(Pfizer)

A white, scored tablet supplied at a strength of 1 mg and used as a DIURETIC to treat fluid retention, high blood pressure.

Dose: ½-4 tablets a day.
Availability: NHS and private prescription.
Side effects: low potassium levels, rash, sensitivity to light, blood changes, gout, tiredness.
Caution: in pregnant women, nursing mothers, and in patients suffering from diabetes, liver or kidney disease, gout. Potassium supplement may be needed.
Not to be used for: children or patients suffering from kidney failure.
Caution needed with: DIGOXIN, LITHIUM, ANTIHYPERTENSIVES.
Contains: POLYTHIAZIDE.
Other preparations:

Nericur
(Schering)

A gel used as an anti-bacterial, skin softener to treat acne.

Dose: wash and dry the affected area, then apply the gel once a day.
Availability: NHS, private prescription, over the counter.
Side effects: irritation, peeling.
Caution: keep out of the eyes, nose, mouth. May bleach fabrics.
Not to be used for: children.
Caution needed with:
Contains: BENZOYL PEROXIDE.
Other preparations: ACETOXYL (Stiefel), ACNECIDE (Galderma), ACNEGEL

N

(Stiefel), BENOXYL (Stiefel), BENZAGEL (Bioglan), PANOXYL (Stiefel), QUINODERM (Quinoderm).

Nerisone
(Schering)

A cream used as a STEROID treatment for skin disorders.

Dose: apply to the affected area 2-3 times a day reducing to once a day as soon as possible.
Availability: NHS and private prescription.
Side effects: fluid retention, suppression of adrenal glands, thinning of the skin may occur.
Caution: do not use for longer than 3 weeks for children under 4 years; do not use for prolonged periods for other patients.
Not to be used for: patients suffering from acne or any other skin infections caused by tuberculosis, ringworm, viruses, or fungi, or continuously especially in pregnant women.
Caution needed with:
Contains: DIFLUCORTOLONE VALERATE.
Other preparations: Nerisone Oily Cream, Nerisone Ointment, Nerisone Forte.

Neulactil
(Rhone-Poulenc Rorer)

A yellow, scored tablet supplied at strengths of 2.5 mg, 10 mg, 25 mg and used as a sedative to treat behavioural and character problems, schizophrenia, anxiety, tension, agitation.

Dose: elderly 15-30 mg a day at first; adults 15-75 mg a day at first; children as advised by physician.
Availability: NHS and private prescription.
Side effects: muscle spasms, restlessness, hands shaking, constipation, blurred vision, dry mouth, urine retention, palpitations, low blood pressure, weight gain, changes in libido, low body temperature, breast swelling, menstrual changes, jaundice, blood and skin changes, drowsiness, rarely fits.
Caution: in pregnant women, nursing mothers.
Not to be used for: unconscious patients, the elderly, or for patients suffering from heart failure, bone marrow depression, liver or kidney disorder, epilepsy, Parkinson's disease, underactive thyroid, glaucoma, enlarged prostate.
Caution needed with: alcohol, tranquillizers, pain killers,

N

ANTIHYPERTENSIVES, antidepressants, anticonvulsants, antidiabetic drugs, LEVODOPA.
Contains: PERICYAZINE.
Other preparations: Neulactil Forte Syrup.

Neutral Insulin *see* **insulin**
(Evans)

Nicabate *see* **Nicotinell**
(Marion Merrell Dow)

---

nicardipine *see* **Cardene**

---

niclosamide *see* **Yomesan**

---

nicofuranose *see* **Bradilan**

Nicorette
(Kabi Pharmacia)

Chewing gum supplied at strengths of 2 mg and used as an alkaloid to end smoking addiction.

Dose: 1 when required.
Availability: private prescription and over the counter.
Side effects: addiction, hiccoughs, indigestion, irritated throat.
Caution: in patients suffering from coronary disease, angina, gastritis, stomach ulcer.
Not to be used for: children or pregnant women.
Caution needed with:
Contains: NICOTINE.
Other preparations: Nicorette Plus 4 mg (only available on private prescription), Nicorette patches, NICOTINELL TTS (Ciba-Geigy).

---

nicotinamide *see* **Abidec, Allbee with C, Apisate, BC 500, BC**

500 with Iron, Becosym, Calcimax, Concavit, Fefol-Vit Spansule, Fesovit Spansule, Fesovit Z Spansule, Galfervit, Givitol, Ketovite, Lipoflavonoid, Lipotriad, Octovit, Orovite, Orovite 7, Polyvite, Pregnavite Forte F, Surbex T, Tonivitan B, Verdiviton, Villescon, vitamins capsules BPC

---

nicotine *see* **Nicabate, Nicorette, Nicotinell**

Nicotinell
(Geigy)

A patch supplied at sizes 10 cm, 20 cm, 30 cm, and used to treat nicotine addiction as an aid to giving up smonking.

Dose: apply a patch to a clean, non-hairy dry area of skin on upper arm or trunk. Change daily. Patch size depends on number of cigarettes smoked. Reduce patch size at monthly intervals. Maximum daily dose 30 cm. Maximum treatment period 3 months.
Availability: private prescription and over the counter.
Side effects: skin reactions.
Caution: in patients suffering from high blood pressure, angina, blood vessel disease, heart failure, overactive thyroid, diabetes, kidney or liver disorder, stomach ulcer. Stop smoking completely when starting treatment. Dispose of patches carefully.
Not to be used for: pregnant women, nursing mothers, children under 18 years, or for patients suffering from heart attack, untreated angina, severe heart rhythm disorder, recent stroke, skin disease. Also not suitable for occasional smokers.
Caution needed with: THEOPHYLLINE, WARFARIN, and other drugs previously affected by NICOTINE in the blood.
Contains: NICOTINE.
Other preparations: NICABATE, NICORETTE (Kabi Pharmacia).

---

nicotinic acid *see* **nicotine acid tablets, Tonivitan**

---

nicotinic acid tablets

Tablets supplied at a strength of 50 mg and used as a lipid-lowering agent to treat high blood lipid levels.

Dose: adults, 2-4 tablets 3 times a day, increased if necessary to 20-40

tablets 3 times a day.
Availability: NHS, private prescription, over the counter.
Side effects: flushing, dizziness, headache, irregular heartbeat, itching, nausea, vomiting, liver disorder, rash.
Caution: in patients suffering from diabetes, gout, liver disease, stomach ulcer.
Not to be used for: pregnant women, nursing mothers.
Caution needed with:
Contains: nicotinic acid.
Other preparations:

---

nicotinyl alcohol tartrate *see* **Ronicol**

---

nicoumalone *see* **Sinthrome**

---

nifedipine *see* **Adalat, Adalat Retard, Beta Adalat, Tenif**

Nifensar XL *see* **Adalat Retard**
(Rhone-Poulenc Rorer)

Niferex
(Tillomed)

An elixir used as an iron supplement to treat iron-deficiency anaemia.

Dose: adults treatment 5 ml 1-2 times a day, prevention 2.5 ml a day; children 0-2 years 1 drop per 0.45 kg bodyweight a day, 2-6 years 2.5 ml a day, 6-12 years 5 ml a day.
Availability: NHS, private prescription, and over the counter.
Side effects:
Caution: in patients with a history of stomach ulcer.
Not to be used for:
Caution needed with: TETRACYCLINES.
Contains: POLYSACCHARIDE-IRON COMPLEX.
Other preparations: Niferex-150 Capsules, Niferex Paediatric Elixir, Niferex Tablets (now discontinued).

N

Nilstim — a bulking agent to treat obesity. Product now discontinued.

---

nimodipine *see* **Nimatop**

---

nimorazole *see* **Naxogin 500**

Nimotop
(Bayer)

A white tablet supplied at a strength of 30 mg and used to treat symptoms following stroke.

Dose: 2 tablets every 4 hours for 21 days.
Availability: NHS and private prescription.
Side effects: low blood pressure, flushing, headache, changes in heart rate.
Caution: in pregnant women and in patients suffering from fluid retention or high blood pressure in the brain, kidney damage.
Not to be used for: children.
Caution needed with: ß-BLOCKERS, other similar drugs.
Contains: NIMODIPINE.
Other preparations: Nimotop Infusion.

Nitoman
(Roche)

A yellow/buff, scored tablet supplied at a strength of 25 mg and used as a sedative to treat Huntington's chorea, hemiballismus, senile chorea (movement disorders)

Dose: 1 tablet 3 times a day at first increasing if needed by 1 tablet a day every 3-4 days to a maximum of 8 tablets a day.
Availability: NHS and private prescription.
Side effects: drowsiness, depression, low blood presure on standing, tremor, rigidity.
Caution: in pregnant women.
Not to be used for: children or for nursing mothers.
Caution needed with: RESERPINE, LEVODOPA, MAOIs.
Contains: TETRABENAZINE.
Other preparations:

N

Nitrados *see* **Mogadon.** Product now discontinued.

---

nitrate

a drug used to treat poor blood supply to the heart muscle (angina). Nitrates reduce the work which the heart has to do. Example GLYCERYL TRINITRATE *see* Suscard Buccal.

---

nitrazepam *see* **Mogadon, Nitrados**

Nitro-Dur *see* **Deponit**
(Schering Plough)

Nitrocontin Continus
(Asta)

A pink tablet supplied at strengths of 2.6 mg, 6.4 mg and used as a NITRATE to treat angina.

Dose: 2.6-6.4 mg a day.
Availability: NHS, private prescription, over the counter.
Side effects: passing headache.
Caution:
Not to be used for: children.
Caution needed with:
Contains: GLYCERYL TRINITRATE.
Other preparations: CORO-NITRO (Boehringer Mannheim), DEPONIT (Schwartz), GLYTRIN (Sanofi Winthrop), NITRO-DUR (Schering Plough), NITROLINGUAL (Lipha), PERCUTOL (Cusi), SUSCARD BUCCAL (Pharmax), SUSTAC (Pharmax), TRANSIDERM NITRO (Ciba).

---

nitrofurantoin *see* **Furadantin**

---

nitrofurazone *see* **Furacin**

N

Nitrolingual
(Lipha)

An aerosol used as a NITRATE for the prevention and treatment of angina.

Dose: 1-2 sprays under the tongue for each attack up to a maximum of 3 sprays.
Availability: NHS, private prescription, over the counter.
Side effects: headache, flushes, dizziness
Caution: do not inhale spray.
Not to be used for: children.
Caution needed with:
Contains: GLYCERYL TRINITRATE.
Other preparations: CORO-NITRO (Boehringer Mannheim), DEPONIT (Schwartz), GLYTRIN (Sanofi Winthrop), NITROCONTIN CONTINUS (Asta), NITRO-DUR (Schering Plough), PERCUTOL (Cusi), SUSCARD BUCCAL (Pharmax), SUSTAC (Pharmax), TRANSIDERM NITRO (Ciba).

Nivaquine
(Rhone-Poulenc Rorer)

A yellow tablet supplied at a strength of 200 mg and used as an antimalarial drug for the prevention and treatment of malaria, and to treat rheumatoid arthritis.

Dose: prevention of malaria adults 2 tablets on the same day once a week; treatment as advised by the physician; Children use Nivaquine Syrup. Rheumatoid arthritis, adults 1 tablet a day.
Availability: NHS, private prescription, and over the counter if for prevention of malaria.
Side effects: headache, stomach upset, skin eruptions, hair loss, eye disorders, blood disorders, loss of pigment, allergy.
Caution: in pregnant women, nursing mothers, or in patients suffering from porphyria (a rare blood disorder), kidney or liver disease, severe gastro-intestinal, nervous, or blood disorder, psoriasis or history of epilepsy. The eyes should be tested before and during prolonged treatment.
Not to be used for:
Caution needed with:
Contains: CHLOROQUINE sulphate.
Other preparations: AVOCLOR (ICI), Nivaquine Syrup, Nivaquine Injection.

Nivemycin
(Boots)

A tablet supplied at a strength of 500 mg and used as an aminoglycoside antibiotic for preparation before bowel surgery, and as an additional treatment in liver disease coma.

Dose: adults 2 tablets every hour for 4 hours, then 2 tablets every 4 hours for 2-3 days; children under 5 years use elixir, 6-12 years ½-1 tablet every 4 hours for 2-3 days, over 12 years 2 tablets every 4 hours for 2-3 days.
Availability: NHS and private prescription.
Side effects: stomach disturbances.
Caution: in patients suffering from kidney or liver damage, Parkinson's disease, damaged hearing.
Not to be used for: patients suffering from a blockage of the intestine.
Caution needed with:
Contains: NEOMYCIN sulphate.
Other preparations: Nivemycin Elixir.

---

nizatidine *see* Axid

Nizoral
(Janssen)

A white scored tablet supplied at a strength of 200 mg and used as an anti-fungal treatment for severe fungus infections, chronic vaginal thrush which does not respond to other treatment.

Dose: adults 1-2 tablets a day with meals; children 3 mg per kg body weight a day.
Availability: NHS and private prescription
Side effects: hepatitis, hypersensitivity, stomach upset, rash, headache, blood changes, rarely breast enlargement.
Caution: liver should be checked regularly.
Not to be used for: pregnant women, patients with any form of liver disorder, or hypersensitivity to ketoconazole or other imidazoles.
Caution needed with: ANTICHOLINERGICS, ANTACIDS, ASTEMIZOLE, CIMETIDINE, RANITIDINE, and some other treatments for stomach ulcer, anticoagulants, PHENYTOIN, RIFAMPICIN, CYCLOSPORIN A.
Contains: KETOCONAZOLE.
Other preparations: Nizoral Suspension, Nizoral Cream.

Nizoral Cream
(Janssen)

A cream used as an antifungal treatment for fungus infections, skin thrush, seborrhoeic dermatitis.

N

Dose: apply to the affected area 1-2 times a day.
Availability: NHS and private prescription.
Side effects: irritation.
Caution:
Not to be used for:
Caution needed with:
Contains: KETOCONAZOLE.
Other preparations: Nizoral Shampoo.

Nobrium
(Roche)

A yellow/orange capsule supplied at a strength of 5 mg, and used as a sleeping tablet for the short-term treatment of anxiety.

Dose: elderly 5-20 mg a day in divided doses; adults 15-40 mg a day in divided doses.
Availability: private prescription only.
Side effects: drowsiness, confusion, unsteadiness, low blood pressure, rash, changes in vision, changes in libido, retention of urine. Risk of addiction increases with dose and length of treatment. May impair judgement.
Caution: in the elderly, pregnant women, nursing mothers, in women during labour, and in patients suffering from lung disorders, kidney or liver disorders. Avoid long-term use and withdraw gradually.
Not to be used for: children, or for patients suffering from acute lung diseases, some chronic lung diseases, some obsessional and psychotic diseases.
Caution needed with: alcohol, other tranquillizers, anticonvulsants.
Contains: MEDAZEPAM.
Other preparations:

Noctec
(Squibb)

A liquid-filled, red capsule supplied at a strength of 500 mg and used as a sedative to treat sleeplessness.

Dose: usually 1-2 capsules taken with water 15-30 minutes before going to bed; maximum dose 4 capsules a day.
Availability: NHS and private prescription.
Side effects: stomach irritation, headache, excitement, delirium, skin allergies, ketones in the urine.
Caution: in nursing mothers and for patients suffering from porphyria (a

N

rare blood disorder). Patients should be warned of reduced judgement and abilities.
Not to be used for: children, pregnant women, or for patients suffering from severe heart, liver, or kidney disease, or gastric inflammation.
Caution needed with: alcohol, sedatives, anticoagulants.
Contains: CHORAL HYDRATE.
Other preparations: WELLDORM (SNP).

Noltam *see* **Nolvadex-D**
(Lederle)

Noludar — sedative to treat sleeplessness. Product now discontinued.

Nolvadex-D
(ICI)

A white, eight-sided tablet supplied at a strength of 20 mg and used as an anti-oestrogen treatment for infertility in women caused by failure of ovulation or breast cancer.

Dose: 1 tablet a day for 4 days beginning on the fourth day of the period. If needed increase to 2 tablets a day then 4 tablets a day for further courses. For breast cancer 1 tablet a day increasing to 2 tablets a day if needed.
Availability: NHS and private prescription.
Side effects: hot flushes, bleeding from the vagina, stomach upset, dizziness, disturbed vision.
Caution:
Not to be used for: children or pregnant women.
Caution needed with: WARFARIN.
Contains: TAMOXIFEN citrate.
Other preparations: Nolvadex Forte, Nolvadex, EMBLON (Berk), NOLTAM (Lederle), OESTRIFEN (Ashbourne), TAMOFEN (Farmitalia CE).

---

non-steroidal anti-inflammatory drug (NSAID)

an antirheumatic preparation which has pain-killing properties. An NSAID may cause stomach upsets. Example IBUPROFEN *see* Brufen.

---

nonivamide *see* **Finalgon**

N

Noradran — cough remedy for treatment of bronchitis/bronchial asthma. Product now discontinued.

Nordox *see* **Vibramycin, Vibramycin-50**
(Panpharma)

norethisterone *see* **BiNovum, Brevinor, Climagest, Controvlar, Estrapak, Loestrin 20, Menophase, Micronor, Neocon 1/35, Noriday, Norimin, Norinyl-1, Ortho-Novin 1/50, Primolut N, Synphase, Trinovum, Trinovum-ED, Trisequens, Utovlan**

norfloxacin *see* **Noroxin, Utinor**

Norgalax *see* **Fletchers' Enemette**
(Norgine)

norgestimate *see* **Cilest**

Norgeston
(Schering)

A white tablet used as a progesterone contraceptive.

Dose: 1 tablet at the same time every day starting on day 1 of the period.
Availability: NHS and over the counter.
Side effects: irregular bleeding, breast discomfort, acne, headache.
Caution: in patients suffering from high blood pressure, tendency to thrombosis, migraine, liver abnormalities, ovarian cysts. Your doctor may advise regular check-ups.
Not to be used for: pregnant women, or for patients suffering from severe heart or artery disease, benign liver tumours, vaginal bleeding, previous ectopic pregnancy.
Caution needed with: BARBITURATES, PHENYTOIN, PRIMIDONE, CARBAMAZEPINE, CHLORAL HYDRATE, DICHLORALPHENAZONE, ETHOSUXIMIDE, RIFAMPICIN, GLUTETHIMIDE, CHLORPROMAZINE, MEPROBAMATE, GRISEOFULVIN.
Contains: LEVONORGESTREL.
Other preparations: MICROVAL (Wyeth).

N

norgestrel *see* **Neogest, Ovysmen, PC4, Prempak-C**

Noriday
(Syntex)

A white tablet used as a progesterone contraceptive.

Dose: 1 tablet at the same time every day starting on day 1 of the period.
Availability: NHS and private prescription.
Side effects: irregular bleeding, breast discomfort, acne, headache.
Caution: in patients suffering from high blood pressure, tendency to thrombosis, migraine, liver abnormalities, ovarian cysts. Your doctor may advise regular check-ups.
Not to be used for: pregnant women, or for patients suffering from severe heart or artery disease, benign liver tumours, vaginal bleeding, previous ectopic pregnancy.
Caution needed with: BARBITURATES, PHENYTOIN, PRIMIDONE, CARBAMAZEPINE, CHLORAL HYDRATE, DICHLORALPHENAZONE, ETHOSUXIMIDE, RIFAMPICIN, GLUTETHIMIDE, CHLORPROMAZINE, MEPROBAMATE, GRISEOFULVIN.
Contains: NORETHISTERONE.
Other preparations: MICRONOR (Ortho).

Norimin
(Syntex)

A yellow tablet used as an oestrogen, progestogen contraceptive.

Dose: 1 tablet a day for 21 days starting on day 5 of the period.
Availability: NHS and private prescription.
Side effects: enlarged breasts, bloating and fluid retention, cramps, leg pains, mood change, reduction in sexual desire, headaches, nausea, vaginal erosion, discharge, and bleeding, weight gain, skin changes.
Caution: in patients suffering from high blood pressure, diabetes, vascular disorders, asthma, depression, kidney disease, multiple sclerosis, womb diseases. Your doctor may advise you not to smoke, to have regular examinations. You should stop treatment at the first sign of serious symptoms such as severe headache or jaundice. Treatment should be stopped before surgery.
Not to be used for: pregnant women, or for patients suffering from sickle-cell anaemia, history of heart disease or thrombosis, liver disorders, some cancers, undiagnosed vaginal bleeding, some ear, skin, and kidney disorders.
Caution needed with: RIFAMPICIN, TETRACYCLINES, GRISEOFULVIN, BARBITURATES, PHENYTOIN, PRIMIDONE, CARBAMAZEPINE, ETHOSUXIMIDE, CHLORAL HYDRATE,

N

DICHLORALPHENAZONE.
Contains: ETHINYLOESTRADIOL, NORETHISTERONE.
Other preparations: NEOCON 1/35 (Ortho).

Norinyl-1
(Syntex)

A white tablet used as an oestrogen, progestogen contraceptive.

Dose: 1 tablet a day for 21 days starting on day 5 of the period.
Availability: NHS and private prescription.
Side effects: enlarged breasts, bloating and fluid retention, cramps, leg pains, mood change, reduction in sexual desire, headaches, nausea, vaginal erosion, discharge, and bleeding, weight gain, skin changes.
Caution: in patients suffering from high blood pressure, diabetes, vascular disorders, asthma, depression, kidney disease, multiple sclerosis, womb diseases. Your doctor may advise you not to smoke, to have regular examinations. You should stop treatment at the first sign of serious symptoms such as severe headache or jaundice. Treatment should be stopped before surgery.
Not to be used for: pregnant women, or for patients suffering from sickle-cell anaemia, history of heart disease or thrombosis, liver disorders, some cancers, undiagnosed vaginal bleeding, some ear, skin, and kidney disorders.
Caution needed with: RIFAMPICIN, TETRACYCLINES, GRISEOFULVIN, BARBITURATES, PHENYTOIN, PRIMIDONE, CARBAMAZEPINE, ETHOSUXIMIDE, CHLORAL HYDRATE, DICHLORALPHENAZONE.
Contains: MESTRANOL, NORETHISTERONE.
Other preparations: ORTHO NOVIN 1/50 (Ortho).

Normacol
(Norgine)

White granules in 7 g sachets or supplied as as 500 g and used as a bulking agent. to treat constipation caused by lack of fibre in the diet.

Dose: adults 1 sachet or 1 heaped 5 ml spoonful once or twice a day after meals swallowed with liquid; children in proportion to adult dose.
Availability: NHS, private prescription, over the counter.
Side effects:
Caution:
Not to be used for:
Caution needed with:
Contains: STERCULIA.

N

Other preparations: Normacol Plus.

Normasol
(Seton Healthcare)

A solution in a sachet used for washing out eyes, burns, wounds.

Dose: use as needed.
Availability: NHS, private prescription, over the counter.
Side effects:
Caution:
Not to be used for:
Caution needed with:
Contains: SODIUM CHLORIDE.
Other preparations: STERIPOD BLUE (Seton Healthcare).

Normax
(Evans)

A brown capsule used as a stimulant and faecal softener to treat constipation in the elderly, in patients being treated with pain-killers, and those with heart failure or coronary thrombosis.

Dose: adults 1-3 capsules at night as required; children over 6 years 1 capsule at night.
Availability: NHS (when prescribed as a generic) and private prescription.
Side effects:
Caution: in nursing mothers.
Not to be used for: children under 6 years or for patients suffering from an obstruction of the intestine.
Caution needed with:
Contains: DANTHRON, DOCUSATE sodium.
Other preparations:

Normetic *see* **Moduretic.** Product now discontinued.

Normison
(Wyeth)

A yellow capsule supplied at strengths of 10 mg, 20 mg and used as a sleeping tablet to prevent interrupted sleep, and for short-term treatment of sleeplessness when sedation during the day could present difficulty.

N

Dose: elderly 10 mg before going to bed; adults usually 10-30 mg but up to 60 mg before going to bed.
Availability: NHS (when prescribed as a generic) and private prescription.
Side effects: drowsiness, confusion, unsteadiness, low blood pressure, rash, changes in vision, changes in libido, retention of urine. Risk of addiction increases with dose and length of treatment. May impair judgement.
Caution: in the elderly, pregnant women, nursing mothers, in women during labour, and in patients suffering from lung disorders, kidney or liver disorders. Avoid long-term use and withdraw gradually.
Not to be used for: children, or for patients suffering from acute lung diseases, some chronic lung diseases, some obsessional and psychotic diseases.
Caution needed with: alcohol, other tranquillizers, anticonvulsants.
Contains: TEMAZEPAM.
Other preparations: EUHYPNOS (Farmitalia CE), TEMAZEPAM CAPSULES.

Noroxin
(MSD)

Drops used as an anti-infective treatment for bacterial eye infections.

Dose: 1-2 drops into the eye 4 times a day.
Availability: NHS and private prescription.
Side effects: irritation, bitter taste.
Caution: in pregnant women.
Not to be used for:
Caution needed with:
Contains: NORFLOXACIN.
Other preparations:

---

nortriptyline *see* **Allegron, Aventyl, Motipress, Motival**

Norval
(Bencard)

An orange tablet supplied at strengths of 10 mg, 20 mg, 30 mg and used as a tetracyclic anti-depressant to treat depression.

Dose: adults 30-40 mg a day at first increasing gradually after a few days if needed to 30-90 mg in divided doses; elderly up to 30 mg a day.
Availability: NHS and private prescription.
Side effects: drowsiness, bone marrow depression, possible jaundice,

N

hypomania, or convulsions.

Caution: in pregnant women, the elderly or patients suffering from epilepsy, glaucoma, enlarged prostate, heart attack; discontinue if jaundice, hypomania, or convulsions happen. Your doctor may advise that blood tests should be taken once a month for the first 3 months.

Not to be used for: children, nursing mothers, or for patients suffering from mania or severe liver disease.

Caution needed with: MAOIS, alcohol, anticoagulants.

Contains: MIANSERIN hydrochloride.

Other preparations: BOLVIDON (Organon).

Nozinan
(Rhone-Poulenc Rorer)

A white, scored tablet supplied at a strength of 25 mg, and used as a sedative to treat schizophrenia and other mental disorders, and to treat severe pain accompanied by restlessness, distress, or vomiting.

Dose: 25-200 mg a day.

Availability: NHS and private prescription.

Side effects: muscle spasms, restlessness, hands shaking, constipation, blurred vision, dry mouth, urine retention, palpitations, low blood pressure, weight gain, changes in libido, low body temperature, breast swelling, menstrual changes, jaundice, blood and skin changes, drowsiness, fits.

Caution: in pregnant women, nursing mothers, and in patients suffering from cardiovascular disease, liver damage, Parkinson's disease, or epilepsy.

Not to be used for: children, or for patients with bone marrow disorder, or who are in a coma.

Caution needed with: alcohol, tranquillizers, pain killers, ANTIHYPERTENSIVES, antidepressants, anticonvulsants, antidiabetics, LEVODOPA.

Contains: METHOTRIMEPRAZINE.

Other preparations:

Nu-K
(Consolidated)

A blue capsule supplied at a strength of 600 mg and used as a potassium supplement to treat potassium deficiency.

Dose: 1-6 capsules a day in divided doses after food.

Availability: NHS, private prescription, over the counter.

Side effects: ulcers or blockage in the small bowel.

N

Not to be used for: children or patients suffering from advanced kidney disease.
Caution needed with:
Contains: POTASSIUM CHLORIDE.
Other preparations: KAY-CEE-L (Geistlich), SLOW-K (Ciba).

Nu-Seals Aspirin
(Eli Lilly)

A red tablet supplied at a strength of 300 mg, and used as an analgesic to relieve pain, rheumatism, rheumatoid arthritis, and to prevent heart attack, thrombosis.

Dose: adults and children over 12 years 300-900 mg 3-4 times a day to a maximum of 8 g a day; to prevent thrombosis 1 a day.
Availability: NHS, private prescription, over the counter.
Side effects: stomach upsets, allergy, asthma.
Caution: in pregnant women, the elderly, or in patients with a history of allergy to aspirin, asthma, impaired kidney or liver function, indigestion.
Not to be used for: children under 12 years, nursing mothers, or patients suffering from haemophilia, or ulcers.
Caution needed with: anticoagulants, some antidiabetic drugs, anti-inflammatory agents, METHOTREXATE, SPIRONOLACTONE, STEROIDS, some ANTACIDS, some uric acid-lowering drugs.
Contains: ASPIRIN.
Other preparations: ASPIRIN TABLETS, PLATET CLEARTAB (Nicholas).

Nuelin SA *see* Lasma
(3M Healthcare)

Nulacin
(Bencard)

A beige tablet used as an ANTACID to treat dyspepsia, acidity, oesophagitis, hiatus hernia, stomach ulcer.

Dose: adults 1 tablet sucked or chewed between meals and at bedtime (up to 8 a day).
Availability: private prescription and over the counter.
Side effects:
Caution:
Not to be used for: children, or for patients suffering from coeliac dis-

ease.

Caution needed with: tablets which are coated to protect the stomach.
Contains: milk solids with dextrins and MALTOSE, MAGNESIUM OXIDE, MAGNESIUM CARBONATE, MAGNESIUM TRISILICATE.
Other preparations:

Numotac — broncho-dilator to treat bronchial spasm. Product now discontinued.

Nupercainal
(Zyma)

An ointment used as a local anaesthetic and a treatment for haemorrhoids.

Dose: apply sparingly 3 times a day.
Availability: NHS, private prescription, over the counter.
Side effects:
Caution:
Not to be used for:
Caution needed with:
Contains: CINCHOCAINE.
Other preparations:

Nutrizym GR
(Merck)

A green/orange capsule used as a source of pancreatic enzymes to treat cystic fibrosis, steatorrhoea, pancreatic disorders.

Dose: 1-2 capsules with meals.
Availability: NHS, private prescription, over the counter.
Side effects: buccal and perianal irritation.
Caution:
Not to be used for:
Caution needed with:
Contains: PANCREATIN.
Other preparations: Nutrizym 22, COTAZYM (Organon), CREON (Duphar), PANCREASE (Cilag), PANCREX-V (Paines & Byrne).

Nuvelle *see* Cyclo-Progynova
(Schering Health Care)

N

Nycopren *see* **Naprosyn**
(Lundbeck)

Nystadermal
(Princeton)

A cream used as a STEROID and antibacterial treatment for thrush, itch, eczema where there is also inflammation.

Dose: apply to the affected area 2-4 times a day.
Availability: NHS and private prescription.
Side effects: fluid retention, suppression of adrenal glands, thinning of the skin may occur.
Caution: use for short periods of time only
Not to be used for: patients suffering from acne or any other skin infections caused by tuberculosis, ringworm, viruses, or fungi, or continuously especially in pregnant women.
Caution needed with:
Contains: NYSTATIN, TRIAMCINOLONE ACETONIDE.
Other preparations:

Nystaform
(Bayer)

A cream used as an antifungal and antibacterial treatment for skin infections or skin conditions where infection may occur.

Dose: apply freely to the affected area 2-3 times a day until 7 days after the wounds have healed.
Availability: NHS and private prescription.
Side effects:
Caution:
Not to be used for:
Caution needed with:
Contains: NYSTATIN, CHLORHEXIDINE.
Other preparations:

Nystaform-HC
(Bayer)

A cream used as a STEROID and antifungal treatment for skin disorders where there is also infection.

N

Dose: apply to the affected area 2-3 times a day for 7 days after the condition has healed.
Availability: NHS and private prescription.
Side effects: fluid retention, suppression of adrenal glands, thinning of the skin may occur.
Caution: use for short periods of time only.
Not to be used for: patients suffering from acne or any other skin infections caused by tuberculosis, ringworm, viruses, or fungi, or continuously especially in pregnant women.
Caution needed with:
Contains: NYSTATIN, CHLORHEXIDINE, HYDROCORTISONE.
Other preparations: Nystaform-HC Ointment, TIMODINE (Reckitt & Coleman).

Nystan
(Squibb)

A yellow, diamond-shaped pessary or a brown tablet used as an antifungal treatment for vaginal, oral, or intestinal thrush.

Dose: vaginal thrush 1-2 pessaries into the vagina for at least 14 nights; children use cream. Other infections 1-2 tablets 4 times a day.
Availability: NHS and private prescription.
Side effects: irritation and burning, nausea, vomiting, diarrhoea in high doses.
Caution:
Not to be used for:
Caution needed with:
Contains: NYSTATIN.
Other preparations: Nystan Vaginal Cream, Nystan Gel, Nystan Oral Suspension, Nystan Oral Tablets. (Nystan Triple Pack, NYSTAVESCENT — both now discontinued.)

Nystan Cream
(Squibb)

A cream used as an antifungal treatment for thrush of the skin and mucous membranes.

Dose: apply to the affected area 2-4 times a day.
Availability: NHS and private prescription.
Side effects: irritation and burning.
Caution:
Not to be used for:

N

Caution needed with:
Contains: NYSTATIN.
Other preparations: Nystan Ointment, Nystan Gel, Nystan Powder.

Nystan Oral Suspension
(Squibb)

A supension used as an antifungal treatment for thrush.

Dose: hold 1 ml of the supension in contact with the affected area 4 times a day for up to 2 days after the symptoms have abated.
Availability: NHS and private prescription.
Side effects:
Caution:
Not to be used for:
Caution needed with:
Contains: NYSTATIN.
Other preparations: Nystan Granules, Nystan Pastilles, NYSTATIN-DOME SUSPENSION (Lagap).

nystatin *see* **Gregoderm, Mutilind, Nystadermal, Nystaform, Nystaform-HC, Nystan, Nystan Cream, Nystan Oral Suspension, Timodine, Tinaderm-M, Tri-Adcortyl, Tri-Adcortyl Otic, Tri-Cicatrin, Trimovate**

Nystatin-Dome Oral Suspension *see* **Nystan Oral Suspension**
(Lagap)

Nystavescent *see* **Nystan.** Product now discontinued.

oat bran meal *see* **Lejfibre**

Octovit
(S K B)

A maroon, oblong tablet used as a multivitamin treatment for vitamin and mineral deficiencies.

Dose: 1 tablet a day
Availability: private prescription and over the counter.
Side effects:
Caution: in pregnant women.
Not to be used for: children.
Caution needed with: tetracyclines, levodopa.
Contains: VITAMIN A, THIAMINE, RIBOFLAVINE, NICOTINAMIDE, PYRIDOXINE, CYANOCOBALAMIN, ASCORBIC acid, CHOLECALCIFEROL, TOCOPHERYL ACETATE, CALCIUM HYDROGEN PHOSPHATE, FERROUS SULPHATE, MAGNESIUM HYDROXIDE, ZINC.
Other preparations:

Ocusert Pilo
(M & B)

An eye insert used as a cholinergic treatment for glaucoma.

Dose: 1 unit under the eyelid replaced every 7 days.
Availability: NHS and private prescription.
Side effects: irritation, reduced sharpness of vision.
Caution:
Not to be used for: children or for patients suffering from acute eye infection or inflammation.
Caution needed with:
Contains: PILOCARPINE.
Other preparations: ISOPTO-CARPINE (Alcon), OPULETS PILOCARPINE (Alcon), PILOCARPINE EYE DROPS, SNO PILO (SNP),

Ocusol *see* Sulphacetamide Minims. Product now discontinued.

oestradiol *see* Climagest, Climaval, Cyclo-Progynova 1mg, Estraderm, Estrapak, Hormonin, Nuvelle, Progynova, Trisequens, Vagifem, Zumenon

Oestrifen *see* Nolvadex-D
(Ashbourne)

oestriol *see* Hormonin, Ovestin, Trisequens

oestrone *see* **Hormonin**

ofloxacin *see* **Tarivid**

Oilatum Cream
(Stiefel)

A cream used as an emollient to treat dermatitis and other dry itchy skin conditions.

Dose: apply after washing and as required.
Availability: NHS, private prescription, over the counter.
Side effects:
Caution:
Not to be used for:
Caution needed with:
Contains: ARACHIS OIL.
Other preparations: OILATUM EMOLLIENT, Oilatum Shower Gel.

Oilatum Emollient
(Stifel)

A liquid used as a bath emollient to treat dermatitis and dry itchy skin conditions.

Dose: adults 1-3 capsful added to the bath and soak for 10-20 minutes, or rub a small amount on to wet skin, rinse and dry; children as for adults; infants ½-2 capsful added to a wash basin and apply over entire body.
Availability: NHS, private prescription, over the counter.
Side effects:
Caution: bath may become slippery
Not to be used for:
Caution needed with:
Contains: acetylated wool alcohols, LIQUID PARAFFIN.
Other preparations: Oilatum Shower Gel, OILATUM CREAM.

oily cream *see* **hydrous ointment**

Olbetam
(Farmitalia CE)

A red-brown/dark-pink capsule supplied at a strength of 250 mg and used as a lipid-lowering agent to treat elevated lipids.

Dose: 2-3 capsules a day with meals, no more than 1200 mg a day.
Availability: NHS and private prescription.
Side effects: flushes, rash, redness, stomach upset, headache, general feeling of being unwell.
Caution:
Not to be used for: children, pregnant women, nursing mothers, or for patients suffering from stomach ulcer.
Caution needed with:
Contains: ACIPIMOX.
Other preparations:

---

oleyl alcohol *see* **Polytar Liquid**

---

olive oil *see* **Rowachol, Rowatinex**

---

olsalazine sodium *see* **Dipentum**

---

omeprazole *see* **Losec**

---

ondansetron *see* **Zofran**

One-Alpha
(Leo)

A white capsule or a brown capsule according to strengths of 0.25 microgram, 1 microgram. and used as a source of vitamin D to treat bone disorders due to kidney disease, rickets, over-or underactive parathyroid glands, low calcium levels in newborn infants, other bone disorders.

Dose: adults and children over 20 kg body weight 1 microgram a day at first adjusting as neded; children under 20 kg 0.05 micrograms per kg a day at first.

Availability: NHS and private prescription.
Side effects:
Caution: in nursing mothers. Your doctor may advise that calcium levels should be checked regularly.
Not to be used for:
Caution needed with: BARBITURATES, anticonvulsants.
Contains: ALFACALCIDOL.
Other preparations: One-Alpha Solution.

Ophthaine
(Squibb)

Drops used as a local anaesthetic for eye procedures.

Dose: 1-2 drops into the eye.
Availability: NHS and private prescription.
Side effects: irritation, rarely severe sensitivity.
Caution: in patients with a history of allergy, heart disease, or overactive thyroid. Do not use over extended periods.
Not to be used for:
Caution needed with:
Contains: PROXYMETACAINE hydrochloride.
Other preparations:

Opilon
(Parke-Davis)

A yellow tablet supplied at a strength of 40 mg and used as a vasodilator to treat Raynaud's syndrome (a condition caused by spasms of arteries in the hand).

Dose: 1 tablet 4 times a day, increasing if necessary to 2 tablets 4 times a day.
Availability: NHS and private prescription.
Side effects: nausea, diarrhoea, vertigo, headache.
Caution: in patients suffering from diabetes, angina, recent heart attack.
Not to be used for: children, pregnant women, nursing mothers, or for patients who are sensitive to THYMOXAMINE.
Caution needed with: TRICYCLIC antidepressants, ANTIHYPERTENSIVES.
Contains: THYMOXAMINE hydrochloride.
Other preparations:

Opticrom
(Fisons)

Drops used as an anti-allergy agent to treat allergic conjunctivitis.

Dose: 1-2 drops into the eyes 4 times a day.
Availability: NHS and private prescription.
Side effects: temporary smarting.
Caution:
Not to be used for: patients who wear contact lenses.
Caution needed with:
Contains: SODIUM CROMOGLYCATE.
Other preparations: Opticrom Eye Ointment.

Optimax — antidepressant. Product now discontinued.

Optimine
(Schering Plough)

A white, scored tablet supplied at a strength of 1 mg and used as an ANTIHISTAMINE and serotonin antagonist (hormone blocker) to treat bites and stings, itch, allergic rhinitis, urticaria.

Dose: adults 1-2 tablets twice a day; children over 1 year use syrup.
Availability: NHS, private prescription, over the counter.
Side effects: drowsiness, reduced reactions, greater appetite, anorexia, nausea, headache, ANTICHOLINERGIC effects.
Caution:
Not to be used for: infants under 1 year or for patients suffering from prostate enlargement, retention of urine, glaucoma, stomach ulcer causing blockage.
Caution needed with: sedatives, MAOIS, alcohol.
Contains: AZATADINE MALEATE.
Other preparations: Optimine Syrup.

Opulets Atropine *see* **Atropine Eye Drops.** Product now discontinued.

Opulets Benoxinate — local anaesthetic eye drops. Product now discontinued.

Opulets Cyclopentolate *see* **Mydrilate.** Product now discontinued.

Opulets Pilocarpine *see* **pilocarpine eye drops.** Product now discontinued.

Opulets Saline *see* **Minims Saline.** Product now discontinued.

Orabase
(Convatec)

An ointment used as a mucoprotectant to protect lesions in the mouth and on moist body surfaces.

Dose: apply to the affected area without rubbing in.
Availability: NHS, private prescription, over the counter.
Side effects:
Caution:
Not to be used for:
Caution needed with:
Contains: CARMELLOSE SODIUM, PECTIN, GELATIN.
Other preparations:

Orabet *see* Glucophage
(Lagap)

Oradexon *see* **Decadron.** Product now discontinued.

Oralcer
(Vitabiotics)

A green pellet used as an antibacterial, antifungal treatment for mouth ulcers.

Dose: adults allow 6-8 pellets to dissolve slowly near the ulcer on the first day, reducing to 4-6 pellets on the second day; children 3-4 pellets a day.
Availability: NHS, private prescription, over the counter.
Side effects: local irritation.
Caution: do not use for extended periods.

Not to be used for: for patients suffering from kidney or liver disease, overactive thyroid, intolerance to IODINE.
Caution needed with:
Contains: CLIOQUINOL, ASCORBIC ACID.
Other preparations:

Oraldene
(Warner-Lambert)

A solution used as an antiseptic rinse to treat thrush, gingivitis, ulcers, bad breath, stomatitis.

Dose: rinse out the mouth or gargle with 15 ml 2-3 times a day.
Availability: NHS, private prescription, over the counter.
Side effects: local irritation.
Caution:
Not to be used for: children under 6 years.
Caution needed with:
Contains: HEXETIDINE.
Other preparations:

Oramorph
(Boehringer Ingelheim)

A solution used as an opiate to control severe pain.

Dose: adults 10-20 mg every 4 hours; children 1-5 years up to 5 mg every 4 hours, 6-12 years up to 5-10 mg every 4 hours.
Availability: controlled drug; NHS and private prescription.
Side effects: tolerance, addiction, constipation, nausea, vomiting, sedation.
Caution: in the elderly, nursing mothers, after surgery, and in patients suffering from underactive thyroid, liver or kidney disease, reduced respiratory reserve, adrenal gland problems, enlarged prostate shock.
Not to be used for: pregnant women, alcoholics, or for patients suffering from respiratory depression, blocked airways, acute liver disease, head injury, coma, convulsions, or raised intracranial pressure.
Caution needed with: MAOIS, sedatives, alcohol.
Contains: MORPHINE sulphate
Other preparations: Oramorph Concentrated, MST CONTINUS (Napp), NEPENTHE (Evans), SEVREDOL (Napp), SRM-RHOTARD (Farmitalia CE).

Orap
(Janssen)

A white, scored tablet or a green, scored tablet according to strengths of 2 mg, 4 mg, 10 mg and used as a sedative to treat schizophrenia.

Dose: 2-20 mg a day.
Availability: NHS and private prescription.
Side effects: muscle spasms, restlessness, hands shaking, blurred vision, constipation, dry mouth, urine retention, palpitations, low blood pressure, weight gain, abnormal heart rhythm, changes in libido, low body temperature, breast swelling, menstrual changes, jaundice, blood and skin changes, drowsiness, rarely fits.
Caution: in pregnant women and in patients suffering from endogenous depression, Parkinson's disease, epilepsy, kidney or liver damage, electrolyte disturbance.
Not to be used for: children or for patients suffering from some heart disorders.
Caution needed with: alcohol, tranquillizers, pain killers, ANTIHYPERTENSIVES, antidepressants, anticonvulsants, antidiabetic drugs, LEVODOPA, some heart drugs, some tranquillizers.
Contains: PIMOZIDE.
Other preparations:

Orbenin
(Beecham)

An orange/black capsule supplied at strengths of 250 mg, 500 mg and used as a penicillin to treat infections.

Dose: adults 500 mg every 6 hours; children over 2 years half adult dose.
Availability: NHS and private prescription.
Side effects: allergy, stomach disturbances.
Caution:
Not to be used for: children under 2 years (except by injection), or for patients suffering from penicillin allergy.
Caution needed with:
Contains: CLOXACILLIN.
Other preparations: Orbenin Injection, Orbenin Syrup (now discontinued).

orciprenaline sulphate *see* Alupent

Orimeten
(Ciba)

An off-white, scored tablet supplied at a strength of 250 mg and used as a STEROID synthesis inhibitor (hormone blocker). to treat breast cancer, prostate cancer, Cushing's syndrome.

Dose: breast or prostate cancer 1 tablet a day increasing by 1 tablet a day every week to 3-4 tablets for prostate or breast cancer; Cushing's syndrome 1 tablet a day increasing to up to 8 a day if needed.
Availability: NHS and private prescription.
Side effects: sedation, stomach disturbances, rash, blood changes, thyroid failure, allergy affecting the lungs.
Caution: STEROIDS may need to be given. Your doctor may advise regular blood tests.
Not to be used for: children, pregnant women, nursing mothers.
Caution needed with: anticoagulants, antidiabetics taken by mouth, artificial glucocorticoids (STEROIDS).
Contains: AMINOGLUTETHIMIDE.
Other preparations:

Orlept *see* Epilim
(CP Pharm)

Orovite
(SKB)

A maroon tablet used as a source of vitamins B and C and used to treat vitamin B and C deficiency.

Dose: 1 tablet 3 times a day.
Availability: private prescription and over the counter.
Side effects: occasionally flushing of the face.
Caution:
Not to be used for:
Caution needed with: LEVODOPA.
Contains: THIAMINE, RIBOFLAVINE, PYRIDOXINE, NICOTINAMIDE, ASCORBIC ACID.
Other preparations: Orovite Syrup (now discontinued).

Orovite 7
(SKB)

Granules in a sachet used as a multivitamin treatment for vitamin deficiencies.

Dose: 1 sachet in water once a day.
Availability: private prescription, over the counter.
Side effects:
Caution: in pregnant women.
Not to be used for: for children under 5 years.
Caution needed with: LEVODOPA.
Contains: VITAMIN A PALMITATE, CALCIFEROL, THIAMINE, RIBOFLAVINE, PYRIDOXINE, NICOTINAMIDE, ASCORBIC ACID.
Other preparations:

---

orphenadrine *see* Biorphen, Disipal

Ortho Dienoestrol
(Cilag)

A cream with applicator used as an oestrogen treatment for atrophic inflammation of the vagina, other disease of the vulva or painful inter-course.

Dose: 1-2 applications into the vagina once a day for 1-2 weeks reducing to half that dose for 1-2 weeks, then 1 application 1-3 times a week.
Availability: NHS and private prescription.
Side effects: tender breasts, headaches, nausea, vaginal bleeding, weight gain, skin changes, rashes, liver function disorders, sodium retention, vomiting.
Caution: in patients suffering from high blood pressure, diabetes, vascular disorders, asthma, kidney disease, heart disease, epilepsy, migraine, thyrotoxicosis, womb diseases. Your doctor may advise you to have regular examinations.
Not to be used for: children, pregnant women, nursing mothers, or for patients suffering from sickle-cell anaemia, thrombosis, liver disorders, some cancers, undiagnosed vaginal bleeding, some ear, skin, and kidney disorders, porphyria (a rare blood disorder), brain blood vessel disease.
Caution needed with: DIURETICS, ANTIHYPERTENSIVES, and drugs that change liver enzymes (eg BARBITURATES, CARBAMAZEPINE, PHENYTOIN).
Contains: DIENOESTROL.
Other preparations:

Ortho-Gynest
(Cilag)

A pessary supplied at a strength of 0.5 mg and used as an oestrogen treatment for atrophic inflammation of the vagina, other disease of the vulva or painful intercourse.

Dose: 1 pessary inserted into the vagina each evening at first, then 1 pessary twice a week.
Availability: NHS and private prescription.
Side effects: tender breasts, fluid retention, headaches, nausea, vaginal bleeding, weight gain, skin changes, rashes, liver function disorders, sodium retention, vomiting.
Caution: in patients suffering from high blood pressure, diabetes, vascular disorders, asthma, kidney disease, heart disease, epilepsy, migraine, thyrotoxicosis, womb diseases. Your doctor may advise you to have regular examinations.
Not to be used for: children, pregnant women, nursing mothers, or for patients suffering from sickle-cell anaemia, thrombosis, liver disorders, some cancers, undiagnosed vaginal bleeding, some ear, skin, and kidney disorders, porphyria (a rare blood disorder), brain blood vessel disease.
Caution needed with: DIURETICS, ANTIHYPERTENSIVES, and drugs that change liver enzymes (eg BARBITURATES, CARBAMAZEPINE, PHENYTOIN).
Contains: OESTRIOL.
Other preparations: Ortho-Gynest Cream.

Ortho-Novin 1/50
(Cilag)

A white tablet used as an oestrogen, progestogen contraceptive.

Dose: 1 tablet a day for 21 days starting on day 5 of the period.
Availability: NHS and private prescription.
Side effects: enlarged breasts, bloating and fluid retention, cramps, leg pains, mood change, reduction in sexual desire, headaches, nausea, vaginal erosion, discharge, and bleeding, weight gain, skin changes.
Caution: in patients suffering from high blood pressure, diabetes, vascular disorders, asthma, depression, kidney disease, multiple sclerosis, womb diseases. Your doctor may advise you not to smoke, to have regular examinations. You should stop treatment at the first sign of serious symptoms such as severe headache or jaundice. Treatment should be stopped before surgery.
Not to be used for: pregnant women, or for patients suffering from sickle-cell anaemia, history of heart disease or thrombosis, liver disorders, some cancers, undiagnosed vaginal bleeding, some ear, skin, and kidney disorders.
Caution needed with: RIFAMPICIN, TETRACYCLINES, GRISEOFULVIN, BARBITURATES, PHENYTOIN, PRIMIDONE, CARBAMAZEPINE, ETHOSUXIMIDE, CHLORAL HYDRATE, DICHLORALPHENAZONE.

Contains: MESTRANOL, NORETHISTERONE.
Other preparations: NORINYL-I (Syntex).

Orudis
(Rhone-Poulenc Rorer)

A green/purple capsule or a pink capsule according to strengths of 50 mg, 100 mg and used as a NON-STEROID ANTI-INFLAMMATORY DRUG to treat rheumatoid arthritis, osteoarthritis, ankylosing spondylitis, acute articular and joint disorders, painful periods.

Dose: 50-100 mg twice a day with food.
Availability: NHS and private prescription.
Side effects: stomach intolerance, rash.
Caution: in the elderly, pregnant women and in patients suffering from kidney, heart, or liver disease.
Not to be used for: children or for patients suffering from severe kidney disease, stomach ulcer or a history of recurring ulcer, asthma, allergy to ASPIRIN/NON-STEROID ANTI-INFLAMMATORY DRUGS, inflammation of the anus or rectum.
Caution needed with: anticoagulants, sulphonamide antibiotics, hydantoins, METHOTREXATE.
Contains: KETOPROFEN.
Other preparations: ALRHEUMAT (Bayer), ORUVAIL (Rhone-Poulenc Rorer).

Oruvail *see* Orudis
(Rhone-Poulenc Rorer)

Ossopan 800
(Sanofi Winthrop)

A buff-coloured tablet supplied at a strength of 830 mg and used as a calcium-phosphorus supplement to treat osteoporosis, rickets, osteomalacia (bone disorders).

Dose: adults 4-8 tablets a day in divided doses before food; children as advised by the physician.
Availability: NHS, private prescription, over the counter.
Side effects:
Caution: in patients suffering from kidney disease, severe loss of movement, immobility, or a history of kidney stones.
Not to be used for: patients suffering from elevated blood or urine calcium.

Caution needed with:
Contains: HYDROXYAPATITE compound.
Other preparations: Ossopan Powder

Otomize
(Stafford-Miller)

A suspension supplied in a pump spray, and used as an antibiotic and STEROID to treat outer ear conditions.

Dose: 1 spray 3 times a day until 2 days after symptoms disappear.
Availability: NHS and private prescription.
Side effects: stinging or burning.
Caution: in pregnant women.
Not to be used for: patients suffering from perforated ear drum.
Caution needed with:
Contains: NEOMYCIN, DEXAMETHASONE.
Other preparations:

Otosporin
(Wellcome)

Drops used as an antibiotic, STEROID treatment for bacterial infections and inflammation of the outer ear.

Dose: 3 drops into the ear 3-4 times a day.
Availability: NHS and private prescription.
Side effects: additional infection.
Caution: in infants and in patients suffering from perforated ear drum — do not use over extended periods.
Not to be used for:
Caution needed with:
Contains: POLYMYXIN B SULPHATE, NEOMYCIN sulphate, HYDROCORTISONE.
Other preparations:

Otrivine
(Zyma)

A spray and drops used as a SYMPATHOMIMETIC preparation to clear blocked nose.

Dose: adults 2-3 drops or 1 spray into each nostril 2-3 times a day; children use paediatric drops.
Availability: NHS (when prescribed as a generic), private prescription,

over the counter.
Side effects: itching nose, headache, sleeplessness, rapid heart rate.
Caution: in pregnant women; do not use for extended periods.
Not to be used for: infants under 3 months.
Caution needed with: MAOIS.
Contains: XYLOMETAZOLINE hydrochloride.
Other preparations: Otrivine Paediatric.

Otrivine-Antistin — nasal spray/drops as a SYMPATHOMIMETIC/ANTIHISTAMINE treatment for hay fever/allergic rhinitis. Product now discontinued.

Otrivine-Antistin Eye Drops
(Zyma)

Drops used as a SYMPATHOMIMETIC, ANTIHISTAMINE treatment for allergic conjunctivitis and other eye inflammations.

Dose: adults 1-2 drops into the eye 2-3 times a day; children over 5 years 1 drop 2-3 times a day.
Availability: NHS, private prescription, over the counter.
Side effects: temporary smarting, headache, drowsiness, blurred vision.
Caution: in patients suffering from high blood pressure, overactive thyroid, dry eyes, coronary disease, diabetes.
Not to be used for: children under 5 years, or for patients suffering from glaucoma or who wear contact lenses.
Caution needed with: MAOIS.
Contains: XYLOMETAZOLINE hydrochloride.
Other preparations:

Ovestin
(Organon)

A white tablet supplied at a strength of 0.25 mg, and used as an oestrogen for treating genital or urinary complaints caused by oestrogen deficiency, and some cases of infertility.

Dose: genital/urinary complaints, 0.5-3 mg a day for 1 month then 0.5-1 mg a day. Infertility, 0.25-1 mg on days 6-15 of cycle.
Availability: NHS and private prescription.
Side effects: enlarged breasts, fluid retention, headaches, nausea, vaginal bleeding, weight gain, skin changes, rash, liver disorder, jaundice, vomiting.
Caution: in patients suffering from high blood pressure, heart disease,

diabetes, vascular disorders, asthma, kidney disease, womb disease, migraine, thyroid disorder, epilepsy.

Not to be used for: pregnant women, nursing mothers, or for patients suffering from sickle-cell anaemia, thrombosis, liver disorders, some cancers, undiagnosed vaginal bleeding, some ear, skin, and kidney disorders, brain blood vessel disease, porphyria (a rare blood disorder)

Caution needed with: DIURETICS, ANTIHYPERTENSIVES, drugs which induce liver enzymes (eg BARBITURATES, CARBAMAZEPINE, PHENYTOIN, PRIMIDONE, RIFAMPICIN).

Contains: OESTRIOL.

Other preparations: OVESTIN CREAM, (used to treat vaginal conditions requiring oestrogen therapy).

Ovestin Cream
(Organon)

A cream used as an oestrogen treatment for atrophic inflammation of the vagina, itch, as a treatment before vaginal surgery, other diseases of the vulva.

Dose: 1 application a day for 3 weeks, then 1 application twice a week.
Availability: NHS and private prescription.
Side effects: tender breasts, fluid retention, headaches, nausea, vaginal bleeding, weight gain, skin changes, rashes, vomiting, sodium retention, liver disorder, jaundice.
Caution: in patients suffering from high blood pressure, diabetes, vascular disorders, asthma, kidney disease, womb diseases, heart disease, epilepsy, migraine. Your doctor may advise you to have regular examinations.
Not to be used for: children, pregnant women, nursing mothers, or for patients suffering from sickle-cell anaemia, brain blood vessel disease, thrombosis, liver disorders, some cancers, undiagnosed vaginal bleeding, some ear, skin, and kidney disorders, porphyria (a rare blood disorder).
Caution needed with: DIURETICS, ANTIHYPERTENSIVES, and drugs that change liver enzymes (eg BARBITURATES, CARBAMAZEPINE, PHENYTOIN).
Contains: OESTRIOL.
Other preparations: Ovestin Tablets.

Ovran
(Wyeth)

A white tablet used as an oestrogen, progestogen contraceptive.

Dose: 1 tablet a day for 21 days starting on day 5 of the period.

Availability: NHS and private prescription.
Side effects: enlarged breasts, bloating and fluid retention, cramps, leg pains, mood change, reduction in sexual desire, headaches, nausea, vaginal erosion, discharge, and bleeding, weight gain, skin changes.
Caution: in patients suffering from high blood pressure, diabetes, vascular disorders, asthma, depression, kidney disease, multiple sclerosis, womb diseases. Your doctor may advise you not to smoke, to have regular examinations. You should stop treatment at the first sign of serious symptoms such as severe headache or jaundice. Treatment should be stopped before surgery.
Not to be used for: pregnant women, or for patients suffering from sickle-cell anaemia, history of heart disease or thrombosis, liver disorders, some cancers, undiagnosed vaginal bleeding, some ear, skin, and kidney disorders.
Caution needed with: RIFAMPICIN, TETRACYCLINES, GRISEOFULVIN, BARBITURATES, PHENYTOIN, PRIMIDONE, CARBAMAZEPINE, ETHOSUXIMIDE, CHLORAL HYDRATE, DICHLORALPHENAZONE.
Contains: ETHINYLOESTRADIOL, LEVONORGESTREL.
Other preparations: Ovran 30 (lower-strength preparation).

Ovranette
(Wyeth)

A white tablet used as an oestrogen, progestogen contraceptive.

Dose: 1 tablet a day for 21 days starting on day 5 of the period.
Availability: NHS and private prescription.
Side effects: enlarged breasts, bloating and fluid retention, cramps, leg pains, mood change, reduction in sexual desire, headaches, nausea, vaginal erosion, discharge, and bleeding, weight gain, skin changes.
Caution: in patients suffering from high blood pressure, diabetes, vascular disorders, asthma, depression, kidney disease, multiple sclerosis, womb diseases. Your doctor may advise you not to smoke, to have regular examinations. You should stop treatment at the first sign of serious symptoms such as severe headache or jaundice. Treatment should be stopped before surgery.
Not to be used for: pregnant women, or for patients suffering from sickle-cell anaemia, history of heart disease or thrombosis, liver disorders, some cancers, undiagnosed vaginal bleeding, some ear, skin, and kidney disorders.
Caution needed with: RIFAMPICIN, TETRACYCLINES, GRISEOFULVIN, BARBITURATES, PHENYTOIN, PRIMIDONE, CARBAMAZEPINE, ETHOSUXIMIDE, CHLORAL HYDRATE, DICHLORALPHENAZONE.
Contains: ETHINYLOESTRADIOL, LEVONORGESTREL.
Other preparations: MICROGYNON-30 (Schering).

Ovysmen
(Cilag)

A white tablet used as an oestrogen, progestogen contraceptive.

Dose: 1 tablet a day for 21 days starting on day 5 of the period.
Availability: NHS and private prescription.
Side effects: enlarged breasts, bloating and fluid retention, cramps, leg pains, mood change, reduction in sexual desire, headaches, nausea, vaginal erosion, discharge, and bleeding, weight gain, skin changes.
Caution: in patients suffering from high blood pressure, diabetes, vascular disorders, asthma, depression, kidney disease, multiple sclerosis, womb diseases. Your doctor may advise you not to smoke, to have regular examinations. You should stop treatment at the first sign of serious symptoms such as severe headache or jaundice. Treatment should be stopped before surgery.
Not to be used for: pregnant women, or for patients suffering from sickle-cell anaemia, history of heart disease or thrombosis, liver disorders, some cancers, undiagnosed vaginal bleeding, some ear, skin, and kidney disorders.
Caution needed with: RIFAMPICIN, TETRACYCLINES, GRISEOFULVIN, BARBITURATES, PHENYTOIN, PRIMIDONE, CARBAMAZEPINE, ETHOSUXIMIDE, CHLORAL HYDRATE, DICHLORALPHENAZONE.
Contains: ETHINYLOESTRADIOL, NORGESTREL.
Other preparations: BREVINOR (Syntex).

---

oxamniquine *see* Vansil

Oxanid *see* Oxazepam. Product now discontinued.

---

oxatomide *see* Tinset

---

oxazepam

A tablet supplied at strengths of 10 mg, 15 mg, 30 mg and used as a sedative to treat anxiety.

Dose: elderly 10-20 mg 3-4 times a day; adults 15-30 mg 3-4 times a day increasing to 60 mg 3 times a day if needed.
Availability: NHS and private prescription.
Side effects: drowsiness, confusion, unsteadiness, low blood pressure,

rash, changes in vision, changes in libido, retention of urine. Risk of addiction increases with dose and length of treatment. May impair judgement.

Caution: in the elderly, pregnant women, nursing mothers, in women during labour, and in patients suffering from lung disorders, kidney or liver disorders. Avoid long-term use and withdraw gradually.

Not to be used for: children, or for patients suffering from acute lung diseases, some chronic lung diseases, some obsessional and psychotic diseases.

Caution needed with: alcohol, other tranquillizers, anticonvulsants.

Contains:

Other preparations: oxazepam capsules, OXANID.

---

oxerutins *see* **Paroven**

---

oxethazaine *see* **Mucaine**

---

oxitropium bromide *see* **Oxivent**

Oxivent
(Boehringer)

An aerosol supplied at a strength of 100 micrograms per dose, and used as an ANTICHOLINERGIC treatment for asthma and other diseases associated with breathing obstruction.

Dose: 2 puffs 2-3 times a day.
Availability: NHS and private prescription.
Side effects: irritation, nausea, dry mouth, ANTICHOLINERGIC effects.
Caution: in patients suffering from glaucoma, enlarged prostate, wheezing, or coughing. Avoid the eyes.
Not to be used for: children, pregnant women, nursing mothers, or for patients sensitive to ATROPINE or IPRATROPIUM BROMIDE.
Caution needed with:
Contains: OXITROPIUM BROMIDE.
Other preparations:

---

oxpentifylline *see* **Trental**

oxprenolol *see* **Slow-Trasicor, Trasicor, Trasidrex**

oxybuprocaine hydrochloride *see* **Opulets Benoxinate**

oxybutynin *see* **Ditropan, Cystrin**

oxymetazoline hydrochloride *see* **Afrazine**

oxymetholone *see* **Anapolon**

Oxymycin *see* **Tetracycline**
(DDSA)

oxypertine *see* **Integrin**

oxyphenbutazone *see* **Tanderil**

Oxyprenix 160-SR *see* **Slow-Trasicor**
(Ashbourne)

oxytetracycline hydrochloride *see* **Terra-Cortril, Terra-Cortril Spray;** *see also* **Tetracycline**

Oxytetramix-250 *see* **Tetracycline**
(Ashbourne)

p-aminobenzoic acid *see* **Labiton**

Pacitron — antidepressant. Product now discontinued.

Paedialyte RS — treatment for dehydration. Product now discontinued.

Palaprin Forte
(Nicholas)

An orange, oval, scored tablet supplied at a strength of 600 mg and used as a NON-STEROID ANTI-INFLAMMATORY DRUG to treat rheumatoid arthritis, osteoarthritis, spondylitis.

Dose: 1 tablet per 6.5 kg body weight a day in divided doses dispersed in water, sucked, chewed, or swallowed whole.
Availability: NHS, private prescription, over the counter.
Side effects: stomach upsets, allergy, asthma.
Caution: in pregnant women, the elderly, or in patients with a history of allergy to aspirin, asthma, impaired kidney or liver function, indigestion.
Not to be used for: children, nursing mothers, or patients suffering from haemophilia, or ulcers.
Caution needed with: anticoagulants (blood-thinning drugs), some antidiabetic drugs, anti-inflammatory agents, METHOTREXATE, SPIRONOLACTONE, STEROIDS, some uric acid-lowering drugs, ANTACIDS.
Contains: ALOXIPRIN.
Other preparations:

Paldesic *see* Calpol Infant
(RP Drugs)

Palfium
(Boehringer Mannheim)

A white, scored tablet or a peach, scored tablet according to strengths of 5 mg, 10 mg and used as an opiate to control severe and prolonged pain.

Dose: adults up to 5 mg initially, and then as advised by physician; children 88 micrograms per kg body weight or as advised by the physician.
Availability: controlled drug; NHS and private prescription.
Side effects: tolerance, addiction, dizziness, sweating, nausea.
Caution: in the elderly, in pregnant women, and in patients suffering from liver disease, underactive thyroid gland.
Not to be used for: women in labour or for patients suffering from respiratory depression or blocked airways.
Caution needed with: MAOIS, sedatives.
Contains: DEXTROMORAMIDE tartrate.

Other preparations: Palfium Injection, Palfium Suppositories.

Paludrine
(ICI)

A white, scored tablet supplied at a strength of 100 mg and used as an antimalarial drug for the prevention of malaria.

Dose: adults and children over 14 years 2 tablets a day after meals; children under 1 year ¼ tablet, 1-4 years ½ tablet, 5-8 years 1 tablet, 9-12 years 1½ tablets after meals.
Availability: NHS, private prescription, over the counter.
Side effects: stomach upset, skin reactions, hair loss, mouth ulcers.
Caution: in patients suffering from severe kidney failure.
Not to be used for:
Caution needed with:
Contains: PROGUANIL hydrochloride.
Other preparations:

Pameton
(Sanofi Winthrop)

A white tablet used as an ANALGESIC to relieve pain and reduce fever, especially where misuse of PARACETAMOL may occur.

Dose: adults 2 tablets up to 4 times a day; children 6-12 years ½-1 tablet every 4 hours to a maximum of 4 doses a day.
Availability: private prescription and over the counter.
Side effects:
Caution: in pregnant women and in patients suffering from liver disease.
Not to be used for: children under 6 years.
Caution needed with: levodopa, other medicines containing PARACETAMOL.
Contains: PARACETAMOL, METHIONINE.
Other preparations:

Panadeine
(Sterling Winthrop)

A white, scored tablet used as an ANALGESIC to relieve pain and reduce fever.

Dose: adults 2 tablets up to 4 times a day; children 7-12 years ½ -1 tablet up to 4 times a day.
Availability: NHS (when prescribed as a generic), private prescription,

over the counter.

Side effects:
Caution: in patients suffering from liver or kidney disease.
Not to be used for: children under 7 years.
Caution needed with: other medicines containing PARACETAMOL.
Contains: PARACETAMOL, CODEINE PHOSPHATE.
Other preparations: CO-CODAMOL, PARACODOL (Fisons), (Panadeine Soluble, Panadeine Forte — both now discontinued.)

Panadol *see* **paracetamol tablets**
(Sterling Health)

Panaleve *see* **Calpol Infant**
(Pinewood)

Pancrease
(Cilag)

A white capsule used as a source of pancreatic enzymes to treat pancreatic exocrine insufficiency as in cystic fibrosis and chronic pancreatitis.

Dose: 1-2 capsules during meals or 1 capsule with a snack
Availability: NHS, private prescription, over the counter.
Side effects: perianal irritation.
Caution:
Not to be used for:
Caution needed with:
Contains: PANCREATIN.
Other preparations: COTAZYME, CREON (Duphar), NUTRIZYM GR (Merck), PANCREX V (Paines & Byrne).

---

pancreatin *see* **Cotazym, Creon, Nutrizym GR, Pancrease, Pancrex V Forte Tablets**

Pancrex V Forte Tablets
(Paines & Byrne)

A white tablet used as a source of pancreatic enzymes to treat cystic fibrosis, steatorrhoea, pancreatic enzyme deficiency states due to pancreatic disease.

Dose: 6-10 tablets before each meal.
Availability: NHS, private prescription, over the counter.
Side effects: irritation of the mouth or anus.
Caution:
Not to be used for:
Caution needed with:
Contains: PANCREATIN.
Other preparations: Pancrex V Capsules, Pancrex V Capsules, Pancrex V Powder, Pancrex Granules, Pancrex V Tablets, COTAZYME, CREON (Duphar), NUTRIZYM GR (Merck), PANCREASE (Cilag)..

Panoxyl
(Stiefel)

A gel used as an antibacterial, skin softener to treat acne.

Dose: wash and dry the affected area, then apply once a day.
Availability: NHS, private prescription, over the counter.
Side effects: irritation, peeling.
Caution: keep out of the eyes, nose, mouth. May bleach fabrics.
Not to be used for:
Caution needed with:
Contains: BENZOYL PEROXIDE.
Other preparations: Panoxyl Aquagel, Panoxyl Wash, ACETOXYL (Stiefel), ACNECIDE (Galderma), ACNEGEL (Stiefel), BENOXYL (Stiefel), BENZAGEL (Bioglan), NERICUR (Schering), QUINODERM (Quinoderm).

---

panthenol *see* **Lipoflavonoid, Lipotriad**

---

papaveretum *see* **Aspav**

---

papaverine *see* **APP, Brovon, Rybarvin**

---

para-aminosalicylic acid *see* **Cytacon**

---

paracetamol *see* **Alvedon, Cafadol, Calpol Infant, Co-Codamol,**

co-dydramol, co-proxamol, Disprol Paed, Femerital, Fortagesic, Lobak, Medised Suspension, Medocodene, Midrid, Migraleve, Pameton, Panadeine, paracetamol tablets, Paracodol, Parahypon, Parake, Paramax, Paramol, Pardale, Propain, Remedeine, Solpadol, Salzone, Solpadeine, Syndol, Tylex, Uniflu and Gregovite C

---

paracetamol paediatric elixir *see* **Calpol**

---

paracetamol tablets

A tablet supplied at a strength of 500 mg and used as an ANALGESIC to relieve pain and reduce fever.

Dose: adults 1-2 tablet 4 times a day; children 6-12 years ½-1 tablet 4 times a day.
Availability: NHS, private prescription, over the counter.
Side effects:
Caution: in patients suffering from kidney or liver disease.
Not to be used for: children under 6 years.
Caution needed with: other medicines containing PARACETAMOL.
Contains: PARACETAMOL.
Other preparations: paracetamol soluble, paracetamol elixir, PANADOL (Sterling Health), RIMADOL (Rima).

Paracodol
(Fisons)

A white, effervescent tablet used as an ANALGESIC to relieve pain.

Dose: adults 1-2 tablets in water every 4-6 hours to a maximum of 8 tablets in 24 hours; children 6-12 years ½-1 tablet to a maximum of 4 doses in 24 hours.
Availability: NHS (when prescribed as a generic), private presciption, over the counter.
Side effects:
Caution: in patients with kidney or liver disease or who are on a limited consumption of salt.
Not to be used for: children under 6 years.
Caution needed with: other medicines containing PARACETAMOL.
Contains: PARACETAMOL, CODEINE PHOSPHATE (CO-CODAMOL).
Other preparations: CO-CODAMOL TABLETS, PANADEINE (Sterling Health).

paradichlorobenzene *see* **Cerumol**

---

paraffin, liquid *see* **Agarol**

Parahypon *see* **co-codamol tablets.** Product now discontinued.

Parake
(Galen)

A white tablet used as an ANALGESIC to relieve pain and reduce fever.

Dose: 2 tablets every 4 hours to a maximum of 8 tablets in 24 hours.
Availability: NHS (when prescribed as a generic), private prescription, over the counter.
Side effects:
Caution: in patients suffering from liver or kidney disease.
Not to be used for: children.
Caution needed with: other medicines containing PARACETAMOL.
Contains: PARACETAMOL, CODEINE PHOSPHATE (CO-CODAMOL).
Other preparations:

Paramax
(Bencard)

A white, scored tablet used as an ANALGESIC, anti-emetic treatment for migraine.

Dose: adults over 20 years 2 tablets at the beginning of the attack, then 2 tablets every 4 hours to a maximum of 6 tablets in 24 hours; 15-19 years and with a body weight over 60 kg, 2 tablets at the beginning of the attack to a maximum of 5 tablets in 24 hours; children 12-14 years and body weight over 30 kg 1 tablet at the beginning to a maximum of 3 tablets in 24 hours.
Availability: NHS and private prescription.
Side effects: extrapyramidal reactions (shaking and rigidity), drowsiness, diarrhoea.
Caution: pregnant women, nursing mothers, and in patients suffering from liver or kidney disease.
Not to be used for: children under 12 years.
Caution needed with: ANTICHOLINERGICS, sedatives, other medicines containing PARACETAMOL.

Contains: PARACETAMOL, METOCLOPRAMIDE hydrochloride.
Other preparations: Paramax Sachets.

Paramol *see* **Co-dydramol.**

Pardale *see* **co-codamol.** Product now discontinued.

Parfenac
(Lederle)

A cream used as a NON-STEROID ANTI-INFLAMMATORY treatment for inflammation in dermatitis and itching.

Dose: apply sparingly and rub in 2-3 times a day.
Availability: NHS and private prescription.
Side effects:
Caution:
Not to be used for:
Caution needed with:
Contains: BUFEXAMAC.
Other preparations:

Paritane *see* **Trasicor.** Product now discontinued.

Parlodel
(Sandoz)

A white, scored tablet supplied at strengths of 1 mg, 2.5 mg and used as a hormone blocker to treat Parkinson's disease, inappropriate lactation, infertility, cyclical benign breast disease, elevated prolactin.

Dose: 1-1.25 mg at night with food at first, increasing after 7 days to 2.5 mg at night, then after 14 days to 2.5 mg twice a day with food. Increase if needed every 3-14 days by 2.5 mg a day to 10-40 mg a day in 3 divided doses.
Availability: NHS and private prescription.
Side effects: low blood pressure on standing, brain and stomach disturbances, nausea, vomiting, constipation, headache, drowsiness, poor circulation, movement disorders, dry mouth, leg cramps, lung changes, dizziness, convulsions.

490

Caution: in women, patients suffering from a history of mental disorder, severe cardiovascular disease. Your doctor may advise regular examinations.
Not to be used for: children, women with complications of pregnancy, or for patients suffering from allergy to ERGOTAMINE.
Caution needed with: alcohol, ERYHTROMYCIN, ERGOTAMINE, drugs affecting blood pressure.
Contains: BROMOCRIPTINE MESYLATE.
Other preparations: Parlodel Capsules

Parmid *see* **Maxolon**
(Lagap)

Parnate
(S K B)

A red tablet used as an MAOI antidepressant to treat depression.

Dose: 1 tablet twice a day at first, increasing after 7 days if necessary to 1 tablet 3 times a day, then usually 1 tablet a day.
Availability: NHS and private prescription.
Side effects: severe high blood pressure reactions with certain foods, sleeplessness, low blood pressure, dizziness, drowsiness, weakness, dry mouth, constipation, stomach upset, blurred vision, urinary difficulties, ankle swelling, rash, jaundice, weight gain, confusion, sexual desire changes.
Caution: in the elderly and in patients suffering from epilepsy.
Not to be used for: children, or for patients suffering from liver disease, blood changes, heart disease, phaeochromocytoma, overactive thyroid, brain artery disease.
Caution needed with: amphetamines or similar SYMPATHOMIMETIC drugs, TRICYCLIC antidepressants, PETHIDINE and other similar ANALGESICS, some cough mixtures and appetite supressants containing SYMPATHOMIMETICS. BARBITURATES, sedatives, alcohol, and antidiabetics may be enhanced. ANTICHOLINERGIC side effects are increased. Cheese, Bovril, Oxo, meat extracts, broad beans, banana, Marmite, yeast extracts, wine, beer, other alcohol, pickled herrings, vegetable proteins. (Up to 14 days after cessation.)
Contains: TRANYLCYPROMINE sulphate.
Other preparations:

Paroven
(Zyma)

A yellow capsule supplied at a strength of 250 mg and used as a vein constrictor to treat ankle swelling, varicose veins.

Dose: 2 capsules twice a day.
Availability: NHS, private prescription, over the counter.
Side effects: stomach disturbances, flushes, headache.
Caution:
Not to be used for: children.
Caution needed with:
Contains: OXERUTINS.
Other preparations:

---

paroxetene *see* **Seroxat**

Parstelin
(S K B)

A green tablet used as an MAOI to treat depression with anxiety.

Dose: 1 tablet twice a day at first, increasing to 1 tablet 3 times a day if needed after 7 days, then usually 1 tablet a day.
Availability: NHS and private prescription.
Side effects: severe high blood pressure reactions with certain foods, low blood pressure, muscle spasms, restlessness, low body temperature, breast swelling, menstrual changes, sleeplessness, low blood pressure, dizziness, drowsiness, weakness, dry mouth, constipation, stomach upset, blurred vision, urinary difficulties, ankle swelling, rash, blood and skin changes, jaundice, weight gain, confusion, sexual desire changes.
Caution: in the elderly, pregnant women, nursing mothers, and in patients suffering from epilepsy. Your doctor may advise regular blood and liver checks.
Not to be used for: children, or for patients suffering from liver disease, blood changes, heart disease, phaeochromocytoma, overactive thyroid, brain artery disease, Parkinson's disease.
Caution needed with: amphetamines or similar SYMPATHOMIMETIC drugs, tricyclic antidepressants, tranquillizers, LEVODOPA, PETHIDINE and other similar analgesics, some cough mixtures and appetite supressants containing SYMPATHOMIMETICS. BARBITURATES, sedatives, alcohol, and antidiabetics may be enhanced. ANTICHOLINERGIC side effects are increased. Cheese, Bovril, Oxo, meat extracts, broad beans, banana, Marmite, yeast extracts, wine, beer, other alcohol, pickled herrings, vegetable proteins.

(Up to 14 days after cessation.)
Contains: TRANYLCYPROMINE sulphate, TRIFLUOPERAZINE.
Other preparations:

Parvolex
(Evans)

An ampoule used to supply amino acid for the treatment of PARACETAMOL overdose.

Dose: as advised by doctor. Commence within 15 hours of PARACETAMOL ingestion.
Availability: NHS and private prescription.
Side effects: rash, allergy.
Caution: in patients with a history of asthma. Blood should be checked regularly.
Not to be used for:
Caution needed with: rubber, metals.
Contains: ACETYLCYSTEINE.
Other preparations:

Pavacol-D
(Boehringer Ingelheim)

A mixture containing opiate and demulcents used to treat cough.

Dose: adults 5-10 ml as needed; children 1-2 years 2.5 ml 3-4 times a day,3-5 years 5 ml 3 times a day, 6-12 years 5 ml 4-5 times a day.
Availability: NHS, private prescription, over the counter.
Side effects: constipation.
Caution: patients suffering from asthma
Not to be used for: for infants under 1 year or for patients suffering from liver disease.
Caution needed with: MAOIS.
Contains: PHOLCODINE, aromatic oils.
Other preparations: GALENPHOL (Galen), PHOLCODINE LINCTUS, PHOLCOMED-D (Medo).

Paxofen *see* **Brufen.** Product now discontinued.

Paynocil *see* **aspirin tablets.** Product now discontinued.

PC4
(Schering)

A white tablet used as an oestrogen, progestogen contraceptive in an emergency within 72 hours of intercourse where no other precautions have been taken.

Dose: 2 tablets within 72 hours of intercourse, then a further 2 tablets 12 hours later.
Availability: NHS and private prescription.
Side effects: vomiting, nausea.
Caution: in patients with a history of depression, diabetes, high blood pressure, epilepsy, porphyria (a rare blood disorder), tetanus, liver and kidney disease, gallstones, cardiovascular disease.
Not to be used for: women whose menstrual bleeding is overdue.
Caution needed with: RIFAMPICIN, TETRACYCLINES, GRISEOFULVIN, BARBITURATES, PHENYTOIN, PRIMIDONE, CARBAMAZIPINE, MEPROBAMATE, GLUTETHIMIDE, CHORAL HYDRATE, DICHLORALPHENAZONE, ETHOSUXIMIDE, CHLORPROMAZINE.
Contains: ETHINYLOESTRADIOL, NORGESTREL.
Other preparations:

Pecram *see* Phyllocontin
(Zyma)

---

pectin *see* Orabase

---

pemoline *see* Volital

Penbritin
(Beecham)

A black/red capsule supplied at strengths of 250 mg, 500 mg and used as a penicillin to treat respiratory, ear, nose, and throat infections, gonorrhoea, soft tissue infections, urinary infections.

Dose: adults 250 mg-1 g every 6 hours; children 125-250 mg every 6 hours.
Availability: NHS and private prescription.
Side effects: allergy, stomach disturbances.
Caution: in patients suffering from glandular fever.
Not to be used for: patients suffering from penicillin allergy.

Caution needed with:
Contains: AMPICILLIN.
Other preparations: AMPICILLIN, AMPILAR, RIMACILLIN (Rima), VIDOPEN (Berk).

penbutolol *see* Lasipressin

Pendramine
(Asta)

A white, oblong, scored tablet supplied at strengths of 125 mg, 250 mg and used as an anti-rheumatic drug to treat severe rheumatoid arthritis, and to assist in liver disease, Wilson's disease, some cases of poisoning, cystinuria where metallic compounds need to be bound.

Dose: adults 125-250 mg a day for the first 4-8 weeks, increasing by similar amounts at no less than 4-week intervals to a maximum of 2 g a day; children 15-20 mg per kg body weight a day starting at a lower dose and increasing at 4-week intervals over a period of 3-6 months.
Availability: NHS and private prescription.
Side effects: nausea, anorexia, fever, rash, loss of taste, blood changes, blood or protein in the urine, myasthenia gravis (a muscle disease), systemic lupus erythematosus (a multisystem disorder).
Caution: in patients suffering from kidney disease or who are sensitive to penicillin.
Not to be used for: pregnant women, nursing mothers, or for patients suffering from systemic lupus erythematosus (a multisystem disorder), low platelet levels, agranulocytosis (low white count).
Caution needed with: gold salts, antimalaria or cytotoxic drugs, PHENYLBUTAZONE.
Contains: PENICILLAMINE.
Other preparations: DISTAMINE (Dista).

penicillamine *see* Distamine, Pendramine

penicillin V potassium *see* Distaquaine V-K, Stabillin V-K, V-Cil-K

Penidural
(Wyeth)

A suspension used as a penicillin antibiotic to treat infections.

Dose: adults 10 ml every 6-8 hours; children half adult dose.
Availability: NHS and private prescription.
Side effects: allergic reactions, stomach upset.
Caution: in patients suffering from kidney damage.
Not to be used for:
Caution needed with:
Contains: BENZATHINE PENICILLIN.
Other preparations: Penidural Oral Drops — now discontinued.

Penmix *see* **insulin**
(Novo Nordisk)

---

pentaerythritol *see* **Cardiacap**

---

pentaerythritol tetranitrate *see* **Mycardol**

Pentasa *see* **Asacol**
(Brocades)

---

pentazocine *see* **Fortagesic, Fortral**

Penthiazide *see* **Trasidrex**

Pentran *see* **Epanutin**
(Berk)

Pepcid
(Morson)

A brown, square tablet supplied at strengths of 20 mg, 40 mg and used as an H_2 blocker in the prevention and treatment of duodenal and gastric ulcers, Zollinger-Ellison syndrome (high acid production).

Dose: adults prevention 20 mg at night, otherwise 40 mg at night and up to 800 mg a day.
Availability: NHS and private prescription.
Side effects: headache, dizziness, constipation, diarrhoea, dry mouth, nausea, rash, bowel discomfort, loss of appetite, fatigue.
Caution: in pregnant women, nursing mothers, and in patients suffering from impaired kidney function. Stomach cancer should be excluded as a diagnosis.
Not to be used for: children.
Caution needed with:
Contains: FAMOTIDINE.
Other preparations:

---

peppermint oil *see* Carbellon, Colpermin, Mintec, Tercoda

---

pepsin *see* Muripsin

Peptard — ANTICHOLINERGIC treatment for stomach ulcer/irritable bowel syndrome/sweating. Product now discontinued.

Peptimax *see* Tagamet
(Ashbourne)

Percutol
(Cusi)

An ointment used as a NITRATE for the prevention of angina.

Dose: apply every 3-4 hours or as advised.
Availability: NHS, private prescription, over the counter.
Side effects: headache.
Caution:
Not to be used for: children.
Caution needed with:
Contains: GLYCERYL TRINITRATE.
Other preparations: CORO-NITRO (Boehringer Mannheim), DEPONIT (Schwarz), GLYTRIN (Sanofi Winthrop), NITRO-DUR (Schering Plough), NITROCONTIN (Asta), NITROLINGUAL (Lipha), SUSCARD BUCCAL (Pharmax), SUSTAC (Pharmax), TRANSIDERM-NITRO (Ciba).

pergolide mesylate *see* **Celance**

Periactin
(MSD)

A white, scored tablet supplied at a strength of 4 mg and used as an
ANTIHISTAMINE, serotonin antagonist (hormone blocker) to improve
appetite,and to treat allergies, itchy skin conditions, migraine.

Dose: adults 1 tablet 3-4 times a day; children reduced doses.
Availability: NHS, private prescription, over the counter.
Side effects: ANTICHOLINERGIC effects, reduced reactions, drowsiness.
Caution: in pregnant women and in patients suffering from bronchial
asthma, raised eye pressure, overactive thyroid, cardiovascular disease,
high blood pressure.
Not to be used for: children under 2 years, nursing mothers, the elderly,
or patients suffering from glaucoma, enlarged prostate, bladder obstruc-
tion, retention of urine, stomach blockage, stomach ulcer, or debilitation.
Caution needed with: MAOIS, alcohol, sedatives.
Contains: CYPROHEPTADINE hydrochloride.
Other preparations: Periactin Syrup.

---

pericyazine *see* **Neulactil**

---

perindoprol *see* **Coversyl**

---

permethrin *see* **Lyclear**

Permitabs *see* potassium permanganate
(Bioglan)

---

perphenazine *see* **Fentazin, Triptafen**

Persantin
(Boehringer Ingelheim)

An orange tablet or a white tablet according to strengths of 25 mg, 100 mg and used as an anti-platelet drug in addition to oral anticoagulants or ASPIRIN to prevent thrombosis.

Dose: adults 300-600 mg a day in 3-4 doses before meals; children 5 mg per kg body weight a day in divided doses.
Availability: NHS and private prescription.
Side effects: headache, dizziness, stomach upset, rash.
Caution: care in patients suffering from rapidly worsening angina, and some other heart conditions.
Not to be used for:
Caution needed with: ANTACIDS.
Contains: DIPYRIDAMOLE.
Other preparations: CEREBROVASE (Ashbourne), VASYROL (Shire).

Pertofran
(Ciba Geigy)

A pale-pink tablet supplied at a strength of 25 mg and used as a TRICYCLIC antidepressant to treat depression.

Dose: adults 1 tablet 3 times a day at first increasing to 2 tablets 3-4 times a day; elderly 1 tablet a day at first.
Availability: NHS and private prescription.
Side effects: dry mouth, constipation, urine retention, blurred vision, palpitations, drowsiness, sleeplessness, dizziness, hands shaking, low blood presure, weight change, skin reactions, jaundice or blood changes, loss of libido may occur.
Caution: in nursing mothers or in patients suffering from heart disease, thyroid disease, epilepsy, diabetes, glaucoma, adrenal tumour, urinary retention, some other psychiatric conditions. Your doctor may advise regular blood tests.
Not to be used for: children, pregnant women, or for patients suffering from heart attacks, liver disease, heart block.
Caution needed with: alcohol, ANTICHOLINERGICS, ADRENALINE, MAOIS, BARBITU-RATES, other antidepressants, ANTIHYPERTENSIVES, CIMETIDINE, oestrogens.
Contains: DESIPRAMINE HYDROCHLORIDE.
Other preparations:

Peru balsam *see* Anugesic-HC, Anusol, Anusol HC

Pethidine hydrochloride *see* pethidine tablets

pethidine tablets
(Roche)

Tablets supplied at strengths of 50 mg and used as an ANALGESIC to treat moderate to severe pain.

Dose: 1-3 tablets every 4 hours; children 0.5-2 mg/kg body weight.
Availability: controlled drug; NHS and private prescription.
Side effects: nausea, vomiting, constipation, drowsiness, low blood pressure, breathing difficulties, difficulty passing urine, dry mouth, sweating, flushing, vertigo, slow or irregular heart beat, loss of body temperature, hallucinations, mood change, addiction, constricted pupils, rash, itching.
Caution: in pregnant women, nursing mothers, and in patients suffering from low blood pressure, underactive thyroid, asthma and breathing problems, liver and kidney damage. Withdraw slowly at end of treatment.
Not to be used for: patients suffering from raised pressure in the head, or head injury.
Caution needed with: MEXILETINE, MAOIS, sedatives, tranquillizers, CISAPRIDE, DOMPERIDONE, METOCLOPRAMIDE, SELEGILINE, CIMETIDINE.
Contains: PETHIDINE HYDROCHLORIDE.
Other preparations:

Petrolagar No 1
(Whitehall)

An emulsion used as a lubricant to treat constipation.

Dose: adults 10 ml night and morning or after meals; children over 3 years 5 ml once or twice a day.
Availability: private prescription and over the counter.
Side effects:
Caution: in patients suffering from swallowing difficulty; avoid using for prolonged treatment.
Not to be used for: children under 3 years.
Caution needed with:
Contains: liquid PARAFFIN, light liquid paraffin.
Other preparations:

Pevaryl
(Cilag)

A cream used as an antifungal treatment for inflammation of the penis, inflammation of the vulva, thrush-like nappy rash, other skin infections such as tinea or nail infections.

Dose: massage gently into the affected area 2-3 times a day.
Availability: NHS, private prescription, over the counter.
Side effects: irritation.
Caution:
Not to be used for:
Caution needed with:
Contains: econazole nitrate.
Other preparations: Pevaryl Lotion, Pevaryl Spray Powder, GYNO PEVARYL. Also Pevaryl TC (with STEROID for inflamed conditions).

---

phaeochromocytoma

a tumour of the adrenal gland which produces excess adrenaline-like hormones.

Phanodorm — BARBITURATE to treat sleeplessness. Product now discontinued.

Phasal
(Lagap)

A white tablet supplied at a strength of 300 mg and used as a LITHIUM salt to treat acute manic or hypomanic disorders, prevention of manic depression and recurring depression.

Dose: to maintain blood level in a given range.
Availability: NHS and private prescription.
Side effects: nausea, diarrhoea, hand tremor, muscular weakness, brain and heart changes, weight gain, swelling, under- or overactive thyroid, thirst and excessive urination, kidney changes, skin reactions, intoxication.
Caution: treatment should be started in hospital and a careful check on the functioning of the kidneys and thyroid should be made, as well as ensuring that there is an adequate consumption of salt and fluid. Your doctor may advise blood tests to gauge dose.
Not to be used for: for children, pregnant women, nursing mothers, or for patients suffering from disturbed sodium balance, Addison's disease, kidney or heart disease, or underactive thyroid.
Caution needed with: DIURETICS, NON-STEROID ANTI-INFLAMMATORY DRUGS, CARBAMAZEPINE, FLUPENTHIXOL, METHYLDOPA, PHENYTOIN, HALOPERIDOL, TETRACYCLINES.
Contains: LITHIUM CARBONATE.

Other preparations: CAMCOLIT (Norgine), LISKONUM (SKB), PRIADEL (Delandale).

phenazocine hydrobromide *see* Narphen

phenazone *see* Auralgicin, Auraltone

phenazopyridine hydrochloride *see* Uromide

phenelzine sulphate *see* Nardil

Phenergan
(Rhone-Poulenc Rorer)

A blue tablet supplied at strengths of10 mg, 25 mg and used as an ANTIHISTAMINE treatment for allergies, nausea, vomiting, and for sedation (if recommended by a doctor).

Dose: adults 10-20 mg 2-3 times a day; children 1-5 years 5-15 mg a day, over 5 years 10-25 mg a day.
Availability: NHS, private prescription, over the counter.
Side effects: drowsiness, reduced reactions, dizziness, disorientation, sensitivity to light, ANTICHOLINERGIC effects, extrapyramidal reactions (shaking and rigidity).
Caution:
Not to be used for: infants under 1 year.
Caution needed with: sedatives, MAOIS, alcohol.
Contains: PROMETHAZINE hydrochloride.
Other preparations: Phenergan Elixir, Phenergan Injection, PHENHALAL (Halal).

phenethicillin *see* Broxil

Phenhalal *see* Phenergan
(Halal)

phenindamine tartrate *see* **Thephorin**

---

phenindione *see* **Dindevan**

---

pheniramine *see* **Daneral SA**

---

phenobarbitone tablets

A white tablet supplied at strengths of 15 mg, 30 mg, 60 mg, 100 mg, and used as a BARBITURATE to treat epilepsy.

Dose: adults, 60-180 mg at night; children 5-8 mg/kg body weight a day.
Availability: controlled drug; NHS and private prescription.
Side effects: drowsiness, lethargy, depression, lack of co-ordination, skin rash, excitement, restlessness, confusion, anaemia.
Caution: in the elderly, pregnant women, nursing mothers, physically weak patients, and in patients suffering from liver or kidney damage, porphyria (a rare blood disease), or breathing difficulty. Withdrawal should be gradual.
Not to be used for:
Caution needed with: DISOPYRAMIDE, QUINIDINE, CHLORAMPHENICOL, DOXYCYCLINE, METRONIDAZOLE, NICOUMALONE, WARFARIN, ANTIDEPRESSANTS, other anti-epileptics, sedatives, FELODIPINE, ISRAPIDINE, NICARDIPINE, NIFEDIPINE, DIGITOXIN, STEROIDS, GESTRINONE, TIBOLONE, the contraceptive pill, THEOPHYLLINE, THYROXINE, VITAMIN D.
Contains: PHENOBARBITONE.
Other preparations: Luminal (now discontinued).

---

phenol *see* **Chloraseptic, magnesium sulphate paste.**

---

phenolphthalein *see* **Agarol, Alophen, Kest**

---

phenothrin *see* **Full Marks**

---

phenoxybenzamine *see* **Dibenyline**

phenoxymethylpenicillin *see* **Penicillin-V**

---

phenoxypropanol *see* **Phytocil**

Phensedyl
(Rhone-Poulenc Rorer)

A linctus used as an ANTIHISTAMINE, opiate, treatment for cough.

Dose: adults 5-10 ml 2-3 times a day; children 1-5 years 2.5 ml 2-3 times a day, 6-12 years 2.5-5 ml 2-3 times a day.
Availability: private prescription and over the counter.
Side effects: constipation, drowsiness, reduced reactions.
Caution: in patients suffering from asthma.
Not to be used for: children under 1 year or for patients suffering from liver disease.
Caution needed with: MAOIS, alcohol, sedatives.
Contains: PROMETHAZINE hydrochloride, CODEINE PHOSPHATE.
Other preparations:

---

phentermine *see* **Duromine, Ionamin**

Phenylephrine Minims
(SNP)

Drops used as a SYMPATHOMIMETIC pupil dilator.

Dose: 1 drop into the eye as needed.
Availability: NHS, private prescription, over the counter.
Side effects:
Caution:
Not to be used for: patients suffering from narrow angle glaucoma, high blood pressure coronary disease, overactive thyroid, diabetes.
Caution needed with: MAOIS, TRICYCLIC antidepressants, ß-blockers.
Contains: PHENYLEPHRINE.
Other preparations: Phenylephrine Eye Drops.

---

phenylephrine *see* **Betnovate Rectal, Bronchilator, Dimotapp LA, Duo-Autohaler, Hayphryn, Isopto Frin, Medihaler-Duo, Neophryn, Phenylephrine Minims, Uniflu and Gregovite C,**

Vibrocil

phenylethyl alcohol *see* **Ceanel Concentrate**

phenylpropanolamine *see* **Dimotapp LA, Eskornade Spansule**

phenyltoloxamine *see* **Pholtex**

phenytoin *see* **Epanutin**

pHiso-Med
(Sterling)

A solution used as a disinfectant to treat acne, and for disinfecting infants' skin, cleansing and disinfecting skin before surgery.

Dose: use as a liquid soap.
Availability: NHS, private prescription, over the counter.
Side effects:
Caution: in newborn infants dilute 10 times. Avoid ears and eyes.
Not to be used for:
Caution needed with:
Contains: CHLORHEXIDINE GLUCONATE.
Other preparations: HIBISCRUB (ICI), HIBISOL (ICI), HIBITANE (ICI), UNISEPT (Seton Healthcare).

pholcodine *see* **Copholco, Copholcoids, Davenol, Expulin, Galenphol, Pavacol-D, Pholcomed-D, Pholtex**

pholcodine linctus *see* **Galenphol**

Pholcomed-D
(Medo)

A linctus used as an opiate to treat dry irritating cough.

Dose: adults 10-15 ml 3 times a day, children 1-2 years 2.5 ml 3 times a day, 2-12 years 5 ml 3 times a day.
Availability: NHS, private prescription, over the counter.
Side effects: constipation.
Caution: in patients suffering from asthma
Not to be used for: children under 1 year, or for patients suffering from liver disease.
Caution needed with: MAOIS.
Contains: PHOLCODINE.
Other preparations: Pholcomed, Pholcomed Pastilles, GALENPHOL (Galen), PAVACOL-D (Boehringer-Ingelheim). (Pholcomed Capsules, Pholcomed Forte, Pholcomed Forte Diabetic, Pholcomed Expectorant — all now discontinued.)

Pholtex — opiate/ANTIHISTAMINE treatment for dry cough. Product now discontinued.

Phosphate-Sandoz
(Sandoz)

A white, effervescent tablet used as a phosphate supplement to treat elevated calcium levels and low phosphate levels.

Dose: adults and children over 5 years up to 6 tablets a day; children under 5 years half adult dose.
Availability: NHS, private prescription, over the counter.
Side effects: diarrhoea, nausea.
Caution: in patients suffering from kidney disease or those on a low sodium diet.
Not to be used for:
Caution needed with: ANTACIDS.
Contains: SODIUM ACID PHOSPHATE, SODIUM BICARBONATE, POTASSIUM BICARBONATE.
Other preparations:

Phospholine-Iodide — drops to treat glaucoma. Product now discontinued.

---

phosphorylcolamine *see* **Fosfor**

Phyllocontin Continus
(Napp)

A pale-yellow tablet supplied at a strength of 225 mg and used as a broncho-dilator to treat left ventricular or congestive heart failure, bronchial spasm associated with asthma, chronic bronchitis, emphysema.

Dose: 1 tablet twice a day for 7 days then 2 tablets twice a day; children used reduced doses.
Availability: NHS, private prescription, over the counter.
Side effects: nausea, stomach upset, headache, brain stimulation.
Caution: in pregnant women, nursing mothers, and in patients suffering from other forms of heart disease, liver disease, stomach ulcer.
Not to be used for:
Caution needed with: CIMETIDINE, ERYTHROMYCIN, CIPROFLOXACIN, INTERFERON, STEROIDS, DIURETICS, some other bronchodilators.
Contains: AMINOPHYLLINE.
Other preparations: Phyllocontin Forte, Phyllocontin Paediatric, AMNIVENT (Ashbourne), PECRAM (Zyma)..

Physeptone
(Wellcome)

A white, scored tablet supplied at a strength of 5 mg and used as an opiate to control severe pain.

Dose: 1-2 tablets every 6-8 hours.
Availability: controlled drug; NHS and private prescription.
Side effects: tolerance, addiction, euphoria, dizziness, sedation, nausea.
Caution: in pregnant women and in patients suffering from liver disease or underactive thyroid.
Not to be used for: children, in obstetrics, for ambulant patients, or for patients with breathing difficulty or blocked airways.
Caution needed with: MAOIS, sedatives.
Contains: METHADONE hydrochloride.
Other preparations: Physeptone Injection.

---

physostigmine *see* physostigmine eye drops

---

physostigmine eye drops

Eye drops supplied at strengths of 0.25%, 0.5%, and used to treat glaucoma.

Dose: adults apply 2-6 times a day
Availability: NHS and private prescription.
Side effects: blurred vision, sweating, slow heart beat, intestinal pain, excess saliva, breathing spasm.
Caution:
Not to be used for:
Caution needed with:
Contains: PHYSOSTIGMINE SULPHATE.
Other preparations: PHYSOSTIGMINE and PILOCARPINE eye drops.

Phytex
(Pharmax)

A paint used as an antifungal treatment for skin and nail infections.

Dose: paint on to the affected area morning and evening and after bathing until 2-3 weeks after the symptoms have gone.
Availability: NHS, private prescription, over the counter.
Side effects:
Caution:
Not to be used for: children under 5 years or pregnant women.
Caution needed with:
Contains: TANNIC ACID, BORIC ACID, SALICYLIC ACID, METHYL SALICYLATE, ACETIC ACID.
Other preparations:

Phytocil
(Fisons)

A cream used as an antifungal treatment for tinea infections.

Dose: apply to the affected area twice times a day.
Availability: NHS, private prescription, over the counter.
Side effects:
Caution:
Not to be used for:
Caution needed with:
Contains: PHENOXYPROPANOL, CHLOROPHENOXYETHANOL, SALICYLIC ACID, MENTHOL.
Other preparations: Phytocil Powder.

---

phytomenadione *see* **Konakion**

Picolax
(Ferring)

Powder supplied in sachets and used as a stimulant and laxative for the evacuation of bowels prior to surgery etc.

Dose: adults 1 sachet dissolved in water before breakfast, repeated 6-8 hours later if required; children 2-4 years ½ sachet morning and afternoon, children 4-9 years 1 sachet in morning, ½ sachet in afternoon, children over 9 years adult dose.
Availability: NHS, private prescription, over the counter.
Side effects:
Caution: low residue food should be eaten and plenty of water drunk during treatment. Special care should be taken for patients suffering from inflammatory bowel disease.
Not to be used for:
Caution needed with: antibiotics.
Contains: SODIUM PICOSULPHATE, MAGNESIUM CITRATE.
Other preparations: LAXOBERAL (Windsor), SODIUM PICOSULPHATE.

Pilocarpine Minims
(SNP)

Drops used as a pupil constrictor to treat glaucoma.

Dose: 1 drop into the eye every 5 minutes until constriction is achieved.
Availability: NHS and private prescription.
Side effects:
Caution:
Not to be used for:
Caution needed with:
Contains: PILOCARPINE nitrate.
Other preparations: CARPINE (Alcon), OCUSERT (M&B), OPULETS PILOCARPINE, SNO PILO (SNP).

pilocarpine *see* **Isopto Carpine, Ocusert Pilo, Opulets Pilocarpine, Pilocarpine, Sno Pilo**

Pimafucin Pessaries — treatment for vaginal thrush and trichomonal infections. Product now discontinued.

Pimafucin 2½% Suspension — antibiotic treatment for respiratory infections. Product now discontinued.

Pimafucin Cream — antifungal treatment for skin and nail infections. Product now discontinued.

pimozide *see* **Orap**

pindolol *see* **Viskaldix, Visken**

pinene *see* **Rowatinex**

pipenzolate bromide *see* **Piptal**

piperazine oestrone sulphate *see* **Harmogen**

piperazine *see* **Antepar, Expelix, Pripsen**

Piptal
(Boehringer Mannheim)

An orange tablet supplied at a strength of 5 mg and used as an anti-spasm, ANTICHOLINERGIC treatment for excess stomach acid, overactive intestine.

Dose: 1 tablet 3 times a day and 1-2 tablets at night.
Availability: NHS and private prescription.
Side effects: blurred vision, confusion, dry mouth, nausea, sleeplessness, constipation, urinary retention, rapid heart rate, dizziness.
Caution: in patients suffering from glaucoma, enlarged prostate, urinary retention.
Not to be used for: children, pregnant women, nursing mothers, or for patients suffering from inflammatory bowel disease, intestinal obstruction, other gastro-intestinal disorders, rapid heart rate, untreated angina, liver or

kidney disease, myaesthenia gravis.
Caution needed with: TRICYCLIC antidepressants, some sedatives, ANTIHIS-
TAMINES.
Contains: PIPENZOLATE BROMIDE.
Other preparations: Piptalin (with DIMETHICONE).

Piptalin see Piptal
(Boehringer Mannheim)

---

pirbuterol see Exirel

---

pirenzepine see Gastrozepin

---

piretanide see Arelix

Piriton
(A & H)

A cream-coloured tablet supplied at a strength of 4 mg and used as an
ANTIHISTAMINE treatment for allergies.

Dose: adults 1 tablet every 4-6 hours up to 6 tablets a day; children 6-12
years ½ tablet every 4-6 hours up to 3 tablets a day, under 6 years use
syrup.
Availability: NHS, private prescription, over the counter.
Side effects: drowsiness, reduced reactions, dizziness, excitation.
Caution: in pregnant women and nursing mothers.
Not to be used for:
Caution needed with: sedatives, MAOIS, alcohol.
Contains: CHLORPHENIRAMINE maleate.
Other preparations: Piriton Syrup, Piriton Injection, RIMARIN (Rima),
(Piriton Spandets — now discontinued.)

---

piroxicam see Feldene

Pirozip *see* **Feldene**
(Ashbourne)

---

pivampicillin *see* **Miraxid, Pondocillin**

---

pivmecillinam *see* **Selexid**

---

pizotifen hydrogen malate *see* **Sanomigran**

Plaquenil
(Sanofi Winthrop)

An orange tablet supplied at a strength of 200 mg and used as an anti-arthritic drug to treat rheumatoid arthritis, lupus erythomatosus (a multisystem disease).

Dose: adults 2 tablets a day with food at first, then 1-2 tablets a day or up to 6.5 mg per kg body weight per day for no more than 6 months; children as advised by the physician.
Availability: NHS and private prescription.
Side effects: eye disorders, skin reactions, bleached hair, alopecia, stomach intolerance.
Caution: in nursing mothers, and in patients suffering from porphyria (a rare blood disorder), kidney or liver disease, psoriasis, history of stomach, neurological, or blood disorders. The eyes should be checked regularly.
Not to be used for: pregnant women, or for patients suffering from maculopathy (eye disease).
Caution needed with: ANTACIDS, aminoglycoside ANTIBIOTICS, any drugs likely to cause eye damage.
Contains: HYDROXYCHLOROQUINE sulphate.
Other preparations:

Platet
(Nicholas)

A white, effervescent tablet supplied at strengths of 100 mg, 300 mg and used as an anti-platelet drug to reduce risk of heart attack, stroke, or blockage of grafted blood vessels.

Dose: 1 tablet a day dissolved in water. 100 mg strength used after heart surgery.

Availability: NHS and private prescription.

Side effects: bronchospasm, stomach bleeding.

Caution: in patients who are allergic to ASPIRIN or anti-inflammatory drugs, and who are suffering from kidney or liver disease, or a history of bronchospasm.

Not to be used for: nursing mothers or for patients with stomach ulcer or any bleeding conditions.

Caution needed with: oral anticoagulants, antidiabetics, NON-STEROID ANTI-INFLAMMATORY DRUGS, uric acid lowering agents, METHOTREXATE, STEROIDS, SPIRONOLACTONE.

Contains: ASPIRIN.

Other preparations: ASPIRIN TABLETS, NU-SEALS ASPIRIN (Lilly).

Plendil
(Schwarz)

Tablets supplied at strengths of 5 mg, 10 mg, and used to treat high blood pressure.

Dose: initially 5 mg a day at first, increasing if needed to a maximum of 20 mg a day.

Availability: NHS and private prescription.

Side effects: fluid retention of the ankles, dizziness, tiredness, headache, flushing, palpitations, rash, mild gum swelling.

Caution: in patients suffering from severe liver disorder or recent coronary heart disease.

Not to be used for: children, pregnant women, nursing mothers.

Caution needed with: CIMETIDINE, PHENYTOIN, CARBAMAZEPINE, PHENOBARBITONE.

Contains: FELODIPINE.

Other preparations:

Plesmet
(Napp)

A syrup used as an iron supplement to treat iron-deficiency anaemia.

Dose: adults 5-10 ml 3 times a day; children 2.5-5 ml 2-3 times a day.

Availability: NHS, private prescription, over the counter.

Side effects:

Caution:

Not to be used for:

Caution needed with: TETRACYCLINES.

Contains: FERROUS GLYCINE SULPHATE.

Other preparations: FERROCONTIN (Asta).

podophyllotoxin *see* **Condyline, Warticon**

podophyllum resin *see* **Posalfilin**

poldine methylsulphate *see* **Nacton Forte**

poloxamer 188 *see* **Codalax**

Polyalk — ANTACID liquid. Product now discontinued.

Polybactrin
(Wellcome)

A powder supplied in an aerosol used as an aminoglycoside antibiotic to treat burns and wounds, and in surgery.

Dose: spray lightly on to the affected area.
Availability: NHS and private prescription.
Side effects: ear damage, kidney damage, allergy.
Caution: in patients with large areas of affected skin.
Not to be used for:
Caution needed with:
Contains: NEOMYCIN SULPHATE, POLYMYXIN B SULPHATE, BACITRACIN ZINC.
Other preparations: TRIBIOTIC (3M Healthcare).

Polycrol Forte Gel *see* **Asilone.** Product now discontinued.

Polycrol *see* **Asilone.** Product now discontinued.

polyethylene glycol *see* **Dioctyl Ear Drops, Hypotears**

polyethylene granules *see* Ionax

Polyfax
(Cusi)

An ointment or eye ointment used as an antibiotic to treat styes, conjunctivitis, other eye inflammations, skin infections.

Dose: apply at least twice a day.
Availability: NHS and private prescription.
Side effects: kidney damage, allergy.
Caution: in patients suffering from large open wounds.
Not to be used for:
Caution needed with:
Contains: POLYMYXIN B SULPHATE, BACITRACIN.
Other preparations:

---

polymyxin B sulphate *see* Gregoderm, Maxitrol, Neosporin, Otosporin, Polybactrin, Polyfax, Polytrim, Terra-Cortril, Tribiotic, Uniroid

---

polynoxylin *see* Anaflex, Ponoxylan

---

polysaccharide-iron complex *see* Niferex

---

polysorbate *see* coal tar and salicylic acid ointment, Ung Merck

---

Polytar Emollient
(Stiefel)

A liquid bath emollient used to treat psoriasis, eczema, and other skin conditions.

Dose: 2-4 capsful added to a 20 cm deep bath. Soak for 15-20 minutes. Pat dry.
Availability: NHS, private prescription, over the counter.
Side effects:

Caution:
Not to be used for:
Caution needed with:
Contains: TAR, CADE OIL, COAL TAR, ARACHIS OIL, LIGHT LIQUID PARAFFIN.
Other preparations:

Polytar Liquid
(Stiefel)

A liquid used as an antipsoriatic treatment for psoriasis of the scalp, dandruff, seborrhoea, eczema.

Dose: shampoo once or twice a week.
Availability: NHS, private prescription, over the counter.
Side effects:
Caution:
Not to be used for:
Caution needed with:
Contains: TAR, CADE OIL, COAL TAR, ARACHIS OIL, COAL TAR EXTRACT, OLEYL ALCOHOL.
Other preparations: Polytar Plus.

polythiazide *see* Nephril

Polytrim
(Cusi)

Drops used as an antibacterial treatment for eye infections.

Dose: 1 drop into the eye 4 times a day until 2 days after the symptoms have gone.
Availability: NHS and private prescription.
Side effects:
Caution:
Not to be used for:
Caution needed with:
Contains: TRIMETHOPRIM, POLYMYXIN B SULPHATE.
Other preparations: Polytrim Ointment.

polyvinyl alcohol *see* Hypotears, Kerecid, Liquifilm Tears, Sno Tears

Polyvite — multivitamin. Product now discontinued.

Ponderax Pacaps
(Servier)

A blue/clear capsule supplied at a strength of 60 mg and used as an appetite suppressant to treat obesity.

Dose: 1 capsule a day.
Availability: NHS and private prescription.
Side effects: nervousness, sedation, diarrhoea, dry mouth, frequent urination, depression if the drug is withdrawn suddenly.
Caution: in patients with a history of mental illness.
Not to be used for: children, epileptics, or patients with a history of alcoholism, drug addiction, or depression.
Caution needed with: MAOIS, ANTIHYPERTENSIVES, antidepressants, antidiabetic drugs, sedatives, alcohol, other obesity drugs.
Contains: FENFLURAMINE HYDROCHLORIDE.
Other preparations:

Pondocillin
(Leo)

A white, egg-shaped tablet supplied at a strength of 500 mg and used as a penicillin to treat bronchitis, pneumonia, ear, nose, and throat infections, skin, soft tissue infections, urine infections, gonorrhoea.

Dose: adults 1 tablet twice a day with food or drink; children use suspension or sachets.
Availability: NHS and private prescription.
Side effects: allergy, stomach disturbances.
Caution: in patients suffering from kidney disease.
Not to be used for: patients suffering from glandular fever.
Caution needed with:
Contains: PIVAMPICILLIN.
Other preparations: Pondocillin Suspension, Pondocillin Sachets, Pondocillin Plus.

Ponoxylan — antibacterial treatment for skin. Product now discontinued.

Ponstan Forte
(Parke-Davis)

A yellow tablet supplied at a strength of 500 mg and used as a NON-STEROID ANTI-INFLAMMATORY DRUG to relieve pain in rheumatoid arthritis including Still's disease, osteoarthritis, and to treat headache, period pain, excessively heavy periods.

Dose: 1 tablet 3 times a day (children use suspension).
Availability: NHS and private prescription.
Side effects: diarrhoea, rash, kidney damage, low platelet levels.
Caution: in the elderly, in pregnant women, and in patients suffering from bronchial asthma, allergy, heart failure.
Not to be used for: patients suffering from kidney or liver disease, gastro-intestinal ulceration, inflammatory bowel disease.
Caution needed with: anticoagulants, antidiabetics, anticonvulsants.
Contains: MEFENAMIC ACID.
Other preparations: Ponstan, Ponstan Dispersible, Ponstan Paediatric Syrup, DYSMAN-500 (Ashbourne).

Posalfilin
(Norgine)

An ointment used as a skin softener to treat warts.

Dose: protect healthy skin, apply the ointment to the wart, and cover; repeat 2-3 times a week.
Availability: NHS, private prescription, over the counter.
Side effects: pain when the ointment is first applied.
Caution: do not use on healthy skin.
Not to be used for: pregnant women or on warts on the face or anal and genital areas.
Caution needed with:
Contains: SALICYLIC ACID, PODOPHYLLUM RESIN.
Other preparations:

Potaba
(Glenwood)

A powder in a 3 g sachet used as a fibrous tissue dissolver to treat scleroderma (thickened skin), Peyronie's disease.

Dose: 1 sachet with food 4 times a day.
Availability: NHS and private prescription.
Side effects: anorexia, nausea.

Caution: in patients suffering from kidney disease.
Not to be used for: for children.
Caution needed with: sulphonamide antibiotics.
Contains: POTASSIUM P-AMINOBENZOATE.
Other preparations: Potaba Tablets, Potaba Capsules.

potassium benzoate *see* **Kloref**

potassium bicarbonate *see* **Algicon, Effercitrate, Kloref, Phosphate, Sando-K, Sandocal**

potassium chloride *see* **Burinex K, Centyl-K, Diarrest, Dioralyte, Diumide-K Continus, Esidrex K, Glandosane, Hygroton K, Kloref, Lasikal, Lasix + K, Leo K, Navidrex-K, Neo-Naclex-K, Nu-K, Rehidrat, Sando-K, Selora, Slow-K**

potassium glycerophosphate *see* **Metatone, Verdiviton**

potassium hydroxyquinolone sulphate *see* **Auralgicin, Quinocort, Quinoderm Cream, Quinoped**

potassium p-aminobenzoate *see* **Potaba**

potassium permanganate

A solution used to cleanse and deodorize weeping eczema and wounds.

Dose: apply as a wet dressing, or soak the affected part.
Availability: NHS, private prescription, over the counter.
Side effects: irritation of mucous membrane.
Caution: stains skin and clothing.
Not to be used for:
Caution needed with:
Contains: potassium permanganate.
Other preparations: PERMITABS (Bioglan).

povidone-iodine *see* **Betadine, Betadine Gargle and Mouthwash, Betadine Ointment, Betadine Scalp and Skin Cleanser, Betadine Spray, Disadine DP, Videne Powder**

Pragmatar
(Bioglan)

A cream used as an anti-itch, antiseptic, skin softener to treat scaly skin, scalp seborrhoea and similar disorders.

Dose: apply weekly, or daily in severe cases, to wet hair.
Availability: NHS, private prescription, over the counter.
Side effects: irritation.
Caution: dilute the cream first when using for infants. Avoid eyes, groin, or inflamed areas.
Not to be used for:
Caution needed with:
Contains: CETYL ALCOHOL/COAL TAR DISTILLATE, SULPHUR, SALICYLIC ACID.
Other preparations:

Pramidex *see* **Rastinon.** Product now discontinued.

---

pramoxine hydrochloride *see* **Anugesic-HC**

---

pramoxine *see* **Epifoam**

Pranoxen *see* **Naprosyn**
(Napp)

---

pravastatin *see* **Lipostat**

Praxilene
(Lipha)

A pink capsule supplied at a strength of 100 mg and used as a blood vessel dilator to treat cerebral and peripheral vascular problems

Dose: 1-2 capsules 4 times a day.
Availability: NHS and private prescription.
Side effects: nausea, stomach pain.
Caution:
Not to be used for: children.
Caution needed with:
Contains: NAFTIDROFURYL OXALATE.
Other preparations: Praxilene Forte (restricted to hospitals).

---

prazosin *see* **Hypovase**

Precortisyl
(Roussel)

A white tablet or a white, scored tablet according to strengths of 1 mg, 5 mg and used as a STEROID treatment for allergies and rheumatic conditions.

Dose: adults 20-40 mg a day at first reducing by 2.5 or 5 mg every 3-4 days to 5-20 mg a day as needed; children 1-7 years quarter to half adult dose, 7-12 years half to three-quarters adult dose.
Availability: NHS and private prescription.
Side effects: high blood sugar, thin bones, mood changes, ulcers.
Caution: in pregnant women, in patients who have had recent bowel surgery, or who are suffering from inflamed veins, psychiatric disorders, virus infections, some cancers, some kidney diseases, thinning of the bones, ulcers, tuberculosis, other infections, high blood pressure, glaucoma, epilepsy, diabetes, underactive thyroid, liver disease, stress. Withdraw gradually.
Not to be used for:
Caution needed with: PHENYTOIN, PHENOBARBITONE, EPHEDRINE, RIFAMPICIN, DIURETICS, ANTICHOLINESTERASES, DIGOXIN, antidiabetic agents, anticoagulants, NON-STEROID ANTI-INFLAMMATORY DRUGS.
Contains: PREDNISOLONE.
Other preparations: Precortisyl Forte, DELTACORTRIL (Pizer), DELTASTAB (Boots), PREDNESOL (Glaxo), SINTISONE (Farmitalia CE).

Pred Forte
(Allergan)

Drops used as a STEROID treatment for inflammation of the eye where no infection is present.

Dose: 1-2 drops into the eye 2-4 times a day or 2 drops every hour for the

first two days if needed.
Availability: NHS and private prescription.
Side effects: rise in eye pressure, secondary fungal or viral infections, thinning cornea, cataract.
Caution: in infants and pregnant women.
Not to be used for: patients suffering from glaucoma, viral, fungal, tubercular, or weeping eye infections, dendritic ulcer, or for patients who wear soft contact lenses.
Caution needed with:
Contains: PREDNISOLONE acetate.
Other preparations: PREDSOL EYE DROPS (Evans).

Predenema *see* Predsol Enema
(Pharmax)

Predfoam *see* Predsol Enema
(Pharmax)

Prednesol
(Glaxo)

A pink, scored tablet supplied at a strength of 5 mg and used as a STEROID treatment for allergies, rheumatic and inflammatory conditions.

Dose: adults 2-20 tablets a day in water in divided doses at first reducing to the minimum effective dose; children 1-7 years quarter to half adult dose, 7-12 years half to three-quarters adult dose.
Availability: NHS and private prescription.
Side effects: high blood sugar, thin bones, mood changes, ulcers.
Caution: in pregnant women, in patients who have had recent bowel surgery, or who are suffering from inflamed veins, psychiatric disorders, virus infections, some cancers, some kidney diseases, thinning of the bones, ulcers, tuberculosis, other infections, high blood pressure, glaucoma, epilepsy, diabetes, underactive thyroid, liver disease, stress. Withdraw gradually.
Not to be used for:
Caution needed with: PHENYTOIN, PHENOBARBITONE, EPHEDRINE, RIFAMPICIN, DIURETICS, ANTICHOLINESTERASES, DIGOXIN, antidiabetic agents, anticoagulants, NON-STEROID ANTI-INFLAMMATORY DRUGS.
Contains: PREDNISOLONE disodium phosphate.
Other preparations: DELTACORTRIL (Pfizer), DELTASTAB (Boots), PRECORTISYL (Roussel), SINTISONE (Farmitalia CE).

Prednisolone Minims
(SNP)

Drops used as a STEROID treatment for inflammation of the eye where no infection is present.

Dose: 1-2 drops as needed.
Availability: NHS and private prescription.
Side effects: rise in eye pressure, fungal infection, cataract, thinning cornea.
Caution: in infants — do not use for extended periods.
Not to be used for: pregnant women or for patients suffering from glaucoma, viral, fungal, tubercular, or acute weeping infections.
Caution needed with:
Contains: PREDNISOLONE sodium phosphate.
Other preparations: PRED-FORTE (Allergan), PREDSOL EYE DROPS (Glaxo).

---

prednisolone *see* **Deltacortril, Precortisyl, Pred Forte, Prednesol, Prednisolone Minims, Predsol Enema, Predsol Drops, Scheriproct, Sintisone**

---

prednisone *see* **Decortisyl**

Predsol Enema
(Glaxo)

An enema supplied at a strength of 20 mg and used as a STEROID treatment for ulcerative colitis.

Dose: 1 at night for 2-4 weeks.
Availability: NHS and private prescription.
Side effects: systemic corticosteroid effects (*see* Precortisyl).
Caution: in pregnant women. Do not use for prolonged periods.
Not to be used for: children.
Caution needed with:
Contains: PREDNISOLONE.
Other preparations: Predsol Suppositories, PREDSOL DROPS, PREDFOAM (Pharmax), PREDENEMA (Pharmax).

Predsol Drops
(Glaxo)

Drops used as a STEROID treatment for inflammation of the ear or eye where no infection is present.

Dose: 2-3 drops into the ear every 2-3 hours or 1-2 drops into the eye every 1-2 hours.
Availability: NHS and private prescription.
Side effects: allergy, resistance to NEOMYCIN (in Predsol-N), rise in eye pressure, thinning cornea, cataract.
Caution: do not use unless necessary, and avoid use over extended periods for infants or pregnant women.
Not to be used for: patients suffering from viral, fungal, tubercular, or weeping infections, dendritic ulcer, glaucoma or for patients who wear soft contact lenses; patients with perforated ear drum (Predsol-N)
Caution needed with:
Contains: PREDNISOLONE sodium phosphate.
Other preparations: Predsol-N (contains NEOMYCIN, for infected conditions), PRED-FORTE (Allergan).

Preferid
(Brocades)

A cream used as a STEROID to treat eczema, psoriasis, and dermatitis.

Dose: apply sparingly 2-3 times a day.
Availability: NHS and private prescription.
Side effects: fluid retention, suppression of adrenal glands, thinning of the skin.
Caution: use for short periods of time only.
Not to be used for: continuously, especially for pregnant women or for patients suffering from acne or any other tubercular, viral, fungal, or ringworm skin infections.
Caution needed with:
Contains: BUDESONIDE.
Other preparations:

Prefil
(Norgine)

Brown granules used as a bulking agent to treat obesity.

Dose: 1-2 sachets swallowed with water ½-1 hour before eating.
Availability: NHS, private prescription, over the counter.
Side effects:
Caution:
Not to be used for: patients suffering from a blocked intestine.

Caution needed with:
Contains: STERCULIA.
Other preparations: NORMACOL (Norgine).

Pregaday
(Evans)

A brownish-red tablet used as an iron and folic acid supplement prevention of iron and FOLIC ACID deficiency in pregnancy.

Dose: 1 tablet a day.
Availability: NHS, private prescription, over the counter.
Side effects: stomach upset, allergy.
Caution: in patients with a history of stomach ulcer or who are in the first three months of pregnancy.
Not to be used for: patients suffering from vitamin B$_{12}$ deficiency.
Caution needed with: TETRACYCLINES, ANTACIDS, anticonvulsant drugs, CO-TRIMOXAZOLE.
Contains: FERROUS FUMARATE, FOLIC ACID.
Other preparations: FOLEX-350 (Rybar), GALFER FA (Galen), METERFOLIC (Sinclair).

Pregnavite Forte F
(Bencard)

A lilac-coloured tablet used as an iron, folic acid, and vitamin supplement to treat iron and vitamin deficiencies. Also given to pregnant women who have previously had handicapped babies to reduce the risk of deformity in the foetus.

Dose: 1 tablet 3 times a day after meals starting at least 1 month before conception and continuing at least until the second missed period date.
Availability: NHS (for cenrtain conditions only), private prescription, over the counter.
Side effects: stomach upset.
Caution:
Not to be used for: children or for patients suffering from megaloblastic anaemia.
Caution needed with: TETRACYCLINES, LEVODOPA.
Contains: FERROUS SULPHATE, FOLIC ACID, CALCIFEROL, THIAMINE hydrochloride, RIBOFLAVINE, PYRIDOXINE hydrochloride, NICOTINAMIDE, ASCORBIC ACID, CALCIUM PHOSPHATE.
Other preparations:

Premarin
(Wyeth)

A maroon, oval tablet, yellow, oval tablet, or purple, oval tablet according to strengths of 0.625 mg, 1.25 mg, 2.5 mg and used as an oestrogen for hormone replacement during and after the menopause, and to treat atrophic inflammation of the vagina, inflammation of the urethra, certain kinds of breast cancer, and to prevent thinning of the bones.

Dose: menopause 0.625-1.25 mg a day for 21 days starting on the fifth day of the period if present, then 7 days without tablets. Other, as advised by the physician.
Availability: NHS and private prescription.
Side effects: enlarged breasts, fluid retention, nausea, vaginal bleeding, weight gain, skin changes, liver disorders, jaundice, rashes, vomiting.
Caution: in patients suffering from high blood pressure, diabetes, heart disease, vascular disorders, asthma, kidney disease, epilepsy, womb diseases, thyroid disorder. Your doctor may advise you to have regular examinations.
Not to be used for: children, pregnant women, nursing mothers or for patients suffering from sickle-cell anaemia, thrombosis, liver disorders, some cancers, undiagnosed vaginal bleeding, some ear, skin, and kidney disorders, jaundice, porphyria (a rare blood disorder), brain blood vessel disease.
Caution needed with: DIURETICS, ANTIHYPERTENSIVES, and drugs that change liver enzymes (eg BARBITURATES, CARBAMAZEPINE, PHENYTOIN).
Contains: conjugated oestrogens.
Other preparations: Premarin Vaginal Cream.

Prempak-C
(Wyeth)

A maroon, oval tablet or yellow, oval tablet according to strengths of 0.625 mg, 1.25 mg plus a brown tablet 0.15 mg and used as an oestrogen, progestogen for hormone replacement during and after the menopause, and treatment of post-menopausal osteoporosis, atrophic inflammation of the vagina, inflammation of the urethra.

Dose: beginning on the first day of the period if present,1 maroon or yellow tablet a day for 16 days then 1 maroon or yellow tablet plus 1 brown tablet a day for 12 days.
Availability: NHS and private prescription.
Side effects: enlarged breasts, bloating and fluid retention, cramps, leg pains, mood change, reduction in sexual desire, headaches, nausea, vaginal erosion, discharge, and bleeding, weight gain, skin changes.
Caution: in patients suffering from high blood pressure, diabetes, vascular

disorders, asthma, depression, kidney disease, multiple sclerosis, womb diseases. Your doctor may advise you not to smoke, to have regular examinations. You should stop treatment at the first sign of serious symptoms such as severe headache or jaundice. Treatment should be stopped before surgery.

Not to be used for: children, pregnant women, or for patients suffering from sickle-cell anaemia, history of heart disease or thrombosis, liver disorders, some cancers, undiagnosed vaginal bleeding, some ear, skin, and kidney disorders.

Caution needed with: RIFAMPICIN, GRISEOFULVIN, BARBITURATES, PHENYTOIN, PRIMIDONE, CARBAMAZEPINE, ETHOSUXIMIDE, CHLORAL HYDRATE, DICHLORALPHENAZONE.

Contains: conjugated oestrogens plus NORGESTREL.
Other preparations:

Prepulsid
(Janssen)

A white tablet supplied at a strength of 10 mg and used as a stomach-emptying drug to treat gastric reflux and to encourage emptying of the stomach in conditions where the nerve supply is impaired.

Dose: 1 tablet 3-4 times a day for 6-12 weeks.
Availability: NHS and private prescription.
Side effects: abdominal cramps, stomach rumbling, diarrhoea, occasionally headaches and convulsions.
Caution: in the elderly, nursing mothers, and in patients suffering from kidney or liver impairment.
Not to be used for: pregnant women or for patients suffering from stomach block, perforation, or bleeding.
Caution needed with: sedatives, anticoagulants, ANTICHOLINERGICS.
Contains: CISAPRIDE.
Other preparations: Prepulsid Suspension, ALIMIX (Janssen).

Prescal
(Ciba)

A yellow scored tablet supplied at a strength of 2.5 mg and used as a calcium antagonist to treat high blood pressure.

Dose: adults 1 tablet morning and evening, increasing after 3-4 weeks to 2 tablets twice a day if needed, up to a maximum of 4 tablets twice a day; lower doses for the elderly.
Availability: NHS and private prescription.

Side effects: weight gain, palpitations, rapid heart rate, swelling, head-ache, flushing, dizziness, tiredness, abdominal pain, skin rash, liver enzyme changes, rise in liver enzymes.
Caution: pregnant women, nursing mothers, and in patients suffering from some rare heart conditions.
Not to be used for: children.
Caution needed with: anticonvulsants.
Contains: ISRADIPINE.
Other preparations:

Prestim
(Leo)

A white, scored tablet used as a ß-BLOCKER/thiazide DIURETIC combination to treat high blood pressure.

Dose: 1-4 tablets a day.
Availability: NHS and private prescription.
Side effects: cold hands and feet, sleep disturbance, slow heart rate, tiredness, wheezing, heart failure, stomach upset, sensitivity to light, weakness, blood changes, gout, dry eyes, rash.
Caution: in pregnant women, nursing mothers, and in patients suffering from diabetes, kidney or liver disorders, asthma, gout. May need to be withdrawn before surgery. Withdraw gradually. Your doctor may advise additional treatment with DIURETICS or DIGOXIN.
Not to be used for: children, or for patients suffering from heart block or failure, severe kidney disease.
Caution needed with: VERAPAMIL, CLONIDINE withdrawal, some anti-arrhythmic drugs and anaesthetics, RESERPINE, some ANTIHYPERTENSIVES, ERGOTAMINE, CIMETIDINE, sedatives, SYMPATHOMIMETICS, INDOMETHACIN, LITHIUM, DIGOXIN.
Contains: TIMOLOL MALEATE, BENDROFLUAZIDE.
Other preparations: Prestim Forte

Priadel
(Delandale)

A white, scored tablet supplied at strengths of 200 mg, 400 mg and used as a LITHIUM salt to treat mania, manic depression, recurring depression, agression, and self-injuring behaviour.

Dose: to keep blood levels in a given range.
Availability: NHS and private prescription.
Side effects: nausea, diarrhoea, hand tremor, muscular weakness, brain

and heart disturbances, weight gain, fluid retention, under- or overactive thyroid, thirst and excessive urination, skin reactions. Your doctor may advise blood tests to gauge dose.

Caution: treatment should start in hospital. Kidney, heart, and thyroid function should be checked regularly. Salt and fluid consumption should be maintained.

Not to be used for: children, pregnant women, nursing mothers, or for patients suffering from Addison's disease, weak kidneys or heart, underactive thyroid, disturbed sodium balance.

Caution needed with: DIURETICS, NON-STEROID ANTI-INFLAMMATORY DRUGS, PHENYTOIN, CARBAMAZEPINE, FLUPENTHIXOL, HALOPERIDOL, DIAZEPAM, METHYLDOPA, TETRACYCLINES.

Contains: LITHIUM CARBONATE.

Other preparations: CAMCOLIT (Norgine), LISKONUM (SKB), PHASAL (Lagap).

Primalan
(Rhone-Poulenc Rorer)

A white tablet supplied at a strength of 5 mg and used as an ANTIHISTAMINE treatment for allergy, itch, hay fever, rhinitis.

Dose: 1 tablet twice a day.
Availability: NHS and private prescription.
Side effects: drowsiness, reduced reactions, ANTICHOLINERGIC effects, extrapyramidal reactions (shaking and rigidity).
Caution:
Not to be used for: children, pregnant women, or for patients suffering from epilepsy, enlarged prostate, liver disease.
Caution needed with: sedatives, MAOIS, SYMPATHOMIMETICS, alcohol.
Contains: MEQUITAZINE.
Other preparations:

---

primaquine tablets
(ICI)

A brown tablet supplied at a strength of 7.5 mg and used to treat malaria.

Dose: 2 tablets a day for 14-21 days, given after a course of chloroquine; children 250 micrograms/kg body weight a day.
Availability: NHS, private prescription, over the counter.
Side effects: nausea, vomiting, stomach pain, blood changes.
Caution: in pregnant women, nursing mothers, and in patients suffering from rheumatoid arthritis, lupus erythematosus (a skin disorder), or some blood enzyme deficiencies.

Not to be used for:
Caution needed with: MEPACRINE.
Contains: primaquine.
Other preparations:

---

primidone see Mysoline

Primolut N
(Schering)

A white tablet supplied at a strength of 5 mg and used as a progestogen treatment for postponing menstruation, and for other menstrual and womb disorders.

Dose: usually 1 tablet 3 times a day.
Availability: NHS and private prescription.
Side effects: liver disturbances, masculinization.
Caution: in patients suffering from epilepsy or migraine.
Not to be used for: children, pregnant women, or patients suffering from severe liver disease, a history of itch or idiopathic jaundice, Dubin-Johnson and Rotor syndromes during pregnancy.
Caution needed with:
Contains: NORETHISTERONE.
Other preparations: MENZOL (Schwarz), SH420 (Schering), UTOVLAN (Syntex).

Primperan see Maxolon
(Berk)

Prioderm
(Napp Consumer)

A lotion used as a pediculicide, scabicide to treat scabies, lice of the head and pubic areas.

Dose: rub in and shampoo after 2-12 hours; repeat after 7-9 days.
Availability: NHS, private prescription, over the counter.
Side effects:
Caution: keep out of the eyes.
Not to be used for:
Caution needed with:

Contains: MALATHION.
Other preparations: Prioderm Cream Shampoo, DERBAC-M (Napp), SULEO-M (Napp).

Pripsen
(Reckitt & Colman)

A sachet used to treat worms.

Dose: adults and children over 6 years1 sachet and then a second dose of 1 sachet after 14 days; infants 3 months-1 year ⅓ sachet then a second dose after 14 days; children 1-6 years ⅔ sachet then a second dose after 14 days.
Availability: NHS, private prescription, over the counter.
Side effects: rarely sight disorders, vertigo.
Caution: care in nursing mothers and in patients suffering from nervous disorders.
Not to be used for: patients suffering from epilepsy, liver or kidney disease.
Caution needed with:
Contains: PIPERAZINE phosphate, SENNOSIDE.
Other preparations: EXPELIX (Cupal).

Pro-Actidil
(Wellcome)

A white tablet supplied at a strength of 10 mg and used as an ANTIHISTAMINE treatment for allergies.

Dose: 1 tablet a day 5-6 hours before going to bed.
Availability: NHS, private prescription, over the counter.
Side effects: drowsiness, reduced reactions, rarely skin eruptions.
Caution: in nursing mothers and in patients suffering from liver or kidney disease.
Not to be used for: children.
Caution needed with: sedatives, MAOIS, alcohol.
Contains: TRIPROLIDINE hydrochloride.
Other preparations:

Pro-banthine
(Baker-Norton)

A pink tablet supplied at a strength of 15 mg and used as an anti-spasm,

ANTICHOLINERGIC treatment for ulcers, irritable bowel syndrome, bed wetting.

Dose: adults up to 8 daily individual doses.
Availability: NHS and private prescription.
Side effects: blurred vision, confusion, dry mouth.
Caution: in the elderly and in patients suffering from ulcerative colitis, heart disease, autonomic neuropathy, kidney and liver disease, overactive thyroid.
Not to be used for: children or for patients suffering from glaucoma, obstructive bowel disease, obstructive disease of the urinary tract.
Caution needed with: DIGOXIN.
Contains: PROPANTHELINE bromide.
Other preparations:

Pro-Vent *see* Lasma
(Wellcome)

Pro-Viron
(Schering)

A white, scored tablet supplied at a strength of 25 mg and used as an androgen to treat low androgen levels, infertility in men.

Dose: 1 tablet 3-4 times a day for several months, then 2-3 tablets a day.
Availability: NHS and private prescription.
Side effects: fluid retention, weight gain, raised calcium levels, increased bone growth, erect penis, premature closure of epiphyses (bone ends), reduced fertility in males, masculinization of women, inflammation of the prostate in the elderly.
Caution: in patients suffering from heart, kidney, or liver impairment, high blood pressure, epilepsy, migraine.
Not to be used for: children, or for patients suffering from prostate or breast cancer, kidney damage, raised calcium levels, heart disease, untreated heart failure.
Caution needed with: liver-enzyme inducing drugs such as BARBITURATES, CARBAMAZEPINE, PHENYTOIN, PRIMIDONE, RIFAMPICIN.
Contains: MESTEROLONE.
Other preparations:

---

probenecid *see* Benemid

probucol *see* **Lurselle**

Procainamide Durules
(Astra)

A pale yellow tablet supplied at a strength of 500 mg and used as a heart rhythm regulator to treat abnormal heart rhythm, some muscle disorders.

Dose: to maintain correct blood levels.
Availability: NHS and private prescription.
Side effects: SLE, stomach and brain disturbance, blood changes.
Caution: in patients suffering from kidney, liver, or heart failure. Your doctor may advise regular blood tests.
Not to be used for: for children or for patients suffering from heart block, SLE (a multisystem disorder), myasthenia gravis, asthma.
Caution needed with:
Contains: PROCAINAMIDE hydrochloride.
Other preparations: PRONESTYL (Squibb).

---

procainamide *see* **Procainamide Durules, Pronestyl**

---

prochlorperazine *see* **Buccastem, Stemetil**

Proctofibe
(Roussel)

A beige tablet used as a bulking agent to treat diverticular disease, irritable colon, constipation because of a diet low in fibre.

Dose: adults and children over 3 years 4-12 tablets a day in divided doses.
Availability: private prescription only.
Side effects:
Caution:
Not to be used for: children under 3 years or for patients suffering from intestinal obstruction.
Caution needed with:
Contains: GRAIN FIBRE, CITRUS FIBRE.
Other preparations:

Proctofoam HC
(Stafford-Miller)

Foam supplied in an aerosol with an applicator and used as a STEROID, local anaesthetic treatment for haemorrhoids, bowel inflammation, fissures.

Dose: in the rectum 1 application 2-3 times a day and after passing motions; around the anus apply as required.
Availability: NHS and private prescription.
Side effects: systemic corticosteroid effects (*see* Precortisyl).
Caution: in pregnant women; do not use for prolonged periods.
Not to be used for: children or for patients suffering from tuberculous, fungal and viral infections.
Caution needed with:
Contains: HYDROCORTISONE acetate, PROXAMINE hydrochloride.
Other preparations:

Proctosedyl
(Roussel)

Suppositories used as a STEROID, local anaesthetic treatment for haemorrhoids, anal fissure, inflammation, itch.

Dose: 1 suppository night and morning and after passing motions.
Availability: NHS and private prescription.
Side effects: systemic corticosteroid effects (*see* Precortisyl).
Caution: in pregnant women; do not use for prolonged periods.
Not to be used for: patients suffering from tuberculous, fungal or viral infections.
Caution needed with:
Contains: HYDROCORTISONE, CINCHOCAINE hydrochloride.
Other preparations: Proctosedyl ointment.

---

procyclidine *see* **Arpicolin, Kemadrin**

---

proflavine cream BPC

A cream used to treat minor cuts and abrasions.

Dose: apply as necessary,
Availability: NHS, private prescription, over the counter.
Side effects:
Caution: stains clothing.

Not to be used for:
Caution needed with:
Contains: proflavine cream BPC.
Other preparations:

Proflex Cream
(Zyma)

A cream used as a NON-STEROID ANTI-INFLAMMATORY to treat rheumatic and muscular pain, sprains, strains.

Dose: 4-10 cm cream applied to the affected area 3-4 times a day.
Availability: NHS, private prescription, over the counter.
Side effects: reddening of skin.
Caution: in pregnant women, nursing mothers. Avoid broken skin, lips, and eyes.
Not to be used for: children, or for patients suffering from allergy to ASPIRIN or anti-inflammatories.
Caution needed with:
Contains: ibuprofen.
Other preparations: Proflex Tablets, IBUGEL (Dermal), Ibuleve (Dendron).

Progesic *see* Fenopron
(Eli Lilly)

progesterone *see* Cyclogest

proguanil hydrochloride *see* Paludrine

Progynova
(Schering)

A beige tablet or a blue tablet according to strengths of 1 mg, 2 mg and used as an oestrogen for the short-term treatment of the menopause.

Dose: initially 1 mg a day for 21 days then 7 or more days without tablets.
Availability: NHS and private prescription.
Side effects: enlarged breasts, fluid retention, headaches, nausea, vaginal bleeding, weight gain, skin changes, liver disorders, jaundice, rashes, vomiting.

Caution: in patients suffering from high blood pressure, diabetes, vascular disorders, asthma, kidney disease, womb diseases, heart disease, epilepsy, migraine. Your doctor may advise you to have regular examinations.

Not to be used for: pregnant women, nursing mothers, or for patients suffering from sickle-cell anaemia, history of heart disease or thrombosis, liver disorders, some cancers, undiagnosed vaginal bleeding, some ear, skin, and kidney disorders, jaundice, porphyria (a rare blood disorder), brain blood-vessel disease.

Caution needed with: DIURETICS, ANTIHYPERTENSIVES, and drugs that change liver enzymes, such as BARBITURATES, CARBAMAZEPINE, PHENYTOIN.

Contains: OESTRADIOL valerate.

Other preparations: CLIMAVAL (Sandoz), ZUMENON (Duphar).

---

prolintane *see* **Villescon**

---

promazine *see* **Sparine**

---

promethazine *see* **Avomine, Medised Suspension, Phenergan, Phensedyl, Sominex**

Prominal
(Sanofi Winthrop)

A white tablet supplied at strengths of 30 mg, 60 mg, 200 mg and used as a BARBITURATE to treat epilepsy.

Dose: adults 100-600 mg a day; children 5-15 mg per kg body weight a day.

Availability: controlled drug; NHS and private precription.

Side effects: drowsiness, hangover, dizziness, allergies, headache, confusion, excitement, addiction, lack of co-ordination.

Caution: in patients suffering from kidney or lung disease. Dependence (addiction) may develop.

Not to be used for: children, young adults, pregnant women, nursing mothers, the elderly, patients with a history of drug or alcohol abuse, or suffering from porphyria (a rare blood disorder), or in the management of pain.

Caution needed with: anticoagulants, alcohol, other tranquillizers, STEROIDS, the contraceptive pill, GRISEOFULVIN, RIFAMPICIN, PHENYTOIN,

METRONIDAZOLE, CHLORAMPHENICOL.
Contains: METHYLPHENOBARBITONE.
Other preparations:

Prondol
(Wyeth)

A yellow tablet supplied at strengths of 15 mg, 30 mg and used as a TRICYCLIC antidepressant to treat depression.

Dose: adults 15-30 mg 3 times a day at first, to a maximum of 60 mg 3 times a day; elderly 15 mg 3 times a day at first.
Availability: NHS and private prescription.
Side effects: dry mouth, constipation, urine retention, blurred vision, palpitations, drowsiness, sleeplessness, dizziness, hands shaking, low blood pressure, weight change, skin reactions, jaundice or blood changes, loss of libido may occur.
Caution: in nursing mothers or in patients suffering from heart disease, thyroid disease, epilepsy, diabetes, liver disorders, glaucoma, retention of urine, some other psychiatric conditions. Your doctor may advise regular blood tests.
Not to be used for: children, pregnant women, or for patients suffering from heart attacks, liver disease, heart block.
Caution needed with: alcohol, ANTICHOLINERGICS, ADRENALINE, MAOIS, BARBITURATES, other antidepressants, ANTIHYPERTENSIVES.
Contains: IPRINDOLE hydrochloride.
Other preparations:

Pronestyl
(Squibb)

A white, scored tablet supplied at a strength of 250 mg and used as an anti-arryhthmic drug to treat abnormal heart rhythm.

Dose: 50 mg per kg body weight a day in divided doses every 3-6 hours.
Availability: NHS and private prescription.
Side effects: SLE (a multi-system disorder), stomach and brain disturbance, blood changes.
Caution: in the elderly, pregnant women, and in patients suffering from kidney, liver, or heart failure, myaesthenia gravis. Your doctor may advise regular blood tests.
Not to be used for: for children or for patients suffering from heart block, SLE (a multi-system disorder).
Caution needed with:

Contains: PROCAINAMIDE hydrochloride.
Other preparations: Pronestyl Injection, PROCAINAMIDE DURULES (Astra).

Propaderm
(Glaxo)

A cream used as a STEROID treatment for skin disorders.

Dose: rub in a small quantity to the affected area twice a day.
Availability: NHS and private prescription.
Side effects: fluid retention, suppression of adrenal glands, thinning of the skin may occur.
Caution: use for short periods of time only.
Not to be used for: patients suffering from acne or any other skin infections caused by tuberculosis, ringworm, viruses, or fungi, or continuously especially in pregnant women.
Caution needed with:
Contains: BECLOMETHASONE DIPROPRIONATE.
Other preparations: Propaderm Ointment, (Propaderm-A — now discontinued).

propafenone *see* Arhythmol

Propain
(Panpharma)

A yellow, scored tablet used as an ANALGESIC, ANTIHISTAMINE treatment for headache, migraine, muscle pain, period pain.

Dose: 1-2 tablets every 4 hours to a maximum of 10 tablets in 24 hours.
Availability: private prescription and over the counter.
Side effects: drowsiness.
Caution: in patients suffering from kidney or liver disease.
Not to be used for: children.
Caution needed with: alcohol, sedatives, other medicines containing PARACETAMOL.
Contains: CODEINE PHOSPHATE, DIPHENHYDRAMINE HYDROCHLORIDE, PARACETAMOL, CAFFEINE.
Other preparations:

Propanix *see* **Inderal**
(Ashbourne)

---

propantheline bromide *see* **Pro-banthine**

Propine
(Allergan)

Drops used as a SYMPATHOMIMETIC treatment for glaucoma, hypertension of the eye.

Dose: 1 drop into the eye every 12 hours.
Availability: NHS and private prescription.
Side effects: temporary smarting, redness, allergy, rarely raised blood pressure.
Caution: in patients suffering from narrow-angle glaucoma, absence of the lens.
Not to be used for: children or for patients suffering from closed angle glaucoma or who wear soft contact lenses.
Caution needed with:
Contains: DIPIVEFRIN HYDROCHLORIDE.
Other preparations:

---

propranolol hydrochloride *see* **Inderal, Inderal LA, Inderetic**

---

propyl salicylate *see* **Monphytol**

---

propyl undecoanate *see* **Monphytol**

---

propylene glycol *see* **Aserbine, Malatex, Unguentum Merck**

---

propylthiouracil tablets

A tablet supplied at a strength of 50 mg and used to treat overactive thyroid.

Dose: adults 6-12 tablets a day, reducing gradually to 1-3 tablets a day.

Availability: NHS and private prescription.
Side effects: nausea, headache, rash, itching, joint pains, hair loss, blood changes, bleeding tendency.
Caution: in pregnant women, nursing mothers, and in patients suffering from large goitre, or kidney damage.
Not to be used for:
Caution needed with:
Contains: propylthiouracil.
Other preparations:

Prosaid *see* Naprosyn
(BHR)

Proscar
(MSD)

A blue, apple-shaped tablet supplied at a strength of 5 mg and used to treat enlarged prostate gland.

Dose: 1 tablet a day for at least 6 months. If then found to be beneficial, treatment should be continued long-term.
Availability: NHS and private prescription.
Side effects: impotence, decreased libido, decreased volume of ejaculate.
Caution: in patients suffering from urine outflow obstruction or prostate cancer. Your doctor may advise regular tests before and during treatment. Female partners of patients being treated who are or who may become pregnant should not handle the tablets and avoid exposure to semen by using a condom.
Not to be used for: children.
Caution needed with:
Contains: FINASTERIDE.
Other preparations:

Prostigimin
(Roche)

A white, scored tablet supplied at a strength of 15 mg and used as an anti-cholinesterase to treat urinary retention following surgery, bowel paralysis, myasthenia gravis (a muscle disorder).

Dose: adults bowel paralysis 1-2 tablets as required; children ⅙-1 tablet as required. Adults myasthenia gravis 5-20 tablets a day in divided doses; infants 1-5 mg every 4 hours, children 15-90 mg a day in divided doses;

after surgery adults 1-2 tablets; children ⅙-1 tablet.
Availability: NHS and private prescription.
Side effects: nausea, diarrhoea, colic, salivation, vomiting.
Caution: in patients suffering from bronchial asthma, heart disease, epilepsy, Parkinson's disease.
Not to be used for: patients suffering from intestinal or urinary obstruction.
Caution needed with: some drugs used in anaesthesia.
Contains: NEOSTIGMINE bromide.
Other preparations: Prostigimin Injection.

P

Protaphane *see* insulin
(Novo Nordisk)

Prothiaden
(Boots)

A red/brown capsule supplied at a strength of 25 mg and used as a TRICYCLIC antidepressant to treat depression, anxiety.

Dose: 3-6 capsules a day.
Availability: NHS and private prescription.
Side effects: dry mouth, constipation, urine retention, blurred vision, palpitations, drowsiness, sleeplessness, dizziness, hands shaking, low blood presure, weight change, skin reactions, jaundice or blood changes, loss of libido may occur, weakness, lack of co-ordination, convulsions, stomach upset, heart irregularities.
Caution: in nursing mothers or in patients suffering from heart disease, thyroid disease, epilepsy, diabetes, retention of urine, liver disorder, adrenal tumour, some other psychiatric conditions. Your doctor may advise regular blood tests.
Not to be used for: children, pregnant women, or for patients suffering from heart attacks, liver disease, heart block.
Caution needed with: alcohol, ANTICHOLINERGICS, ADRENALINE, MAOIS, BARBITURATES, other antidepressants, ANTIHYPERTENSIVES, CIMETIDINE, oestrogens.
Contains: DOTHIEPIN hydrochloride.
Other preparations: Prothiaden Tablets, DOTHAPAX (Ashbourne).

---

protriptyline *see* Concordin

Provera
(Upjohn)

A white, scored tablet supplied at strengths of 5 mg, 10 mg, 100 mg, 200 mg, 400 mg and used as a progestogen treatment for abnormal bleeding of the uterus, secondary absence of periods, endometriosis, hormone-dependent disorders such as breast cancer.

Dose: abnormal bleeding 2.5-10 mg a day for 5-10 days, repeated on 2-3 consecutive menstrual cycles; breast cancer 400-800 mg a day; other cancers 200-400 mg a day; endometriosis 10 mg 3 times a day.
Availability: NHS and private prescription.
Side effects: nausea; on high doses breast pain, lactation, abnormal menstrual bleeding, weight gain, fluid retention.
Caution: in patients with a history of depression, diabetes, epilepsy, migraine, asthma, heart or kidney failure.
Not to be used for: children, pregnant women, or patients suffering from some cancers, liver disease, or a history of thromboembolic disorders.
Caution needed with:
Contains: MEDROXYPROGESTERONE.
Other preparations: (Provera Suspension — now discontinued), FARLUTAL (Farmitalia CE).

---

proxamine *see* Proctofoam HC

---

proxymetacaine hydrochloride *see* Ophthaine

Prozac
(Dista)

A green/off-white capsule supplied at a strength of 20 mg and used as an antidepressant to treat depression, bulimia nervosa (an eating disorder).

Dose: adults 1 capsule a day up to a maximum of 3 capsules.
Availability: NHS and private prescription.
Side effects: nausea, headache, anxiety, sleeplessness, dizziness, rash, weakness, reduced judgement and abilities; rarely convulsions, hypomania, mania.
Caution: in pregnant women and in patients suffering from unstable epilepsy, liver failure, moderate kidney failure, heart disease, diabetes.
Not to be used for: children, nursing mothers, or for patients suffering from severe kidney failure or allergy to FLUOXETINE.

Caution needed with: MAOIS, tryptophan (this is in many health foods), LITHIUM.
Contains: FLUOXETINE.
Other preparations:

---

pseudoephedrine *see* **Actifed Compound, Congesteze, Dimotane Expectorant, Dimotane Plus, Expulin, Galpseud, Galpseud Plus, Sudafed, Sudafed Plus**

Psoradrate
(Norwich Eaton)

A cream used as an anti-psoriatic, drying agent to treat psoriasis.

Dose: wash and dry the area, then apply the cream twice a day.
Availability: NHS, private prescription, over the counter.
Side effects: irritation, hypersensitivity.
Caution:
Not to be used for: patients suffering from pustular psoriasis.
Caution needed with:
Contains: DITHRANOL, UREA.
Other preparations: ALPHODITH (Stafford-Miller), ANTHRANOL (Stiefl), DITHROCREAM (Dermal), EXOLAN (Dermal).

Psoriderm
(Dermal)

An emulsion used as an antipsoriatic to treat psoriasis.

Dose: add 30 ml of the emulsion to the bath water, soak for 15 minutes, dry, then apply the cream to the affected area.
Availability: NHS, private prescription, over the counter.
Side effects: irritation, sensitivity to light.
Caution:
Not to be used for: patients suffering from acute psoriasis.
Caution needed with:
Contains: COAL TAR.
Other preparations: Psoriderm Cream, Psoriderm Scalp Lotion, CARBO-DOME (Lagap), CLINITAR (Shire), GELCOTAR (Quinderm), PSORIGEL (Galderma).

Psorigel
(Galderma)

A gel used as an antipsoriatic treatment for psoriasis, eczema, dermatoses.

Dose: rub into the affected area and allow to dry 1-2 times a day.
Availability: NHS, private prescription, over the counter.
Side effects: irritation, sensitivity to light.
Caution:
Not to be used for: patients suffering from acute psoriasis.
Caution needed with:
Contains: COAL TAR solution.
Other preparations: CARBO-DOME (Lagap), CLINITAR (Shire), GELCOTAR (Quinderm), PSORIDERM (Dermal).

Psorin
(Thames)

An ointment used as an antipsoriatic, skin softener to treat psoriasis.

Dose: apply to the affected areas twice a day.
Availability: NHS, private prescription, over the counter.
Side effects:
Caution: keep out of the eyes, and avoid direct sunlight.
Not to be used for: patients suffering from unstable psoriasis.
Caution needed with:
Contains: COAL TAR, DITHRANOL, SALICYLIC ACID.
Other preparations: DITHROLAN (Dermal).

Pulmadil
(3M Healthcare)

An aerosol supplied at a strength of 0.2 mg and used as a broncho-dilator to treat bronchial spasm brought on by chronic bronchitis, bronchial asthma.

Dose: 1-3 sprays and again after 30 minutes if needed, up to a maximum of 24 sprays in 24 hours.
Availability: NHS and private prescription.
Side effects: headache, dilation of the blood vessels.
Caution: in pregnant women and in patients suffering from abnormal heart rhythms, high blood pressure, overactive thyroid, heart muscle disorders, angina.
Not to be used for:

Caution needed with: SYMPATHOMIMETICS.
Contains: RIMITEROL HYDROBROMIDE.
Other preparations: Pulmadil Auto.

Pulmicort
(Astra)

An aerosol supplied at a strength of 200 micrograms and used as a STEROID to treat bronchial asthma.

Dose: 1 spray twice a day up to a maximum of 8 sprays a day if needed; children reduced doses or use Pulmicort LS.
Availability: NHS and private prescription.
Side effects: hoarseness, thrush of the mouth and throat.
Caution: in pregnant women, in patients suffering from tuberculosis of the lungs, and in those transferring from STEROIDS taken by mouth.
Not to be used for:
Caution needed with:
Contains: BUDESONIDE.
Other preparations: Pulmicort LS, Pulmicort Respules, Pulmicort Turbohaler.

pumilio pine oil *see* Tercoda

Pur-in *see* insulin
(CP Pharmaceuticals)

Pyralvex
(Norgine)

A liquid used as an anti-inflammatory treatment for mouth inflammations.

Dose: apply to the affected area 3-4 times a day.
Availability: NHS, private prescription, over the counter.
Side effects: local irritation.
Caution:
Not to be used for:
Caution needed with:
Contains: ANTHRAQUINONE GLYCOSIDES, SALICYLIC ACID.
Other preparations:

pyrantel *see* **Combantrin**

---

pyrazinamide *see* **Rifater, Zinamide**

---

pyridostigmine *see* **Mestinon**

pyridoxine *see* **Abidec, Allbee with C, Apisate, BC 500, BC 500 with Iron, Becosym, Calcimax, Complement Continus, Fefol-Vit Spansule, Fesovit Spansule, Fesovit Z Spansule, Galfervit, Givitol, Ketovite, Lipoflavonoid, Lipotriad, Octovit, Optimax, Orovite, Orovite 7, Polyvite, Pregnavite Forte F, Surbex T, Tonivitan B, Verdiviton, Villescon**

---

pyrimethamine *see* **Daraprim, Fansidar, Maloprim**

Pyrogastrone *see* **Biogastrone**
(Sanofi Withrop)

Quellada
(Stafford-Miller)

A lotion used as a scabicide to treat scabies.

Dose: apply as directed.
Availability: NHS, private prescription, over the counter.
Side effects:
Caution: keep out of the eyes.
Not to be used for: infants under 1 month.
Caution needed with:
Contains: LINDANE.
Other preparations: Quellada Application PC (for treating lice).

Questran
(Bristol-Myers Squibb)

A powder in a sachet used as a lipid-lowering agent to treat elevated lipids, and to relieve some cases of diarrhoea and itching.

Dose: adults 1-6 sachets a day in divided doses to a maximum of 9 sachets a day; children over 6 years in proportion to dose for 70 kg adult.
Availability: NHS and private prescription.
Side effects: constipation, vitamin K deficiency.
Caution: in pregnant women, nursing mothers, and patients on long-term treatment should take Vitamin A, D, K supplements.
Not to be used for: children under 6 years or for patients suffering from complete biliary blockage.
Caution needed with: DIGOXIN, antibiotics, DIURETICS; allow 1 hour between treatment and any other drugs.
Contains: CHOLESTYRAMINE.
Other preparations: Questran-A (with added sweetener).

Q

---

quinalbarbitone *see* **Seconal Sodium, Tuinal**

---

quinapril *see* **Accupro**

---

quinidine *see* **Kinidin Durules**

---

quinine bisulphate tablets *see* **quinine sulphate tablets**

---

quinine dihydrochloride tablets *see* **quinine sulphate tablets**

---

quinine hydrochloride tablets *see* **quinine sulphate tablets**

---

quinine sulphate tablets

Tablets supplied at strengths of 200 mg, 300 mg, and used to treat malaria and leg cramps at night.

Dose: for cramp, adults 200-300 mg at night. For malaria, adults 600 mg every 8 hours for 7 days; children 10 mg/kg body weight every 8 hours for 7 days.
Availability: NHS and private prescription.

Side effects: noise in the ears, headache, nausea, stomach pain, rash, disturbance of vision, confusion, allergy, blood disorders, kidney failure, low blood sugar.
Caution: in pregnant women, and in patients suffering from some heart conditions and blood enzyme deficiencies.
Not to be used for: patients suffering from some blood disorders or inflammation of the optic nerve.
Caution needed with: MEFLOQUINE, DIGOXIN, CIMETIDINE.
Contains: quinine sulphate.
Other preparations: QUININE HYDROCHLORIDE TABLETS, QUININE DIHYDROCHLORIDE TABLETS, QUININE BISULPHATE TABLETS.

Quinocort
(Quinoderm)

A cream used as a STEROID, antifungal, antibacterial treatment for skin disorders where there is also infection.

Dose: massage into the affected area 2-3 times a day.
Availability: NHS and private prescription
Side effects: fluid retention, suppression of adrenal glands, thinning of the skin may occur.
Caution: use for short periods of time only.
Not to be used for: patients suffering from acne or any other skin infections caused by tuberculosis, ringworm, viruses, or fungi, or continuously especially in pregnant women.
Caution needed with:
Contains: POTASSIUM HYDROXYQUINOLONE SULPHATE, HYDROCORTISONE.
Other preparations:

Quinoderm Cream
(Quinoderm)

A cream used as an antibacterial, skin softener to treat acne, acne-like eruptions, inflammation of the follicles.

Dose: massage into the affected area 1-3 times a day.
Availability: NHS, private prescription, over the counter.
Side effects: irritation, peeling.
Caution: keep out of the eyes, nose, mouth. May bleach fabrics.
Not to be used for:
Caution needed with:
Contains: POTASSIUM HYDROXYQUINOLONE SULPHATE, BENZOYL PEROXIDE.
Other preparations: Quinoderm Cream 5, Quinoderm Lotio-Gel,

Quinoderm Lotio-Gel 5%, Quinoderm with Hydrocortisone (not available over the counter).

Quinoped
(Quinoderm)

A cream used as an antifungal treatment for athlete's foot and similar infections.

Dose: rub lightly into the affected area night and morning.
Availability: NHS, private prescription, over the counter.
Side effects:
Caution: may bleach fabrics.
Not to be used for:
Caution needed with:
Contains: BENZOYL PEROXIDE, POTASSIUM HYDROXYQUINOLONE SULPHATE.
Other preparations:

R

Rabro *see* **Caved-S.** Product now discontinued.

ramipril *see* **Tritace**

ranitidine *see* **Zantac**

Rapitard *see* **insulin**
(Novo Nordisk)

Rastinon
(Hoechst)

A white, scored tablet supplied at a strength of 500 mg and used as an antidiabetic treatment for diabetes.

Dose: 2 tablets a day at first adjust to 1-3 tablets a day as needed.
Availability: NHS and private prescription.
Side effects: allergy including skin rash.
Caution: in the elderly and in patients suffering from kidney failure.
Not to be used for: children, pregnant women, nursing mothers, during

surgery, or for patients suffering from juvenile diabetes, liver or kidney disorders, stress, infections, endocrine disorder.

Caution needed with: ß-BLOCKERS, MAOIS, STEROIDS, DIURETICS, alcohol, anticoagulants, lipid-lowering agents, ASPIRIN, some antibiotics (RIFAMPICIN, sulphonamides, CHLORAMPHENICOL), GLUCAGON, CYCLOPHOSPHAMIDE, the contraceptive pill.

Contains: TOLBUTAMIDE.

Other preparations: PRAMIDEX, GLYCONON (DDSA).

Redoxon
(Roche Nicholas)

A white tablet supplied at strengths of 25 mg, 50 mg, 200 mg, 500 mg and used as a vitamin C treatment for scurvy, and as an additional treatment for wounds and infections.

Dose: adults 500 mg-1 g 2-3 times a day; children under 4 years quarter adult dose, 4-12 years half adult dose, 12-14 years three-quarters adult dose.

Availability: NHS (when prescribed as a generic), private prescription, over the counter.

Side effects: diarrhoea.

Caution:

Not to be used for:

Caution needed with:

Contains: ASCORBIC ACID.

Other preparations: Redoxon Effervescent (not available on NHS).

Refolinon
(Farmitalia CE)

A light-yellow, scored tablet supplied at a strength of 15 mg and used as a folinic acid treatment for megaloblastic anaemia. Also used in emergency treatment of some cases of poisoning.

Dose: for anaemia 1 tablet a day.

Availability: NHS and private prescription.

Side effects:

Caution:

Not to be used for: patients suffering from vitamin B_{12} deficiency anaemia.

Caution needed with:

Contains: CALCIUM FOLINATE.

Other preparations:

Regaine
(Upjohn)

A liquid used as a hair restorer to treat hair loss in men and women.

Dose: 1 ml applied to the scalp twice a day for at least 4 months. Treatment must be continued or hair loss will recur.
Availability: private prescription only.
Side effects: dermatitis.
Caution: in patients suffering from low blood pressure, and on broken skin.
Not to be used for: children.
Caution needed with:
Contains: MINOXIDIL.
Other preparations:

Regulan
(Procter and Gamble)

An effervescent powder supplied in sachets of 3.6 g and used as a bulking agent to treat constipation owing to lack of fibre in the diet.

Dose: adults1 sachet in water 1-3 times a day; children over 6 years 2.5-5 ml 3 times a day.
Availability: NHS, private prescription, over the counter.
Side effects:
Caution:
Not to be used for: children under 6 years and patients suffering from intestinal obstruction.
Caution needed with:
Contains: ISPAGHULA husk.
Other preparations: FYBOGEL (Reckitt & Colman), ISOGEL (Charwell), METAMUCIL (Procter & Gamble).

Rehibin
(Serono)

A white, scored tablet supplied at a strength of 100 mg and used as an anti-oestrogen treatment for infertility due to failure of ovulation caused by impaired hypothalamic-pituitary function.

Dose: 2 tablets morning and evening for 10 days beginning on the third day of the period; continue the treatment for at least 3 cycles.
Availability: NHS and private prescription.
Side effects: hot flushes, nausea, uncomfortable abdomen, jaundice.

Not to be used for: pregnant women or for patients suffering from liver disease, endometrial (womb) cancer, or bleeding from the uterus.
Caution needed with:
Contains: CYCLOFENIL.
Other preparations:

Rehidrat
(Searle)

A lemon and lime, and orange-flavoured powder used to provide electrolytes in fluid and electrolyte loss, and diarrhoea.

Dose: adults and children drink until thirst is quenched; infants substitute for feeds or after breast feeding.
Availability: NHS, private prescription, over the counter.
Side effects:
Caution:
Not to be used for: care in patients suffering from kidney disease, blocked intestine, bowel paralysis.
Caution needed with:
Contains: SODIUM CHLORIDE, POTASSIUM CHLORIDE, SODIUM BICARBONATE, CITRIC ACID, GLUCOSE, SUCROSE, LAEVULOSE.
Other preparations: DIORALYTE (Rhone-Poulenc Rorer), ELECTROLADE (Nicholas), GLUCO-LYTE (Cupal).

Relaxit
(Kabi Pharmacia)

A micro-enema used as a faecal softener to treat constipation.

Dose: 1 enema.
Availability: NHS and private prescription.
Side effects:
Caution:
Not to be used for:
Caution needed with:
Contains: SODIUM CITRATE, SODIUM LAURYL SULPHATE, SORBIC ACID, GLYCEROL, SORBITOL solution.
Other preparations:

Relifex
(Bencard)

A red tablet supplied at a strength of 500 mg and used as a NON-STEROID ANTI-INFLAMMATORY DRUG to treat rheumatoid arthritis, osteoarthritis.

Dose: adults 2 tablets at bed time and, if needed, 1-2 tablets in the morning; elderly 1-2 tablets a day.
Availability: NHS and private prescription.
Side effects: diarrhoea, dyspepsia, nausea, constipation, stomach pain, wind, headache, dizziness, rash, sedation.
Caution: in the elderly and in patients suffering from kidney or liver disease or with a history of stomach ulcer, allergy to ASPIRIN or anti-inflammatories.
Not to be used for: pregnant women, nursing mothers, children, or for patients suffering from stomach ulcer, severe liver disease.
Caution needed with: anticoagulants taken by mouth, hydantoins, anticonvulsants, antidiabetics.
Contains: NABUMETONE.
Other preparations: Relifex Suspension.

Remedeine
(Napp)

A white tablet used as a pain killer to treat pain and fever.

Dose: 1-2 tablets every 4-6 hours to a maximum of 8 tablets a day.
Availability: NHS and private prescription.
Side effects: drowsiness, nausea, vomiting, headache, vertigo, retention of urine, constipation.
Caution: in patients suffering from underactive thyroid, chronic liver disease, severe kidney disease, allergic disorder.
Not to be used for: children, or for patients suffering from breathing difficulty, raised pressure in the brain.
Caution needed with: MAOIS, alcohol, other medicines containing PARA-CETAMOL.
Contains: PARACETAMOL, DIHYDROCODEINE TARTRATE.
Other preparations: Remedeine Forte, CO-DYDRAMOL.

Remnos *see* Mogadon
(DDSA)

---

remoxipride hydrochloride *see* Roxiam

---

reproterol *see* **Bronchodil**

Rescufolin *see* **Refolinon.** Product now discontinued.

reserpine *see* **Serpasil, Serpasil Esidrex**

Resonium-A
(Sanofi Winthrop)

A powder used for ion-exchange to lower potassium levels.

Dose: 15 g 3-4 times a day.
Availability: NHS, private prescription, over the counter.
Side effects: low potassium levels, high sodium levels, impaction of resin
Caution: in patients suffering from heart disease. Potassium and sodium levels should be checked regularly.
Not to be used for:
Caution needed with:
Contains: SODIUM POLYSTYRENE SULPHONATE.
Other preparations:

resorcinol *see* **Dome-Acne, Eskamel**

Respacal *see* **Brelomax**

Restandol
(Organon)

A brown, oval capsule supplied at a strength of 40 mg and used as an androgen to treat hypogonadism and osteoporosis in men caused by low androgen levels.

Dose: 3-4 tablets a day for 2-3 weeks, then 1-3 tablets a day as needed.
Availability: NHS and private prescription.
Side effects: fluid retention, weight gain, raised calcium levels, increased bone growth, erect penis, premature closure of epiphyses (bone ends), reduced fertility in males, masculinization of women, inflammation of the prostate in the elderly.

Caution: in patients suffering from heart, kidney, or liver impairment, high blood pressure, epilepsy, migraine.
Not to be used for: children, or for patients suffering from prostate or breast cancer, kidney damage, raised calcium levels, heart disease, untreated heart failure.
Caution needed with: liver-enzyme inducing drugs (such as CARBAMAZEPINE, PHENYTOIN).
Contains: TESTOSTERONE UNDECANOATE.
Other preparations:

Retcin *see* Erythrocin
(DDSA)

Retin-A
(Cilag)

A lotion used as a VITAMIN A derivative to treat acne where there are comedones, papules, and pustules.

Dose: apply to the affected area 1-2 times a day for at least 8 weeks.
Availability: NHS and private prescription.
Side effects: redness, irritation, loss or gain of skin pigment.
Caution: in pregnant women; avoid direct sunlight or ultra-violet lamps, and keep the lotion away from the eyes, nose, and mouth etc.
Not to be used for: patients suffering from eczema, cuts, abrasion,
Caution needed with: skin softener.
Contains: TRETINOIN.
Other preparations: Retin-A Gel, Retin-A Cream.

Retrovir
(Wellcome)

A white capsule or blue/white capsule according to strengths of 100 mg, 250 mg and used as an anti-viral treatment for serious HIV infections in patients suffering from AIDS, or to delay the onset of AIDS in HIV positive people.

Dose: 500-1500 mg a day in divided doses.
Availability: NHS and private prescription.
Side effects: anaemia, white cell changes, headache, nausea, rash, stomach pain, fever, pins and needles, anorexia, muscle pain, sleeplessness.
Caution: in the elderly, pregnant women, and in patients suffering from

kidney or liver disease. Regular blood tests should be carried out.
Not to be used for: nursing mothers or for patients suffering from low white cell counts.
Caution needed with: ANALGESICS, especially PARACETAMOL, drugs inhibiting liver enzymes (such as CIMETIDINE, CIPROFLOXACIN, ERYTHROMYCIN), cytotoxic drugs, PROBENECID.
Contains: ZIDOVUDINE.
Other preparations: Retrovir Syrup.

Revanil
(Roche)

A white, scored tablet supplied at a strength of 200 micrograms and used as a hormone blocker to treat Parkinson's disease.

Dose: 1 tablet at bedtime with food, gradually increasing to a maximum of 25 tablets a day.
Availability: NHS and private prescription.
Side effects: low blood pressure, nausea, vomiting, dizziness, headache, tiredness, general feeling of being unwell, drowsiness, skin eruptions, abdominal pain , constipation, mental disturbance, blood vessel disease in the hands and feet.
Caution: in pregnant women and in patients with tumour of the pituitary gland.
Not to be used for: children, or for patients suffering from severe disturbance of circulation, heart disease.
Caution needed with: antidepressants, tranquillizers, other similar drugs to treat Parkinson's disease.
Contains: LYSURIDE MALEATE.
Other preparations:

Rheuflex *see* Naprosyn

Rheumox
(Wyeth)

A light/dark orange capsule supplied at a strength of 300 mg and used as a NON-STEROID ANTI-INFLAMMATORY DRUG to treat rheumatoid arthritis, osteoarthritis, ankylosing spondylitis, acute gout.

Dose: adults 4 capsules a day in 2 or 4 divided doses; acute gout 8 capsules in divided doses for 24 hours then 6 capsules a day reducing to 4 capsules a day until symptoms are relieved. Elderly 1 capsule morning

and night increasing to 3 capsules a day if the kidneys function normally.
Availability: NHS and private prescription.
Side effects: sensitivity to light, fluid retention, stomach bleeding, inflammation of the lungs, interference with some blood tests.
Caution: in pregnant women and in patients with a history of stomach ulcer, or suffering from liver disease or heart failure. Patients on long-term treatment should be checked regularly.
Not to be used for: children or for patients suffering from stomach ulcer, history of blood changes, or kidney disease.
Caution needed with: PHENYTOIN, anticoagulants, antidiabetics, sulphonamide antibiotics.
Contains: AZAPROPAZONE.
Other preparations: Rheumox 600 Tablets.

R

Rhinocort
(Astra)

An aerosol supplied at a strength of 50 micrograms and used as a STEROID treatment for rhinitis.

Dose: 2 sprays into each nostril twice a day at first, then 1 spray into each nostril twice a day.
Availability: NHS and private prescription.
Side effects: sneezing.
Caution: in pregnant women and in patients suffering from fungal, viral, or tubercular infections of the nose.
Not to be used for: children for prolonged treatment.
Caution needed with:
Contains: BUDESONIDE.
Other preparations: Rhinocort Aqua.

Rhinolast
(ASTA)

A nasal spray used as an ANTIHISTAMINE to treat hay fever and rhinitis.

Dose: 1 spray in each nostril twice a day.
Availability: NHS and private prescription.
Side effects: nasal irritation, taste disturbance.
Caution: in pregnant women and nursing mothers.
Not to be used for: children.
Caution needed with:
Contains: AZELASTINE.
Other preparations:

Rhumalgan *see* **Voltarol**
(Lagap)

---

riboflavine *see* **Abidec, Allbee with C, Apisate, BC 500, BC 500 with Iron, Becosym, Calcimax, Concavit, Fefol-Vit Spansule, Fesovit Spansule, Fesovit Z Spansule, Galfervit, Givitol, Ketovite, Lipoflavonoid, Octovit, Orovite, Orovite 7, Polyvite, Pregnavite Forte F, Surbex T, Tonivitan B, Verdiviton, Villescon, Vitamins Capsules**

Ridaura Tiltab
(Bridge)

A pale-yellow, square tablet supplied at a strength of 3 mg and used as an oral gold salt to treat progressive rheumatoid arthritis which cannot be controlled effectively by NON-STEROID ANTI-INFLAMMATORY DRUGS.

Dose: 1 tablet in the morning and 1 tablet in the evening for the first 3-6 months, then increase to 3 tablets a day if needed for no longer than a further 3 months when the treatment should be discontinued.
Availability: NHS and private prescription.
Side effects: diarrhoea, nausea, stomach pain, ulcerative enterocolitis, rash, itch, mouth inflammation, hair loss, conjunctivitis, disturbance of taste, blood changes, kidney effects, lung fibrosis.
Caution: in patients suffering from kidney or liver disease, inflammatory bowel disease, rash, history of bone marrow depression. Your doctor may advise that blood counts should be checked regularly. Women should take contraceptive measures until 6 months after end of treatment.
Not to be used for: children, pregnant women, nursing mothers, or for patients suffering from severe kidney or liver disease, SLE (a multisystem disorder), history of necrotizing enterocolitis, lung fibrosis, exfoliative dermatitis, bone marrow aplasia, severe blood changes.
Caution needed with:
Contains: AURANOFIN.
Other preparations:

Rifadin
(Marion Merrell Dow)

A red/blue capsule or a red capsule according to strengths of 150 mg, 300 mg and used as an antibiotic in the additional treatment for tuberculosis, and other infections. Used to prevent meningitis in susceptible patients

Dose: as advised by doctor according to condition.
Availability: NHS and private prescription.
Side effects: symptoms similar to influenza, rash, stomach and liver disturbances, orange-coloured urine and faeces.
Caution: in the elderly, pregnant women, nursing mothers, underfed or very young infants, and in patients suffering from liver disease.
Not to be used for: patients suffering from jaundice.
Caution needed with: anticoagulants, DIGOXIN, antidiabetics, contraceptive pill, STEROIDS, CYCLOSPORIN, DAPSONE, PHENYTOIN, QUINIDINE, some ANALGESICS.
Contains: RIFAMPICIN.
Other preparations: Rifadin Syrup, RIMACTANE (Ciba).

---

rifampicin *see* Rifadin, Rifinah, Rimactane

Rifater
(Marion Merrell Dow)

A pink/beige tablet used as an antibiotic combination to treat tuberculosis of the lungs.

Dose: adults under 40 kg body weight 3 tablets a day, 40-49 kg 4 tablets a day, 50-64 kg 5 tablets a day, over 65 kg 6 tablets a day; children as advised by the physician.
Availability: NHS and private prescription.
Side effects: flu-like symptoms, skin reactions, stomach and liver disturbances, change in urine colour, insomnia, muscle twitch, mental disturbance.
Caution: in the elderly, pregnant women, nursing mothers and in patients suffering from liver disease, gout, or coughing blood.
Not to be used for: patients suffering from jaundice.
Caution needed with: anticoagulants, DIGOXIN, QUINIDINE, STEROIDS, the contraceptive pill, DAPSONE, ANALGESICS, antidiabetics taken by mouth, CYCLOSPORIN, PHENYTOIN, some painkillers.
Contains: ISONIAZID, PYRAZINAMIDE, RIFAMPICIN.
Other preparations:

Rifinah
(Marion Merrell Dow)

A pink tablet or an orange, oval-shaped tablet according to strength and used as an antibiotic combination to treat tuberculosis.

Dose: under 50 kg body weight 3 pink tablets once a day before breakfast;

over 50 kg body weight 2 orange tablets once a day before breakfast.
Availability: NHS and private prescription.
Side effects: sleeplessness, muscle twitching, flu-like symptoms, skin reactions, stomach and liver disturbances, orange urine and faeces.
Caution: in pregnant women, nursing mothers, the elderly, and patients suffering from liver disease, or with a history of epilepsy.
Not to be used for: children or for patients suffering from jaundice.
Caution needed with: anticoagulants, DIGOXIN, STEROIDS, the contraceptive pill, antidiabetics, CYCLOSPORIN, DAPSONE, PHENYTOIN, QUINIDINE, some painkillers.
Contains: RIFAMPICIN, ISONIAZID.
Other preparations: RIMACTAZID (Ciba).

Rimacid *see* Indocid
(Rima)

Rimacillin *see* ampicillin
(Rima)

Rimactane
(Ciba)

A red capsule or a brown/red capsule according to strengths of 150 mg, 300 mg and used as an antibiotic in the additional treatment for tuberculosis and other similar infections. Used to prevent meningitis in susceptible patients.

Dose: as advised by doctor according to condition.
Availability: NHS and private prescription.
Side effects: flu-like symptoms, skin reactions, stomach and liver disturbances, orange urine and faeces.
Caution: in the elderly, pregnant women, nursing mothers, or in very young undernourished patients, and in patients suffering from liver disease, porphyria (a rare blood disorder).
Not to be used for: patients suffering from jaundice.
Caution needed with: anticoagulants, contraceptive pill, STEROIDS, DIGOXIN, antidiabetics, CYCLOSPORIN, DAPSONE, PHENYTOIN, QUINIDINE, indigestion remedies, ANTICHOLINERGICS, some painkillers.
Contains: RIFAMPICIN.
Other preparations: Rimactane Syrup, Rimactane Infusion, RIFADIN (Marion Merrell Dow).

Rimactazid *see* **Rifinah**
(Ciba)

Rimadol *see* **paracetamol**
(Rima)

Rimafen *see* **Brufen**
(Rima)

Rimapam *see* **diazepam**
(Rima)

Rimapen *see* **Distaquaine V-K**
(Rima)

Rimapurinol *see* **Zyloric**
(Rima)

Rimarin *see* **Piriton**
(Rima)

Rimasal *see* **Ventolin**
(Rima)

rimiterol hydrobromide *see* **Pulmadil**

Rimoxacillin *see* **Amoxil**
(Rima)

Rimoxyn *see* **Naprosyn**
(Rima)

Rinatec
(Boehringer)

A nasal spray supplied at a strength of 20 micrograms per dose, and used as an ANTICHOLINERGIC to treat nasal discharge associated with rhinitis.

Dose: 1-2 sprays in the nostril(s) up to 4 times a day.
Availability: NHS and private prescription.
Side effects: dry nose, irritation.
Caution: in patients suffering from glaucoma or enlarged prostate.
Not to be used for: children.
Caution needed with:
Contains: IPRATROPIUM BROMIDE.
Other preparations:

---

ritodrine hydrochloride *see* **Yutopar**

Rivotril
(Roche)

A beige tablet or white tablet according to strengths of 0.5 mg, 2 mg and used as an anticonvulsant to treat epilepsy.

Dose: adults 1 mg a day at first, up to 4-8 mg a day; children and the elderly reduced doses.
Availability: NHS and private prescription.
Side effects: drowsiness, confusion, unsteadiness, low blood pressure, rash, changes in vision, changes in libido, retention of urine. Risk of addiction increases with dose and length of treatment. May impair judgement.
Caution: in children, the elderly, pregnant women, nursing mothers, in women during labour, and in patients suffering from lung disorders, kidney or liver disorders. Avoid long-term use and withdraw gradually.
Not to be used for: patients suffering from acute lung diseases, some chronic lung diseases, some obsessional and psychotic diseases.
Caution needed with: alcohol, other tranquillizers, anticonvulsants.
Contains: CLONAZEPAM.
Other preparations: Rivotril Injection.

Ro-A-Vit — VITAMIN A supplement. Product in tablet form now discontinued.
(Roche)

Roaccutane
(Roche)

A white/red capsule used as a VITAMIN A derivative to treat severe acne.

Dose: 0.5 mg per kg body weight a day with food for the first 4 weeks, then adjust according to response for another 8-12 weeks.
Availability: NHS (hospitals only).
Side effects: dryness, erosion of mucous membranes, hair loss, rise in liver enzymes and serum lipids, nausea, headache, sweating, moodiness, seizures, irregular periods, rarely loss of hearing, blood changes, blood vessel inflammation.
Caution: women of child-bearing age must take contraceptive precautions before, during, and after treatment. Your doctor may advise that liver and blood should be checked regularly.
Not to be used for: children, pregnant women, nursing mothers, or for patients suffering from liver or kidney disease.
Caution needed with: VITAMIN A.
Contains: ISOTRETINOIN.
Other preparations: ISOTREX (Stiefel).

R

Robaxin
(Wyeth)

A white, oblong, scored tablet supplied at a strength of 750 mg and used as a muscle relaxant to treat skeletal muscle spasm.

Dose: adults 2 tablets 4 times a day; elderly 1 tablet 4 times a day.
Availability: NHS and private prescription.
Side effects: drowsiness, allergy.
Caution: in pregnant women, nursing mothers, and in patients suffering from kidney or liver disease.
Not to be used for: children or for patients in a coma or suffering from brain damage, epilepsy, myaesthenia gravis.
Caution needed with: alcohol, sedatives and stimulants, ANTICHOLINERGICS.
Contains: METHOCARBAMOL.
Other preparations: Robaxin Injectable.

Robaxisal Forte
(Wyeth)

A pink/white, two-layered, scored tablet used as a muscle relaxant and ANALGESIC to treat skeletal muscle spasm.

Dose: adults 2 tablets 4 times a day; elderly 1 tablet 4 times a day.

Availability: private prescription only.
Side effects: drowsiness, allergy, stomach bleeding.
Caution: in pregnant women, nursing mothers, and in patients suffering from kidney or liver disease, allergy to anti-inflammatory drugs, or a history of bronchospasm.
Not to be used for: children or for patients suffering from coma, brain damage, epilepsy, myasthenia gravis, stomach ulcer, haemophilia.
Caution needed with: alcohol, sedatives and stimulants, ANTICHOLINERGICS, anticoagulants, antidiabetics, HYDANTOINS.
Contains: METHOCARBAMOL, ASPIRIN.
Other preparations:

Rocaltrol
(Roche)

A white/red capsule or a red capsule according to strengths of 0.25 micrograms, 0.5 micrograms and used as a source of VITAMIN D for correcting calcium and phosphate metabolism in patients suffering from kidney osteodystrophy (bone disease due to kidney disorder).

Dose: 1-2 micrograms a day increasing if needed by 0.25-0.5 micrograms at a time to no more than 2-3 micrograms a day.
Availability: NHS and private prescription.
Side effects: increased blood and urine calcium levels.
Caution: in pregnant women. Do not take any other vitamin D preparations. Your doctor may advise that calcium levels should be checked regularly.
Not to be used for: patients suffering from metastatic calcification (laying down of calcium), raised calcium levels.
Caution needed with: other VITAMIN D preparations.
Contains: CALCITRIOL.
Other preparations:

Roccal — disinfectant solution. Product now discontinued.

Rohypnol
(Roche)

A purple, diamond-shaped, scored tablet supplied at a strength of 1 mg and used as a sedative for the short-term treatment of sleeplessness or to bring on sleep at other times.

Dose: elderly ½ tablet before going to bed; adults ½-1 tablet before going to bed.
Availability: private prescription only.
Side effects: drowsiness, confusion, unsteadiness, low blood pressure, rash, changes in vision, changes in libido, retention of urine. Risk of addiction increases with dose and length of treatment. May impair judgement.
Caution: in the elderly, pregnant women, nursing mothers, in women during labour, and in patients suffering from lung disorders, kidney or liver disorders. Avoid long-term use and withdraw gradually.
Not to be used for: children, or for patients suffering from acute lung diseases, some chronic lung diseases, some obsessional and psychotic diseases.
Caution needed with: alcohol, other tranquillizers, anticonvulsants.
Contains: FLUNITRAZEPAM.
Other preparations:

R

Ronicol
(Roche)

A white, scored tablet supplied at a strength of 25 mg and used as a vasodilator to treat poor circulation.

Dose: 1-2 tablets 4 times a day.
Availability: NHS, private prescription, over the counter.
Side effects: flushes.
Caution: care in long-term treatment of diabetics.
Not to be used for: children.
Caution needed with:
Contains: NICOTINYL ALCOHOL TARTRATE.
Other preparations: Ronicol Timespan.

Ronmix *see* Erythrocin
(Ashbourne)

Rose Bengal Minims
(SNP)

Drops used as a dye to stain the eye for finding degenerated cells in dry eye syndrome.

Dose: 1-2 drops into the eye as needed.

Availability: NHS, private prescription, over the counter.
Side effects: severe smarting.
Caution:
Not to be used for: children.
Caution needed with:
Contains: ROSE BENGAL.
Other preparations:

Roter
(Roterpharma)

A pink tablet used as an ANTACID and antibulking agent to treat stomach ulcers, gastritis.

Dose: adults 1-2 tablets 3 times a day.
Availability: private prescription and over the counter.
Side effects: constipation, nerve damage.
Caution:
Not to be used for: for children.
Caution needed with: TETRACYCLINE antibiotics, tablets which are coated to protect the stomach.
Contains: MAGNESIUM CARBONATE, BISMUTH SUBNITRATE, SODIUM BICARBONATE, FRANGULA.
Other preparations:

Rotersept
(Roterpharma)

An aerosol used as a disinfectant for the prevention of mastitis, and to treat cracked nipples.

Dose: spray on to the breast before and after feeding.
Availability: NHS, private prescription, over the counter.
Side effects:
Caution:
Not to be used for: children.
Caution needed with:
Contains: CHLORHEXIDINE GLUCONATE.
Other preparations:

Rowachol
(Monmouth)

A capsule containing essential oils used to treat cholelithiasis (gall stones).

Dose: adults 1-2 capsules 3 times a day before meals.
Availability: NHS and private prescription.
Side effects:
Caution:
Not to be used for: children.
Caution needed with: anticoagulants, contraceptive pill.
Contains: MENTHOL, MENTHONE, ALPHA-BETA-PINENES, CAMPHENE, CINEOLE, BORNEOL, OLIVE OIL.
Other preparations:

Rowatinex
(Monmouth)

A capsule containing volatile oils used to treat urinary stones, kidney disorders, prevention of urinary stones, and mild urine infections

Dose: 1 capsule 3-4 times a day before food.
Availability: NHS and private prescription.
Side effects:
Caution:
Not to be used for: children.
Caution needed with: anticoagulants, contraceptive pill.
Contains: PINENE, CAMPHENE, BORNEOL, ANETHOL, FENCHONE, CINEOLE, OLIVE OIL.
Other preparations:

Roxiam
(Astra)

A blue capsule supplied at strengths of 150 mg, 300 mg, and used to treat schizophrenia.

Dose: initially 300 mg once a day, adjusted to 150-600 mg once a day; elderly 150 mg initially.
Availability: NHS and private prescription.
Side effects: drowsiness, restlessness, tremor, ANTICHOLINERGIC effects, menstrual disorder, rash, high temperature.
Caution: in pregnant women, nursing mothers, and in patients suffering from severe kidney or liver damage, Parkinson's disease, epilepsy, or with a history of breast cancer.
Not to be used for: children
Caution needed with:
Contains: REMOXIPRIDE HYDROCHLORIDE.

Rusyde *see* Lasix
(CP Pharmaceuticals)

Rybarvin — anti-asthmatic inhaler. Product now discontinued.

Rynacrom Spray
(Fisons)

A spray used as an anti-allergy treatment for allergic rhinitis.

Dose: 1 spray into each nostril 4-6 times a day continuously.
Availability: NHS, private prescription, over the counter.
Side effects: temporary itching nose, rarely bronchial spasm.
Caution:
Not to be used for:
Caution needed with:
Contains: SODIUM CROMOGLYCATE.
Other preparations: Rynacrom Nasal Drops, Rynacrom Cartridges, Rynacrom Compound, Rynacrom Capsules.

Rythmodan
(Roussel)

A yellow/green capsule or a white capsule according to strengths of 100 mg, 150 mg and used as an anti-arrhythmic treatment for abnormal heart rhythm

Dose: 300-800 mg a day in divided doses.
Availability: NHS and private prescription.
Side effects: ANTICHOLINERGIC effects, rarely jaundice, mood changes, low blood sugar.
Caution: in pregnant women, and in patients suffering from heart conduction block, heart,liver, and kidney failure, enlarged prostate, glaucoma, urine retention, low potassium levels.
Not to be used for: for patients suffering from severe heart conduction block, heart failure.
Caution needed with: ß-BLOCKERS, DIURETICS, ANTICHOLINERGICS, other anti-arrhythmics.
Contains: DISOPYRAMIDE.

Other preparations: Rythmodan Retard, Rythmodan Injection, DIRYTHMIN (Astra), ISOMIDE (Monmouth).

S.H. 420 *see* Primolut-N
(Schering)

Sabidal SR *see* Lasma
(Zyma)

Sabril
(Marion Merrell Dow)

A white, oval, scored tablet supplied at a strength of 500 mg and used to treat epilepsy.

Dose: adults, 4 tablets a day initially, adjusted to a maximum of 8 tablets a day; children 1-8 tablets a day according to body weight.
Availability: NHS and private prescription.
Side effects: aggression, mental disturbance, tiredness, dizziness, nervousness, irritability, memory and visual disturbances, excitation, agitation, increased frequency of seizures.
Caution: in the elderly, and in patients with a history of mental or behavioural problems, or suffering from kidney damage. Your doctor may recommend regular examinations.
Not to be used for: children under 10 kg body weight, pregnant women, nursing mothers.
Caution needed with:
Contains: VIGABATRIN.
Other preparations: Sabril Sachets.

Salactol
(Dermal)

A paint used as a skin softener to treat warts.

Dose: apply to the wart once a day and rub down with a pumice stone between treatments.
Availability: NHS, private prescription, over the counter.
Side effects:
Caution: do not apply to healthy skin.
Not to be used for: warts on the face or anal and genital areas.

Caution needed with:
Contains: SALICYLIC ACID, LACTIC ACID.
Other preparations: CUPLEX (SNP), DUOFILM (Stiefel), SALATAC (Dermal).

Salatac *see* Salactol
(Dermal)

Salazopyrin
(Kabi Pharmacia)

An orange, scored tablet supplied at a strength of 500 mg and used as a salicylate-sulphonamide treatment for ulcerative colitis, Crohn's disease.

Dose: adults 2-4 tablets 4 times a day for 2-3 weeks; children over 2 years 40-60 mg/kg body weight a day.
Availability: NHS and private prescription.
Side effects: nausea, headache, rash, high temperature, loss of appetite.
Caution: in patients with liver or kidney disease. Your doctor may advise regular blood tests.
Not to be used for: children under 2 years.
Caution needed with: DIGOXIN.
Contains: SULPHASALAZINE.
Other preparations: SALAZOPYRIN-EN TABLETS, Salazopyrin suspension, enema, suppositories.

Salazopyrin-EN Tablets
(Kabi Pharmacia)

An orange, oval tablet supplied at a strength of 500 mg and used as a salicylate-sulphonamide. treatment for rheumatoid arthritis which is not responding to NON-STEROID ANTI-INFLAMMATORY DRUGS. Also used to treat ulcerative colitis and Crohn's disease (*see* Salazopyrin).

Dose: 1 tablet a day for the first 7 days increasing by 1 tablet a day each subsequent 7 days to a maximum of 6 tablets a day in divided doses.
Availability: NHS and private prescription.
Side effects: nausea, headache, rash, fever, loss of appetite.
Caution: in patients suffering from liver or kidney disease. Your doctor may advise that blood should be checked regularly and any other ANALGE-SICS taken at the same time should only be withdrawn after response has been monitored.
Not to be used for: children.

Caution needed with: DIGOXIN.
Contains: SULPHASALAZINE.
Other preparations: SALAZOPYRIN, salazopyrin suspension, enema suppositories.

Salbulin Tablets *see* **Ventolin.** Product now discontinued.

Salbulin Inhaler *see* **Ventolin**
(3M Healthcare)

---

salbutamol *see* **Cobutolin, Salbulin, Ventide, Ventodisks, Ventolin**

Salbuvent *see* **Ventolin**
(Farmitalia CE)

---

salicylamide *see* **Intralgin**

---

salicylic acid *see* **Aserbine, benzoic acid compound ointment, Capasal, coal tar and salicylic acid ointment, Cocois, Cuplex, Diprosalic, Dithrolan, Duofilm, Gelcosal, Ional T, Keralyt, Malatex, Monphytol, Movelat, Phytex, Phytocil, Posalfilin, Pragmatar, Psorin, Pyralvex, Salactol, Verrugon**

Saline Minims
(SNP)

Drops used to irrigate the eyes.

Dose: use as needed.
Availability: NHS, private prescription, over the counter.
Side effects:
Caution:
Not to be used for:
Not to be used with:

Contains: SODIUM CHLORIDE.
Other preparations:

---

salmeterol *see* Serevent

Salofalk *see* Asacol
(Thames)

Salonair
(Eastern)

An aerosol used as an ANALGESIC rub to relieve muscular and rheumatic pain.

Dose: spray on to the affected area 1-2 times a day.
Availability: NHS, private prescription , over the counter.
Side effects: may be irritant.
Caution:
Not to be used for: areas such as near the eyes, on broken or inflamed skin, or on membranes (such as the mouth).
Caution needed with:
Contains: GLYCOL SALICYLATE, MENTHOL, CAMPHOR, SQUALANE, BENZYL NICOTINATE.
Other preparations:

---

salsalate *see* Disalcid

Saluric
(MSD)

A white, scored tablet supplied at a strength of 500 mg and used as a DIURETIC to treat fluid retention, high blood pressure.

Dose: adults fluid retention ½-2 tablets a day or from time to time up to 4 a day, high blood pressure ½-2 a day up to 2 a day if needed; children under 2 years 125-375 mg a day in two doses, 2-12 years 375-1 g a day in two doses.
Availability: NHS and private prescription.
Side effects: low potassium level, rash, sensitivity to light, blood changes, gout, tiredness.

Caution: in pregnant women and in patients suffering from diabetes, kidney or liver disease, gout. Potassium supplements may be needed.
Not to be used for: nursing mothers or for patients suffering from severe kidney failure or liver, Addison's disease, high calcium levels.
Caution needed with: DIGOXIN, LITHIUM, ANTIHYPERTENSIVES, NON-STEROID ANTI-INFLAMMATORY DRUGS, sedatives, ACE INHIBITORS, STEROIDS.
Contains: CHLOROTHIAZIDE.
Other preparations:

Salzone
(Wallace)

A syrup supplied at a strength of 120 mg/5 ml and used as an ANALGESIC to relieve pain and reduce fever.

Dose: children 2.5-10 ml every 4 hours according to age (not more than 4 doses in 24 hours).
Availability: NHS, private prescription, over the counter.
Side effects:
Caution: in children suffering from kidney or liver disease.
Not to be used for:
Caution needed with: other medicines containing PARACETAMOL.
Contains: PARACETAMOL.
Other preparations: CALPOL (Wellcome), DISPROL PAEDIATRIC (Reckitt and Coleman), PALDESIC (RP Drugs), PANALEVE (Pinewood, prescribed as a generic on NHS), PARACETAMOL PAEDIATRIC ELIXIR.

Sandimmun
(Sandoz)

A pink, oval capsule, yellow, oblong capsule, or pink, oblong capsule according to strengths of 25 mg, 50 mg, 100 mg, and used as a treatment for severe psoriasis. Also used to prevent rejection following transplantation or grafts.

Dose: for psoriasis, initially 1.25 mg/kg body weight twice a day, increasing to 5 mg/kg a day. After transplant/graft as advised by doctor.
Availability: NHS and private prescription.
Side effects: kidney or liver disorder, high blood pressure, tremor, stomach upset, swollen gums, burning sensation, high potassium and uric acid levels, fluid retention, convulsions.
Caution: in pregnant women, nursing mothers, and in patients with high potassium or uric acid levels. Your doctor may advise regular tests during

treatment.

Not to be used for: patients suffering from malignant conditions, kidney damage, or uncontrolled high blood pressure or infection.

Caution needed with: antibiotics, some vaccines, PHENYTOIN, KETOCONAZOLE, RIFAMPICIN, ISONIAZID, CARBAMAZEPINE, BARBITURATES, COLCHICINE, drugs affecting the kidneys.

Contains: cyclosporin.

Other preparations: Sandimmun Oral Solution, Sandimmun Infusion.

Sando-K
(Sandoz)

A white, effervescent tablet used as a potassium supplement to treat potassium deficiency.

Dose: 2-4 tablets a day dissolved in water.
Availability: NHS, private prescription, over the counter.
Side effects: stomach upset.
Caution: in patients suffering from kidney disease.
Not to be used for:
Caution needed with:
Contains: POTASSIUM BICARBONATE, POTASSIUM CHLORIDE.
Other preparations:

Sandocal
(Sandoz)

A white, effervescent tablet supplied at strengths of 400 mg, 1 g and used as a calcium supplement in additional treatment for osteoporosis, and where calcium is deficient in the diet or requirements are high.

Dose: adults 400 mg-2 g a day; children 400 mg-1 g a day.
Availability: NHS, private prescription, over the counter.
Side effects: diarrhoea, nausea, flushes.
Caution: in patients suffering from kidney disease, unbalanced electrolyte levels. Your doctor may advise that calcium levels should be checked regularly.
Not to be used for: for patients suffering from raised calcium levels in the blood or urine, kidney stones, galactosaemia.
Caution needed with: THIAZIDES, TETRACYCLINES, VITAMIN D, fluoride.
Contains: CALCIUM LACTATE GLUCONATE, SODIUM BICARBONATE, POTASSIUM BICARBONATE.
Other preparations: Calcium Sandoz Syrup, Calcium Sandoz Injection.

Sanomigran
(Sandoz)

An ivory, scored tablet supplied at strengths of 0.5 mg, 1.5 mg and used as a blood vessel stabilizer to treat migraine or headache.

Dose: adults 1.5 mg a day as a single dose at night or in 3 divided doses to a maximum of 4.5 mg a day in divided doses; children up to 1.5 mg a day in divided doses, or 1 mg at night.
Availability: NHS and private prescription.
Side effects: drowsiness, weight gain, excitement.
Caution: in patients suffering from glaucoma or retention of urine.
Not to be used for:
Caution needed with:
Contains: PIZOTIFEN HYDROGEN MALATE.
Other preparations: Sanomigran Elixir.

Saventrine
(Pharmax)

A white, mottled tablet supplied at a strength of 30 mg and used to treat conduction defects in the heart.

Dose: as advised by physician.
Availability: NHS and private prescription.
Side effects: palpitations, tremor, sweating, headache, diarrhoea.
Caution: in patients suffering from high blood pressure and diabetes.
Not to be used for: patients suffering from some heart diseases and overactive thyroid.
Caution needed with:
Contains: ISOPRENALINE hydrochloride
Other preparations: Saventrine I.V, MEDIHALER-ISO (3M Healthcare).

Savloclens *see* Savlon Hospital Concentrate. Product now discontinued.

Savlodil *see* Savlon Hospital Concentrate. Product now discontinued.

Savlon Hospital Concentrate
(ICI)

A solution used as a disinfectant and general antiseptic.

Dose: adequate amounts.
Availability: NHS, private prescription, over the counter.
Side effects:
Caution:
Not to be used for:
Caution needed with:
Contains: CHLORHEXIDINE gluconate, CETRIMIDE.
Other preparations:

Schering PC4 *see* PC4

Scheriproct
(Schering)

An ointment used as a steroid, local anaesthetic treatment for haemor-rhoids, anal fissure, itch, bowel inflammation.

Dose: apply 2-4 times a day.
Availability: NHS and private prescription.
Side effects: systemic corticosteroid effects (*see* Precortisyl).
Caution: in pregnant women; do not use for prolonged periods.
Not to be used for: patients suffering from tuberculous, fungal, or viral infections
Caution needed with:
Contains: PREDNISOLONE hexanoate, CINCHOCAINE hydrochloride
Other preparations: Scheriproct suppositories.

Scopoderm
(Ciba)

A pink, self-adhesive patch used as an ANTICHOLINERGIC to prevent travel sickness.

Dose: 1 patch applied to clean dry skin behind the ear 5-6 hours before a journey, replacing after 3 days if needed. Remove after journey is completed.
Availability: NHS and private prescription.
Side effects: local skin irritation, rash, dry mouth, drowsiness, dizziness, retention of urine, visual disturbances.
Caution: care in pregnant women, nursing mothers, and in patients

suffering from blocked bladder outflow, bowel obstruction, kidney or liver disease.
Not to be used for: children under 10 years or for patients suffering from glaucoma.
Caution needed with: sedatives, ANTICHOLINERGICS, alcohol.
Contains: HYOSCINE.
Other preparations:

Secadrex
(Rhone-Poulenc Rorer)

A white tablet supplied at a strength of 400 mg and used as a ß-BLOCKER/ THIAZIDE DIURETIC combination to treat high blood pressure.

Dose: 1-2 tablets a day.
Availability: NHS and private prescription.
Side effects: cold hands and feet, sleep disturbance, slow heart rate, rash, gout, blood changes, tiredness, wheezing, heart failure, stomach upset, sensitivity to light, dry eyes.
Caution: in pregnant women, nursing mothers, and in patients suffering from diabetes, gout, kidney or liver disorders, asthma. May need to be withdrawn before surgery. Withdraw gradually. Your doctor may advise additional treatment with DIURETICS or DIGOXIN.
Not to be used for: children, or for patients suffering from heart block or failure, kidney failure.
Caution needed with: VERAPAMIL, CLONIDINE withdrawal, some anti-arrhythmic drugs and anaesthetics, RESERPINE, some ANTIHYPERTENSIVES, ERGOTAMINE, CIMETIDINE, sedatives, SYMPATHOMIMETICS, INDOMETHACIN, LITHIUM, DIGOXIN.
Contains: ACEBUTOLOL hydrochloride, HYDROCHLOROTHIAZIDE.
Other preparations:

Seconal Sodium
(Eli Lilly)

An orange capsule supplied at strengths of 50 mg, 100 mg and used as a BARBITURATE to treat sleeplessness.

Dose: 50-100 mg at night.
Availability: controlled drug; NHS and private prescription.
Side effects: drowsiness, hangover, dizziness, allergies, headache, confusion, excitement.
Caution: in patients suffering from kidney, liver, or lung disease. Depend-

ence (addiction) may develop.

Not to be used for: children, young adults, pregnant women, nursing mothers, the elderly, patients with a history of drug or alcohol abuse, or suffering from porphyria (a rare blood disorder), or in the management of pain.

Caution needed with: anticoagulants, alcohol, other tranquillizers, STEROIDS, the contraceptive pill, GRISEOFULVIN, RIFAMPICIN, PHENYTOIN, METRONIDAZOLE, CHLORAMPHENICOL.

Contains: QUINALBARBITONE sodium.

Other preparations:

Sectral
(Rhone-Poulenc Rorer.)

A buff/white capsule or a buff/pink capsule according to strengths of 100 mg, 200 mg, or a white tablet supplied at a strength of 400 mg and used as a ß-BLOCKER to treat angina, abnormal heart rhythm, or high blood pressure.

Dose: up to 1200 mg a day in divided doses; high blood pressure up to 800 mg a day.

Availability: NHS and private prescription.

Side effects: cold hands and feet, sleep disturbance, slow heart rate, tiredness, wheezing, heart failure, stomach upset, dry eyes, rash.

Caution: in pregnant women, nursing mothers, and in patients suffering from diabetes, kidney or liver disorders, asthma. May need to be withdrawn before surgery. Withdraw gradually. Your doctor may advise additional treatment with DIURETICS or DIGOXIN.

Not to be used for: children or for patients suffering from heart block or failure.

Caution needed with: VERAPAMIL, CLONIDINE withdrawal, some anti-arrhythmic drugs and anaesthetics, RESERPINE, some ANTIHYPERTENSIVES, ERGOTAMINE, CIMETIDINE, sedatives, antidiabetics, SYMPATHOMIMETICS, INDOMETHACIN.

Contains: ACEBUTOLOL hydrochloride.

Other preparations:

Securon
(Knoll)

A white tablet or a white, scored tablet according to strengths of 40 mg, 80 mg, 120 mg, 160 mg and used as a calcium blocker to treat angina, rapid heart beat, high blood pressure.

Dose: up to 120 mg 3 times a day.
Availability: NHS and private prescription.
Side effects: constipation, flushes; occasionally headache, nausea, allergies.
Caution: in pregnant women and in patients suffering from slow heart rate, heart failure, liver or kidney damage, some heart rhythm disturbances.
Not to be used for: children or for patients suffering from severe shock or heart block, heart failure, heart attacks.
Caution needed with: ß-BLOCKERS, DIGOXIN, anti-arrhythmics.
Contains: VERAPAMIL hydrochloride.
Other preparations: SECURON SR, CORDILOX (Baker Norton), BERKATENS (Berk), GEANGIN (Cusi), UNIVER (Rhone-Poulenc Rorer).

Securon SR
(Knoll)

S

A green, scored, oblong tablet supplied at a strength of 240 mg and used as a calcium blocker to treat high blood pressure, angina.

Dose: ½ tablet at first, the usually 1 tablet a day to a maximum of 2 tablets a day if needed.
Availability: NHS and private prescription.
Side effects: constipation, flushes, rarely headaches, nausea, allergies, enlarged breasts, gum disorders, heart disorder, low blood pressure.
Caution: in pregnant women, nursing mothers, and in patients suffering from slow heart rate, heart failure, liver damage, some heart rhythm disturbances.
Not to be used for: children or for patients suffering from severe shock or heart block, heart failure, heart attacks, severe low blood pressure.
Caution needed with: ß-BLOCKERS, DIGOXIN, anti-arrhythmics, CYCLOSPORIN, muscle relaxants, CARBAMAZEPINE, RIFAMPICIN, LITHIUM, other ANTIHYPERTENSIVES, some anaesthetics.
Contains: VERAPAMIL hydrochloride.
Other preparations: Half Securon SR, SECURON, CORDILOX (Baker Norton), BERKATENS (Berk), GEANGIN (Cusi), UNIVER (Rhone-Poulenc Rorer).

---

selegiline *see* **Eldepryl**

---

selenium sulphide *see* **Lenium, Selsun**

Selexid
(Leo)

A white tablet supplied at a strength of 200 mg and used as a penicillin to treat urinary system and other infections.

Dose: 2 tablets immediately followed by 1 or 2 tablets 3 or 4 times a day, up to a maximum of 12 tablets a day; children use reduced doses.
Availability: NHS and private prescription.
Side effects: allergy, stomach disturbances.
Caution: in patients suffering from kidney disease.
Not to be used for:
Caution needed with:
Contains: PIVMECILLINAM hydrochloride.
Other preparations: Selexid Suspension.

Selora — salt substitute. Product now discontinued.

Selsun
(Abbott)

A suspension used as an anti-dandruff treatment for dandruff, tinea versicolor (a scalp condition).

Dose: shampoo twice a week for 2 weeks, then once a week for 2 weeks.
Availability: NHS, private prescription, over the counter.
Side effects:
Caution: keep out of the eyes or broken skin; do not use within 48 hours of using waving or colouring substances.
Not to be used for:
Caution needed with:
Contains: SELENIUM SULPHIDE.
Other preparations: LENIUM (Janssen).

Semitard *see* insulin
(Novo Nordisk)

Semprex
(Wellcome)

A white capsule supplied at a strength of 8 mg and used as an ANTIHISTA-

MINE treatment for allergic rhinitis, other allergies.

Dose: 1 capsule 3 times a day.
Availability: NHS and private prescription
Side effects: rarely drowsiness.
Caution: in pregnant women and nursing mothers.
Not to be used for: children, the elderly, or for patients suffering from kidney failure.
Caution needed with: sedatives, alcohol.
Contains: ACRIVASTINE.
Other preparations:

---

senna tablets

A tablet supplied at a strength of 7.5 mg and used as a stimulant laxative to treat constipation.

Dose: adults 2-4 tablets at bedtime; children 6-12 years half adult dose.
Availability: NHS, private prescription, over the counter.
Side effects:
Caution:
Not to be used for: children under 6 years.
Caution needed with:
Contains: SENNOSIDES.
Other preparations: SENOKOT (Reckitt & Colman).

---

sennoside B *see* Senokot

---

sennosides *see* Manevac, Pripsin, senna tablets

Senokot
(Reckitt & Colman)

A brown tablet supplied at a strength of 7.5 mg and used as a stimulant to treat constipation.

Dose: adults 2-4 tablets at bedtime; children 2-6 years 2.5-5 ml syrup (see below) in morning; children over 6 years half adult dose in morning.
Availability: NHS (when prescribed as a generic), private prescription, over the counter.
Side effects:

S

Caution:
Not to be used for: infants under 2 years.
Caution needed with:
Contains: SENNOSIDE B.
Other preparations: Senokot granules, Senokot syrup, SENNA TABLETS.

Sential (formerly Sential HC)
(Kabi Pharmacia)

A cream used as a STEROID, wetting agent to treat dry eczema.

Dose: apply lightly to the affected area twice a day.
Availability: NHS and private prescription.
Side effects: fluid retention, suppression of adrenal glands, thinning of the skin may occur.
Caution: use for short periods of time only.
Not to be used for: patients suffering from acne or any other skin infections caused by tuberculosis, ringworm, viruses, or fungi, or continuously especially in pregnant women.
Caution needed with:
Contains: HYDROCORTISONE, UREA, SODIUM CHLORIDE.
Other preparations: Sential-E (without HYDROCORTISONE, for dry skin conditions) ALPHADERM (Norwich Eaton), CALMURID HC (Kabi Pharmacia).

Septrin
(Wellcome)

A white tablet or an orange, dispersible tablet used as an antibiotic to treat respiratory, stomach, and skin infections.

Dose: adults 1-3 tablets twice a day; children under 6 years use paediatric syrup, 6-12 years 1 tablet twice a day.
Availability: NHS and private prescription.
Side effects: nausea, vomiting, tongue inflammation, rash, blood changes, folate (vitamin) deficiency, rarely skin changes.
Caution: in the elderly, nursing mothers, and in patients suffering from kidney disease. Your doctor may advise that patients undergoing prolonged treatment should have regular blood tests.
Not to be used for: pregnant women, new-born infants, or for patients suffering from severe kidney or liver disease, or blood changes.
Caution needed with: folate inhibitors, anticoagulants, anticonvulsants, antidiabetics.
Contains: TRIMETHOPRIM, SULPHAMETHOXAZOLE, (CO-TRIMOXAZOLE).

Other preparations: Septrin Adult Suspension, Septrin Paediatric Suspension, Septrin IM Injection, Septrin for Infusion. BACTRIM (Roche), CHEMOTRIM PAEDIATRIC (RP Drugs), COMIXCO (Ashbourne), COMOX, LARATRIM (Lagap).

Serc
(Duphar)

A white tablet supplied at a strength of 8 mg, 16 mg and used as a histamine-type drug to treat vertigo, tinnitus, and hearing loss caused by Ménière's disease.

Dose: 16 mg 3 times a day at first then 24-48 mg tablets a day.
Availability: NHS and private prescription.
Side effects: stomach upset.
Caution: in patients suffering from bronchial asthma, stomach ulcer.
Not to be used for: children or patients suffering from phaeochromocytoma (a disease of the adrenal glands).
Caution needed with:
Contains: BETAHISTINE dihydrochloride.
Other preparations:

S

Serenace
(Baker Norton)

A green/pale-green capsule supplied at a strength of 0.5 mg and used as a sedative for an additional treatment in the short-term management of anxiety. (Serenace Tablets and Liquid used to treat schizophrenia and behavioural disorders.)

Dose: 1 capsule twice a day.
Availability: NHS and private prescription.
Side effects: muscle spasms, restlessness, hands shaking, constipation, blurred vision, dry mouth, urine retention, palpitations, low blood pressure, weight gain, changes in libido, low body temperature, breast swelling, menstrual changes, jaundice, blood and skin changes, drowsiness, rarely fits.
Caution: in pregnant women or in patients suffering from hyperthyroidism, liver or kidney failure, severe cardiovascular disease, tardive dyskinesia (a movement disorder), epilepsy.
Not to be used for: nursing mothers, unconscious patients, or for patients suffering from Parkinson's disease.
Caution needed with: alcohol, tranquillizers, pain killers,

ANTIHYPERTENSIVES, antidepressants, anticonvulsants, antidiabetic drugs, LEVODOPA.

Contains: HALOPERIDOL.

Other preparations: Serenace Liquid, Serenace Tablets, Serenace Injection, DOZIC (R.P. Drugs), HALDOL (Janssen).

Serevent
(Allen and Hanburys)

An aerosol supplied at a strength of 25 micrograms per dose, and used as a broncho-dilator to treat asthma and chronic bronchitis,

Dose: 2-4 puffs twice a day.
Availability: NHS and private prescription.
Side effects: low potassium levels, breathing difficulty, headache, tremor, palpitations.
Caution: in pregnant women and nursing mothers.
Not to be used for: children, or for emergency use.
Caution needed with: SS-BLOCKERS.
Contains: SALMETEROL.
Other preparations: Serevent Diskhaler.

Serophene
(Serono)

A white, scored tablet supplied at a strength of 50 mg and used as a anti-oestrogen treatment for infertility due to failure of ovulation caused by impaired hypothalamic-pituitary function.

Dose: 1 tablet a day for 5 days beginning within 5 days of the start of the period, increased to 2 tablets a day for superovulation.
Availability: NHS and private prescription.
Side effects: enlargement of the ovaries, hot flushes, uncomfortable abdomen, blurred vision.
Caution:
Not to be used for: children, pregnant women, or patients suffering from liver disease, large ovarian cyst, endometrial cancer, bleeding from the uterus.
Caution needed with:
Contains: CLOMIPHENE citrate.
Other preparations: CLOMID (Marion Merrell Dow).

Seroxat
(S. K. B.)

A white, oval, scored tablet or a blue, oval, scored tablet according to strengths of 20 mg, 30 mg, and used as an antidepressant to treat depression and anxiety.

Dose: initially 20 mg once a day in the morning with food, increased to a maximum of 50 mg a day; elderly, 20-40 mg a day only.
Availability: NHS and private prescription.
Side effects: nausea, sleepiness, sweating, tremor, tingling, dry mouth, insomnia, sexual disturbance.
Caution: in pregnant women, nursing mothers, and in patients suffering from severe kidney or liver damage, cardiovascular disease, epilepsy, or a history of mental disturbance.
Not to be used for: children.
Caution needed with: MAOIS, TRYPTOPHAN, LITHIUM, PHENYTOIN, anticonvulsants, drugs affecting liver enzymes (eg BARBITURATES, CARBAMAZEPINE, PRIMIDONE, RIFAMPICIN, ALLOPURINOL, CIPROFLOXACIN, CIMETIDINE, ERYTHROMYCIN).
Contains: PAROXETENE.
Other preparations:

Serpasil — ANTIHYPERTENSIVE drug. Product now discontinued.

Serpasil Esidrex — ANTIHYPERTENSIVE drug. Product now discontinued.

---

sertraline *see* **Lustral**

Sevredol *see* **MST Continus**
(Napp)

---

silicic acid *see* **Unguentum Merck**

Siloxyl *see* **Asilone.** Product now discontinued.

---

silver sulphadiazine *see* **Flamazine**

Simeco *see* **Asilone**
(Wyeth)

---

simple linctus BP

A linctus used to soothe a dry, irritating cough.

Dose: 5 ml 3-4 times a day; children use paediatric simple linctus.
Availability: NHS, private prescription, over the counter.
Side effects:
Caution: in patients suffering from diabetes.
Not to be used for:
Caution needed with:
Contains: CITRIC ACID, concentrated ANISE water, chloroform spirit, ameranth solution, syrup.
Other preparations: paediatric simple linctus.

Simplene
(SNP)

Drops used as a SYMPATHOMIMETIC treatment for primary open angle or secondary glaucoma.

Dose: 1 drop into the eye 1-2 times a day.
Availability: NHS and private prescription.
Side effects: pain in the eye, headache, redness, skin reactions, melanosis, rarely systemic effects.
Caution:
Not to be used for: patients suffering from narrow angle glaucoma, diabetes.
Caution needed with: MAOIS, TRICYCLIC antidepressants, ß-BLOCKERS.
Contains: ADRENALINE.
Other preparations: EPPY (SNP).

---

simple eye ointment *see* **Lubrifilm**

---

simvastatin *see* **Zocor**

Sinemet
(Du Pont)

A blue, scored, oval tablet or a yellow, scored tablet according to strengths of LS 50/12.5 mg, 110 110/10 mg, Plus 100/25 mg, 275 250/25 mg and used as an anti-parkinsonian preparation to treat Parkinson's disease.

Dose: 1 'plus' 3 times a day at first, increasing gradually to a maximum of 8 'plus' a day, or as advised.
Availability: NHS and private prescription.
Side effects: nausea, vomiting, anorexia, low blood pressure on standing, involuntary movements, heart and brain disturbances, discoloration of urine.
Caution: in patients suffering from cardiovascular, liver, kidney, lung, or endocrine disease, stomach ulcer, or glaucoma. Your doctor may advise that blood, liver, kidney, and cardiovascular system should be checked regularly.
Not to be used for: patients under 18 years, pregnant women, nursing mothers, or for patients suffering from severe mental disorders or glaucoma, or for patients with a history of malignant melanoma.
Caution needed with: drugs affecting brain peptides, MAOIS, ANTIHYPERTENSIVES, and SYMPATHOMIMETICS.
Contains: LEVODOPA, CARBIDOPA monohydrate (CO-CARELDOPA).
Other preparations: Sinemet CR.

S

Sinequan
(Pfizer)

A red capsule, blue/red capsule, or blue capsule according to strengths of 10 mg, 25 mg, 50 mg and used as a TRICYCLIC antidepressant to treat depression.

Dose: 10-100 mg 3 times a day or once a day at bedtime.
Availability: NHS and private prescription.
Side effects: dry mouth, constipation, urine retention, blurred vision, palpitations, drowsiness, sleeplessness, dizziness, hands shaking, low blood presure, weight change, skin reactions, jaundice or blood changes, weakness, unsteadiness, convulsions. Loss of sexual desire may occur.
Caution: in the elderly, nursing mothers or in patients suffering from adrenal tumour, urine retention, heart or liver disease, thyroid disease, epilepsy, diabetes, some other psychiatric conditions. Your doctor may advise regular blood tests.
Not to be used for: children, pregnant women, or for patients suffering from heart attacks, severe liver disease, heart block.
Caution needed with: alcohol, ANTICHOLINERGICS, ADRENALINE, MAOIS, BARBITU-

RATES, other antidepressants, CIMETIDINE, oestrogens, ANTIHYPERTENSIVES.
Contains: DOXEPIN hydrochloride
Other preparations:

Sinthrome
(Ciba-Geigy)

White tablets supplied at strengths of 1 mg, 4 mg and used as an antico-agulant drug to treat thrombotic disorders.

Dose: 8-12 mg on the first day, 4-8 mg second day, and then adjust as required.
Availability: NHS and private prescription.
Side effects: bleeding, allergies, liver damage, reversible alopecia, rarely nausea, anorexia, headache, skin necrosis.
Caution: in nursing mothers, the elderly, and in patients suffering from high blood pressure, reduced protein binding, severe heart failure, liver dysfunction, gastro-intestinal disorders.
Not to be used for: children, pregnant women, the unco-operative, and in patients suffering from bleeding conditions, blood changes, damaged kidney or liver function, inflammation of the heart or lungs, very high blood pressure, or within 24 hours of surgery.
Caution needed with: NON-STEROID ANTI-INFLAMMATORY DRUGS, vitamin K, oral antidiabetics, QUINIDINE, antibiotics, PHENFORMIN, CIMETIDINE, STEROIDS, drugs affecting liver chemistry or bleeding.
Contains: NICOUMALONE.
Other preparations:

Sintisone — STEROID tablet. Product now discontinued.

Skinoren
(Schering Health Care)

A cream used to treat acne.

Dose: apply twice a day (once a day if skin is sensitive). Use 2 g a day for the face, or 10 g a day for face, chest, and back. Continue for up to 6 months.
Availability: NHS and private prescription.
Side effects: irritation, sensitivity to light.
Caution: in pregnant women and nursing mothers. Avoid the eyes.
Not to be used for:

Caution needed with:
Contains: AZELAIC ACID.
Other preparations:

Slo-Phyllin *see* Lasma
(Lipha)

Slow Sodium
(Ciba)

A white tablet supplied at a strength of 600 mg and used as a salt supplement to treat salt deficiency.

Dose: adults 4-20 tablets a day, children in proportion to dose for 70 kg adult.
Availability: NHS, private prescription, over the counter.
Side effects:
Caution:
Not to be used for: patients suffering from fluid retention, heart disease, heart failure, adrenal tumour.
Caution needed with: DIURETICS, LITHIUM.
Contains: SODIUM CHLORIDE.
Other preparations:

Slow-Fe
(Ciba)

An off-white tablet supplied at a strength of 160 mg and used as a iron supplement. to treat iron-deficiency anaemia.

Dose: adults 1-2 tablets a day; children 6-12 years 1 tablet a day.
Availability: NHS, private prescription, over the counter.
Side effects: nausea, constipation.
Caution:
Not to be used for: children under 6 years.
Caution needed with: TETRACYCLINES, LEVODOPA, PENICILLAMINE, ZINC, ANTACIDS.
Contains: FERROUS SULPHATE.
Other preparations: FEOSPAN (SKB), FERROGRAD (Abbott).

Slow-Fe Folic
(Ciba)

A cream-coloured tablet used as an iron and folic acid supplement for the prevention of iron and folic acid deficiencies in pregnancy.

Dose: 1-2 tablets a day.
Availability: NHS and private prescription.
Side effects: nausea, constipation.
Caution:
Not to be used for: for children.
Caution needed with: TETRACYCLINES, PENICILLAMINE, ZINC, anticonvulsants, ANTACIDS.
Contains: FERROUS SULPHATE, FOLIC ACID.
Other preparations: FEFOL (SKB), FERROGRAD FOLIC (Abbott).

Slow-K
(Ciba)

An orange tablet supplied at a strength of 600 mg and used as a potassium supplement to treat potassium deficiency.

Dose: adults 2-12 tablets a day or every other day after food.
Availability: NHS, private prescription, over the counter.
Side effects: blocked or ulcerated small bowel.
Caution: in pregnant women, and in patients suffering from kidney disease, stomach ulcer, low magnesium levels.
Not to be used for: children, or for patients suffering from advanced kidney disease, Addison's disease, adrenal disorder, dehydration, metabolic.
Caution needed with: some DIURETICS, CYCLOSPORIN, ACE INHIBITORS, NON-STEROID ANTI-INFLAMMATORY DRUGS.
Contains: POTASSIUM CHLORIDE.
Other preparations: KAY-CEE-L (Geistlich), LEO K (Leo).

Slow-Pren *see* Slow Trasicor. Product now discontinued.

Slow-Trasicor
(Ciba)

A white tablet supplied at a strength of 160 mg and used as a ß-BLOCKER to treat high blood pressure and angina.

Dose: 1 tablet a day in the morning at first, then increase to 2-3 tablets a day if needed.
Availability: NHS and private prescription.
Side effects: cold hands and feet, sleep disturbance, slow heart rate, tiredness, wheezing, heart failure, stomach upset, dry eyes, skin rash.
Caution: in pregnant women, nursing mothers, and in patients suffering from diabetes, kidney or liver disorders, asthma. May need to be withdrawn before surgery. Withdraw gradually. Your doctor may advise additional treatment with DIURETICS or DIGOXIN.
Not to be used for: children or for patients suffering from heart block or failure.
Caution needed with: VERAPAMIL, CLONIDINE withdrawal, some anti-arrhythmic drugs and anaesthetics, RESERPINE, some ANTIHYPERTENSIVES, ERGOTAMINE, CIMETIDINE, sedatives, antidiabetics, SYMPATHOMIMETICS, INDOMETHACIN.
Contains: OXPRENOLOL hydrochloride.
Other preparations: SLOW-PREN, OXYPRENIX 160-SR (Ashbourne).

S

Sno Phenicol *see* Chloromycetin Eye Ointment
(SNP)

Sno Pilo
(SNP)

Drops used as a cholinergic treatment for glaucoma.

Dose: 1-2 drops into the eye 4 times a day.
Availability: NHS and private prescription.
Side effects: temporary reduction of visual sharpness.
Caution:
Not to be used for: patients suffering from acute iritis or who wear soft contact lenses.
Caution needed with:
Contains: PILOCARPINE.
Other preparations: CARPINE (Alcon), OCUSERT PILO (M&B), OPULETS PILOCARPINE, PILOCARPINE EYE DROPS.

Sno Tears
(SNP)

Drops used to lubricate the eyes.

Dose: 1 or more drops into the eye as needed.
Availability: NHS, private prescription, over the counter.
Side effects: transient stinging, blurred vision.
Caution:
Not to be used for: patients who wear soft contact lenses.
Caution needed with:
Contains: POLYVINYL ALCOHOL.
Other preparations: LIQUIFILM TEARS (Allergan), HYPOTEARS (Iolab).

soap spirit BP

A liquid used as a soap to remove crusts from the skin.

Dose: apply as needed.
Availability: NHS, private prescription, over the counter.
Side effects:
Caution:
Not to be used for:
Caution needed with:
Contains: soap spirit BP.
Other preparations:

sodium acid phosphate (anhydrous) *see* Carbalax, Fletchers' Phosphate, Phosphate

sodium alginate *see* Gaviscon

sodium alkylsulphoacetate *see* Micralax

Sodium Amytal
(Eli Lilly)

A blue capsule supplied at strengths of 60 mg, 200 mg and used as a BARBITURATE to treat sleeplessness, status epilepticus (severe epilepsy).

Dose: 60-200 mg at night. Status epilepticus use injection.
Availability: controlled drug; NHS and private prescription.
Side effects: drowsiness, hangover, dizziness, allergies, headache, confusion, excitement, unsteadiness, breathing difficulty.

Caution: in patients suffering from liver, kidney, or lung disease. Dependence (addiction) may develop.

Not to be used for: children, young adults, pregnant women, nursing mothers, the elderly, patients with a history of drug or alcohol abuse, or suffering from porphyria (a rare blood disorder), or in the management of pain.

Caution needed with: anticoagulants, alcohol, other tranquillizers, STEROIDS, the contraceptive pill, GRISEOFULVIN, RIFAMPICIN, PHENYTOIN, METRONIDAZOLE, CHLORAMPHENICOL.

Contains: AMYLOBARBITONE sodium.

Other preparations: Sodium Amytal Tablets (now discontinued), Sodium Amytal Vials, AMYTAL (Eli Lilly).

---

sodium bicarbonate *see* Carbalax, Caved-S, Dioralyte, Gastrocote, Gastron, Gaviscon, magnesium carbonate aromatic mixture, Mictral, Phosphate, Rehidrat, Roter, Sandocal, sodium bicarbonate ear drops BP

---

sodium bicarbonate ear drops BP

Ear drops used to remove ear wax.

Dose: use as needed. Lie down with treated ear uppermost for 5-10 minutes after inserting the drops.

Availability: NHS, private prescription, over the counter.

Side effects:

Caution:

Not to be used for:

Caution needed with:

Contains: SODIUM BICARBONATE, GLYCEROL.

Other preparations:

---

sodium cellulose *see* Calcisorb

---

sodium chloride *see* Diarrest, Dioralyte, Glandosane, Minims Saline, Normasol, Opulets Saline, Rehidrat, Sential, Slow Sodium, Topiclens

---

sodium citrate *see* **Benylin Expectorant, Diarrest, Guanor, Histalix, Micolette, Micralax, Mictral, Relaxit, Urisal**

sodium cromoglycate *see* **Intal, Intal Compound, Nalcrom, Opticrom, Rynacrom Spray**

sodium docusate *see* **Molcer, Soliwax**

sodium fluorescein *see* **Lignocaine and Fluorescein**

sodium fusidate *see* **Fucidin, Fucidin H**

sodium glycerophosphate *see* **Verdiviton**

sodium hydrogen tartrate *see* **Bocasan**

sodium hypochlorite *see* **Chlorasol**

sodium iron edetate *see* **Sytron**

sodium lauryl sulphate *see* **Relaxit**

sodium lauryl sulphoacetate *see* **Micolette**

sodium nedocromil *see* **Tilade**

sodium oleate *see* **Alcos-Anal**

sodium perborate *see* **Bocasan**

---

sodium phenolate *see* **Chloraseptic**

---

sodium phosphate *see* **Fletchers' Phosphate**

---

sodium picosulphate

A stimulant laxative used to treat constipation, and to clear the bowels before medical procedures.

Dose: adults 5-15 ml at night; children 0-5 years 2.5 ml at night; children 5-10 years 5 ml at night.
Availability: NHS and private prescription.
Side effects:
Caution: in patients suffering from inflammatory bowel disease.
Not to be used for:
Caution needed with: antibiotics.
Contains:
Other preparations: LAXOBERAL (Windsor), PICOLAX (Ferring).

---

sodium polystyrene sulphonate *see* **Resonium-A**

---

sodium *see* **Metatone**

---

sodium sulphacetamide *see* **Cortucid, Sulphacetamide**

---

sodium sulphosuccinated undecylenic monoalkylolamide *see* **Genisol, Synogist**

---

sodium thyroxine *see* **Eltroxin**

---

sodium valproate *see* **Epilim**

S

Sofradex Drops
(Roussel)

Drops used as an aminoglycoside antibiotic, STEROID treatment for inflammation of the outer ear or eye.

Dose: 2-3 drops into the ear 3-4 times a day, or 1-2 drops into the eye up to 6 times a day.
Availability: NHS and private prescription.
Side effects: rise in eye pressure, fungal infection, thinning cornea, cataract.
Caution: in pregnant women and infants — do not use over extended periods.
Not to be used for: patients suffering from perforated ear drum, glaucoma, viral, fungal, tubercular, or weeping infections.
Caution needed with:
Contains: FRAMYCETIN sulphate, DEXAMETHASONE, GRAMICIDIN.
Other preparations: SOFRADEX OINTMENT.

Sofradex Ointment
(Roussel)

An ointment used as a STEROID, aminoglycoside antibiotic treatment for inflammation of the outer ear or eye.

Dose: apply to the eye 2-3 times a day and at night, apply to the ear once or twice a day.
Availability: NHS and private prescription.
Side effects: rise in eye pressure, fungal infection, thinning cornea, cataract.
Caution: in pregnant women and infants — do not use for extended periods.
Not to be used for: patients suffering from glaucoma, viral, fungal, tubercular, or weeping infections, perforated ear drum.
Caution needed with:
Contains: DEXAMETHASONE, FRAMYCETIN sulphate, GRAMICIDIN.
Other preparations: SOFRADEX.

Soframycin Tablets — antibiotic. Product now discontinued.

Soframycin Cream — antibiotic treatment for skin infections. Product now discontinued.

Soframycin Drops
(Roussel)

Drops used as an aminoglycoside antibiotic treatment for conjunctivitis, styes, eyelid inflammation

Dose: 1-2 drops into the eye 3-4 times a day.
Availability: NHS and private prescription.
Side effects:
Caution:
Not to be used for:
Caution needed with:
Contains: FRAMYCETIN sulphate.
Other preparations: SOFRAMYCIN OINTMENT.

Solis *see* **Valium.** Product now discontinued.

S

Soliwax — softener for ear wax. Product now discontinued.

Solpadeine
(Sterling Research Laboratories)

A white, effervescent tablet used as an ANALGESIC to relieve rheumatic, muscle, bone pain, headache, sinusitis, influenza.

Dose: adults 2 tablets in water 3-4 times a day; children 7-12 years ½ -1 tablet 3-4 times a day.
Availability: private prescription and over the counter.
Side effects: constipation.
Caution: in patients with liver or kidney disease, or who have a restricted salt consumption.
Not to be used for: children under 7 years.
Caution needed with: other medicines containing PARACETAMOL.
Contains: PARACETAMOL, CODEINE PHOSPHATE, CAFFEINE.
Other preparations: CO-CODAMOL, PANADEINE (Sterling Health), PARACODOL (Fisons).

Solpadol
(Sanofi Winthrop)

A white, scored, effervescent tablet used as an ANALGESIC to treat severe pain.

Dose: 2 tablets dissolved in water every 4 hours to a maximum of 8 tablets in 24 hours.
Availability: NHS and private prescription.
Side effects: tolerance and addiction, constipation, dizziness, sedation, nausea, dry mouth, blurred vision.
Caution: in the elderly, during labour, and in patients suffering from underactive thyroid, kidney or liver damage.
Not to be used for: children, pregnant women, nursing mothers, or for patients suffering from breathing difficulty.
Caution needed with: MAOIS, sedatives, other medicines containing PARACETAMOL.
Contains: PARACETAMOL, CODEINE PHOSPHATE.
Other preparations: Solpadol Caplets.

Solprin *see* **aspirin tablets.** Product now discontinued.

Solvazinc
(Thames)

An off-white, effervescent tablet supplied at a strength of 200 mg and used as a zinc supplement to treat zinc deficiency.

Dose: adults and children over 30 kg body weight 1 tablet dissolved in water 1-3 times a day after food; children under 10 kg body weight ½ tablet in water once a day after food, 10-30 kg half adult dose.
Availability: NHS, private prescription, over the counter.
Side effects: stomach upset.
Caution: in patients suffering from kidney failure.
Not to be used for:
Caution needed with: TETRACYCLINES.
Contains: ZINC SULPHATE.
Other preparations: ZINCOMED (Medo), ZINCOSOL (Bioceuticals), Z-SPAN (SKB).

Sominex
(S K B)

A white, scored tablet supplied at a strength of 20 mg and used as an ANTIHISTAMINE treatment for occasional sleeplessness.

Dose: 1 tablet immediately before or up to 1 hour after going to bed.
Availability: NHS, private prescription, over the counter.
Side effects: ANTICHOLINERGENIC effects, brain and stomach upsets, allergies, blood disorders, allergy.
Caution: in patients suffering from glaucoma, enlarged prostate, epilepsy, liver disease. Patients should be warned of drowsiness and should not drive or carry out any functions requiring alertness.
Not to be used for: children under 16 years.
Caution needed with: alcohol, sedatives, ANTICHOLINERGICS.
Contains: PROMETHAZINE hydrochloride.
Other preparations:

Somnite *see* Mogadon
(Norgine)

Soneryl
(Rhone-Poulenc Rorer)

A pink, scored tablet supplied at a strength of 100 mg and used as a BARBITURATE to treat sleeplessness.

Dose: 1-2 tablets before going to bed.
Availability: controlled drug; NHS and private prescription.
Side effects: drowsiness, hangover, dizziness, allergies, headache, confusion, excitement, unsteadiness, breathing difficulty.
Caution: patients suffering from kidney or lung disease. Dependence (addiction) may develop.
Not to be used for: children, young adults, pregnant women, nursing mothers, the elderly, patients with a history of drug or alcohol abuse, or suffering from porphyria (a rare blood disorder), or in the management of pain.
Caution needed with: anticoagulants, alcohol, other tranquillizers, STEROIDS, the contraceptive pill, GRISEOFULVIN, RIFAMPICIN, PHENYTOIN, METRONIDAZOLE, CHLORAMPHENICOL.
Contains: BUTOBARBITONE.
Other preparations:

Soni-Slo
(Lipha)

A pink/clear capsule or a yellow/clear capsule according to strengths of 20 mg, 40 mg, and containing off-white pellets used as a NITRATE for the prevention of angina.

Dose: 40-120 mg a day in 2-3 divided doses.
Availability: NHS, private prescription, over the counter.
Side effects: flushes, headache, dizziness.
Caution:
Not to be used for: children.
Caution needed with:
Contains: ISOSORBIDE DINITRATE.
Other preparations: CEDOCARD RETARD (Farmitalia CE), IMTACK (Astra), ISOKET RETARD (Schwarz), ISORDIL (Monmouth), SORBICHEW (Stuart), SORBID-SA (Stuart), SORBITRATE (Stuart), VASCARDIN (Nicholas).

S

sorbic acid *see* **Micralax, Relaxit, Unguentum Merck**

Sorbichew
(Stuart)

A green, scored tablet supplied at a strength of 5 mg and used as a NITRATE to treat acute angina attacks.

Dose: 1-2 tablets chewed thoroughly.
Availability: NHS, private prescription, over the counter.
Side effects: flushes, headache, dizziness.
Caution:
Not to be used for: children.
Caution needed with:
Contains: ISOSORBIDE DINITRATE.
Other preparations: CEDOCARD RETARD (Farmitalia CE), IMTACK (Astra), ISOKET RETARD (Schwarz), ISORDIL (Monmouth), SONI-SLO (Lipha), SORBID-SA (Stuart), SORBITRATE (Stuart), VASCARDIN (Nicholas).

Sorbid SA
(Stuart)

A red/yellow capsule or a red/clear capsule according to strengths of 20 mg, 40 mg and used as a NITRATE for the prevention of angina.

Dose: 20-80 mg twice a day.
Availability: NHS, private prescription, over the counter.
Side effects: flushes, headache, nausea.

Caution:
Not to be used for: children.
Caution needed with:
Contains: ISOSORBIDE DINITRATE.
Other preparations: CEDOCARD RETARD (Farmitalia CE), IMTACK (Astra), ISOKET RETARD (Schwarz), ISORDIL (Monmouth), SONI-SLO (Lipha) SORBICHEW (Stuart), SORBITRATE (Stuart), VASCARDIN (Nicholas).

---

sorbitol *see* Glandosane, Relaxit

Sorbitrate
(Stuart)

A yellow, oval, scored tablet or a blue, oval scored tablet according to strengths of 10 mg, 20 mg and used as a NITRATE for the prevention of angina.

Dose: 10-40 mg 3-4 times a day.
Availability: NHS, private prescription, over the counter.
Side effects: flushes, headache, dizziness.
Caution:
Not to be used for: children.
Caution needed with:
Contains: ISOSORBIDE DINITRATE.
Other preparations: CEDOCARD RETARD (Farmitalia CE), IMTACK (Astra), ISOKET RETARD (Schwarz), ISORDIL (Monmouth), SONI-SLO (Lipha) SORBICHEW (Stuart), SORBID-SA (Stuart), VASCARDIN (Nicholas).

Sotacor
(Bristol-Myers Squibb)

A pink tablet or a blue tablet according to strengths of 80 mg, 160 mg and used as a ß-BLOCKER to treat angina, abnormal heart rhythm, high blood pressure, and for the prevention of heart attacks.

Dose: angina 160 mg a day in single or divided doses; for other uses higher doses.
Availability: NHS and private prescription.
Side effects: cold hands and feet, sleep disturbance, slow heart rate, tiredness, wheezing, heart failure, stomach upset, dry eyes, skin rash.
Caution: in pregnant women, nursing mothers, and in patients suffering from diabetes, kidney or liver disorders, asthma. May need to be with-

drawn before surgery. Withdraw gradually. Your doctor may advise additional treatment with DIURETICS or DIGOXIN.

Not to be used for: children, or for patients suffering from heart block or failure.

Caution needed with: VERAPAMIL, CLONIDINE withdrawal, some anti-arrhythmic drugs and anaesthetics, RESERPINE, some ANTIHYPERTENSIVES, ERGOTAMINE, CIMETIDINE, sedatives, antidiabetics, SYMPATHOMIMETICS, INDOMETHACIN.

Contains: SOTALOL hydrochloride.

Other preparations: Sotacor Injection, BETA-CARDONE (Evans).

---

sotalol *see* **Beta-Cardone, Sotacor, Sotazide, Tolerzide**

Sotazide
(Bristol-Myers Squibb)

A blue, oblong, scored tablet used as a ß-BLOCKER to treat high blood pressure.

Dose: 1 tablet a day at first increasing to 2 tablets a day if needed.
Availability: NHS and private prescription.
Side effects: cold hands and feet, sleep disturbance, slow heart rate, tiredness, wheezing, heart failure, stomach upset, dry eyes, skin rash.
Caution: in pregnant women, nursing mothers, and in patients suffering from diabetes, kidney or liver disorders, asthma. May need to be with-drawn before surgery. Withdraw gradually. Your doctor may advise additional treatment with DIURETICS or DIGOXIN.
Not to be used for: children or for patients suffering from heart block or failure.
Caution needed with: VERAPAMIL, CLONIDINE withdrawal, some anti-arrhythmic drugs and anaesthetics, RESERPINE, some ANTIHYPERTENSIVES, ERGOTAMINE, CIMETIDINE, sedatives, antidiabetics, SYMPATHOMIMETICS, INDOMETHACIN.
Contains: SOTALOL hydrochloride, HYDROCHLOROTHIAZIDE.
Other preparations: TOLERZIDE (Bristol-Myers Squibb).

---

soya oil *see* **Balneum, Balneum Plus, Balneum with Tar**

Sparine
(Wyeth)

A suspension used as a sedative to treat agitation or restlessness in the elderly, additional short-term treatment for psychomotor agitation and severe hiccup.

Dose: adults 10-20 ml 4 times a day; elderly half adult dose or 2.5-5 ml for restlessness.
Availability: NHS and private prescription.
Side effects: muscle spasms, restlessness, hands shaking, dry mouth, urine retention, palpitations, low blood pressure, weight gain, changes in libido, low body temperature, breast swelling, menstrual changes, jaundice, blood and skin changes, drowsiness, rarely fits.
Caution: in pregnant women, nursing mothers, and in patients suffering from liver disease, Parkinson's disease, or cardiovascular disease.
Not to be used for: children or for patients suffering from bone marrow depression or in an unconscious state
Caution needed with: alcohol, tranquillizers, pain killers, ANTIHYPERTENSIVES, antidepressants, anticonvulsants, antidiabetic drugs, LEVODOPA.
Contains: PROMAZINE embonate.
Other preparations: Sparine Injection, Promazine Tablets.

S

Spasmonal
(Norgine)

A blue/grey capsule supplied at a strength of 60 mg and used as an anti-spasmodic treatment for irritable bowel syndrome and period pain.

Dose: adults 1-2 tablets 1-3 times a day; children 1 tablet 3 times a day.
Availability: NHS, private prescription, over the counter.
Side effects:
Caution:
Not to be used for: children under 8 years.
Caution needed with:
Contains: ALVERINE CITRATE.
Other preparations:

Spiretic *see* Aldactone
(DDSA)

Spiroctan
(Boehringer Mannheim)

A blue tablet or a green tablet according to strengths of 25 mg, 50 mg and used as a potassium-sparing DIURETIC to treat congestive heart failure, liver cirrhosis, fluid retention, kidney and adrenal gland disorders.

Dose: adults 50-200 mg a day to a maxium of 600 mg a day; children 1.5-3 mg per kg of bodyweight a day.
Availability: NHS and private prescription.
Side effects: enlarged breasts, stomach upset, drowsiness, headache, confusion, rash.
Caution: in pregnant women , young patients, and in patients suffering from kidney or liver disease.
Not to be used for: nursing mothers and for patients suffering from severe or progressive kidney failure, raised potassium levels, Addison's disease.
Caution needed with: potassium supplements, potassium-sparing DIURETICS, CARBENOXOLONE, ANTIHYPERTENSIVES, ACE INHIBITORS.
Contains: SPIRONOLACTONE.
Other preparations: Spiroctan Capsules, Spiroctan-M.

Spirolone *see* Aldactone
(Berk)

---

spironolactone *see* Aldactide 50, Aldactone, Diatensic, Lasilactone, Spiroctan

---

Spirospare *see* Aldactone
(Ashbourne)

Sporanox
(Janssen)

A blue/pink capsule supplied at a strength of 100 mg and used as an antifungal treatment for skin, vaginal, or mouth infections.

Dose: 1-2 capsules a day for 1-30 days, or 2 capsules twice a day for 1 day.
Availability: NHS and private prescription.
Side effects: headache, indigestion, nausea, stomach pain.
Caution: in patients suffering from liver disease.
Not to be used for: pregnant women, nursing mothers.

Caution needed with: CYCLOSPORIN, ANTACIDS, some treatments for stomach ulcer, ASTEMIZOLE, TERFENADINE.
Contains: ITRACONAZOLE.
Other preparations:

---

squalane *see* **Dermalex, Salonair**

SRM-Rhotard *see* **MST Continus**
(Farmitalia CE)

Stabillin V-K
(Boots)

A tablet supplied at a strength of 250 mg and used as a penicillin treatment for infections.

Dose: adults 2-8 tablets a day in divided doses; children under 1 year 62.5 mg every 6 hours, 1-5 years 125 mg every 6 hours, 6-12 years 250 mg every 6 hours.
Availability: NHS and private prescription.
Side effects: allergy, stomach upset.
Caution: in patients suffering from kidney disease.
Not to be used for:
Caution needed with:
Contains: PENICILLIN V-POTASSIUM.
Other preparations: Stabillin V-K Elixi, DISTAQUAINE V-K (Dista), V-CIL-K, RIMAPEN (Rima).

Stafoxil
(Brocades)

A brown/cream capsule supplied at strengths of 250 mg, 500 mg and used as a penicillin treatment for infections.

Dose: adults 250 mg 4 times a day 1 hour before food; children over 2 years half adult dose.
Availability: NHS and private prescription.
Side effects: allergy, stomach upset.
Caution:
Not to be used for: children under 2 years.

Caution needed with:
Contains: FLUCLOXACILLIN sodium.
Other preparations: FLOXAPEN (Beecham Research), FLUCLOMIX (Ashbourne), LADROPEN (Berk).

---

stanozolol *see* **Stromba**

Staphlipen *see* **Floxapen**. Product now discontinued.

---

starch *see* **Arobon**

S

Staril
(Squibb)

A white, diamond-shaped tablet supplied at strengths of 10 mg, 20 mg, and used as an ACE-INHIBITOR, to treat high blood pressure.

Dose: 10-40 mg once a day. Discontinue any DIURETIC several days before starting treatment; re-introduce later if needed.
Availability: NHS and private prescription.
Side effects: dizziness, cough, stomach upset, palpitations, chest pain, rash, muscle/bone pain, tiredness, taste disturbance, severe allergy.
Caution: in patients suffering from liver or kidney damage, congestive heart failure, salt or body fluid depletion.
Not to be used for: children, pregnant women, nursing mothers.
Caution needed with: some DIURETICS, potassium supplements, NON-STEROID ANTI-INFLAMMATORY DRUGS, ANTACIDS, LITHIUM, ANTIHYPERTENSIVES.
Contains: FOSINOPRIL SODIUM.
Other preparations:

Stelazine
(S K B)

A blue tablet supplied at strengths of 1 mg, 5 mg and used as a sedative to treat anxiety, depression, agitation, schizophrenia, mental disorders, severe agitation, dangerous impulsive behaviour, nausea, vomiting.

Dose: anxiety etc, adults 2-4 mg up to a maximum of 6 mg a day in divided doses; children 3-5 years up to 1 mg a day, 6-12 up to 4 mg a

day.For schizophrenia etc, adults 5 mg twice a day increasing after 7 days to 15 mg; children up to 5 mg a day. For nausea and vomiting adults 2-6 mg a day; children 3-5 years up to 1 mg a day, 6-12 up to 4 mg a day.
Availability: NHS and private prescription.
Side effects: brain disturbances, dry mouth, blurred vision, ECG and hormone changes, allergies, impaired judgement and ability, rarely extrapyramidal symptoms (shaking and rigidity).
Caution: in the elderly, pregnant women, nursing mothers, and in patients suffering from undiagnosed vomiting, epilepsy, cardiovascular disease or Parkinson's disease. Your doctor may advise you to watch for loss of dexterity.
Not to be used for: patients in an unconscious state or patients suffering from liver disease, bone marrow depression.
Caution needed with: sedatives, alcohol, ANALGESICS, ANTIHYPERTENSIVES.
Contains: TRIFLUOPERAZINE hydrochloride.
Other preparations: Stelazine Syrup, Stelazine Spansules, Stelazine Concentrate, Stelazine Injection.

S

Stemetil
(Rhone-Poulenc Rorer)

A cream tablet or a cream, scored tablet according to strengths of 5 mg, 25 mg and used as a anti-sickness medication for minor mental and emotional problems, schizophrenia and other mental disorders, vertigo caused by Ménière's disease, severe nausea, vomiting.

Dose: 15-20 mg a day in divided doses up to a maximum of 40 mg a day for minor problems, 75-100 mg a day for schizophrenia.
Availability: NHS and private prescription.
Side effects: brain disturbances, ANTICHOLINERGIC effects, ECG and hormone changes, allergies, reduced judgement and abilities, rarely extrapyramidal effects, jaundice, blood disorder.
Caution: in the elderly, nursing mothers, and in patients suffering from cardiovascular disease, undiagnosed or prolonged vomiting.
Not to be used for: patients in an unconscious state, pregnant women, or patients suffering from bone marrow depression, liver or kidney disease, Parkinson's disease.
Caution needed with: sedatives, alcohol, ANALGESICS, ANTIHYPERTENSIVES, antidepressants, ANTICHOLINERGICS, anticonvulsants, antidiabetics.
Contains: PROCHLORPERAZINE maleate.
Other preparations: Stemetil Syrup, Stemetil Effervescent Powders, Stemetil Suppositories, Stemetil Injection, BUCCASTEM (Reckitt & Colman), VERTIGON (SKB).

Ster-Zac Bath Concentrate
(Hough, Hoseason)

A liquid used as an antibacterial treatment for skin infections.

Dose: add 28.5 ml to the bath water.
Availability: NHS, private prescription, over the counter.
Side effects:
Caution: keep out of the eyes.
Not to be used for:
Caution needed with:
Contains: TRICLOSAN.
Other preparations:

Ster-Zac DC
(Hough, Hoseason)

A cream used as a disinfectant for cleansing and disinfecting the hands before surgery.

Dose: 3-5 ml used as a liquid soap.
Availability: NHS and private prescription.
Side effects:
Caution: in children under 2 years.
Not to be used for:
Caution needed with:
Contains: HEXACHLOROPHANE.
Other preparations:

Ster-Zac Powder
(Hough, Hoseason.)

A powder used as a disinfectant for the prevention of infections in new-born infants, and to treat recurring skin infections.

Dose: adults apply to the affected area once a day; infants dust the affected area at each change of nappy.
Availability: NHS, private prescription, over the counter.
Side effects:
Caution: in patients where the skin is broken.
Not to be used for:
Caution needed with:
Contains: HEXACHLOROPHANE.
Other preparations:

sterculia *see* **Normacol, Prefil**

Steri-neb Cromogen *see* **Intal**
(Baker Norton)

Steri-neb Salamol *see* **Ventolin**
(Baker Norton)

Steripod Blue *see* **Normasol**
(Seton)

Steripod Yellow *see* **Unisept**
(Seton)

---

steroid

A preparation which supplements the hormones naturally produced by the adrenal gland. Corticosteroids (example PREDNISOLONE *see* Precortisyl) are used to suppress inflammatory or allergic disorders, such as asthma, rheumatic conditions, or eczema. High doses may cause patients to develop a 'moon face' appearance. After long treatment periods, the drug should be withdrawn gradually. Anabolic steroids (example STANOZOLOL *see* Stromba) are used to treat vascular disorders, thinning of the bones, and some bone marrow disorders. They may be abused by some athletes because of their body-building properties.

Stesolid *see* **Valium**
(CP Pharmaceuticals)

Stiedex
(Stiefel)

An oily cream used as a STEROID treatment for skin disorders.

Dose: massage a small quantity into the affected area 2-3 times a day.

Availability: NHS and private prescription.
Side effects: fluid retention, suppression of adrenal glands, thinning of the skin may occur.
Caution: use for short periods of time only.
Not to be used for: patients suffering from acne or any other skin infections caused by tuberculosis, ringworm, viruses, or fungi, or continuously especially in pregnant women.
Caution needed with:
Contains: DESOXYMETHASONE.
Other preparations: Stiedex LP, Stiedex Lotion (for psoriasis).

Stiemycin
(Stiefel)

A solution used as an antibiotic treatment for acne.

Dose: wash and dry the affected area and apply twice a day.
Availability: NHS and private prescription.
Side effects: irritation, dryness.
Caution:
Not to be used for:
Caution needed with:
Contains: ERYTHROMYCIN.
Other preparations:

---

stilboesterol *see* Tampovagan

Stromba
(Sanofi Winthrop)

A white, quarter-scored tablet supplied at a strength of 5 mg and used as an anabolic STEROID to treat vascular disorders.

Dose: adults vascular complications 1 tablet twice a day, angio-oedema ½-2 tablets a day at first reducing as appropriate; children use reduced doses.
Availability: NHS and private prescription.
Side effects: masculinization, liver poisoning, dyspepsia, cramp, headache.
Caution: in children (avoid long-term use), women before the menopause, and in patients suffering from heart or kidney disease. Your doctor may advise blood tests for liver function.

Not to be used for: for pregnant women or for patients suffering from prostate cancer, liver disease, porphyria (a rare blood disorder).
Caution needed with: anticoagulants taken by mouth.
Contains: STANOZOLOL.
Other preparations:

Stugeron
(Janssen)

A white, scored tablet supplied at a strength of 15 mg and used as an ANTIHISTAMINE treatment for vestibular disorders, travel sickness.

Dose: vestibular disorders adults, 2 tablets 3 times a day; travel sickness 2 tablets 2 hours before journey, then 1 every 8 hours during the journey. Children 5-12 years half adult dose.
Availability: NHS, private prescription, over the counter.
Side effects: drowsiness, reduced reactions, rarely skin eruptions.
Caution: in pregnant women, nursing mothers, and in patients suffering from liver or kidney disease, glaucoma, epilepsy, or enlarged prostate.
Not to be used for: children under 5 years.
Caution needed with: alcohol, sedatives, some antidepressants (MAOIS), ANTICHOLINERGICS.
Contains: CINNARIZINE.
Other preparations:

S

Stugeron Forte
(Janssen)

An orange/cream capsule supplied at a strength of 75 mg and used as an ANTIHISTAMINE treatment for peripheral vascular disease including intermittent claudication and Raynaud's syndrome (a disease of the arteries of the hands).

Dose: 1 capsule 3 times a day.
Availability: NHS and private prescription.
Side effects: drowsiness, rash.
Caution: in patients suffering from low blood pressure.
Not to be used for: children.
Caution needed with: alcohol, sedatives.
Contains: CINNARIZINE.
Other preparations:

---

sucralfate *see* **Antepsin**

sucrose *see* **Rehidrat**

Sudafed
(Wellcome)

A red tablet supplied at a strength of 60 mg and used as a SYMPATHOMIMETIC treatment to relieve congestion of the nose, sinuses, and upper respiratory tract.

Dose: adults 1 tablet 3 times a day; children use elixir.
Availability: NHS, private prescription, over the counter.
Side effects: rapid or abnormal heart rate, dry mouth, brain stimulation.
Caution: in patients suffering from diabetes.
Not to be used for: patients suffering from cardivascular disorders, overactive thyroid.
Caution needed with: MAOIS, TRICYCLICS.
Contains: PSEUDOEPHEDRINE.
Other preparations: Sudafed Elixir, Sudafed SA (not available over the counter), Sudafed-Co, Sudafed Expectorant, GALPSEUD (Galen).

Sudafed Plus
(Wellcome)

A white, scored tablet used as an ANTIHISTAMINE, SYMPATHOMIMETIC treatment for allergic rhinitis.

Dose: adults 1 tablet 3 times a day; children over 2 years use syrup.
Availability: NHS, private prescription, over the counter.
Side effects: drowsiness, rash, disturbed sleep, rarely hallucinations.
Caution: in patients suffering from raised eye pressure, enlarged prostate.
Not to be used for: infants under 2 years or for patients suffering from severe high blood pressure, coronary artery disease, overactive thyroid.
Caution needed with: MAOIS, SYMPATHOMIMETICS, FURAZOLIDONE, alcohol.
Contains: TRIPROLIDINE hydrochloride, PSEUDOEPHEDRINE hydrochloride.
Other preparations: Sudafed Plus Syrup, ACTIFED (Wellcome — not available on NHS).

sulconazole *see* **Exelderm**

Suleo-C
(Napp)

A lotion used as a pediculicide to treat head lice.

Dose: rub into the scalp as directed. Shampoo off after 12 hours
Availability: NHS, private prescription, over the counter.
Side effects:
Caution: keep out of the eyes.
Not to be used for:
Caution needed with:
Contains: CARBARYL.
Other preparations: Suleo-C Shampoo, CARYLDERM (Napp), CLINICIDE (De Witt), DERBAC-C (Napp).

Suleo-M
(Napp)

A lotion used as a pediculicide to treat head lice.

Dose: rub into the scalp as directed. Shampoo off after 12 hours.
Availability: NHS, private prescription, over the counter.
Side effects:
Caution: keep out of the eyes.
Not to be used for:
Caution needed with:
Contains: MALATHION.
Other preparations: DERBAC-M (Napp), PRIODERM (Napp).

---

sulfadoxine *see* **Fansidar**

---

sulfametopyrazine *see* **Kelfizine W**

---

sulindac *see* **Clinoril**

---

sulphabenzamide *see* **Sultrin**

---

sulphacarbamide *see* **Uromide**

Sulphacetamide Minims

(SNP)

Drops used as a sulphonamide antibiotic treatment for eye infections.

Dose: 1 drop into the eye every 2 hours.
Availability: NHS and private prescription.
Side effects: transient irritation.
Caution:
Not to be used for:
Caution needed with:
Contains: SODIUM SULPHACETAMIDE.
Other preparations: OCUSOL, ALBUCID (Nicholas).

---

sulphacetamide sodium *see* Albucid, Ocusol, Sultrin, Sulphacetamide

---

sulphadiazine tablets

Tablets supplied at a strength of 500 mg, and used as an antibiotic to treat meningococcal meningitis

Dose: as directed by doctor.
Availability: NHS and private prescription.
Side effects: nausea, vomiting, tongue inflammation, rash, blood changes.
Caution: in the elderly, nursing mothers, and in patients suffering from kidney damage or sensitivity to light. A reasonable fluid intake must be maintained. Your doctor may advise regular blood tests.
Not to be used for: infants under 6 weeks, pregnant women, or for patients suffering from jaundice, blood disorders, or kidney or liver failure.
Caution needed with: anticoagulants, antidiabetics, PYRIMETHAMINE, CYCLOSPORIN.
Contains: sulphadiazine.
Other preparations:

---

sulphadimidine tablets

Tablets supplied at a strength of 500 mg and used as an antibiotic to treat infections of the urinary system, and meningococcal meningitis.

Dose: initially 4 tablets, then 1-2 tablets every 6-8 hours; children use reduced doses.

Availability: NHS and private prescription.
Side effects: nausea, vomiting, tongue inflammation, rash, blood changes.
Caution: in the elderly, nursing mothers, and in patients suffering from kidney damage or sensitivity to light. A reasonable fluid intake must be maintained. Your doctor may advise regular blood tests.
Not to be used for: infants under 6 weeks, pregnant women, or for patients suffering from jaundice, blood disorders, or kidney or liver failure.
Caution needed with: anticoagulants, antidiabetics, PYRIMETHAMINE, CYCLOSPORIN.
Contains: sulphadimidine.
Other preparations:

---

sulphamethoxazole *see* **Septrin**

---

sulphasalazine *see* **Salazopyrin, Salazopyrin EN-tablets**

---

sulphathiazole *see* **Sultrin**

---

sulphinpyrazone *see* **Anturan**

---

sulphur *see* **Actinac, Cocois, Dome-Acne, Eskamel, Medrone Lotion, Neo-Medrone Lotion, Pragmatar**

---

sulpiride *see* **Dolmatil, Sulpitil**

Sulpitil
(Farmitalia CE)

A white, scored tablet supplied at a strength of 200 mg and used as a sedative to treat schizophrenia.

Dose: elderly ¼-½ a tablet twice a day at first increasing to adult dose; adults over 14 years 1-2 tablets twice a day up to a maximum of 9 tablets a day.

Availability: NHS and private prescription.
Side effects: muscle spasms, restlessness, hands shaking, constipation, blurred vision, dry mouth, urine retention, palpitations, low blood pressure, weight gain, changes in libido, low body temperature, breast swelling, menstrual changes, jaundice, blood and skin changes, drowsiness, rarely fits.
Caution: in pregnant women and in patients suffering from hypertension, kidney disease, hypomania, or epilepsy
Not to be used for: children under 14 years or for patients suffering from phaeochromocytoma (a disease of the adrenal glands).
Caution needed with: alcohol, tranquillizers, pain killers, ANTIHYPERTENSIVES, antidepressants, anticonvulsants, antidiabetic drugs, LEVODOPA.
Contains: SULPIRIDE.
Other preparations: DOLMATIL (Squibb).

---

sultamicillin *see* Unasyn

Sultrin
(Cilag)

A white, lozenge-shaped vaginal tablet used as a sulphonamide antibacterial treatment for bacterial inflammation of the vagina or cervix, and for care after surgery.

Dose: 1 tablet into the vagina twice a day for 10 days.
Availability: NHS and private prescription.
Side effects: allergy.
Caution:
Not to be used for: children or patients suffering from kidney disease.
Caution needed with:
Contains: SULPHATHIAZOLE, SULPHACETAMIDE, SULPHABENZAMIDE.
Other preparations: Sultrin Cream.

---

sumatriptan *see* Imigran

Suprax
(Lederle)

A white tablet supplied at a strength of 200 mg and used as a cephalosporin antibiotic to treat infections of the respiratory and urinary tract.

Dose: adults, 200-400 mg a day for 7-14 days; children use suspension.
Availability: NHS and private prescription.
Side effects: stomach upset, headache, dizziness, colitis.
Caution: in pregnant women, nursing mothers, and in patients suffering from severe kidney damage or allergy to this type of antibiotic.
Not to be used for: infants under 6 months.
Caution needed with:
Contains: CEFIXIME.
Other preparations: Suprax Paediatric Suspension.

Suprecur
(Hoechst)

A nasal spray with metered dose pump, used as a synthetic hormone to treat endometriosis.

Dose: 1 application in each nostril 3 times a day for up to 6 months. Start treatment on 1st or 2nd day of cycle.
Availability: NHS and private prescription.
Side effects: hot flushes, vaginal dryness, loss of sexual desire, emotional upset, headache, breast tenderness, alteration of breast size, ovarian cyst, nasal irritation.
Caution: in patients who may later develop thinning of the bones, and in depressed patients. A non-hormonal method of contraception must be used throughout treatment.
Not to be used for: children, pregnant women, nursing mothers, or patients suffering from undiagnosed vaginal bleeding or some cancers.
Caution needed with: decongestant sprays for the nose.
Contains: BUSERELIN.
Other preparations:

Suprefact
(Hoechst)

A nasal spray used as a hormone treatment for prostate cancer.

Dose: 1 spray into each nostril 6 times a day.
Availability: NHS and private prescription.
Side effects: hot flushes, loss of sex drive, temporary irritation of the nose.
Caution:

Not to be used for: tumours which are not sensitive to hormones, or following removal of a testicle.
Caution needed with:
Contains: BUSERELIN.
Other preparations: Suprefact Injection.

Surbex T — multivitamin. Product now discontinued.

Surem *see* **Mogadon.** Product now discontinued.

Surgam SA
(Roussel)

A maroon/pink capsule supplied at a strength of 300 mg and used as a NON-STEROID ANTI-INFLAMMATORY DRUG to treat rheumatoid arthritis, osteoarthritis, ankylosing spondylitis, lumbago, acute bone or muscular problems.

Dose: 2 capsules once a day.
Availability: NHS and private prescription.
Side effects: stomach upset, headache, drowsiness, rash, bladder irritation.
Caution: in the elderly, pregnant women, nursing mothers, and in patients suffering from severe kidney or liver disease, asthma, allergy to ASPIRIN/ NON-STEROID ANTI-INFLAMMATORY DRUGS.
Not to be used for: children or for patients suffering from stomach ulcer or with a history of stomach ulcer.
Caution needed with: anticoagulants, antidiabetics, hydantoins, sulphonamide antibiotics, DIURETICS.
Contains: TIAPROFENIC ACID.
Other preparations: Surgam Tablets, Surgam Sachets (now discontinued).

Surmontil
(Rhone-Poulenc Rorer)

A white tablet supplied at strengths of 10 mg, 25 mg and used as a TRICYCLIC antidepressant to treat depression, anxiety, sleep disturbance, agitation.

Dose: 50-75 mg 2 hours before going to bed for at least 3 weeks, increasing to up to 300 mg a day.
Availability: NHS and private prescription.
Side effects: dry mouth, constipation, urine retention, blurred vision, palpitations, drowsiness, sleeplessness, dizziness, hands shaking, low blood presure, weight change, skin reactions, unsteadiness, convulsions, jaundice or blood changes. Loss of sexual desire may occur.
Caution: in nursing mothers or in patients suffering from adrenal tumour, heart or liver disease, thyroid disease, epilepsy, diabetes, some other psychiatric conditions. Your doctor may advise regular blood tests.
Not to be used for: children, pregnant women, or for patients suffering from heart attacks, liver disease, heart block.
Caution needed with: alcohol, ANTICHOLINERGICS, ADRENALINE, MAOIS, BARBITURATES, other antidepressants, ANTIHYPERTENSIVES, CIMETIDINE, oestrogens.
Contains: TRIMIPRAMINE maleate.
Other preparations: Surmontil Capsules.

S

Suscard Buccal
(Pharmax)

A white tablet supplied at strengths of 1 mg, 2 mg, 3 mg, 5 mg and used as a NITRATE to treat angina, acute heart failure, congestive heart failure.

Dose: for heart failure 5 mg 3 times a day at first or repeated until symptoms are relieved, allowing tablet to dissolve between upper lip and gum. For angina 2 mg as required or 2 mg 3 times a day increasing strength and frequency as needed.
Availability: NHS, private prescription, over the counter.
Side effects: headache, flushes.
Caution:
Not to be used for: for children.
Caution needed with:
Contains: GLYCERYL TRINITRATE.
Other preparations: CORO-NITRO (Boehringer Mannheim), DEPONIT (Schwarz), GLYTRIN (Sanofi Winthrop), NITRODUR (Schering-Plough), NITROCONTIN (Asta), NITROLINGUAL (Lipha), PERCUTOL (Cusi), SUSTAC (Pharmax), TRANSIDERM-NITRO (Ciba).

Sustac
(Pharmax)

A pink, mottled tablet supplied at strengths of 2.6 mg, 6.4 mg, 10 mg and used as a NITRATE for the prevention of angina.

Dose: 2.6-12.8 mg 2-3 times a day.
Availability: NHS, private prescription, over the counter.
Side effects: headache, flushes.
Caution:
Not to be used for: children.
Caution needed with:
Contains: GLYCERYL TRINITRATE.
Other preparations: CORO-NITRO (Boehringer Mannheim), DEPONIT (Schwarz), GLYTRIN (Sanofi Winthrop), NITRODUR (Schering-Plough), NITROCONTIN (Asta), NITROLINGUAL (Lipha), PERCUTOL (Cusi), SUSCARD BUCCAL (Pharmax), TRANSIDERM-NITRO (Ciba).

Sustamycin *see* Tetracycline
(Boehringer Mannheim)

Symmetrel
(Ciba-Geigy)

A brownish-red capsule supplied at a strength of 100 mg and used as an anti-parkinsonian/antiviral drug to treat Parkinson's disease, virus infections.

Dose: for Parkinson's disease1 tablet a day for 7 days then 1 tablet twice a day; virus infections 1 tablet twice a day.
Availability: NHS and private prescription.
Side effects: skin changes, fluid retention, rash, sight, brain and stomach disturbances.
Caution: in pregnant women, confused patients, and in patients suffering from liver or kidney disease or congestive heart failure.
Not to be used for: patients suffering from severe kidney disease or with a history of convulsions or stomach ulcers.
Caution needed with: ANTICHOLINERGICS, LEVODOPA, stimulants.
Contains: AMANTADINE hydrochloride.
Other preparations: Symmetrel Syrup.

---

sympathomimetic

A drug which functions like ADRENALINE and causes narrowing of the blood vessels but which may open other organs, such as the bronchial tubes. Example PSEUDOEPHEDRINE *see* Sudafed.

Synalar
(ICI)

An ointment used as a STEROID treatment for skin disorders.

Dose: apply to the affected area 2-3 times a day.
Availability: NHS and private prescription.
Side effects: fluid retention, suppression of adrenal glands, thinning of the skin may occur.
Caution: use for short periods of time only.
Not to be used for: patients suffering from acne or any other skin infections caused by tuberculosis, ringworm, viruses, or fungi, or continuously especially in pregnant women.
Caution needed with:
Contains: FLUOCINOLONE ACETONIDE.
Other preparations: Synalar Cream, Synalar 1:4, Synalar Cream, Synalar Gel 1:10; also Synalar C and Synalar N (for infected conditions).

Syndol
(Marion Merrell Dow)

A yellow, scored tablet used as an ANALGESIC, ANTIHISTAMINE treatment for tension headache after dental or other surgery.

Dose: 1-2 tablets every 4-6 hours up to a maximum of 8 tablets in 24 hours.
Availability: over the counter and private prescription only.
Side effects: drowsiness, constipation.
Caution: in patients suffering from liver or kidney disease.
Not to be used for: children.
Caution needed with: alcohol, sedatives, other medicines containing PARACETAMOL.
Contains: PARACETAMOL, CODEINE PHOSPHATE, DOXYLAMINE SUCCINATE, CAFFEINE.
Other preparations:

Synflex
(Syntex)

An orange tablet supplied at a strength of 275 mg and used as a NON-STEROID ANTI-INFLAMMATORY DRUG to treat period pain, migraine, pain after surgery, bone or muscle problems including sprains, strains, and lumbosacral pain.

Dose: for pain 2 tablets immediately, then 1 tablet every 6-8 hours as needed to a maximum of 4 tablets a day after the first day; migraine 3 tablets immediately then 1-2 tablets as needed (up to 5 a day); for muscle/ bone disorder 2 tablets twice a day.

Availability: NHS and private prescription.
Side effects: rash, stomach intolerance, headache, tinnitus, vertigo, blood changes.
Caution: in pregnant women, nursing mothers, the elderly, and in patients with a history of gastro-intestinal lesions, or suffering from kidney or liver disease.
Not to be used for: patients under 16 years, or for patients suffering from stomach ulcer, ASPIRIN or anti-inflammatory induced allergy.
Caution needed with: anticoagulants, hydantoins, some antidiabetics, LITHIUM, ß-BLOCKERS, METHOTREXATE, PROBENECID, FRUSEMIDE.
Contains: NAPROXEN sodium
Other preparations: ARTHROSIN (Ashbourne), ARTHROXEN (CP Pharm), NAPRATEC (Searle), NAPROSYN (Syntex), NYCOPREN (Lundbeck), PRANOXEN (Napp), PROSAID (BHR), RHEUFLEX (Goldcrest), RIMOXYN (Rima), VALROX (Shire).

Synkavit
(Cambridge)

A white, scored tablet supplied at a strength of 10 mg and used as vitamin K to prevent bleeding, and to treat jaundice.

Dose: adults 1-4 tablets a day; children ½-2 tablets a day.
Availability: NHS, private prescription, over the counter.
Side effects: anaemia, jaundice.
Caution:
Not to be used for: childern under 5 years.
Caution needed with: anticoagulants.
Contains: MENADIOL DIPHOSPHATE.
Other preparations:

Synogist — shampoo to treat seborrhoea. Product now discontinued.

Synphase
(Syntex)

White tablets and yellow tablets used as an oestrogen, progestogen contraceptive.

Dose: 1 tablet a day for 21 days starting on day 5 of the period.
Availability: NHS and private prescription.
Side effects: enlarged breasts, bloating and fluid retention, cramps, leg pains, mood change, reduction in sexual desire, headaches, nausea, vaginal erosion, discharge, and bleeding, weight gain, skin changes.
Caution: in patients suffering from high blood pressure, diabetes, vascular disorders, asthma, depression, kidney disease, multiple sclerosis, womb diseases. Your doctor may advise you not to smoke, to have regular examinations. You should stop treatment at the first sign of serious symptoms such as severe headache or jaundice. Treatment should be stopped before surgery.
Not to be used for: pregnant women, or for patients suffering from sickle-cell anaemia, history of heart disease or thrombosis, liver disorders, some cancers, undiagnosed vaginal bleeding, some ear, skin, and kidney disorders.
Caution needed with: RIFAMPICIN, TETRACYCLINES, GRISEOFULVIN, BARBITURATES, PHENYTOIN, PRIMIDONE, CARBAMAZEPINE, ETHOSUXIMIDE, CHLORAL HYDRATE, DICHLORALPHENAZONE.
Contains: ETHINYLOESTRADIOL, NORETHISTERONE.
Other preparations:

S

Syntaris
(Syntex)

A spray supplied at a strength of 25 micrograms and used as a STEROID treatment for rhinitis, hay fever.

Dose: adults 2 sprays into each nostril 2-3 times a day at first reducing according to response; children over 5 years 1 spray into each nostril 3 times a day.
Availability: NHS and private prescription.
Side effects: temporary itching.
Caution: in pregnant women, and in patients suffering from ulcerated nose, trauma, or who have undergone nasal surgery, or who are being transferred from STEROIDS taken by mouth or injected.
Not to be used for: children under 5 years or for patients suffering from untreated nose or eye infections.
Caution needed with:
Contains: FLUNISOLIDE.
Other preparations:

Syntex Menophase *see* Menophase

Syntopressin
(Sandoz)

A nasal spray used as a hormone treatment for diabetes insipidus (a condition causing excess thirst and urination).

Dose: adults 1-2 sprays into one or both nostrils 3-7 times a day; children as advised by the physician.
Availability: NHS and private prescription.
Side effects: nausea, stomach pain, desire to defaecate, blocked nose and ulceration.
Caution: in pregnant women and in patients suffering from epilepsy, or heart failure, high blood pressure, circulation disorders.
Not to be used for: patients suffering from coronary heart disease.
Caution needed with: CARBAMAZEPINE, LITHIUM, CLOFIBRATE, CHLORPROPAMIDE, some anaesthetics.
Contains: LYPRESSIN.
Other preparations:

S

Synuretic *see* Moduretic
(DDSA)

Syraprim *see* Monotrim. Product now discontinued.

Sytron
(Parke-Davis)

An elixir used as an iron supplement to treat iron-deficiency anaemia.

Dose: adults 5 ml 3 times a day at first increasing gradually to 10 ml 3 times a day; children 0-1 year 2.5 ml twice a day, 1-5 years 2.5 ml 3 times a day, 6-12 years 5 ml 3 times a day.
Availability: NHS, private prescription, over the counter.
Side effects: nausea, diarrhoea.
Caution:
Not to be used for:
Caution needed with: TETRACYCLINES.
Contains: SODIUM IRON EDETATE.
Other preparations:

T Gel
(Neutrogena)

A shampoo used as an anti-psoriatic treatment for dandruff, seborrhoea, and psoriasis of the scalp.

Dose: shampoo 1-2 times a week.
Availability: NHS, private prescription, over the counter.
Side effects: irritation.
Caution:
Not to be used for: patients suffering from acute psoriasis.
Caution needed with:
Contains: COAL TAR EXTRACT.
Other preparations: ALPHOSYL SHAMPOO (Stafford-Miller), CLINITAR SHAMPOO (Shire), GELCOTAR LIQUID (Quinoderm), POLYTAR LIQUID (Stiefel), PSORIDERM SCALP LOTION (Dermal), PSORIGEL (Galderma).

Tachyrol — vitamin D tablets. Product now discontinued.

Tagamet
(S K B)

A green tablet supplied at strengths of 200 mg, 400 mg, 800 mg and used as an H_2 BLOCKER to treat duodenal and gastric ulcers, hiatus hernia, dyspepsia, oesophageal reflux.

Dose: children over 1 year 25-30 mg per 1 kg body weight a day, adults 800 mg at night or 400 mg twice a day, maintenance 400 mg at night or 200 mg twice a day.
Availability: NHS and private prescription.
Side effects: diarrhoea, rash, tiredness, dizziness, liver changes, confusion, breast swelling; rarely kidney, pancreas, bone marrow, joint, and muscle problems; headache.
Caution: in pregnant women, nursing mothers and in patients suffering from impaired kidney function. Ensure cancer has not been missed as a diagnosis. Monitor patients on long-term therapy.
Not to be used for:
Caution needed with: oral anticoagulants, PHENYTOIN, THEOPHYLLINE.
Contains: CIMETIDINE.
Other preparations: Tagamet syrup, injections, infusions. ALGITEC (S K B) in combination with alginic acid, DYSPAMET (Bridge), PEPTIMAX (Ashbourne).

---

talampicillin *see* **Talpen**

Talpen — penicillin antibiotic. Product now discontinued.

Tambocor
(3M Healthcare)

A white, scored tablet supplied at strengths of 50 mg, 100 mg and used as an anti-arrhythmic treatment for abnormal heart rhythm.

Dose: ½-1 tablet twice a day at first for 3-5 days (or up to 4 tablets a day), then reduce the dose to the minimum necessary to keep symptoms under control.
Availability: NHS and private prescription.
Side effects: dizziness, disturbed vision, sensitivity to light, nausea, vomiting, liver disturbance, tingling, unsteadiness.
Caution: in pregnant women, patients fitted with pacemakers, and in patients suffering from kidney or liver problems, some heart muscle disorders. Your doctor may advise blood tests to check electrolytes and blood levels.
Not to be used for: children and for patients suffering from some heart disorders.
Caution needed with: DIGOXIN and some other heart drugs.
Contains: FLECAINIDE acetate.
Other preparations: Tambocor Injection.

Tamofen *see* **Nolvadex-D**
(Farmitalia CE)

---

tamoxifen citrate *see* **Nolvadex-D**

Tampovagan
(Norgine)

A pessary used as an oestrogen treatment for atrophic or menopausal inflammation of the vagina.

Dose: 2 pessaries in the vagina at night.
Availability: NHS and private prescription.

626

Side effects: enlarged breasts, fluid retention, headaches, nausea, vaginal bleeding, weight gain, skin changes, liver disorders, jaundice, rashes, vomiting.
Caution: in patients suffering from high blood pressure, diabetes, heart disease, vascular disorders, asthma, kidney disease, epilepsy womb diseases. Your doctor may advise you to have regular examinations.
Not to be used for: children, pregnant women, nursing mothers, or for patients suffering from sickle-cell anaemia, thrombosis, liver disorders, some cancers, undiagnosed vaginal bleeding, some ear, skin, and kidney disorders, jaundice, porphyria (a rare blood disorder), brain blood vessel disease.
Caution needed with: DIURETICS, ANTIHYPERTENSIVES, and drugs that change liver enzymes (BARBITURATES, CARBAMAZEPINE, PHENYTON).
Contains: STILBOESTEROL, LACTIC ACID.
Other preparations:

Tanderil
(Zyma)

An ointment used as a NON-STEROID ANTI-INFLAMMATORY DRUG to treat eye inflammation.

Dose: apply into the eye 2-5 times a day.
Availability: NHS and private prescription.
Side effects: swelling, redness, rarely blood changes
Caution: in patients suffering from glaucoma, weeping infections.
Not to be used for:
Caution needed with:
Contains: OXYPHENBUTAZONE.
Other preparations:

---

tannic acid *see* **Phytex**

---

tar *see* **Gelcosal, Gelcotar, Polytar Liquid**

Tarcortin
(Stafford-Miller)

A cream used as a STEROID, anti-psoriatic treatment for eczema, psoriasis, other skin disorders.

Dose: apply to the affected area at least twice a day.
Availability: NHS and private prescription.
Side effects: fluid retention, suppression of adrenal glands, thinning of the skin may occur.
Caution: use for short periods of time only.
Not to be used for: patients suffering from acne or any other skin infections caused by tuberculosis, ringworm, viruses, or fungi, or continuously especially in pregnant women.
Caution needed with:
Contains: HYDROCORTISONE, COAL TAR EXTRACT.
Other preparations: ALPHOSYL HC (Stafford-Miller).

Tarivid
(Hoechst)

A white, oblong, scored tablet supplied at a strength of 200 mg, and used as an antibiotic to treat urine or lung diseases, or sexually transmitted diseases.

Dose: 2-4 tablets a day depending upon severity and type of condition.
Availability: NHS and private prescription.
Side effects: stomach upset, allergy, skin reactions, convulsions, nerve disorders, colitis, joint and muscle pain, changes in liver or bone marrow.
Caution: in patients suffering from psychiatric disorders or kidney damage, or those exposed to strong sunlight, or who will be driving or operating machinery.
Not to be used for: children, pregnant women, nursing mothers, growing adolescents, or for patients with a history of epilepsy.
Caution needed with: magnesium or aluminium ANTACIDS, iron, NON-STEROID ANTI-INFLAMMATORY DRUGS.
Contains: OFLOXACIN.
Other preparations: Tarivid Infusion.

Tavegil
(Sandoz)

A white, scored tablet supplied at a strength of 1 mg and used as an ANTIHISTAMINE treatment for allergic rhinitis, dermatoses, urticaria, allergy to other drugs.

Dose: adults 1 tablet night and morning; children over 3 years ½-1 tablet night and morning, under 3 years use elixir.
Availability: NHS, private prescription, over the counter.

Side effects: drowsiness, reduced reactions, rarely dizziness, dry mouth, palpitations, gastro-intestinal disturbances, excitement.
Caution: in pregnant women, nursing mothers, and in patients suffering from glaucoma, enlarged prostate, some stomach ulcers.
Not to be used for: children under 1 year.
Caution needed with: sedatives, MAOIS, alcohol.
Contains: CLEMASTINE.
Other preparations: Tavegil Elixir.

Tears Naturale
(Alcon)

Drops used to lubricate dry eyes.

Dose: 1-2 drops into the eye as needed.
Availability: NHS, private prescription, over the counter.
Side effects:
Caution:
Not to be used for: patients who wear soft contact lenses.
Caution needed with:
Contains: DEXTRAN, HYPROMELLOSE.
Other preparations: HYPROMELLOSE EYE DROPS, ISOPTO ALKALINE (Alcon), ISOPTO PLAIN (Alcon),.

Tedral *see* **Theophylline.** Product now discontinued.

Teejel
(Napp)

A gel used as an antiseptic, ANALGESIC treatment for mouth ulcers, stomatitis, gingivitis, glossitis, teething, uncomfortable dentures.

Dose: rub gently into the affected area every 3-4 hours.
Availability: NHS, private prescription, over the counter.
Side effects:
Caution:
Not to be used for: infants under 4 months.
Caution needed with:
Contains: CHOLINE SALICYLATE, CETALKONIUM CHLORIDE.
Other preparations: Bonjela (Reckitt & Colman).

Teflox — antibiotic to treat infections. Product now discontinued.

Tegretol
(Ciba-Geigy)

A white, scored tablet or a white, scored, oblong tablet according to strengths of 100 mg, 200 mg, 400 mg and used as an anticonvulsant, ANALGESIC treatment for manic depression, epilepsy, neuralgia.

Dose: for manic depression 400 mg a day in divided doses at first increasing gradually until symptoms are controlled and up to a maximum of 1.6 g a day. For epilepsy and neuralgia adults 100-200 mg 1-2 times a day at first increasing usually to 800 mg-1.2 g a day up to a maximum of 1.6 g; children up to 1 year 100-200 mg a day, 1-5 years 200-400 mg a day, 5-10 years 400-600 mg a day, 10-15 years 600 mg-1 g a day.
Availability: NHS and private prescription.
Side effects: stomach upset, double vision, dry mouth, drowsiness, dizziness, fluid retention, low blood sodium, blood changes, rash, acute kidney failure, jaundice, hair loss, hepatitis, hypersensitivity.
Caution: in the elderly, pregnant women, nursing mothers, and in patients suffering from severe cardiovascular disease, liver or kidney disease. Your doctor may advise that blood tests should be made regularly.
Not to be used for: patients suffering from heart conduction block.
Caution needed with: anticoagulants taken by mouth, MAOIS, contraceptive pill, ERYTHROMYCIN, ISONIAZID, CIMETIDINE, DEXTROPROPOXYPHENE, DILTIAZEM, VERAPAMIL, VILOXAZINE, STEROIDS, PHENYTOIN, LITHIUM, DOXYCYCLINE.
Contains: CARBAMAZEPINE.
Other preparations: Tegretol Chewtabs, Tegretol Liquid, Tegretol Retard.

temafloxacin *see* Teflox

temazepam capsules

A capsule supplied at strengths of 10 mg, 15 mg, 20 mg, 30 mg and used as a sleeping preparation to treat sleeplessness.

Dose: elderly 5-15 mg before going to bed; adults 10-30 mg before going to bed; in severe cases a maximum of 60 mg may be taken if needed.
Availability: NHS and private prescription.
Side effects: drowsiness, confusion, unsteadiness, low blood pressure, rash, changes in vision, changes in libido, retention of urine. Risk of addiction increases with dose and length of treatment. May impair judgement.

Caution: in the elderly, pregnant women, nursing mothers, in women during labour, and in patients suffering from lung disorders, kidney or liver disorders. Avoid long-term use and withdraw gradually.
Not to be used for: children, or for patients suffering from acute lung diseases, some chronic lung diseases, some obsessional and psychotic diseases.
Caution needed with: alcohol, anticonvulsants, other tranquillizers.
Contains: temazepam.
Other preparations: temazepam elixir, Temazepam Gelthix (Farmitalia CE), EUHYPNOS (Farmitalia CE), NORMISON (Wyeth) — all available on NHS only if prescribed as generic.

Temgesic
(Reckitt & Colman)

A white tablet supplied at strength of 0.2 mg, 0.4 mg and used as a opiate to control pain.

Dose: 0.2-0.4 mg under the tongue every 6-8 hours or as needed; children use reduced doses.
Availability: controlled drug; NHS and private prescription.
Side effects: drowsiness, nausea, sweating, dizziness.
Caution: in pregnant women, women in labour, and in patients suffering from breathing or liver problems, or patients addicted to or with a history of addiction to narcotics.
Not to be used for: children under 16 kg body weight.
Caution needed with: MAOIS or sedatives.
Contains: BUPRENORPHINE hydrochloride.
Other preparations: Temgesic Injection.

Tenavoid — DIURETIC/sedative to treat premenstrual syndrome. Product now discontinued.

Tenif
(Stuart)

A reddish-brown capsule used as a calcium blocker/ß-BLOCKER to treat high blood pressure, angina.

Dose: 1 capsule a day at first increasing to 2 capsules a day if needed; elderly a maximum of 1 capsule a day.
Availability: NHS and private prescription.

Side effects: flushing, headache, dizziness, dry eyes, rash, fluid retention, jaundice, swollen gums.
Caution: in patients suffereing from heart failure, kidney or liver disease, diabetes, or patients undergoing anaesthesia.
Not to be used for: children, pregnant women, nursing mothers, or for patients suffering from heart failure, block, or shock.
Caution needed with: CIMETIDINE, QUINIDINE, heart depressants.
Contains: ATENOLOL, NIFEDIPINE.
Other preparations: BETA-ADALAT (Bayer).

Tenoret 50
(Stuart)

A brown capsule used as a ß-BLOCKER/THIAZIDE DIURETIC to treat high blood pressure especially for the elderly.

Dose: 1 capsule a day.
Availability: NHS and private prescription.
Side effects: cold hands and feet, sleep disturbance, slow heart rate, tiredness, wheezing, heart failure, stomach upset, gout, blood changes, sensitivity to light, weakness, dry eyes, rash.
Caution: in pregnant women, nursing mothers, and in patients suffering from diabetes, gout, kidney or liver disorders, asthma. May need to be withdrawn before surgery. Withdraw gradually. Your doctor may advise additional treatment with DIURETICS or DIGOXIN.
Not to be used for: children or patients suffering from heart block or failure, kidney failure.
Caution needed with: VERAPAMIL, CLONIDINE withdrawal, some anti-arrhythmic drugs and anaesthetics, RESERPINE, some ANTIHYPERTENSIVES, ERGOTAMINE, CIMETIDINE, sedatives, SYMPATHOMIMETICS, INDOMETHACIN, antidiabetics, LITHIUM, DIGOXIN.
Contains: ATENOLOL, CHLORTHALIDONE (CO-TENIDONE).
Other preparations: TENORETIC (Stuart — double strength).

Tenoretic
(Stuart)

A brown tablet used as a ß-BLOCKER/THIAZIDE DIURETIC to treat high blood pressure.

Dose: 1 tablet a day.
Availability: NHS and private prescription.
Side effects: cold hands and feet, sleep disturbance, slow heart rate,

tiredness, wheezing, heart failure, stomach upset, gout, sensitivity to light, blood changes, weakness, dry eyes, rash.

Caution: in pregnant women, nursing mothers, and in patients suffering from diabetes, gout kidney or liver disorders, asthma. May need to be withdrawn before surgery. Withdraw gradually. Your doctor may advise additional treatment with DIURETICS or DIGOXIN.

Not to be used for: children or for patients suffering from heart block or failure, kidney failure.

Caution needed with: VERAPAMIL, CLONIDINE withdrawal, some anti-arrhythmic drugs and anaesthetics, RESERPINE, some ANTIHYPERTENSIVES, ERGOTAMINE, CIMETIDINE, sedatives, antidiabetics, LITHIUM, DIGOXIN, SYMPATHOMIMETICS, INDOMETHACIN.

Contains: ATENOLOL, CHLORTHALIDONE (CO-TENIDONE).

Other preparations: TENORET-50 (Stuart — half strength).

Tenormin
(Stuart)

An orange capsule supplied at a strength of 100 mg and used as a ß-BLOCKER to treat angina, abnormal heart rhythm, high blood pressure.

Dose: 50-100 mg a day.

Availability: NHS and private prescription.

Side effects: cold hands and feet, sleep disturbance, slow heart rate, tiredness, wheezing, heart failure, stomach upset, dry eyes, rash.

Caution: in pregnant women, nursing mothers, and in patients suffering from diabetes, kidney or liver disorders, asthma. May need to be withdrawn before surgery. Withdraw gradually. Your doctor may advise additional treatment with DIURETICS or DIGOXIN.

Not to be used for: children or for patients suffering from heart block or failure.

Caution needed with: VERAPAMIL, CLONIDINE withdrawal, some anti-arrhythmic drugs and anaesthetics, RESERPINE, some ANTIHYPERTENSIVES, ERGOTAMINE, CIMETIDINE, sedatives, antidiabetics, SYMPATHOMIMETICS, INDOMETHACIN.

Contains: ATENOLOL.

Other preparations: Tenormin Injection, Tenormin Syrup, Tenormin 25, Tenormin LS. ANTIPRESSAN (Berk), ATENIX (Ashbourne), TOTAMOL (CP Pharm), VASATEN (Shire).

---

tenoxicam *see* **Mobiflex**

Tensium *see* Valium
(DDSA)

Tenuate Dospan
(Marion Merrell Dow)

A white, oblong, scored tablet supplied at a strength of 75 mg and used as an appetite suppressant to treat obesity.

Dose: 1 tablet a day in the middle of the morning.
Availability: controlled drug; NHS and private prescription.
Side effects: tolerance, addiction, mental disturbances, sleeplessness, nervousness, agitation.
Caution: in patients suffering from high blood pressure, angina, abnormal heart rhythm, stomach ulcer. Do not use for prolonged periods.
Not to be used for: children, pregnant women, nursing mothers, or for patients suffering from hardening of the arteries, overactive thyroid, severe high blood pressure, glaucoma, or with a history of alcoholism or drug addiction.
Caution needed with: MAOIS, SYMPATHOMIMETICS, METHYLDOPA, GUANETHIDINE, sedatives, other obesity drugs.
Contains: DIETHYLPROPION HYDROCHLORIDE.
Other preparations: APISATE (Wyeth).

Teoptic
(Dispersa)

Drops used as a ß-BLOCKER to treat hypertension of the eye, open angle glaucoma, some secondary glaucomas.

Dose: 1 drop into the eye twice a day.
Availability: NHS and private prescription.
Side effects: burning, stinging, and painful sensations of the eye, blurred vision, redness, corneal inflammation.
Caution: in patients suffering from heart conduction block, heart failure, diabetes.
Not to be used for: children, pregnant women, or for patients suffering from heart failure, asthma, chronic obstructive lung disease, or for those who wear contact lenses.
Caution needed with: ß-BLOCKERS taken by mouth or injection.
Contains: CARTEOLOL HYDROCHLORIDE.
Other preparations:

---

terazosin *see* **Hytrin**

terbinafine *see* **Lamisil**

terbutaline *see* **Bricanyl, Bricanyl Expectorant, Monovent**

Tercoda — antitussive/expectorant to treat bronchitis. Product now discontinued.

terfenadine *see* **Triludan**

terodiline hydrochloride *see* **Micturin**

Terolin *see* **Micturin.** Product now discontinued.

Teronac
(Sandoz)

A white, scored tablet supplied at a strength of 2 mg and used as an appetite suppressant to treat obesity.

Dose: 1 tablet a day after breakfast.
Availability: controlled drug; NHS and private prescription.
Side effects: rapid heart rate, nervousness, headache, fainting, dizziness, chills, skin rashes constipation, dry mouth, sweating, sleeplessness, urgent need to urinate and defaecate, impotence.
Caution: care in patients suffering from coronary heart disease, severe agitation, enlarged prostate.
Not to be used for: children, the elderly, pregnant women, nursing mothers, or for patients suffering from stomach ulcer, glaucoma, severe kidney, liver or heart disease, abnormal heart rhythms, severe high blood pressure, or with a history of mental illness alcoholism, or drug addiction.
Caution needed with: MAOIS, GUANETHIDINE, DEBRISOQUINE, thyroid drugs, SYMPATHOMIMETICS, psychostimulants, antidiabetic drugs, alcohol.
Contains: MAZINDOL.

Other preparations:

---

terpin hydrate *see* **Copholco, Copholcoids, Tercoda**

Terpoin
(Hough, Hoseason)

An elixir used as an opiate treatment for dry cough.

Dose: 5 ml every 3 hours.
Availability: private prescription and over the counter.
Side effects: constipation.
Caution: in patients suffering from asthma.
Not to be used for: children, or for patients suffering from liver disease.
Caution needed with: MAOIS.
Contains: CODEINE PHOSPHATE, CINEOLE, MENTHOL.
Other preparations:

Terra-Cortril Ear Suspension
(Pfizer)

Drops used as an antibiotic, STEROID treatment for infections of the outer ear.

Dose: 2-4 drops into the ear 3 times a day for up to 7 days.
Availability: NHS and private prescription.
Side effects: additional infection, rarely allergy.
Caution:
Not to be used for: children, pregnant women, or for patients suffering from perforated ear drum, or viral, fungal, tubercular, or acute weeping infections.
Caution needed with:
Contains: OXYTETRACYCLINE hydrochloride, HYDROCORTISONE acetate, POLYMYXIN B SULPHATE.
Other preparations:

Terra-Cortril Spray
(Pfizer)

A spray used as an antibiotic, STEROID treatment for weeping and infected eczema, insect bites, weeping intertrigo.

Dose: apply to the affected area 2-4 times a day.
Availability: NHS and private prescription.
Side effects: fluid retention, suppression of adrenal glands, thinning of the skin may occur.
Caution: use for short periods of time only.
Not to be used for: children or for patients suffering from acne or any other skin infections caused by tuberculosis, ringworm, viruses, or fungi, or continuously especially in pregnant women.
Caution needed with:
Contains: OXYTETRACYCLINE hydrochloride.
Other preparations: Terra-Cortril Ointment, Terra-Cortril Nystatin (for infected conditions).

Terramycin *see* Tetracycline
(Pfizer)

Tertroxin
(Evans)

A white, scored tablet supplied at a strength of 20 micrograms and used as a thyroid hormone to treat severe thyroid deficiency, to test for thyrotoxicosis.

Dose: adults 10-20 micrograms every 8 hours at first, increasing after 1 week to 60 micrograms a day in 2-3 divided doses; children 5 micrograms a day at first.
Availability: NHS and private prescription.
Side effects: abnormal heart rhythm, chest pain, rapid heart rate, muscle cramp, headache, restlessness, flushing, excitability, sweating, diarrhoea, rapid weight loss.
Caution: in nursing mothers.
Not to be used for: patients suffering from cardiovascular problems or where effort causes anginal pain.
Caution needed with: anticoagulants, TRICYCLICS, PHENYTOIN, CHOLESTYRAMINE.
Contains: LIOTHYRONINE sodium.
Other preparations:

---

testosterone *see* Restandol

Tetmosol

(ICI)

A solution used as a scabicide to treat scabies.

Dose: dilute and apply to the body as directed.
Availability: NHS, private prescription, over the counter.
Side effects:
Caution: keep out of the eyes.
Not to be used for:
Caution needed with: alcohol.
Contains: MONOSULFIRAM.
Other preparations: Tetmosol Soap.

---

tetrabenazine *see* Nitoman

Tetrabid *see* Tetracycline

(Organon)

Tetrachel *see* Tetracycline

(Berk)

Tetracycline Tablets

An orange tablet supplied at a strength of 250 mg and used as an antibiotic treatment for infections.

Dose: 1-2 tablets 4 times a day.
Availability: NHS and private prescription.
Side effects: stomach disturbances, allergy, additional infections.
Caution: in patients suffering from liver or kidney disease.
Not to be used for: children, nursing mothers, or women during the latter half of pregnancy.
Caution needed with: milk, ANTACIDS, mineral supplements, the contraceptive pill.
Contains: TETRACYCLINE HYDROCHLORIDE.
Other preparations: Tetracycline Tablets, Tetracycline
Syrup,Tetracycline Injection, Tetracycline V. ACHROMYCIN (Lederle),
Achromycin Tablets, BERKMYCEN (Berk), CHYMOCYCLAR, DETECLO (Lederle),
ECONOMYCIN (DDSA), IMPERACIN (ICI), MINOCIN (Lederle), MYSTECLIN (Squibb),

OXYMYCIN (DDSA), OXYTETRACYCLINE, SUSTAMYCIN (Boehringer Mannheim) TOPICYCLINE (Norwich Eaton).

tetracycline hydrochloride *see* **Achromycin, Tetracycline, Topicycline**

Tetralysal *see* **Tetracycline**
(Farmitalia CE)

Tetrex *see* **Tetracycline.** Product now discontinued.

thenyldiamine *see* **Hayphryn**

Theo-Dur *see* **Lasma**
(Astra)

Theodrox *see* **Phyllocontin.** Product now discontinued.

theophylline *see* **Biophylline, Franol, lasma**

Thephorin
(Sinclair)

A white tablet supplied at a strength of 25 mg and used as an ANTIHISTAMINE to treat allergies.

Dose: 1-2 tablets 3 times a day before 4.00 in the afternoon.
Availability: NHS, private prescription, over the counter.
Side effects: dry mouth, stomach upset, rarely drowsiness.
Caution:
Not to be used for: children.
Caution needed with: sedatives, MAOIS, ANTICHOLINERGICS, alcohol.
Contains: PHENINDAMINE tartrate.

Other preparations:

Theraderm *see* **Acetoxyl.** Product now discontinued.

thiabendazole *see* **Mintezol**

thiamine *see* **Abidec, Allbee with C, Apisate, BC 500, BC 500 with Iron, Becosym, Benerva, Calcimax, Concavit, Fefol-Vit Spansule, Fesovit Spansule, Fesovit Z Spansule, Galfervit, Ketovite, Labiton, Lipaflavonoid, Lipotriad, Metatone, Multivite, nicotinamide, Octovit, Orovite, Orovite 7, Polyvite, Pregnavite Forte F, Surbex T, Tonivitan, Tonivitan B, Verdiviton, Villescon, vitamins capsules**

thiethylperazine maleate *see* **Torecan**

thioridazine *see* **Melleril**

thurfyl salicylate *see* **Transvasin,**

Thymoxamine Minims — drops used to treat pupil constriction. Product now discontinued.

thymoxamine hydrochloride *see* **Opilon, Thymoxamine**

tiaprofenic acid *see* **Surgam SA**

tibolone *see* **Livial**

Tiempe *see* **Monotrim**
(DDSA)

Tigason
(Roche)

A buff-coloured or a buff/orange capsule according to strengths of 10 mg, 25 mg and used as a vitamin A derivative to treat psoriasis, palmoplantar pustulosis, ichthyosis, Darier's disease (skin disorders).

Dose: 0.75 mg per kg body weight a day in divided doses at first up to a maximum of 75 mg a day according to response.
Availability: NHS (for hospital use only).
Side effects: dryness, erosion of mucous membranes, hair loss, liver poisoning, change in serum lipids, nausea, headache, sweating, anorexia, drowsiness, mood changes, blood changes, bone changes.
Caution: children should only undergo short-term treatment. Women of child-bearing age should take contraceptive precautions for at least 2 years after treatment ceases. Your doctor may advise regular tests and examinations.
Not to be used for: pregnant women or for patients suffering from liver or kidney disease.
Caution needed with: VITAMIN A, METHOTREXATE.
Contains: ETRETINATE.
Other preparations:

Tilade
(Fisons)

An aerosol supplied at a strength of 2 mg and used as a bronchial anti-inflammatory drug to treat blocked airway, bronchial asthma, asthmatic bronchitis, asthma.

Dose: 2 sprays twice a day up to a maximum of 2 sprays 4 times a day if needed.
Availability: NHS and private prescription.
Side effects: headache, nausea.
Caution: in pregnant women.
Not to be used for: children.
Caution needed with:
Contains: SODIUM NEDOCROMIL.
Other preparations:

Tildiem Retard
(Lorax)

A tablet supplied at strengths of 90 mg, 120 mg and used as a calcium antagonist to treat angina and high blood pressure.

Dose: 90-120 mg twice a day increasing as need to up to 480 mg day in divided doses; elderly 60 mg twice a day at first.
Availability: NHS and private prescription.
Side effects: nausea, headache, rash, slow heart rate, ankle swelling, heart conduction block.
Caution: your doctor may advise that the heart rate be measured regularly especially in the elderly and in patients suffering from kidney or liver problems.
Not to be used for: children, pregnant women or for patients suffering from slow heart rate or heart block.
Caution needed with: ß-BLOCKERS, DIGOXIN.
Contains: DILTIAZEM hydrochloride.
Other preparations: Tildiem, Tildiem LA, ADIZEM (Napp), ANGIOZEM (Ashbourne), BRITIAZEM (Thames).

Timodine
(Reckitt & Colman)

A cream used as a STEROID, disinfectant, antifungal treatment for skin disorders, nappy rash with thrush.

Dose: apply a small quantity to the affected area 3 times a day or when the nappy is changed.
Availability: NHS and private prescription.
Side effects: fluid retention, suppression of adrenal glands, thinning of the skin may occur.
Caution: use for short periods of time only.
Not to be used for: patients suffering from acne or any other skin infections caused by tuberculosis, ringworm, viruses, or fungi, or continuously especially in pregnant women.
Caution needed with:
Contains: NYSTATIN, HYDROCORTISONE, BENZALKONIUM CHLORIDE, DIMETHICONE.
Other preparations: NYSTAFORM-HC (Bayer).

timolol *see* Blocadren, Prestim, Timoptol

Timoped — antifungal cream. Product now discontinued.

Timoptol
(MSD)

Drops used as a ß-BLOCKER to treat hypertension of the eye, glaucomas.

Dose: 1 drop into the eye twice a day.
Availability: NHS and private prescription.
Side effects: eye irritation, systemic ß-BLOCKER effects (*see* Blocadren).
Caution: in pregnant women, nursing mothers. Treatment should be withdrawn gradually.
Not to be used for: children or patients suffering from asthma, heart conduction block, heart failure, or for patients who wear soft contact lenses.
Caution needed with: VERAPAMIL, ANTIHYPERTENSIVES, ADRENALINE.
Contains: TIMOLOL maleate.
Other preparations:

T

Tinaderm-M
(Schering-Plough)

A cream used as an antifungal treatment for skin and nail infections

Dose: apply to the affected area 2-3 times a day.
Availability: NHS and private prescription.
Side effects:
Caution:
Not to be used for:
Caution needed with:
Contains: TOLNAFTATE, NYSTATIN.
Other preparations:

Tineafax
(Wellcome)

An ointment used as an antifungal treatment for athlete's foot and similar skin infections.

Dose: apply to the affected area twice a day at first then once a day.
Availability: NHS, private prescription, over the counter.
Side effects:
Caution:

Not to be used for:
Caution needed with:
Contains: ZINC UNDECENOATE, ZINC NAPHTHENATE.
Other preparations: Tineafax Powder (for prevention only).

---

tinidazole *see* Fasigyn

Tinset
(Janssen)

A white, scored tablet supplied at a strength of 30 mg and used as an ANTIHISTAMINE treatment for allergies including rhinitis, urticaria.

Dose: adults 1-2 tablets twice a day; children over 5 years half adult dose.
Availability: NHS and private prescription.
Side effects: drowsiness, reduced reactions.
Caution:
Not to be used for: children under 5 years.
Caution needed with: sedatives, MAOIS, alcohol.
Contains: OXATOMIDE.
Other preparations:

---

tioconazole *see* Trosyl

Tisept
(Seton Healthcare)

A solution in a sachet used as a disinfectant for cleansing and disinfecting wounds and burns, changing dressings, obstetrics.

Dose: use neat as needed.
Availability: NHS, private prescription, over the counter.
Side effects:
Caution:
Not to be used for:
Caution needed with:
Contains: CHLORHEXIDINE GLUCONATE, CETRIMIDE.
Other preparations: SAVLON HOSPITAL CONCENTRATE (ICI).

Titralac
(3M Healthcare)

A white tablet used as a calcium supplement, and to regulate blood phosphate levels in patients with kidney failure.

Dose: to be adjusted for individuals.
Availability: NHS, private prescription, over the counter.
Side effects:
Caution: your doctor may advise regular blood and urine tests.
Not to be used for: patients with high blood phosphate levels or high blood/urine calcium levels.
Caution needed with: TETRACYCLINES, STEROIDS, CHOLECALCIFEROL, some DIURETICS, tablets coated to protect the stomach.
Contains: CALCIUM CARBONATE, GLYCINE.
Other preparations:

Tobralex
(Alcon)

Drops used as an aminoglycoside antibiotic treatment for eye infections.

Dose: 1-2 drops every 4 hours or up to 2 drops every hour in severe infections.
Availability: NHS and private prescription.
Side effects: temporary irritation.
Caution:
Not to be used for:
Caution needed with:
Contains: TOBRAMYCIN.
Other preparations:

---

tobramycin *see* **Tobralex**

---

tocainide *see* **Tonocard**

---

tocopheryl *see* **Ephynal, Ketovite, Octovit, Vita-E**

Tofranil
(Ciba-Geigy)

A red-brown, triangular tablet or red-brown, round tablet according to strengths of 10 mg, 25 mg and used as a tricyclic antidepressant to treat depression, night-time bed wetting in children

Dose: adults 25 mg up to 3 times a day, then increasing to 150-200 a day; elderly 10 mg at night at first increasing to 30-50 mg a day; children 6-7 years 25 mg, 8-11 years 25-50 mg, over 11 years 50-75 mg before going to bed, for 6-8 weeks then withdraw gradually.
Availability: NHS and private prescription.
Side effects: dry mouth, constipation, urine retention, blurred vision, palpitations, drowsiness, sleeplessness, dizziness, hands shaking, low blood presure, weight change, skin reactions, jaundice or blood changes. Loss of sexual desire may occur.
Caution: in nursing mothers or in patients suffering from heart disease, thyroid disease, epilepsy, diabetes, glaucoma, urine retention, some other psychiatric conditions. Your doctor may advise regular blood tests.
Not to be used for: children under 6 years, pregnant women, or for patients suffering from heart attacks, liver disease, heart block.
Caution needed with: alcohol, ANTICHOLINERGICS, ADRENALINE, MAOIS, BARBITURATES, other antidepressants, ANTIHYPERTENSIVES, CIMETIDINE, oestrogens.
Contains: IMIPRAMINE hydrochloride.
Other preparations: Tofranil Syrup.

Tolanase
(Upjohn)

A white, scored tablet supplied at strengths of 100 mg, 250 mg and used as an antidiabetic treatment for diabetes

Dose: 100-250 mg a day in divided doses to a maximum of 1 g a day.
Availability: NHS and private prescription.
Side effects: allergy including skin rash.
Caution: in the elderly and in patients suffering from kidney failure.
Not to be used for: children, pregnant women, nursing mothers, during surgery, or for patients suffering from juvenile diabetes, liver or kidney disorders, stress, infections.
Caution needed with: ß-BLOCKERS, MAOIS, STEROIDS, DIURETICS, alcohol, anticoagulants, lipid-lowering agents, ASPIRIN, some antibiotics (RIFAMPICIN, sulphonamides, CHLORAMPHENICOL), GLUCAGON, CYCLOPHOSPHAMIDE, the contraceptive pill.
Contains: TOLAZAMIDE.
Other preparations:

tolazamide *see* **Tolanase**

---

tolbutamide *see* **Rastinon**

Tolectin
(Cilag)

An orange/ivory capsule or orange capsule supplied at strengths of 200 mg, 400 mg and used as a NON-STEROID ANTI-INFLAMMATORY DRUG to treat rheumatoid arthritis, osteoarthritis, ankylosing spondylitis, other joint dsorders.

Dose: 600-800 mg a day in divided doses; children 20-25 mg/kg a day.
Availability: NHS and private prescription.
Side effects: stomach pain, fluid retention, rash.
Caution: in the elderly, pregnant women, nursing mothers, and in patients suffering from kidney, liver, or heart disease or a history of gastro-intestinal disease.
Not to be used for: patients suffering from stomach ulcer or allergy to ASPIRIN/NON-STEROID ANTI-INFLAMMATORY DRUGS.
Caution needed with:
Contains: TOLMETIN.
Other preparations:

Tolerzide
(Bristol-Myers Squibb)

A lilac tablet used as a ß-BLOCKER/THIAZIDE DIURETIC to treat high blood pressure.

Dose: 1 tablet a day.
Availability: NHS and private prescription.
Side effects: cold hands and feet, sleep disturbance, slow heart rate, tiredness, wheezing, heart failure, stomach upset, gout, sensitivity to light, blood changes, weakness, rash, dry eyes.
Caution: in pregnant women, nursing mothers, and in patients suffering from diabetes, gout, kidney or liver disorders, asthma. May need to be withdrawn before surgery. Withdraw gradually. Your doctor may advise additional treatment with DIURETICS or DIGOXIN.
Not to be used for: children, patients suffering from heart block or failure, kidney failure.
Caution needed with: VERAPAMIL, CLONIDINE withdrawal, some anti-

arrhythmic drugs and anaesthetics, RESERPINE, some ANTIHYPERTENSIVES, ERGOTAMINE, CIMETIDINE, sedatives, SYMPATHOMIMETICS, INDOMETHACIN, LITHIUM, DIGOXIN.
Contains: SOTALOL hydrochloride, HYDROCHLOROTHIAZIDE.
Other preparations: SOTAZIDE (Bristol-Myers Squibb).

---

tolmetin *see* **Tolectin**

---

tolnaftate *see* **Timoped, Tinaderm-M**

Tonivitan — multivitamin capsule. Product now discontinued.

Tonivitan A & D — multivitamin/mineral tonic. Product now discontinued.

Tonivitan B — vitamin B/mineral tonic. Product now discontinued.

Tonocard
(Astra)

A yellow tablet supplied at a strength of 400 mg and used as an anti-arrhythmic drug to treat abnormal heart rhythms.

Dose: 1.2 g a day in 2-3 divided doses to a maximum of 2.4 g a day..
Availability: NHS and private prescription.
Side effects: tremor, dizziness, stomach upset, white cell changes, SLE (a multisystem disorder).
Caution: in the elderly and pregnant women, and in patients suffering from severe liver or kidney disease or uncompensated heart failure.
Not to be used for: children or patients suffering from heart conduction block.
Caution needed with: other anti-arrhythmics.
Contains: TOCAINIDE hydrochloride.
Other preparations: Tonocard Injection — now discontinued.

Topal
(ICI)

A cream tablet used as an ANTACID to treat oesophagitis, heartburn, gastritis, dyspepsia, reflux oesophagitis.

Dose: adults 1-3 tablets 4 times a day after meals and at bedtime, children half adult dose.
Availability: NHS, private prescription, over the counter.
Side effects:
Caution:
Not to be used for: infants.
Caution needed with: TETRACYCLINE antibiotics, tablets which are coated to protect the stomach.
Contains: ALUMINIUM HYDROXIDE, MAGNESIUM CARBONATE, ALGINIC ACID.
Other preparations:

Topiclens — saline solution to wash wounds/eyes etc. Product now discontinued.

Topicycline
(Norwich Eaton)

A solution used as an antibiotic treatment for acne.

Dose: apply freely to the affected area twice a day.
Availability: NHS and private prescription.
Side effects: stinging or burning sensations.
Caution: in pregnant women, nursing mothers, and in patients suffering from kidney disease. Keep out of the eyes, nose, mouth, etc.
Not to be used for: children.
Caution needed with:
Contains: TETRACYCLINE hydrochloride.
Other preparations:

Topilar
(Bioglan)

A cream used as a STEROID treatment for skin disorders, psoriasis.

Dose: apply to the affected area twice a day.
Availability: NHS and private prescription.
Side effects: fluid retention, suppression of adrenal glands, thinning of the

skin may occur.

Caution: use for short periods of time only.

Not to be used for: patients suffering from acne or any other skin infections caused by tuberculosis, ringworm, viruses, or fungi, or continuously especially in pregnant women.

Caution needed with:

Contains: FLUCLOROLONE acetonide.

Other preparations: Topilar Ointment.

Toradol
(Syntex)

A white tablet supplied at a strength of 10 mg and used as a NON-STEROID ANTI-INFLAMMATORY drug to treat pain after surgery.

Dose: 1 tablet every 4-6 hours for up to 7 days, to a maximum of 4 tablets a day or more if transferred from injectable form of the drug. Elderly patients 1 every 6-8 hours.

Availability: NHS and private prescription.

Side effects: stomach upset, ulcers, bleeding, liver abnormalities, drowsiness, kidney failure, swelling.

Caution: in the elderly, and in patients suffering from gastro-intestinal disease, heart, kidney, or liver disease, or allergy.

Not to be used for: children under 16 years, pregnant women, nursing mothers, or for patients suffering from stomach ulcer, allergy to ASPIRIN or anti-inflammatory drugs, blood-clotting disorders, asthma, severe kidney disease.

Caution needed with: LITHIUM, NON-STEROID ANTI-INFLAMMATORY DRUGS, anticoagulants, METHOTHREXATE, PROBENECID, FRUSEMIDE.

Contains: KETEROLAC TROMETAMOL

Other preparations:

Torbetol
(Torbet Laboratories)

A lotion used as an antibacterial treatment for acne.

Dose: apply to the affected area 3 times a day.

Availability: NHS, private prescription, over the counter.

Side effects:

Caution:

Not to be used for:

Caution needed with:

Contains: CETRIMIDE, BENZALKONIUM CHLORIDE.
Other preparations:

Torecan
(Sandoz)

A white tablet supplied at a strength of 6.33 mg and used as an anti-emetic treatment for nausea, vomiting, vertigo.

Dose: 1 tablet 2-3 times a day.
Availability: NHS and private prescription.
Side effects: brain disturbances, ANTICHOLINERGIC symptoms, low blood pressure on standing, drowsiness, movement disorder, heart changes, allergies, rarely liver disturbance.
Caution: in pregnant women, nursing mothers and in patients suffering from liver or kidney disease, cardiovascular disease, bone marrow depression.
Not to be used for: children under 15 years, or for severely depressed or unconscious patients.
Caution needed with: sedatives, alcohol, ANALGESICS, ANTIHYPERTENSIVES, antidepressants, anticonvulsants, antidiabetics.
Contains: THIETHYLPERAZINE MALEATE.
Other preparations: Torecan Suppositories — now discontinued, Torecan Injection.

Totamol *see* Tenormin
(CP Pharm)

---

tramazoline *see* Dexa-Rhinaspray

Trancopal
(Sanofi Winthrop)

A yellow tablet supplied at a strength of 200 mg and used as a tranquillizer in the short-term treatment of sleeplessness, anxiety, and muscle spasm.

Dose: elderly 1 tablet at night or ½ tablet 4 times a day; adults 2 tablets at night or 1 tablet 4 times a day.
Availability: NHS and private prescription.
Side effects: nausea, dry mouth, headache, dizziness, lethargy, rash,

jaundice

Caution: in pregnant women and in patients suffering from kidney or liver disease. Patients should be warned of reduced judgement and abilities.
Not to be used for: children, or for patients suffering from porphyria (a rare blood disorder).
Caution needed with: MAOIS, alcohol, sedatives.
Contains: CHLORMEZANONE.
Other preparations:

Trancoprin — ANALGESIC/muscle relaxant. Product now discontinued.

Trandate
(Duncan, Flockhart)

An orange tablet supplied at strengths of 50 mg, 100 mg, 200 mg, 400 mg and used as an alpha- and ß-BLOCKER to treat angina with high blood pressure, high blood pressure of pregnancy.

Dose: 100 mg twice a day with food at first increasing as needed every 14 days to a maximum of 2.4 g a day in 3-4 divided doses; elderly 50 mg twice a day at first.
Availability: NHS and private prescription.
Side effects: cold hands and feet, sleep disturbance, slow heart rate, tiredness, wheezing, heart failure, stomach upset, dry eyes, skin rash.
Caution: in pregnant women, nursing mothers, and in patients suffering from diabetes, kidney or liver disorders, asthma. May need to be withdrawn before surgery. Withdraw gradually. Your doctor may advise additional treatment with DIURETICS or DIGOXIN.
Not to be used for: children or for patients suffering from heart block or failure.
Caution needed with: VERAPAMIL, CLONIDINE withdrawal, some anti-arrhythmic drugs and anaesthetics, RESERPINE, some ANTIHYPERTENSIVES, ERGOTAMINE, CIMETIDINE, sedatives, antidiabetics, SYMPATHOMIMETICS, INDOMETHACIN.
Contains: LABETALOL hydrochloride.
Other preparations: Trandate Injection, LABROCOL (Lagap).

---

tranexamic acid *see* **Cyklokapron**

Transiderm-Nitro
(Ciba)

Patches supplied at strengths of 5 mg, 10 mg and used as a NITRATE for the prevention of angina and vein inflammation.

Dose: for angina apply a patch to a hairless part of the chest every 24 hours on a different place each time (up to 2 patches may be needed). For other use as advised.
Availability: NHS, private prescription, over the counter.
Side effects: headache, rash, dizziness.
Caution: in patients suffering from heart failure or who have recently had a heart attack. The treatment should be reduced gradually and replaced with decreasing doses of an oral nitrate.
Not to be used for: children, or for patients suffering from low blood pressure, raised pressure in the brain, or heart muscle weakness.
Caution needed with:
Contains: GLYCERYL TRINITRATE.
Other preparations: CORO-NITRO (Boehringer Mannheim), DEPONIT (Schwarz), GLYTRIN (Sanofi Winthrop), NITRO-DUR (Schering-Plough), NITROCONTIN (Asta), NITROLINGUAL (Lipha), PERCUTOL (Cusi), SUSCARD BUCCAL (Pharmax), SUSTAC (Pharmax).

Transvasin
(Seton)

A cream used as an ANALGESIC rub for the relief of rheumatic and muscular pain, strains and sprains.

Dose: massage into the affected area at least twice a day.
Availability: NHS, private prescription, over the counter.
Side effects:
Caution:
Not to be used for:
Caution needed with:
Contains: THURFYL SALICYLATE, ETHYL NICOTINATE, N-HEXYL NICOTINATE, BENZOCAINE.
Other preparations:

Tranxene
(Boehringer Ingelheim)

A pink/grey capsule or a maroon/ grey capsule according to strengths of 15 mg, 7.5 mg and used as a sedative to treat anxiety and depression.

Dose: elderly 7.5 mg a day; adults over 16 years 7.5-22.5 mg a day.
Availability: private prescription only.
Side effects: drowsiness, confusion, unsteadiness, low blood pressure, rash, changes in vision, changes in libido, retention of urine. Risk of addiction increases with dose and length of treatment. May impair judgement.
Caution: in the elderly, pregnant women, nursing mothers, in women during labour, and in patients suffering from lung disorders, kidney or liver disorders. Avoid long-term use and withdraw gradually.
Not to be used for: children under 16 years, or for patients suffering from acute lung diseases, some chronic lung diseases, some obsessional and psychotic diseases.
Caution needed with: alcohol, other tranquillizers, anticonvulsants.
Contains: CLORAZEPATE potassium.
Other preparations:

---

tranylcypromine sulphate *see* Parnate, Parstelin

Trasicor
(Ciba)

A white tablet, a beige tablet, or an orange tablet according to strengths of 20 mg, 40 mg, 80 mg, 160 mg and used as a ß-BLOCKER to treat angina, abnormal heart rhythm, high blood pressure, anxiety.

Dose: for abnormal rhythm adults 20-40 mg 2-3 times a day at first; children 1 mg per kg of bodyweight a day. For angina 40-160 mg 3 times a day to a maximum of 480 mg a day. For high blood pressure 80 mg twice a day at first increasing to 480 mg a day. For anxiety 40-60 mg a day.
Availability: NHS and private prescription.
Side effects: cold hands and feet, sleep disturbance, slow heart rate, tiredness, wheezing, heart failure, stomach upset, dry eyes, skin rash.
Caution: in pregnant women, nursing mothers, and in patients suffering from diabetes, kidney or liver disorders, asthma. May need to be withdrawn before surgery. Withdraw gradually. Your doctor may advise additional treatment with DIURETICS or DIGOXIN.
Not to be used for: patients suffering from heart block or failure.
Caution needed with: VERAPAMIL, CLONIDINE withdrawal, some anti-arrhythmic drugs and anaesthetics, RESERPINE, some ANTIHYPERTENSIVES, ERGOTAMINE, CIMETIDINE, sedatives, antidiabetics, SYMPATHOMIMETICS, INDOMETHACIN.
Contains: OXPRENOLOL hydrochloride.

Other preparations: APSOLOX (APS).

Trasidrex
(Ciba)

A red, coated tablet used as a ß-BLOCKER/thiazide to treat high blood pressure.

Dose: 1 tablet every morning at first, increasing to 3 tablets a day if needed.
Availability: NHS and private prescription.
Side effects: cold hands and feet, sleep disturbance, slow heart rate, tiredness, wheezing, heart failure, stomach upset, dry eyes, skin rash, gout, sensitivity to light, blood changes, weakness.
Caution: in pregnant women, nursing mothers, and in patients suffering from diabetes, kidney or liver disorders, asthma, gout. May need to be withdrawn before surgery. Withdraw gradually. Your doctor may advise additional treatment with DIURETICS or DIGOXIN.
Not to be used for: children, or for patients suffering from heart block or failure, kidney failure.
Caution needed with: VERAPAMIL, CLONIDINE withdrawal, some anti-arrhythmic drugs and anaesthetics, RESERPINE, some ANTIHYPERTENSIVES, ERGOTAMINE, CIMETIDINE, sedatives, antidiabetics, LITHIUM, DIGOXIN, SYMPATHOMIMETICS, INDOMETHACIN.
Contains: OXPRENOLOL hydrochloride, PENTHIAZIDE (CO-PRENOZIDE).
Other preparations:

Travasept 100
(Baxter)

A solution used as an aminoglycocide antibiotic, antibacterial preparation for disinfecting wounds and burns.

Dose: use neat as needed.
Availability: NHS, private prescription, over the counter.
Side effects:
Caution:
Not to be used for:
Caution needed with:
Contains: CHLORHEXIDINE ACETATE, CETRIMIDE.
Other preparations: SAVLON HOSPITAL CONCENTRATE (ICI).

Travogyn
(Schering)

A white, almond-shaped vaginal tablet supplied at a strength of 300 mg and used as an antifungal treatment for thrush or other infections of the vagina.

Dose: 2 tablets inserted together into the vagina as a single dose.
Availability: NHS, private prescription, over the counter.
Side effects: irritation and burning.
Caution:
Not to be used for: children.
Caution needed with:
Contains: ISOCONAZOLE nitrate.
Other preparations: Travogyn Cream — now discontinued.

Traxam
(Lederle)

A clear gel used as a topical NON-STEROID ANTI-INFLAMATORY rub to treat soft tissue injury such as strains, sprains, contusions.

Dose: massage gently into the affected area 2-4 times a day for up to 14 days up to a maximum of 25 g a day.
Availability: NHS and private prescription.
Side effects: mild local redness, dermatitis, itch.
Caution: in pregnant women and nursing mothers. Use only on unbroken skin and keep out of the eyes, nose, mouth etc. It should not be used with covering dressings.
Not to be used for: children or for patients suffering from allergy to ASPIRIN/anti-inflammatory drugs.
Caution needed with:
Contains: FELBINAC.
Other preparations: Traxam Foam.

---

trazodone *see* **Molipaxin**

Tremonil
(Sandoz)

A white, scored tablet supplied at a strength of 5 mg and used as an ANTICHOLINERGIC treatment for Parkinson's disease and senile tremor.

Dose: adults ½ tablet 3 times a day at first increasing gradually to 3-12 tablets a day in divided doses; elderly usually 3-6 tablets a day.
Availability: NHS and private prescription.
Side effects: ANTICHOLINERGIC effects, confusion at high doses, nausea, fatigue, stomach pain.
Caution: in patients with marked disease of the autonomic nervous system. Dose should be reduced slowly.
Not to be used for: children or for patients suffering from enlarged prostate, glaucoma, abnormal heart rhythm, intestinal slowness, tardive dyskinesia (a movement disorder), myasthenia gravis, urine retention.
Caution needed with: ANTIHISTAMINES, antidepressants, ANALGESICS, alcohol, ANTICHOLINERGICS, some sedatives.
Contains: METHIXENE hydrochloride.
Other preparations:

Trental
(Hoechst)

A pink, oblong tablet supplied at a strength of 400 mg and used as a blood cell altering drug to treat peripheral vascular problems.

Dose: 1 tablet 2-3 times a day.
Availability: NHS and private prescription.
Side effects: stomach disturbances, vertigo, flushes.
Caution: in patients suffering from low blood pressure, severe heart artery disease, kidney disease.
Not to be used for: children.
Caution needed with: ANTIHYPERTENSIVES.
Contains: OXPENTIFYLLINE.
Other preparations:

---

tretinoin *see* Retin-A

Tri-Adcortyl
(Princeton)

A cream used as an antifungal, antibacterial, STEROID treatment for skin disorders where there is also inflammation, infection, or thrush.

Dose: apply to the affected area 2-4 times a day.
Availability: NHS and private prescription.
Side effects: fluid retention, suppression of adrenal glands, thinning of the

skin may occur.
Caution: use for short periods of time only
Not to be used for: patients suffering from acne or any other skin infections caused by tuberculosis, ringworm, viruses, or fungi, or continuously especially in pregnant women.
Caution needed with:
Contains: TRIAMCINOLONE acetonide, NYSTATIN, NEOMYCIN, GRAMICIDIN.
Other preparations: Tri-Adcortyl Ointment.

Tri-Adcortyl Otic
(Princeton)

An ointment with an aural applicator used as an antibiotic, antifungal, STEROID treatment for inflammation of the external ear.

Dose: apply the ointment into the ear 2-4 times a day.
Availability: NHS and private prescription.
Side effects: additional infection.
Caution: in infants, pregnant women, and in patients suffering from perforated ear drum — avoid using over extended periods.
Not to be used for: patients suffering from tubercular or viral wounds.
Caution needed with:
Contains: TRIAMCINOLONE acetonide, NEOMYCIN sulphate, GRAMICIDIN, NYSTATIN.
Other preparations:

Tri-Cicatrin
(Wellcome)

An ointment used as a STEROID, antibacterial, antifungal treatment for skin disorders where there is also inflammation, infection, or thrush.

Dose: apply a small quantity to the affected area 1-3 times a day.
Availability: NHS and private prescription.
Side effects: fluid retention, suppression of adrenal glands, thinning of the skin may occur.
Caution: use for short periods of time only.
Not to be used for: patients suffering from acne or any other skin infections caused by tuberculosis, ringworm, viruses, or fungi, or continuously especially in pregnant women.
Caution needed with:
Contains: HYDROCORTISONE, NEOMYCIN, ZINC BACITRACIN, NYSTATIN.
Other preparations:

Tri-Minulet
(Wyeth)

Beige, brown, and white tablets used as an oestrogen, progestogen contraceptive.

Dose: 1 tablet a day, starting on day 1 of menstruation, for 21 days, then 7 days without tablets.
Availability: NHS and private prescription.
Side effects: enlarged breasts, bloating and fluid retention, cramps, leg pains, mood change, reduction in sexual desire, headaches, nausea, vaginal erosion, discharge and bleeding, weight gain, skin changes.
Caution: in patients suffering from high blood pressure, diabetes, vascular disorders, asthma, depression, kidney disease, multiple sclerosis, womb diseases. Your doctor may advise you not to smoke, to have regular examinations. You should stop treatment at the first sign of serious symptoms such as severe headache or jaundice. Treatment should be stopped before surgery.
Not to be used for: pregnant women, or for patients suffering from sickle-cell anaemia, history of heart disease or thrombosis, liver disorders, some cancers, undiagnosed vaginal bleeding, some ear, skin and kidney disorders.
Caution needed with: RIFAMPICIN, TETRACYCLINES, GRISEOFULVIN, BARBITURATES, PHENYTOIN, PRIMIDONE, CARBAMAZEPINEM, ETHOSUXIMIDE, CHLORAL HYDRATE, DICHLORALPHENAZONE.
Contains: ETHINYLOESTRADIOL, GESTODENE.
Other preparations:

---

tri-potassium dicitrato bismuthate *see* **De-Nol**

Triadene *see* **Tri-minulet**
(Schering)

Triamaxco *see* **Dyazide**
(Ashbourne)

---

triamcinolone acetonide *see* **Adcortyl, Adcortyl in Orabase, Audicort, Aurecort, Ledercort, Ledercort Cream, Nystadermal, Tri-Adcortyl, Tri-Adcortyl Otic**

Triamco *see* **Dyazide**
(Baker Norton)

---

triamterene *see* **Dyazide, Dytac, Dytide, Frusene, Kalspare**

---

triazolam *see* **Halcion.** Product now discontinued.

Tribiotic
(3M Healthcare)

An aerosol used as an aminoglycoside antibiotic, antibacterial preparation to prevent and treat infection in surgery.

Dose: apply sparingly up to 1 aerosol per day for up to 7 days.
Availability: NHS and private prescription.
Side effects: ear and kidney damage, sensitization.
Caution: in pregnant women, nursing mothers, and in patients with large areas of affected skin, or hearing loss.
Not to be used for: treating burns.
Caution needed with: other similar antibiotics
Contains: NEOMYCIN sulphate, BACITRACIN zinc, POLYMYXIN B SULPHATE.
Other preparations: POLYBACTRIN (Wellcome).

---

triclosan *see* **Aquasept, Manusept, Ster-Zac Bath Concentrate, Timoped, Triclosept**

Triclosept — disinfectant solution. Product now discontinued.

---

tricyclic antidepressant

a drug used to treat depression but which may cause sedation and dryness of the mouth. Example AMITRYPTILINE *see* Tryptizol.

Tridesilon — STEROID treatment cream. Product now discontinued.

---

trifluoperazine *see* **Parstelin, Stelazine**

---

trifluperidol *see* **Triperidol**

Trifyba
(Sanofi Winthrop)

A powder used as a bulking agent to treat constipation, diverticular disease, irritable colon, haemorrhoids, and fissures.

Dose: adults, 1 sachet 2-3 times a day; children ½-1 sachet once or twice a day.
Availability: NHS, private prescription, over the counter.
Side effects:
Caution: adequate fluids must be taken.
Not to be used for: patients suffering from blocked intestine.
Caution needed with:
Contains: concentrated extract of WHEAT HUSK.
Other preparations:

Trilisate
(Napp)

An orange, oblong, scored tablet supplied at a strength of 500 mg and used as a salicylate to treat rheumatoid arthritis, osteoarthritis.

Dose: 2-3 tablets twice a day.
Availability: NHS, private prescription, over the counter.
Side effects: stomach upsets, allergy, asthma.
Caution: in pregnant women, the elderly, or in patients with a history of allergy to aspirin, asthma, impaired kidney or liver function, indigestion.
Not to be used for: children, nursing mothers, or patients suffering from haemophilia, or ulcers.
Caution needed with: anticoagulants, some antidiabetic drugs, anti-inflammatory agents, METHOTREXATE, SPIRONOLACTONE, STEROIDS, some uric acid-lowering drugs.
Contains: CHOLINE MAGNESIUM TRISALICYLATE.
Other preparations:

---

trilostane *see* **Modrenal**

Triludan
(Merion Merrell Dow)

A white, scored tablet supplied at a strength of 60 mg and used as an ANTIHISTAMINE treatment for allergies including hay fever and rhinitis.

Dose: adults 1 tablet twice a day or 2 tablets once a day; children 6-12 years ½ tablet twice a day, 3-6 years use suspension.
Availability: NHS, private prescription, over the counter.
Side effects: rash, sweating, headache, mild stomach disturbances, rapid heart beat.
Caution: in patients suffering from liver disease or some heart irregularities.
Not to be used for: children under 3 years.
Caution needed with: KETOCONAZOLE, ERYTHROMYCIN, ITRACONAZOLE.
Contains: TERFENADINE.
Other preparations: Triludan Forte, Triludan Suspension.

---

trimeprazine *see* Vallergan

---

trimethoprim *see* Monotrim, Polytrim, Septrin, Syraprim, Trimopan

---

trimipramine maleate *see* Surmontil

Trimogal *see* Monotrim
(Lagap)

Trimopan
(Berk)

A white, scored tablet supplied at strengths of 100 mg, 200 mg and used as an antibiotic treatment for infections.

Dose: adults 200 mg twice a day; children use suspension.
Availability: NHS and private prescription.
Side effects: stomach disturbances, skin reactions, folate (vitamin) deficiency.
Caution: in the elderly, nursing mothers, and in patients suffering from

kidney disease or folate deficiency. Your doctor may advise that patients undergoing prolonged treatment should have regular blood tests.

Not to be used for: infants under 4 months, pregnant women, or for patients suffering from severe kidney disease where blood tests cannot be carried out regularly.

Caution needed with:

Contains: TRIMETHOPRIM.

Other preparations: Trimopan Suspension, MONOTRIM (Duphar), TIEMPE (DDSA), TRIMOGAL (Lagap).

Trimovate
(Glaxo)

A cream used as an antibiotic, antifungal, STEROID treatment in skin disorders in moist or covered places where there is also thrush or infection.

Dose: apply to the affected area 1-4 times a day.

Availability: NHS and private prescription.

Side effects: fluid retention, suppression of adrenal glands, thinning of the skin may occur.

Caution: use for short periods of time only.

Not to be used for: patients suffering from acne or any other skin infections caused by tuberculosis, ringworm, viruses, or fungi, or continuously especially in pregnant women.

Caution needed with:

Contains: CLOBETASONE BUTYRATE, NYSTATIN, CALCIUM OXYTETRACYCLINE.

Other preparations: Trimovate Ointment — now discontinued.

Trinordiol
(Wyeth)

Brown, white, and ochre tablets used as an oestrogen, progestogen contraceptive.

Dose: 1 tablet a day for 21 days starting on day 1 of the period.

Availability: NHS and private prescription.

Side effects: enlarged breasts, bloating and fluid retention, cramps, leg pains, mood change, reduction in sexual desire, headaches, nausea, vaginal erosion, discharge, and bleeding, weight gain, skin changes.

Caution: in patients suffering from high blood pressure, diabetes, vascular disorders, asthma, depression, kidney disease, multiple sclerosis, womb diseases. Your doctor may advise you not to smoke, to have regular examinations. You should stop treatment at the first sign of serious symptoms such as severe headache or jaundice. Treatment should be stopped before surgery.

Not to be used for: pregnant women, or for patients suffering from sickle-cell anaemia, history of heart disease or thrombosis, liver disorders, some cancers, undiagnosed vaginal bleeding, some ear, skin, and kidney disorders.

Caution needed with: RIFAMPICIN, TETRACYCLINES, GRISEOFULVIN, BARBITURATES, PHENYTOIN, PRIMIDONE, CARBAMAZEPINE, ETHOSUXIMIDE, CHLORAL HYDRATE, DICHLORALPHENAZONE.

Contains: ETHINYLOESTRADIOL, LEVONORGESTREL.

Other preparations: LOGYNON (Schering).

Trinovum
(Cilag)

White tablets, pale peach tablets, and peach-coloured tablets used as an oestrogen, progestogen contraceptive.

Dose: 1 tablet a day for 21 days starting on day 1 of the period.

Availability: NHS and private prescription.

Side effects: enlarged breasts, bloating and fluid retention, cramps, leg pains, mood change, reduction in sexual desire, headaches, nausea, vaginal erosion, discharge, and bleeding, weight gain, skin changes.

Caution: in patients suffering from high blood pressure, diabetes, vascular disorders, asthma, depression, kidney disease, multiple sclerosis, womb diseases. Your doctor may advise you not to smoke, to have regular examinations. You should stop treatment at the first sign of serious symptoms such as severe headache or jaundice. Treatment should be stopped before surgery.

Not to be used for: pregnant women, or for patients suffering from sickle-cell anaemia, history of heart disease or thrombosis, liver disorders, some cancers, undiagnosed vaginal bleeding, some ear, skin, and kidney disorders.

Caution needed with: RIFAMPICIN, TETRACYCLINES, GRISEOFULVIN, BARBITURATES, PHENYTOIN, PRIMIDONE, CARBAMAZEPINE, ETHOSUXIMIDE, CHLORAL HYDRATE, DICHLORALPHENAZONE.

Contains: ETHINYLOESTRADIOL, LEVONORGESTREL.

Other preparations:

Trinovum-ED
(Cilag)

White, light-peach, peach, and green tablets used as an oestrogen, progestogen contraceptive.

Dose: 1 tablet a day starting on day 1 of menstruation.
Availability: NHS and private prescription.
Side effects: enlarged breasts, bloating and fluid retention, cramps, leg pains, mood change, reduction in sexual desire, headaches, nausea, vaginal erosion, discharge and bleeding, weight gain, skin changes.
Caution: in patients suffering from high blood pressure, diabetes, vascular disorders, asthma, depression, kidney disease, multiple sclerosis, womb diseases. You should stop treatment at the first sign of serious symptoms such as severe headache or jaundice. Treatment should be stopped before surgery.
Not to be used for: pregnant women or for patients suffering from sickle-cell anaemia, history of heart disease or thrombosis, liver disorders, some cancers, undiagnosed vaginal bleeding, some ear, skin and kidney disorders.
Caution needed with: RIFAMPICIN, TETRACYCLINES, GRISEOFULVIN, BARBITURATES, PHENYTOIN, PRIMIDONE, CARBAMAZEPINEM, ETHOSUXIMIDE, CHLORAL HYDRATE, DICHLORALPHENAZONE.
Contains: ETHINYLOESTRADIOL, NORETHISTERONE, LACTOSE.
Other preparations:

Triperidol
(Lagap)

A tablet supplied at strengths of 0.5 mg, 1 mg and used as a sedative to treat manic agitation.

Dose: adults up to 8 mg a day; children 5-12 years up to 2 mg a day.
Availability: NHS and private prescription.
Side effects: muscle spasms, restlessness, hands shaking, constipation, blurred vision, dry mouth, urine retention, palpitations, low blood pressure, weight gain, changes in libido, low body temperature, breast swelling, menstrual changes, jaundice, blood and skin changes, drowsiness, rarely fits.
Caution: in pregnant women, nursing mothers and in patients suffering from severe liver disease, pyramidal or extrapyramidal symptoms (tremor and rigidity).
Not to be used for: patients suffering from severe clinical depression.
Caution needed with: alcohol, tranquillizers, pain killers, ANTIHYPERTENSIVES, antidepressants, anticonvulsants, antidiabetic drugs, LEVODOPA.
Contains: TRIFLUPERIDOL.

Other preparations:

---

triprolidine hydrochloride *see* **Actidil, Actifed Compound, Pro-Actidil, Sudafed Plus**

Triptafen
(Evans)

A pink tablet used as a TRICYCLIC antidepressant to treat depression with anxiety.

Dose: 1 tablet 3 times a day with 1 tablet at bed time if needed.
Availability: NHS and private prescription.
Side effects: dry mouth, constipation, urine retention, blurred vision, palpitations, drowsiness, sleeplessness, dizziness, hands shaking, low blood presure, weight change, skin reactions, jaundice or blood changes. Loss of sexual desire may occur.
Caution: in nursing mothers and in patients suffering from Parkinson's disease, heart or liver disease, thyroid disorder, adrenal tumour, diabetes, glaucoma, urine retention, epilepsy.
Not to be used for: children or for patients suffering from bone marrow depression, heart attack, heart block, severe liver disease.
Caution needed with: alcohol, ANTICHOLINERGICS, ADRENALINE, MAOIS, BARBITURATES, other antidepressants, ANTIHYPERTENSIVES, CIMETIDINE, oestrogens.
Contains: AMITRYPTILINE hydrochloride, PERPHENAZINE.
Other preparations: Triptafen-M.

Trisequens
(Novo-Nordisk)

Twelve blue tablets, 10 white tablets, and 6 red tablets used as a oestrogen, progestogen treatment for menopausal symptoms, and to prevent bone thinning after the menopause.

Dose: 1 tablet a day starting on the fifth day of the period if present, beginning with the blue tablets and continuing in sequence without a break.
Availability: NHS and private prescription.
Side effects: enlarged breasts, bloating and fluid retention, cramps, leg pains, mood change, reduction in sexual desire, headaches, nausea, vaginal erosion, discharge, and bleeding, weight gain, skin changes.
Caution: in patients suffering from high blood pressure, diabetes, vascular

disorders, asthma, depression, kidney disease, multiple sclerosis, womb diseases. Your doctor may advise you not to smoke, to have regular examinations. You should stop treatment at the first sign of serious symptoms such as severe headache or jaundice. Treatment should be stopped before surgery.

Not to be used for: children, pregnant women, or for patients suffering from sickle-cell anaemia, history of heart disease or thrombosis, liver disorders, some cancers, undiagnosed vaginal bleeding, some ear, skin, and kidney disorders.

Caution needed with: DIURETICS, ANTIHYPERTENSIVES, and drugs that change liver enzymes, RIFAMPICIN, TETRACYCLINES, GRISEOFULVIN, BARBITURATES, PHENYTOIN, PRIMIDONE, CARBAMAZEPINE, ETHOSUXIMIDE, CHLORAL HYDRATE, DICHLORALPHENAZONE.

Contains: OESTRADIOL, OESTRIOL, NORETHISTERONE acetate.

Other preparations: Trisequens Forte.

Tritace
(Hoechst)

A yellow/white capsule, orange/white capsule or crimson/white capsule according to strengths 1.25 mg, 2.5 mg and 5 mg, and used as an ACE INHIBITOR to treat high blood pressure.

Dose: initially 1.25 mg a day, increasing to a maximum of 10 mg a day. Stop any DIURETIC 2-3 days before starting treatment.

Availability: NHS and private prescription.

Side effects: nausea, vomiting, tiredness, headache, abdominal pain, low blood pressure, diarrhoea, cough, severe allergy, fainting, kidney damage.

Caution: in patients suffering from congestive heart failure, liver or kidney damage.

Not to be used for: children, pregnant women, nursing mothers, or for patients suffering from heart abnormalities, or with a history of severe allergy.

Caution needed with: ANTIHYPERTENSIVES, some DIURETICS, LITHIUM, potassium supplements.

Contains: RAMIPRIL.

Other preparations:

Tropicamide Minims
(SNP)

Drops used as an ANTICHOLINERGIC, short-acting pupil dilator.

Dose: 2 drops with 5 minutes between each drop, then 1-2 drops 30 minutes later if needed.
Availability: NHS and private prescription.
Side effects: temporary smarting.
Caution: care in infants.
Not to be used for: for patients suffering from narrow angle glaucoma.
Caution needed with:
Contains: TROPICAMIDE.
Other preparations:

---

tropicamide *see* Mydriacyl, Tropicamide

Tropium *see* Librium
(DDSA)

Trosyl
(Novex Pharma)

A solution used as an antifungal treatment for infections of the nails.

Dose: apply to the affected areas every 12 hours for 6-12 months.
Availability: NHS and private prescription.
Side effects: mild irritation.
Caution:
Not to be used for: pregnant women.
Caution needed with:
Contains: TIOCONAZOLE.
Other preparations: Trosyl Cream (also available over the counter).

---

trypsin *see* Chymoral Forte

Tryptizol
(Morson)

A blue tablet, yellow tablet, or brown tablet according to strengths of 10 mg, 25 mg, 50 mg and used as a TRICYCLIC antidepressant to treat depression, bed wetting in children.

Dose: adults 75 mg a day in divided doses, increasing if needed to 150 mg a day; children 6-10 years 10-20 mg a day; 11-16 years 25-50 mg a day.

Availability: NHS and private prescription.

Side effects: dry mouth, constipation, urine retention, blurred vision, palpitations, drowsiness, sleeplessness, dizziness, hands shaking, low blood presure, weight change, skin reactions, jaundice or blood changes. Loss of sexual desire may occur.

Caution: in nursing mothers or in patients suffering from heart disease, thyroid disease, epilepsy, diabetes, urine retention, adrenal tumour, glaucoma, some other psychiatric conditions. Your doctor may advise regular blood tests.

Not to be used for: children under 6 years, pregnant women, or for patients suffering from heart attacks, liver disease, heart block.

Caution needed with: alcohol, ANTICHOLINERGICs, ADRENALINE, MAOIS, BARBITURATES, other antidepressants, ANTIHYPERTENSIVES CIMETIDINE, oestrogens.

Contains: AMITRIPTYLINE hydrochloride.

Other preparations: Tryptizol Capsules, Tryptizol Syrup, Tryptizol Injection, DOMICAL (Berk), ELAVIL (DDSA), LENTIZOL (Parke-Davis).

T

---

tryptophan *see* **Optimax, Pacitron**

Tuinal
(Eli LIlly)

An orange/blue capsule used as a BARBITURATE to treat sleeplessness in patients with barbiturate habit.

Dose: 1-2 tablets before going to bed.

Availability: controlled drug; NHS and private prescription.

Side effects: drowsiness, hangover, dizziness, allergies, headache, confusion, excitement, unsteadiness, breathing difficulty.

Caution: in patients suffering from kidney, liver, or lung disease. Dependence (addiction) may develop.

Not to be used for: children, young adults, pregnant women, nursing mothers, the elderly, patients with a history of drug or alcohol abuse, or suffering from porphyria (a rare blood disorder), or in the management of pain.

Caution needed with: anticoagulants, alcohol, other tranquillizers, STEROIDS, the contraceptive pill, GRISEOFULVIN, RIFAMPICIN, PHENYTOIN, METRONIDAZOLE, CHLORAMPHENICOL.

Contains: QUINALBARBITONE sodium, AMYLOBARBITONE sodium.

Other preparations:

---

tulobuterol *see* **Brelomax, Respacal**

Tylex
(Cilag)

A red/white capsule used as an ANALGESIC to relieve severe pain.

Dose: 1-2 tablets every 4 hours to a maximum of 8 tablets in 24 hours.
Availability: NHS and private prescription.
Side effects: tolerance, addiction, constipation, dizziness, sedation, nausea, dry mouth, blurred vision.
Caution: in the elderly, women in labour, and in patients suffering from underactive thyroid, or kidney or liver disease.
Not to be used for: children, pregnant women, nursing mothers, or for patients suffering from breathing difficulty or blocked airways.
Caution needed with: MAOIS, sedatives, other medicines containg PARA-CETAMOL.
Contains: PARACETAMOL, CODEINE PHOSPHATE.
Other preparations:

---

tyrothricin *see* **Tyrozets**

Tyrozets
(MSD)

A pink lozenge used as an antibiotic and local anaesthetic to treat mild mouth and throat disorders.

Dose: allow 1 lozenge to dissolve in the mouth every 3 hours to a maxi-mum of 8 lozenges in 24 hours.
Availability: NHS, private prescription, over the counter.
Side effects: additional infection, blackening or soreness of mouth and tongue.
Caution:
Not to be used for:
Caution needed with:
Contains: TYROTHRICIN, BENZOCAINE.
Other preparations:

Ubretid Tablets
(Rhone-Poulenc Rorer)

A white, scored tablet supplied at a strength of 5 mg and used as an ANTICHOLINESTERASE to treat myasthenia gravis, post-operative bladder or intestine problems.

Dose: adults myasthenia gravis 1 tablet a day ½ hour before breakfast at first adjusting every 3-4 days up to 4 tablets a day; children up to 2 tablets a day. Otherwise 1 tablet a day or alternate days.
Availability: NHS and private prescription.
Side effects: nausea, vomiting, colic, diarrhoea, salivation.
Caution: in patients suffering from bronchial asthma, heart disease, stomach ulcer, epilepsy, Parkinson's disease.
Not to be used for: pregnant women, or for patients suffering from bowel or urinary blockage, or with weak circulation or in shock after surgery.
Caution needed with: some medicines used during anaesthesia.
Contains: DISTIGMINE bromide.
Other preparations: Ubretid Injection.

Ucerax *see* Atarax
(UCB Pharma)

Ultrabase *see* Diprobase
(Schering Healthcare)

Ultradil Plain Cream
(Schering)

A cream used as a STEROID treatment for skin disorders, eczema.

Dose: apply to the affected area 3 times a day at first, then reduce as soon as possible to once a day.
Availability: NHS and private prescription.
Side effects: fluid retention, suppression of adrenal glands, thinning of the skin may occur.
Caution: use for short periods of time only.
Not to be used for: patients suffering from acne or any other skin infections caused by tuberculosis, ringworm, viruses, or fungi, or continuously especially in pregnant women.
Caution needed with:
Contains: FLUOCORTOLONE PIVALATE, FLUOCORTOLONE HEXANOATE.

Other preparations: Ultradil Plain Ointment.

Ultralanum Plain Cream
(Schering)

A cream used as a STEROID treatment for skin disorders.

Dose: apply to the affected area 2-3 times a day at first reducing to once a day as soon as possible.
Availability: NHS and private prescription.
Side effects: fluid retention, suppression of adrenal glands, thinning of the skin may occur.
Caution: use for short periods of time only.
Not to be used for: patients suffering from acne or any other skin infections caused by tuberculosis, ringworm, viruses, or fungi, or continuously especially in pregnant women.
Caution needed with:
Contains: FLUOCORTOLONE PIVALATE, FLUOCORTOLONE HEXANOATE.
Other preparations: Ultralanum Plain Ointment.

Ultraproct
(Schering)

A suppository supplied at a strength of 1 mg and used as a STEROID, local anaesthetic, ANTIHISTAMINE treatment for haemorrhoids, anal fissure, proctitis, anal itch.

Dose: 1 suppository 1-3 times a day after passing motions.
Availability: NHS and private prescription.
Side effects: systemic corticosteroid effects (*see* Precortisyl).
Caution: do not use for prolonged periods; care in pregnant women.
Not to be used for: children, or for patients suffering from tuberculous, fungal, or viral infections.
Caution needed with:
Contains: FLUOCORTOLONE PIVALATE, FLUOCORTOLONE HEXANOATE, CINCHOCAINE HYDROCHLORIDE,
Other preparations: Ultraproct ointment.

Ultratard *see* insulin
(Novo Nordisk)

Unasyn
(Pfizer)

A white capsule-shaped tablet supplied at a strength of 375 mg, and used as an antibiotic to treat respiratory, urinary tract, skin, and soft tissue infections, kidney infection or venereal disease.

Dose: adults and children over 30 kg, 1-2 tablets twice a day for 5-14 days. For venereal disease, as directed by the doctor.
Availability: NHS and private prescription.
Side effects: stomach upset, rash, itching, drowsiness, tiredness, headache.
Caution: in pregnant women, nursing mothers, and in patients suffering from glandular fever or severe kidney damage.
Not to be used for: children under 30 kg body weight.
Caution needed with: ALLOPURINOL.
Contains: SULTAMICILLIN
Other preparations: Unasyn Injection.

---

undecenoic acid *see* Audicort, Ceanel

Unguentum Merck
(Merck)

A cream used as an emollient to treat dermatitis, nappy rash, and dry, scaly skin.

Dose: apply thinly 3 times a day or as required.
Availability: NHS, private prescription, over the counter.
Side effects:
Caution:
Not to be used for:
Caution needed with:
Contains: SILICIC ACID, LIQUID PARAFFIN, WHITE SOFT PARAFFIN, CETOSTEARYL ALCOHOL, POLYSORBATE-40, GLYCEROL MONOSTEARATE, saturated neutral oil, SORBIC ACID, PROPYLENE GLYCOL.
Other preparations:

Unicap M
(Upjohn)

A yellow tablet used as an iron and vitamin supplement.

Dose: 1 tablet a day.
Availability: NHS, private prescription, over the counter.
Side effects: stomach upset.
Caution:
Not to be used for:
Caution needed with: TETRACYCLINES, ANTACIDS, LEVODOPA, PENICILLAMINE.
Contains: FERROUS FUMARATE, VITAMIN A, VITAMIN B group, VITAMIN C, VITAMIN D, minerals.
Other preparations: UNICAP T.

Unicap T
(Upjohn)

A yellow tablet used as an iron and vitamin supplement in cases of vitamin deficiency, severe chronic disease, food absorption disorders, etc.

Dose: 1 tablet a day.
Availability: NHS, private prescription, over the counter.
Side effects: stomach upset.
Caution:
Not to be used for:
Caution needed with: TETRACYCLINES, ANTACIDS, LEVODOPA, PENICILLAMINE.
Contains: FERROUS FUMARATE, VITAMIN A, VITAMIN B group, VITAMIN C, VITAMIN D, minerals.
Other preparations: UNICAP M.

Uniflu & Gregovite C
(Unigreg)

A red, oblong tablet and a yellow tablet used as an ANALGESIC, opiate, cough suppressant, xanthine, and ANTIHISTAMINE treatment for cold and flu symptoms.

Dose: 1 each of the tablets every 4 hours up to a maximum of 4 of each tablets in 24 hours.
Availability: private prescription and over the counter.
Side effects: constipation, drowsiness, reduced reactions, anxiety, hands shaking, irregular or rapid heart rate, dry mouth, excitement, rarely skin eruptions.
Caution: in patients suffering from asthma, kidney disease, diabetes.
Not to be used for: children, or for patients suffering from liver disease, heart or thyroid disorders.
Caution needed with: MAOIS, alcohol, sedatives, TRICYCLICS, other medi-

cines containing PARACETAMOL.
Contains: PARACETAMOL, CODEINE PHOSPHATE, CAFFEINE, DIPHENHYDRAMINE HYDROCHLORIDE, PHENYLEPHRINE HYDROCHLORIDE; ASCORBIC ACID.
Other preparations:

Unigest *see* Asilone
(Unigreg)

Unimycin *see* Tetracycline
(Unigreg)

Uniphyllin Continus *see* Lasma
(Napp)

Uniroid-HC
(Unigreg)

An ointment used as a STEROID and local anaeesthetic treatment for pain, irritation, and itching associated with haemorrhoids and other itchy anal conditions.

Dose: apply a small amount 3 times a day and after each bowel movement, for a maximum of 7 days.
Availability: NHS and private prescription.
Side effects: allergy, systemic corticosteroid effects (*see* Precortisyl).
Caution:
Not to be used for: children under 12 years, pregnant women, nursing mothers, or for patients suffering from tuberculous, fungal, or viral infections, or allergy to any ingredient.
Caution needed with:
Contains: HYDROCORTISONE, CINCHOCAINE HYDROCHLORIDE.
Other preparations: Uniroid — now discontinued, Uniroid-HC Suppositories.

Unisept
(Seton-Healthcare)

A solution used as a disinfectant and general antiseptic.

Dose: use neat as needed.
Availability: NHS, private prescription, over the counter.
Side effects:
Caution:
Not to be used for:
Caution needed with:
Contains: CHLORHEXIDINE gluconate.
Other preparations: HIBISCRUB (ICI), HIBISOL (ICI), PHISOMED (Sterling).

Unisomnia *see* **Mogadon**
(Unigreg)

Univer *see* **Cordilox**
(Rhone-Poulenc Rorer)

Urantoin *see* **Furadantin**
(DDSA)

---

urea hydrogen peroxide *see* **Exterol**

---

urea *see* **Alphaderm, Calmurid HC, Psoradrate, Sential**

Uriben *see* **Negram**
(RP Drugs)

Urisal — sodium citrate treatment for cystitis. Product now discontinued.

Urispas
(Syntex)

A white tablet supplied at a strength of 100 mg and used as an anti-spasmodic treatment for incontinence, abnormally frequent or urgent urination, bed wetting, painful urination.

Dose: 2 tablets 3 times a day.
Availability: NHS and private prescription.
Side effects: headache, nausea, tiredness, diarrhoea, blurred vision, dry mouth.
Caution: in pregnant women, and in patients suffering from glaucoma.
Not to be used for: children or for patients suffering from obstruction of the urinary or gastro-intestinal tracts.
Caution needed with:
Contains: FLAVOXATE HYDROCHLORIDE.
Other preparations:

Uromide — antibiotic/anaesthetic treatment for urinary infections. Product now discontinued.

---

ursodeoxycholic acid *see* **Destolit**

Ursofalk *see* **Destolit, Lithofalk**
(Thames)

Uticillin — penicillin treatment for urinary tract infections. Product now discontinued.

Utovlan
(Syntex)

A white, scored tablet supplied at a strength of 5 mg and used as a progestogen for postponing menstruation, and to treat premenstrual syndrome, abnormal uterine bleeding, breast cancer, uterine and menstrual disorders.

Dose: normally 1 tablet 3 times a day for 10 days.
Availability: NHS and private prescription.
Side effects: liver disturbances, masculinization.
Caution: in patients suffering from migraine, epilepsy, diabetes.
Not to be used for: children, pregnant women, or for patients suffering from certain types of breast cancer, liver disease, abnormal vaginal bleeding, a history of thromboembolic disorders, severe itching, herpes.
Caution needed with:

Contains: NORETHISTERONE.
Other preparations: MENZOL (Schwarz), PRIMOLUT-N (Schering), S.H.420 (Schering).

V-Cil-K — penicillin antibiotic. Product now discontinued.

Vagifem
(Novo Nordisk)

Pessaries supplied with applicators, and used as an oestrogen treatment for atrophic inflammation of the vagina.

Dose: 1 pessary inserted into the vagina daily for 2 weeks, then twice a week for 3 months.
Availability: NHS and private prescription.
Side effects: enlarged breasts, fluid retention, headaches, nausea, vaginal bleeding, weight gain, skin changes, liver disorders, jaundice, rashes, vomiting.
Caution: in patients suffering from high blood pressure, diabetes, heart disease, vascular disorders, asthma, kidney disease, epilepsy, migraine, womb disease, thyroid disorder. Your doctor may advise you to have regular examinations.
Not to be used for: pregnant women, nursing mothers, or for patients suffering from sickle-cell anaemia, history of heart disease or thrombosis, liver disorders, some cancers, undiagnosed vaginal bleeding, some ear, skin and kidney disorders, jaundice, porphyria (a rare blood disease), brain blood vessel disorder.
Caution needed with: DIURETICS, ANTIHYPERTENSIVES, drugs which induce liver enzymes (eg BARBITURATES, CARBAMAZEPINE, PHENYTOIN, PRIMIDONE, RIFAMPICIN).
Contains: OESTRADIOL.
Other preparations:

Vaginyl *see* **Flagyl**
(DDSA)

Valenac *see* **Voltarol**
(Shire)

Valium
(Roche)

A white tablet, yellow tablet, or blue tablet according to strengths of 2 mg, 5 mg, 10 mg and used as a sedative to treat anxiety, acute alcohol withdrawal, and for the short-term treatment of sleeplessness where sedation during the day is not a difficulty, fear and sleepwalking at night in children, muscle spasm.

Dose: elderly 1-30 mg a day; adults 2-60 mg a day; children 2-40 mg a day.
Availability: NHS (when prescribed as a generic) and private prescription.
Side effects: drowsiness, reduced reactions, .
Caution: in the elderly, pregnant women, nursing mothers, and in patients suffering from chronic lung weakness, kidney or liver disease. Avoid long-term treament and withdraw gradually.
Not to be used for: patients with acute lung weakness, some mental disorders.
Caution needed with: alcohol, sedatives, anticonvulsants.
Contains: DIAZEPAM.
Other preparations: Valium Syrup, Valium Suppositories — now discontinued, Valium Injection, ALUPRAM, ATENSINE (Berk), DIALAR, (Lagap), DIAZEPAM TABLETS/suppositories, RIMAPAM (Rima), SOLIS, STESOLID (CP Pharmaceuticals), TENSIUM (DDSA)

Vallergan
(Rhone-Poulenc Rorer)

A blue tablet supplied at a strength of 10 mg and used as an ANTIHISTAMINE treatment for itch, allergy.

Dose: adults 1 tablet 2-3 times a day or up to 10 a day if needed; children over 2 years use syrup.
Availability: NHS and private prescription.
Side effects: drowsiness, reduced reactions, rash, elation, depression, convulsions on high doses, extrapyramidal reactions (shaking and rigidity), stomach disturbances, ANTICHOLINERGIC effects, heart disturbances, breathing difficulty, blood changes, jaundice, sensitivity to light.
Caution:
Not to be used for: infants under 2 years.
Caution needed with: sedatives, MAOIS, SYMPATHOMIMETICS, alcohol, antidiabetics, ANTIHYPERTENSIVES, ANTICHOLINERGICS.
Contains: TRIMEPRAZINE tartrate.
Other preparations: Vallergan Syrup, Vallergan Forte Syrup.

V

Valoid
(Wellcome)

A white, scored tablet supplied at a strength of 50 mg and used as an ANTIHISTAMINE treatment for vomiting, nausea, vertigo, inner ear disorders.

Dose: adults and children over 10 years 1 tablet 3 times a day; children 1-10 years ½ tablet 3 times a day.
Availability: NHS, private prescription, over the counter.
Side effects: drowsiness, reduced reactions, ANTICHOLINERGIC reactions, allergy, blood disorders, rarely skin eruptions.
Caution: in nursing mothers, and in patients suffering from liver or kidney disease, glaucoma, epilepsy, enlarged prostate.
Not to be used for: infants under 1 year, pregnant women.
Caution needed with: alcohol, sedatives, ANTICHOLINERGICS.
Contains: CYCLIZINE hydrochloride.
Other preparations: Valoid Injection (not available over the counter).

Valrox *see* Naprosyn
(Shire)

Vansil
(Pfizer)

A capsule supplied at a strength of 250 mg and used to treat some worm infestations in the intestine.

Dose: from 15 mg/kg body weight as a single dose to 60 mg/kg body weight given over 2-3 days.
Availability: NHS and private prescription.
Side effects: convulsions.
Caution:
Not to be used for:
Caution needed with:
Contains: OXAMNIQUINE.
Other preparations:

Variclene
(Dermal)

A gel used as an antiseptic treatment for skin ulcers.

Dose: apply to the affected area and cover; repeat no later than 7 days

after.
Availability: NHS, private prescription, over the counter.
Side effects:
Caution:
Not to be used for:
Caution needed with:
Contains: BRILLIANT GREEN, LACTIC ACID.
Other preparations:

Vasaten *see* Tenormin
(Shire)

Vascace
(Roche)

Tablets supplied at strengths of 0.25 mg, 0.5 mg, 1.0 mg, 2.5 mg, 5 mg and used as an ACE-INHIBITOR to treat high blood pressure, including that associated with kidney disease.

Dose: initially 1 mg a day, increasing to up to 5 mg a day. Stop DIURETICS 2-3 days before starting treatment. Lower doses used for the elderly, and for patients with kidney involvement.
Availability: NHS and private prescription.
Side effects: headache, dizziness, tiredness, stomach discomfort, nausea, rash, cough, severe allergy, blood changes.
Caution: in patients suffering from kidney or liver damage, congestive heart failure, salt or body fluid depletion, or undergoing surgery or anaesthesia.
Not to be used for: children, pregnant women, nursing mothers, or for patients suffering from some heart defects or fluid in the abdomen.
Caution needed with: some DIURETICS, NON-STEROID ANTI-INFLAMMATORY DRUGS.
Contains: CILAZAPRIL.
Other preparations:

Vascardin
(Nicholas)

A white, scored tablet supplied at a strength of 10 mg, 30 mg and used as a NITRATE treatment for angina, and as an additional treatment for congestive heart failure.

Dose: for heart failure 10-30 mg 4 times a day increasing according to response. For angina 5-10 mg under the tongue for an acute attack and 30-120 mg in divided doses or as required to prevent attacks.
Availability: NHS, private prescription, over the counter.
Side effects: headache, flushes.
Caution:
Not to be used for: children.
Caution needed with:
Contains: ISOSORBIDE DINITRATE.
Other preparations: CEDOCARD (Farmitalia CE), CEDOCARD RETARD (Farmitalia CE), ISOKET RETARD (Schwarz), ISORDIL (Monmouth), SONI-SLO (Lipha), SORBICHEW (Stuart), SORBID-SA (Stuart), SORBITRATE (Stuart), IMTACK (Astra).

Vasetic *see* Moduretic
(Shire)

Vasocon-A
(Iolab)

Drops used as an ANTIHISTAMINE, SYMPATHOMIMETIC treatment for allergic conjunctivitis and other eye inflammations.

Dose: adults 1-2 drops into the eye every 3-4 hours; children over 2 years as advised by the physician.
Availability: NHS and private prescription.
Side effects: temporary smarting, headache, sleeplessness, rapid heart rate, drowsiness, congestion.
Caution: in patients suffering from diabetes, coronary disease, high blood pressure, overactive thyroid gland.
Not to be used for: infants under 2 years, patients suffering from glaucoma, or for those who wear soft contact lenses.
Caution needed with:
Contains: ANTAZOLINE phosphate, NAPHAZOLINE hydrochloride.
Other preparations:

Vasyrol *see* Persantin
(Shire)

Velosef
(Squibb)

A blue/orange capsule or a blue capsule according to strengths of 250 mg, 500 mg and used as a cephalosporin antibiotic to treat infections, and for the prevention of infections in surgery.

Dose: adults 1-2 g a day in 2-4 divided doses up to a maximum of 4 g a day; children 25-50 mg per kg body weight a day in 2-4 divided doses.
Availability: NHS and private prescription.
Side effects: allergy, stomach disturbances thrush, blood changes, change in liver, rise in urea level, interference with some blood test results.
Caution: in patients suffering from kidney disease or who are sensitive to penicillin.
Not to be used for:
Caution needed with: aminoglycoside antibiotics.
Contains: CEPHRADINE.
Other preparations: Velosef Syrup, Velosef Injection.

Velosulin *see* insulin
(Novo Nordisk)

Ventide
(A & H)

An aerosol supplied at a strength of 100 micrograms and used as a broncho-dilator and STEROID to treat asthma.

Dose: adults 2 sprays 3-4 times a day; children 1-2 sprays 2-4 times a day.
Availability: NHS and private prescription.
Side effects: hand shaking, nervous tension, headache, hoarseness, thrush, dilation of the blood vessels.
Caution: in pregnant women, and in patients suffering from overactive thyroid gland, heart muscle disease, abnormal heart rhythms, angina, high blood pressure, tuberculosis of the lungs, or in those transferring from STEROIDS taken by mouth.
Not to be used for:
Caution needed with: SYMPATHOMIMETICS.
Contains: SALBUTAMOL, BECLOMETHASONE diproprionate.
Other preparations: Ventide Rotacaps, Ventide Paediatric Rotacaps.

Ventodisks
(A & H)

A pale-blue disc or a dark-blue disc according to strengths of 200 micrograms, 400 micrograms. and used as a broncho-dilator to treat bronchial spasm brought on by bronchial asthma, bronchitis, emphysema.

Dose: adults 200-400 micrograms as a single dose or 400 micrograms 3-4 times a day; children 200 micrograms or 200 micrograms 3-4 times a day.
Availability: NHS and private prescription.
Side effects: hand shaking, nervous tension, headache, dilation of the blood vessels.
Caution: in pregnant women and in patients suffering from high blood pressure, abnormal heart rhythms, angina, overactive thyroid gland, heart muscle disease.
Not to be used for:
Caution needed with: SYMPATHOMIMETICS.
Contains: SALBUTAMOL sulphate.
Other preparations: AEROLIN (3M Healthcare), ASMAVEN (APS), CYCLOHALER (Pharbita), MAXIVENT (Ashbourne), RIMASAL (Rima), SALBULIN (3M Healthcare), SALBUVENT (Farmitalia CE), STERI-NEB SALAMOL (Baker Norton), VENTOLIN (A & H), VOLMAX (Duncan Flockhart).

Ventolin
(A & H)

A pink tablet supplied at strengths of 2 mg, 4 mg and used as a broncho-dilator to treat bronchial spasm brought on by bronchial asthma, chronic bronchitis, emphysema. Also used to stop premature labour.

Dose: adults 2-4 mg 3-4 times a day; children 2-6 years 1-2 mg 3-4 times a day, 6-12 years 2 mg 3-4 times a day.
Availability: NHS and private prescription.
Side effects: rapid heart rate, anxiety, rise in blood sugar level, shaking of the hands, nervous tension, dilation of the blood vessels, headache.
Caution: in patients suffering from thyrotoxicosis, diabetes, or cardiovascular disease. Heart rate of mother and foetus should be monitored carefully when used for treatment of premature labour.
Not to be used for: children under 2 years, or for patients suffering from antepartum haemorrhage, toxaemia of pregnancy, cord compression, threatened abortion, or conditions where prolonging the pregnancy may be dangerous.
Caution needed with: ß-BLOCKERS, other broncho-dilators, SYMPATHOMIMETICS.
Contains: SALBUTAMOL sulphate.

Other preparations: Ventolin Infusion, Ventolin CR, Ventolin Inhaler, Ventolin Spandets — now discontinued, Ventolin Rotacaps, Ventolin Injection, Ventolin Respirator Solution, Ventolin Nebules, AEROLIN (3M Healthcare), ASMAVEN (APS), CYCLOHALER (Pharbita), MAXIVENT (Ashbourne), RIMASAL (Rima), SALBULIN (3M Healthcare), SALBUVENT (Farmitalia CE), STERI-NEB SALAMOL (Baker Norton), VENTODISKS (A & H), VOLMAX (Duncan Flockhart).

Veractil *see* **Nozinon**. Product now discontinued.

Veracur
(Typharm)

A gel used as a skin softener to treat warts.

Dose: apply to the wart twice a day and cover, rubbing down with a pumice stone between treatments.
Availability: NHS, private prescription, over the counter.
Side effects:
Caution: do not apply to healthy skin.
Not to be used for: warts on the face or anal and genital areas.
Caution needed with:
Contains: FORMALDEHYDE.
Other preparations: formaldehyde lotion.

---

verapamil *see* **Cordilox, Cordilox 160, Glauline, Securon, Securon SR**

Verdiviton — vitamin B complex supplement. Product now discontinued.

Vermox
(Janssen)

A suspension used as a vermicide to treat worms.

Dose: adults and children over 2 years 5 ml morning and evening for 3 days or 5 ml repeated after 2-3 weeks according to the type of infestation.
Availability: NHS and private prescription.
Side effects: stomach upset.
Caution:

Not to be used for: children under 2 years or pregnant women.
Caution needed with:
Contains: MEBENDAZOLE.
Other preparations: Vermox Tablets, (Ovex Tablets available over the counter).

Verrugon
(Pickles)

An ointment with corn rings and plasters used as a skin softener to treat warts.

Dose: protect healthy skin, apply the ointment to the wart, and cover with a plaster, rubbing down with a pumice stone between treatments.
Availability: NHS, private prescription, over the counter.
Side effects:
Caution: do not apply to healthy skin.
Not to be used for: warts on the face or anal and genital areas.
Caution needed with:
Contains: SALICYLIC ACID.
Other preparations:

Vertigon Spansule *see* Stemetil
(S K B)

Verucasep
(Galen)

A gel used as a virucidal, anhidrotic treatment for viral warts.

Dose: apply twice a day, paring down any hard skin around the wart.
Availability: NHS, private prescription, over the counter.
Side effects: stains the skin.
Caution: do not apply to healthy skin.
Not to be used for: warts on the face or anal and genital areas.
Caution needed with:
Contains: GLUTARALDEHYDE.
Other preparations: GLUTAROL (Dermal).

Vibramycin
(Invicta)

A green capsule supplied at a strength of 100 mg and used as a tetracycline treatment for pneumonia, respiratory, stomach, soft tissue, eye, and urinary infections.

Dose: adults 2 capsules with food or drink on the first day then 1-2 capsules a day.
Availability: NHS and private prescription.
Side effects: stomach disturbances, allergy, additional infections, oesophagitis, allergy, raised blood pressure in the brain.
Caution: in patients suffering from liver disease.
Not to be used for: children, nursing mothers, women in the last half of pregnancy, or even for pregnant women at all unless no other treatment is possible.
Caution needed with: ANTACIDS, mineral supplements, BARBITURATES, CARBAMAZEPINE, PHENYTOIN.
Contains: DOXYCYCLINE hydrochloride.
Other preparations: Vibramycin-D Tablets, DEMIX-100 (Ashbourne), DOXYLAR (Lagap), NORDOX (Panpharma).

Vibramycin 50
(Pfizer)

A green/cream capsule supplied at a strength of 50 mg and used as an antibiotic treatment for acne.

Dose: 1 capsule a day with food or drink for 6-12 weeks.
Availability: NHS and private prescription.
Side effects: stomach disturbances, allergies, oesophagitis, additional infection, raised blood pressure in the brain.
Caution: in patients suffering from liver disease.
Not to be used for: nursing mothers or women in the last half of pregnancy.
Caution needed with: ANTACIDS, mineral supplements, BARBITURATES, PHENYTOIN, CARBAMAZEPINE.
Contains: DOXYCYCLINE hydrochloride.
Other preparations:

Vibrocil
(Zyma)

A spray, drops, or gel used as an ANTIHISTAMINE, antibiotic, SYMPATHOMIMETIC treatment for rhinitis, hay fever, sinusitis.

Dose: adults 3 sprays, 3-4 drops, or a little gel into each nostril 3-4 times a

V

day; children under 6 years 1-2 drops or a little gel into each nostril 3-4 times a day, 6-12 years 3-4 drops or a little gel into each nostril 3-4 times a day.
Availability: NHS and private prescription.
Side effects:
Caution: in patients suffering from cardiovascular disease, high blood pressure overactive thyroid gland. Do not use for extended periods.
Not to be used for:
Caution needed with: MAOIS.
Contains: DIMETHINDENE maleate, PHENYLEPHRINE, NEOMYCIN sulphate.
Other preparations:

---

vidarabine *see* **Vira-A**

Videne Powder
(Beta Medical Products)

A powder used as an antiseptic treatment for skin.

Dose: dust the affected area lightly with the powder.
Availability: NHS, private prescription, over the counter.
Side effects: rarely sensitivity.
Caution: in pregnant women, nursing mothers, and in patients suffering from thyroid disorder, kidney disease, or broken skin.
Not to be used for:
Caution needed with:
Contains: POVIDONE-IODINE.
Other preparations: (Videne Solution, Videne Tincture, Videne Surgical Scrub — all now discontinued), BETADINE DRY POWDER SPRAY (Napp).

Vidopen
(Berk)

A pink/red capsule supplied at a strength of 250 mg, 500 mg and used as a penicillin to treat respiratory, eye, nose, and throat, soft tissue, and urinary infections.

Dose: adults and children over 20 kg body weight 250 mg-1 g 4 times a day; children under 20 kg body weight 200 mg per kg a day in divided doses.
Availability: NHS and private prescription.
Side effects: allergy, stomach disturbances.

Caution: in patients suffering from kidney disease or glandular fever.
Not to be used for: patients suffering from penicillin allergy
Caution needed with:
Contains: AMPICILLIN trihydrate.
Other preparations: Vidopen Syrup, AMFIPEN (Brocades), AMPICILLIN CAPSULES, PENBRITIN (Beecham), RIMACILLIN (Rima).

---

vigabatrin *see* **Sabril**

Villescon
(Boehringer Ingelheim)

A liquid used as a tonic.

Dose: adults 10 ml after breakfast and 10 ml before 4 pm each day for 1-2 weeks; children 5-12 years 2.5-10 ml twice a day.
Availability: private prescription only.
Side effects: rapid heart rate, nausea, colic, sleeplessness.
Caution:
Not to be used for: children under 5 years or for patients suffering from thyrotoxicosis, epilepsy.
Caution needed with: MAOIS, LEVODOPA.
Contains: PROLINTANE hydrochloride, THIAMINE mononitrate, RIBOFLAVINE, PYRIDOXINE hydrochloride, NICOTINAMIDE, ASCORBIC ACID.
Other preparations: Villescon Liquid.

---

viloxazine hydrochloride *see* **Vivalan**

Vioform-Hydrocortisone
(Zyma)

A cream used as a STEROID, antibacterial, antifungal treatment for skin disorders, infected skin in the anal and genital areas.

Dose: apply to the affected area 1-3 times a day.
Availability: NHS and private prescription.
Side effects: fluid retention, suppression of adrenal glands, thinning of the skin may occur.
Caution: use for short periods of time only.
Not to be used for: patients suffering from acne or any other skin infec-

tions caused by tuberculosis, ringworm, viruses, or fungi, or continuously especially in pregnant women.
Caution needed with:
Contains: CLIOQUINOL, HYDROCORTISONE.
Other preparations: Vioform-Hydrocortisone Ointment, Vioform Powder (without steroid).

Vira-A — antiviral eye treatment. Product now discontinued.

Virudox
(Bioglan)

A transparent, colourless solution used as an antiviral treatment for herpes, shingles.

Dose: apply 4 times a day for 4 days within 2-3 days of the appearance of the rash.
Availability: NHS and private prescription.
Side effects: local stinging, taste change.
Caution: keep away from eyes, mucous membranes, and clothing.
Not to be used for: children, pregnant women, nursing mothers.
Caution needed with:
Contains: IDOXURIDINE, DIMETHYL SULPHOXIDE.
Other preparations: HERPID (Boehringer Ingelheim), IDURIDIN (Ferring).

Visclair
(Sinclair)

A yellow tablet supplied at a strength of 100 mg and used as a mucus softener to treat bronchitis, phlegm.

Dose: adults 2 tablets 3-4 times a day for 6 weeks then 2 tablets twice a day; children over 5 years 1 tablet 3 times a day.
Availability: private prescription and over the counter.
Side effects: stomach upset.
Caution:
Not to be used for: children under 5 years.
Caution needed with:
Contains: METHYLCYSTEINE HYDROCHLORIDE.
Other preparations:

Viskaldix
(Sandoz)

A white, scored tablet used as a ß-BLOCKER and DIURETIC to treat high blood pressure.

Dose: 1 tablet in the morning at first, then increase to 2-3 tablets a day after 2-3 weeks.
Availability: NHS and private prescription.
Side effects: cold hands and feet, sleep disturbance, slow heart rate, tiredness, wheezing, heart failure, stomach upset, dry eyes, skin rash, gout, sensitivity to light, blood changes, weakness.
Caution: in pregnant women, nursing mothers, and in patients suffering from diabetes, gout, kidney or liver disorders, asthma. May need to be withdrawn before surgery. Withdraw gradually. Your doctor may advise additional treatment with DIURETICS or DIGOXIN.
Not to be used for: children or for patients suffering from heart block or failure, kidney failure.
Caution needed with: VERAPAMIL, CLONIDINE withdrawal, some anti-arrhythmic drugs and anaesthetics, RESERPINE, other ANTIHYPERTENSIVES, ERGOTAMINE, CIMETIDINE, sedatives, LITHIUM, DIGOXIN, SYMPATHOMIMETICS, INDOMETHACIN.
Contains: PINDOLOL, CLOPAMIDE.
Other preparations:

Visken
(Sandoz)

A white, scored tablet supplied at stregths of 5 mg, 15 mg and used as a ß-BLOCKER to treat angina, high blood pressure.

Dose: angina 2.5-5 mg up to 3 times a day. High blood pressure 10-15 mg a day at first increasing if needed at weekly intervals to 45 mg a day.
Availability: NHS and private prescription.
Side effects: cold hands and feet, sleep disturbance, slow heart rate, tiredness, wheezing, heart failure, stomach upset, dry eyes, skin rash.
Caution: in pregnant women, nursing mothers, and in patients suffering from diabetes, kidney or liver disorders, asthma. May need to be withdrawn before surgery. Withdraw gradually. Your doctor may advise additional treatment with DIURETICS or DIGOXIN.
Not to be used for: children or for patients suffering from heart block or failure.
Caution needed with: VERAPAMIL, CLONIDINE withdrawal, some anti-arrhythmic drugs and anaesthetics, RESERPINE, other ANTIHYPERTENSIVES, ERGOTAMINE, CIMETIDINE, sedatives, antidiabetics, SYMPATHOMIMETICS,

V

691

INDOMETHACIN.
Contains: PINDOLOL.
Other preparations:

Vista-Methasone
(Daniel)

Drops used as a STEROID treatment for inflammation of the ears, nasal passages, or eyes where there is no infection present.

Dose: 2-3 drops into each nostril twice a day, 2-3 drops into the ear every 3-4 hours, or 1-2 drops into the eye every 2 hours at first then as needed.
Availability: NHS and private prescription.
Side effects: additional infection, rise in eye pressure, thinning of the cornea, fungal infection, cataract.
Caution: in infants and pregnant women — avoid using over extended periods.
Not to be used for: patients suffering from viral, fungal, or tubercular infections of the nose, perforated ear drum, glaucoma, or for those who wear soft contact lenses.
Caution needed with:
Contains: BETAMETHASONE sodium phosphate.
Other preparations: Vista-Methasone N (for infected conditions), BETNESOL (Evans).

V

Vita-E Capsules
(Bioglan)

A yellow, oval capsule, yellow, oblong capsule, or red, oblong capsule according to strengths of 75 units, 200 units, 400 units, and used as a vitamin E supplement to treat blood vessel spasm in the legs.

Dose: 400-1600 units a day with meals.
Availability: NHS, private prescription, over the counter.
Side effects:
Caution:
Not to be used for: children or for patients suffering from overactive thyroid.
Caution needed with: fish oils, iron, DIGOXIN, INSULIN.
Contains: D-ALPHA-TOCOPHERYL ACETATE.
Other preparations: Vita-E Gelucaps, Vita-E Succinate.

Vita-E Ointment
(Bioglan)

An ointment used as an anti-oxidant to treat wounds, bed sores, burns, skin ulcers.

Dose: apply to the affected area as needed.
Availability: NHS, private prescription, over the counter.
Side effects:
Caution:
Not to be used for: patients suffering from overactive thyroid gland.
Caution needed with: fish liver oils, DIGOXIN, INSULIN, iron.
Contains: D-ALPHA-TOCOPHERYL ACETATE.
Other preparations:

---

vitamin A *see* **Concavit, Ketovite, Halycitrol, Multivite, Octovit, Orovite 7, Polyvite, Ro-A-Vit, Tonivitan, Tonivitan A & D, Unicap-M, vitamins capsules**

---

vitamin C (ascorbic acid) *see* **Abidec, Allbee with C, BC 500, BC 500 with Iron, Concavit, Dalivit Drops, Fefol-Vit Spansule, Ferrograd C, Fesovit Spansule, Fesovit 2 Spansule, Galfervit, Givitol, Irofol C, Lipoflavonoid, Multivite, Octovit, Optimax, Oralcer, Orovite, Orovite 7, Polyvite, Pregnavite Forte F, Redoxon, Surbex T, Tonivitan, Unicap-M, Uniflu & Gregovite C, Villescon, vitamins capsules**

---

vitamin D *see* **Halycitrol, Ketovite, Unicap-M, vitamins capsules**

---

vitamin E *see* **Concavit, Ephynal, Vita-E**

---

vitamins capsules

Capsules used as a multivitamin supplement.

Dose: as advised by the doctor.
Availability: NHS, private prescription, over the counter.
Side effects:

Caution: in pregnant women.
Not to be used for:
Caution needed with:
Contains: ASCORBIC ACID, NICOTINAMIDE, RIBOFLAVINE, THIAMINE, VITAMIN A, VITAMIN D.
Other preparations:

Vivalan
(ICI)

A yellow tablet supplied at a strength of 50 mg and used as an anti-depressant to treat depression, especially in patients for whom sedation is not required.

Dose: adults usually 6 tablets a day in divided doses up to a maximum of 8 tablets a day; elderly 2 tablets a day at first.
Availability: NHS and private prescription.
Side effects: vomiting, headache, impaired reactions, ANTICHOLINERGIC effects, jaundice, convulsions.
Caution: in pregnant women and in patients with suicidal tendencies, or suffering from heart disease including congestive heart failure, heart block, epilepsy.
Not to be used for: children, nursing mothers, or patients suffering from mania, severe liver disease, history of stomach ulcer, recent heart attack.
Caution needed with: MAOIS, alpha blockers, CLONIDINE, PHENYTOIN, LEVODOPA, sedatives, CARBAMAZEPINE, THEOPHYLLINE.
Contains: VILOXAZINE hydrochloride.
Other preparations:

Volital
(LAB)

A white, scored tablet supplied at a strength of 20 mg and used as a brain stimulant to treat movement disorders in children.

Dose: children 6-12 years 1 tablet a day in the morning, increasing if necessary to 6 a day.
Availability: NHS and private prescription.
Side effects: dizziness, sweating, palpitations, headache, irritability, dry mouth, loss of appetite and weight.
Caution:
Not to be used for: children under 6 years or for adults.
Caution needed with: MAOIS.

Contains: PEMOLINE.
Other preparations:

Volmax *see* Ventolin
(Duncan, Flockhart)

Volraman *see* Voltarol
(Eastern)

Voltarol
(Ciba-Geigy)

A yellow tablet or brown tablet according to strengths of 25 mg, 50 mg and used as a NON-STEROID ANTI-INFLAMMATORY DRUG to treat bone or muscular problems, rheumatoid arthritis, osteoarthritis, ankylosing spondylitis, acute gout, chronic juvenile arthritis.

Dose: adults 75-150 mg a day in 2-3 divided doses; children 1-3 mg per kg body weight a day in divided doses.
Availability: NHS and private prescription.
Side effects: passing stomach pain, nausea, headache, rash, fluid retention, rarely blood changes, stomach ulcer, abnormal liver or kidney function.
Caution: in pregnant women, nursing mothers, the elderly, or patients suffering from kidney, liver, or heart weakness, blood abnormalities, history of gastro-intestinal lesions. Your doctor may advise regular check-ups.
Not to be used for: patients suffering from asthma, stomach ulcer, or allergy to ASPIRIN/NON-STEROID ANTI-INFLAMMATORY DRUGS, rectal inflammation.
Caution needed with: SALICYLATES, METHOTREXATE, LITHIUM, DIGOXIN, DIURETICS, CYCLOSPORIN.
Contains: DICLOFENAC sodium.
Other preparations: Voltarol Retard, Voltarol SR, Voltarol Suppositories, DICLOZIP (Ashbourne), RHUMALGAN (Lagap), VALENAC (Shire), VOLRAMAN (Eastern).

---

warfarin *see* Marevan

Warticon
(Janssen)

A solution with applicators used as a cell softener and remover to treat warts on the penis.

Dose: apply twice a day for 3 days and repeat after 7 days if needed.
Availability: NHS and private prescription.
Side effects: irritation.
Caution:
Not to be used for: children.
Caution needed with:
Contains: PODOPHYLLOTOXIN.
Other preparations: CONDYLINE (Brocades).

Waxsol
(Norgine)

Drops used as a wax softener to remove ear wax.

Dose: fill the ear with the solution for 2 nights before they are to be syringed.
Availability: NHS, private prescription, over the counter.
Side effects: temporary irritation.
Caution:
Not to be used for: patients suffering from inflammation of the ear or perforated ear drum.
Caution needed with:
Contains: sodium DOCUSATE.
Other preparations: DIOCTYL (Medo).

W

Welldorm
(SNP)

A purple, oval tablet supplied at a strength of 707 mg and used as a sedative-hypnotic to treat sleeplessness or to sedate children when elixir is used.

Dose: 1-2 tablets before going to bed.
Availability: NHS and private prescription.
Side effects: nausea, vomiting, headache, rash, rarely blood changes, excitement, abdominal enlargement, wind.
Caution:
Not to be used for: pregnant women, nursing mothers, or for patients

suffering from acute intermittent porphyria (a rare blood disorder), severe kidney, liver, or heart disease, stomach inflammation.
Caution needed with: alcohol, sedatives, ANTICHOLINERGICS, anticoagulants.
Contains: CHLORAL HYDRATE.
Other preparations: NOCTEC (Squibb).

---

wheat husk *see* **Trifyba**

---

white soft paraffin *see* **calamine and coal tar ointment, coal tar and salicyic acid ointment, Diprobase, Lipobase, Unguentum Merck**

Whitfields Ointment *see* **benzoic acid compound ointment**

---

wool fat *see* **calamine and coal tar ointment, Lubrifilm**

---

xamoterol *see* **Corwin**

Xanax
(Upjohn)

A white, oval, scored tablet or a pink, oval, scored tablet according to strengths of 0.25 mg, 0.5 mg and used as a sedative for the short-term treatment of anxiety and depression.

Dose: elderly 0.25 mg 2-3 times a day; adults 0.25-0.5 mg 3 times a day to a maximum of 3 mg a day.
Availability: private prescription only.
Side effects: drowsiness, confusion, unsteadiness, low blood pressure, rash, changes in vision, changes in libido, retention of urine. Risk of addiction increases with dose and length of treatment. May impair judgement.
Caution: in the elderly, pregnant women, nursing mothers, in women during labour, and in patients suffering from lung disorders, kidney or liver disorders. Avoid long-term use and withdraw gradually.

Not to be used for: children, or for patients suffering from acute lung diseases, some chronic lung diseases, some obsessional and psychotic diseases.
Caution needed with: alcohol, other tranquillizers, anticonvulsants.
Contains: ALPRAZOLAM.
Other preparations:

Xanthomax *see* **Zyloric**
(Ashbourne)

---

xipamide *see* **Diurexan**

Xuret *see* **Metenix**
(Galen)

Xylocaine
(Astra)

An ointment used to anaesthetize the skin or mucous membranes.

Dose: as advised by your doctor.
Availability: NHS, private prescription, over the counter.
Side effects:
Caution: in patients suffering from epilepsy.
Not to be used for:
Caution needed with:
Contains: LIGNOCAINE.
Other preparations: Xylocaine Gel, Xylocaine Antiseptic Gel, Xylocaine Topical, Xylocaine Pump Spray, Xylocaine Injection.

---

xylometazoline hydrochloride *see* **Otrivine, Otrivine-Antistin**
(Zyma)

Xyloproct
(Astra)

A suppository used as a local anaesthetic and STEROID treatment for haemorrhoids, anal itch, anal fissure and fistula.

Dose: 1 at night and after passing motions.
Availability: NHS and private prescription.
Side effects: systemic corticosteroid effects (*see* Precortisyl).
Caution: do not use for prolonged periods; care in pregnant women.
Not to be used for: patients suffering from tuberculous, fungal, or viral infections
Caution needed with:
Contains: LIGNOCAINE, ALUMINIUM ACETATE, ZINC OXIDE, HYDROCORTISONE acetate.
Other preparations: Xyloproct ointment.

---

yellow soft paraffin *see* **Lubrifilm**

Yomesan — treatment for tapeworm. Product now discontinued.

Yutopar
(Duphar)

A buff, scored tablet supplied at a strength of 10 mg and used as a ß-agonist to treat premature labour, foetal asphyxiation in labour.

Dose: 1 tablet about 30 minutes before ending intravenous treatment, 1 tablet every 2 hours for 24 hours, and then 1-2 tablets every 4-6 hours.
Availability: NHS and private prescription.
Side effects: rapid heart rate, anxiety, rise in blood sugar level.
Caution: in patients suffering from diabetes, cardiovascular disease, or maternal thyrotoxicosis. The heart rate of mother and foetus should be checked carefully.
Not to be used for: children or for patients suffering from antepartum bleeding, toxaemia of pregnancy, cord compression, threatened abortion, or where prolonging the pregnancy might be dangerous.
Caution needed with: MAOIS, ß-BLOCKERS, other ß-agonists.
Contains: RITODRINE hydrochloride.
Other preparations: Yutopar Injection.

Z Span Spansule
(S K B)

A blue/clear capsule used as a zinc supplement for the prevention and treatment of zinc deficiency.

Dose: adults and children over 1 year 1 capsule 1-3 times a day.
Availability: NHS, private prescription, over the counter.
Side effects: stomach upset.
Caution: in patients suffering from kidney failure.
Not to be used for: infants under 1 year.
Caution needed with: TETRACYCLINES.
Contains: ZINC SULPHATE MONOHYDRATE.
Other preparations: SOLVAZINC (Thames), ZINCOMED (Medo), ZINCOSOL (Bioceuticals).

Zaditen
(Sandoz)

A white, scored tablet supplied at a strength of 1 mg and used as an ANTIHISTAMINE preparation for the prevention of bronchial asthma, and the treatment of allergic rhinitis, conjunctivitis.

Dose: adults 1-2 tablets twice a day with food; children over 2 years 1 tablet twice a day with food.
Availability: NHS and private prescription.
Side effects: drowsiness, reduced reactions, dizziness, dry mouth, excitement, weight gain.
Caution:
Not to be used for: children under 2 years, pregnant women, nursing mothers.
Caution needed with: alcohol,sedatives, antidiabetics taken by mouth, other ANTIHISTAMINES.
Contains: KETOTIFEN.
Other preparations: Zaditen Capsules, Zaditen Elixir.

Zadstat *see* Flagyl
(Lederle)

Zantac
(Glaxo)

A peach or white tablet supplied at strengths of 150 mg, 300 mg and used as an H_2 blocker to treat duodenal and gastric ulcers, oesophagitis, dyspepsia, reduction of gastric acid.

Dose: children over 8 years up to 150 mg twice a day, adults 150 mg twice a day or 300 mg at bedtime for 28 days, 150 mg at bedtime thereafter.
Availability: NHS and private prescription.
Side effects: headache, dizziness, occasionally hepatitis, low platelet counts, low white blood cell counts, allergy, confusion, breast symptoms.
Caution: exclude malignant disease. Care in pregnant women, nursing mothers, and in patients suffering from impaired kidney function.
Not to be used for:
Caution needed with:
Contains: RANITIDINE.
Other preparations: Zantac dispensible, Zantac syrup, Zantac injection.

Zarontin
(Parke-Davis)

An orange capsule supplied at a strength of 250 mg and used as an anticonvulsant to treat epilepsy.

Dose: adults and children over 6 years 2 tablets a day increasing as needed by 1 tablet a day every 4-7 days up to 8 tablets a day; children under 6 years 1 tablet a day at first increasing according to response.
Availability: NHS and private prescription.
Side effects: stomach and brain disturbances, rash, blood changes, SLE (a multisystem disorder).
Caution: in pregnant women, nursing mothers, and in patients suffering from kidney or liver disease. Dose should be decreased gradually.
Not to be used for:
Caution needed with:
Contains: ETHOSUXIMIDE.
Other preparations: Zarontin Syrup, EMESIDE (LAB).

Zestoretic *see* Carace Plus
(ICI)

Zestril
(ICI)

A white, pink, or red tablet according to strengths of 2.5 mg, 5 mg, 10 mg, 20 mg and used as an ACE INHIBITOR to treat congestive heart failure in addition to DIURETICS and DIGOXIN, high blood pressure.

Z

Dose: 2.5 mg once a day at first increasing over 2-4 weeks to 5-20 mg once a day, or up to 40 mg a day for high blood pressure.
Availability: NHS and private prescription.
Side effects: low blood pressure, kidney failure, rash, dizziness,diarrhoea, cough, tiredness, palpitations, chest pain, weakness, headache, nausea, severe allergy.
Caution: in nursing mothers and in patients suffering from kidney disease, congestive heart failure.
Not to be used for: children, pregnant women, or for patients suffering from some heart diseases or previous ellergy to ACE INHIBITORS.
Caution needed with: DIURETICS, potassium supplements, INDOMETHACIN, ANTIHYPERTENSIVES.
Contains: LISINOPRIL.
Other preparations: CARACE (Morson).

---

zidovudine *see* Retrovir

Zimovane
(Rhone-Poulenc Rorer)

A white, scored tablet supplied at a strength of 7.5 mg and used as a sedative to treat sleeplessness.

Dose: 1-2 at bedtime; elderly ½ tablet only.
Availability: NHS and private prescription.
Side effects: metallic aftertaste, stomach upset, minor mental disturbance, allergy, drowsiness, impaired judgement.
Caution: in patients suffering from liver disorder.
Not to be used for: pregnant women, nursing mothers, children.
Caution needed with: alcohol, other sedatives, TRIMIPRAMINE.
Contains: ZOPICLONE.
Other preparations:

Zinamide
(MSD)

A white, scored tablet supplied at a strength of 500 mg and used as an anti-tubercular drug in the additional treatment for tuberculosis.

Dose: 20-35 mg per kg body weight to a maximum of 3 g a day in divided doses.
Availability: NHS and private prescription.

Side effects: hepatitis.
Caution: in patients with a history of gout or diabetes. Your doctor may advise that liver function and blood should be checked regularly.
Not to be used for: children or for patients suffering from liver disease.
Caution needed with:
Contains: PYRAZINAMIDE.
Other preparations:

---

zinc acetate *see* Zineryt

---

zinc bacitracin *see* hydroderm

---

zinc and castor oil ointment BP *see* zinc cream

---

zinc and coal tar paste *see* coal tar paste

---

zinc cream BP

A cream used as an emollient to treat nappy and urine rashes, and eczema.

Dose: apply as needed.
Availability: NHS, private prescription, over the counter.
Side effects:
Caution:
Not to be used for:
Caution needed with:
Contains: ZINC OXIDE.
Other preparations: ZINC OINTMENT BP, ZINC AND CASTOR OIL OINTMENT BP.

---

zinc naphthenate *see* Tineafax

---

zinc ointment BP *see* zinc cream

Z

zinc oxide *see* **Anugesic-HC, Anusol, Anusol HC, calamine and coal tar ointment, coal tar paste, Mutilind, Xyloproct, zinc cream**

---

zinc sulphate eye drops

Eye drops supplied at a strength of 0.25% and used as an astringent to treat excessive tear production.

Dose: as advised by doctor.
Availability: NHS, private prescription, over the counter.
Side effects:
Caution:
Not to be used for:
Caution needed with:
Contains: ZINC SULPHATE.
Other preparations:

---

zinc sulphate monohydrate *see* **Efalith, Fefol Z Spansule, Fesovit Z Spansule, Octovit, Solvazinc, Z Span Spansule, zinc sulphate eye drops**

---

zinc undecenoate *see* **Tineafax**

Zincomed *see* Z-span
(Medo)

Zincosol *see* Z-Span
(Bioceuticals)

Zineryt
(Brocades)

A solution used as an antibiotic to treat acne.

Dose: apply twice a day.
Availability: NHS and private prescription.

Side effects: irritation.
Caution: avoid eyes and mucous membrane.
Not to be used for:
Caution needed with:
Contains: ERYTHROMYCIN, ZINC ACETATE.
Other preparations:

Zinnat
(Glaxo)

A white tablet supplied at strengths of 125 mg, 250 mg and used as a cephalosporin antibiotic to treat respiratory, ear, nose, and throat, skin, soft tissue, and urinary infections.

Dose: adults usually 250-500 mg twice a day, urinary infections 125 mg twice a day, gonorrhoea 1 g as one dose; children 3 months-2 years 125 mg twice a day, over 2 years 250 mg twice a day.
Availability: NHS and private prescription.
Side effects: stomach disturbances, allergy, colitis, blood changes, thrush, change in liver chemistry, headache, interference with some blood tests.
Caution: in pregnant women, nursing mothers, and in patients who are sensitive to penicillin.
Not to be used for:
Caution needed with:
Contains: CEFUROXIME AXETIL.
Other preparations:

Zirtek
(UCB Pharma)

A white, oblong, scored tablet supplied at a strength of 10 mg and used as an ANTIHISTAMINE treatment for rhinitis, allergy.

Dose: 1 tablet a day in the morning.
Availability: NHS and private prescription
Side effects: drowsiness, dizziness, headache, agitation, stomach disturbances, dry mouth.
Caution: in pregnant women and in patients suffering from kidney disease.
Not to be used for: children, nursing mothers.
Caution needed with: sedatives, alcohol.
Contains: CETIRIZINE DIHYDROCHLORIDE.

Z

Zithromax
(Richborough)

A white capsule supplied at a strenth of 250 mg, and used as an antibiotic to treat respiratory, soft tissue, skin, ear, and genital infections.

Dose: adults, 2 capsules a day for 3 days, or 2 capsules initially, than 1 capsule a day for 4 days. For genital infection 4 capsules as a single dose. Children use suspension.
Availability: NHS and private prescription.
Side effects: stomach upset, liver changes.
Caution: in pregnant women, nursing mothers, and in patients with kidney damage.
Not to be used for: children under 15 kg body weight, or for patients suffering from liver disease.
Caution needed with: ERGOTAMINE, ANTACIDS, CYCLOSPORIN.
Contains: AZITHROMYCIN.
Other preparations: Zithromax Suspension.

Zocor
(MSD)

A peach-coloured, oval tablet or a tan, oval tablet according to strengths of 10 mg, 20 mg and used as a lipid-lowering agent to treat raised cholesterol.

Dose: 10-40 mg taken at night.
Availability: NHS and private prescription.
Side effects: headache, indigestion, diarrhoea, tiredness, rash, constipation, wind, nausea, muscle weakness.
Caution: in patients suffering from liver disease. Your doctor may advise liver and eye checks.
Not to be used for: pregnant women, nursing mothers, or for patients suffering from liver disease.
Caution needed with: DIGOXIN, some anticoagulants, CYCLOSPORIN, GEMIFIBROZIL, NICOTINIC ACID.
Contains: SIMVASTATIN.
Other preparations:

Z

Zofran
(Glaxo)

Yellow, oval tablets supplied at strengths 4 mg, 8 mg, and used to treat nausea and vomiting associated with cancer treatment or surgical operation.

Dose: as advised by doctor.
Availability: NHS and private prescription.
Side effects: constipation, headache, flushing, liver changes, allergy.
Caution: in pregnant women.
Not to be used for: nursing mothers.
Caution needed with:
Contains: ONDANSETRON.
Other preparations: Zofran Injection.

---

zopiclone *see* Zimovane

Zovirax
(Wellcome)

A blue, shield-shaped tablet supplied at strengths of 200 mg, 400 mg, 800 mg and used as an antiviral treatment for genital herpes, other skin herpes, shingles.

Dose: adults shingles1 800 mg tablet 5 times a day every 4 hours for 7 days; other herpes infections 200 mg 5 times a day for 5 days; reduced doses for prevention or in children.
Availability: NHS and private prescription.
Side effects: irritation (local use).
Caution: in patients suffering from kidney damage; drink plenty of fluids.
Not to be used for:
Caution needed with: PROBENECID.
Contains: ACYCLOVIR.
Other preparations: Zovirax Suspension, Zovirax Cream, Zovirax Infusion.

Zovirax Eye Ointment
(Wellcome)

An ointment used as an antiviral treatment for herpes simplex infection of the cornea.

Z

Dose: insert 1 cm length of ointment into the corner of the eye 5 times a day every 4 hours for at least 3 days after healing.
Availability: NHS and private prescription.
Side effects: mild smarting, superficial punctate inflammation of the cornea.
Caution:
Not to be used for:
Caution needed with:
Contains: ACYCLOVIR.
Other preparations:

---

zuclopenthixol *see* Clopixol

Zumenon *see* Climaval
(Duphar)

Zyloric
(Wellcome)

A white tablet supplied at a strength of 100 mg, 300 mg and used as an enzyme blocker to treat gout, and for the prevention of uric acid and calcium oxalate stones.

Dose: 100-300 mg a day at first, then 200-600 mg a day.
Availability: NHS and private prescription.
Side effects: skin reactions, nausea, acute gout.
Caution: in pregnant women, the elderly, and in patients suffering from kidney or liver disease. Be sure to drink plenty of fluids.
Not to be used for: children or for patients suffering from acute gout.
Caution needed with: anticoagulants, CHLORPROPAMIDE, MERCAPTOPURINE, AZATHIOPRINE.
Contains: ALLOPURINOL.
Other preparations: ALORAL, ALULINE, CAPLENAL (Berk), COSURIC (DDSA), HAMARIN (Nicholas), RIMAPURINOL (Rima), XANTHOMAX (Ashbourne).

Z

For each of the medicines described in detail in this book, there is a paragraph headed 'Not to be used with'. This paragraph includes other medicines, groups of medicines, substances such as alcohol, or even foods which should not be taken at the same time as the drug described. This is because the medicine may interact with one or more of the substances mentioned in an unpleasant, harmful, or potentially dangerous way. On the other hand, for an individual patient, there may be no serious interaction at all.

The purpose of the chart set out below is to depict, using a simple and familiar technique, whether or not major 'families' of medicines have been found to interact with one another in any way. It does not attempt to show the degree of interaction. To work out whether or not a medicine you have been prescribed is likely to interact with any other substance, just pick out the family to which it belongs in the vertical column, and trace it horizontally across the chart. Where a '●' occurs, trace down the chart and you will find the name of the substance with which it may interact.

For detailed information concerning interactions, you should, of course, refer to the 'Not to be used with' paragraph for the particular medicine you have been prescribed.

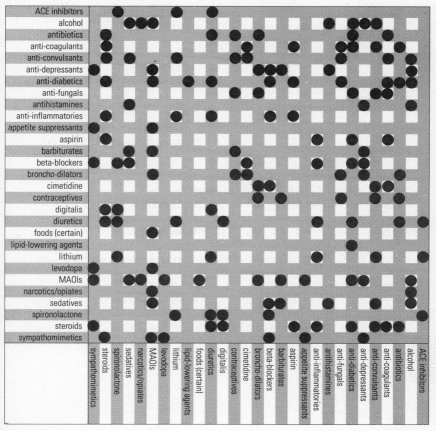